The Heart

Physiology, Metabolism, Pharmacology and Therapy

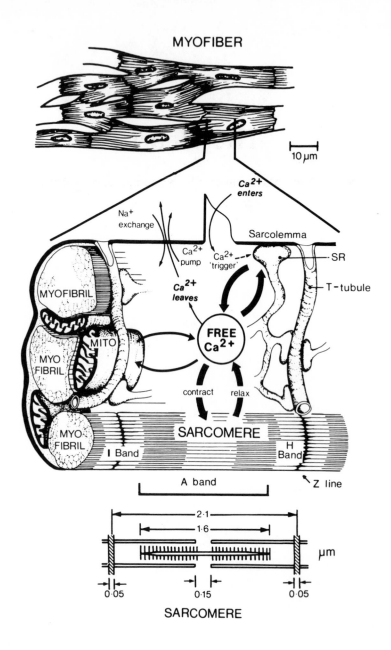

MYOFIBER

10 μm

Ca²⁺ enters

Na⁺ exchange

Sarcolemma

Ca²⁺ pump

Ca²⁺ 'trigger'

SR

Ca²⁺ leaves

MYOFIBRIL

T-tubule

FREE Ca²⁺

MITO

MYO FIBRIL

contract   relax

MYO FIBRIL

SARCOMERE

I Band

H Band

A band

Z line

2·1

1·6

μm

0·05   0·15   0·05

SARCOMERE

Frontispiece The modern view is that the changing concentration of calcium ions in the myocardial cell plays a predominant role in the physiological regulation of cardiac contraction. Calcium ions are schematically shown as entering via the slow phase of an action potential which travels along the sarcolemma to ''trigger'' the release of more calcium from the sarcoplasmic reticulum (SR) and thereby to initiate a contraction–relaxation cycle. Eventually the small amount of calcium that has entered the cell will leave predominantly by a sodium–calcium mechanism with a lesser role for the sarcolemmal calcium pump. The upper panel is reproduced with permission from Braunwald E, et al. (1976). Mechanisms of Contraction of the Normal and Failing Heart, 2nd ed, Little Brown, Boston. The lower panel is from Jewell BR (1977). Circ Res 40: 221, by courtesy of the author and the American Heart Association. The dimensions shown are for frog skeletal muscle. The middle panel is from Opie LH (1984). Calcium Antagonists and Cardiovascular Disease, Raven Press, New York, with permission.

The Heart

Physiology, Metabolism, Pharmacology and Therapy

Lionel H. Opie

M.D., D.Phil, F.R.C.P., F.R.S.(SA)

Professor of Medicine (Cardiac), University of Cape Town, South Africa;
Director, Ischemic Heart Disease Research Unit, Medical Research Council of South Africa;
Consultant Professor, Cardiology Division, Stanford University Medical Center, California, U.S.A.

Biochemical Consultant: *Wieland Gevers* M.B., Ch.B., D.Phil., F.R.S. (SA)
Professor of Medical Biochemistry, University of Cape Town, South Africa; Director, Muscle Research Unit, Medical Research Council of South Africa; Previously Visiting Professor, Department of Pathology, Pritzker School of Medicine, University of Chicago, U.S.A.

Pharmacological Consultant: *Winifred G. Nayler* Ph.D.
Principal Research Investigator, Department of Medicine, Austin Hospital, University of Melbourne, Australia

Contributor: *Radovan Zak* Ph.D.
Professor, Cardiology Section of the Department of Medicine and Department of Pharmacology and Physiological Sciences, University of Chicago, U.S.A.

Introduction by: *Richard J. Bing* M.D.
Professor Emeritus, University of Southern California, U.S.A.

GRUNE & STRATTON, INC.
Harcourt Brace Jovanovich, Publishers
London Orlando San Diego New York Boston
San Francisco Tokyo Sydney Toronto

GRUNE & STRATTON LTD.
24/28 Oval Road, London NW1 7DX

United States edition published by
GRUNE & STRATTON INC.
Orlando, Florida 32887

British Library Cataloguing in Publication Data
Opie, Lionel H.
  The heart
  1. Heart — Diseases
  I. Title
  616.1′2   RC681

ISBN 0-8089-1668-8

Second printing, revised
1986
Printed in the United States of America
86 87 88 89   10 9 8 7 6 5 4 3 2

Preface

The majority of books concerning the heart have been written either entirely from its clinical or its physiological aspect. I have tried to combine the two points of view, for it so happens that my methods have been those of the physiologist and biochemist, whereas my interest in the subject and manner of approach to its problems have been entirely those of a clinician.

Tinsley Harrison (1935). *Failure of the Circulation*

This book is intended to explain the principles of **cardiac function in health and disease** to a wide range of potential readers, including fellows in cardiology, interns and residents, medical registrars, as well as students of physiology, pharmacology or medicine. It is not a conventional textbook of cardiology; rather it strives to emphasize the principles of physiology, metabolism and pharmacological therapy. The diagrams and metabolic schemes have been carefully designed to allow a simple visual approach to teaching or learning so complex a subject. It is anticipated that the result will appeal both to teachers and to those taught—those whose highest standards require a thorough understanding of one of the most important organs of the body.

The first section deals with the **cellular basis of the physiology** of the heart, including the ultrastructure and the biochemical function of organelles. Thereafter, the normal ionic balance is described with particular reference to the role of the sodium pump and the regulation of sodium and calcium channels, the opening and closing of which results in the normal action potential. The conduction of the wave of excitation is traced from the sinus node, through the atria to the atrioventricular node, along the His bundle and the bundle branches via the Purkinje fibers to the contracting ventricular cells. The fundamental role of calcium ions lies in the regulation of excitation–contraction coupling and contractility. This process is controlled in turn by catecholamine beta-adrenergic stimulation by means of intracellular messengers.

The second section on **energy metabolism and ventricular function** traces the metabolic pathways converting carbohydrates and lipid fuels to the 2-carbon fragments, which ultimately provide adenosine triphosphate (ATP) through oxidation in the mitochondria. The energy thus produced is used largely for contraction and the associated movements of ions. Increased heart work and exercise alter the myocardial energy production and utilization. When an excessive load on the heart is maintained for a long time, myocardial hypertrophy is then required to alter the wall stress favorably in order to cope with the increased oxygen demand. Thus myocardial mechanical function is the basis of the control of the energy metabolism of the heart. The link between oxygen demand and oxygen supply is the coronary circulation and its complex regulation.

The third section outlines the **pharmacological properties** of those therapeutic agents in daily cardiological use. For example, every cardiologist requires an appreciation of the most important facet of the metabolism of the heart—its oxygen uptake. Patients with angina pectoris are treated with beta-adrenergic receptor blocking agents, so that the oxygen uptake of the heart during exercise decreases and the anginal point is not reached. Beta-adrenergic receptor blocking agents are known to decrease three of the most important determinants of the oxygen uptake of the heart: heart rate, blood pressure and contractility, thereby altering myocardial oxygen metabolism. Newly developed calcium (slow channel) antagonist agents alter the oxygen metabolism of the heart favorably in patients with angina pectoris, both by increasing the oxygen supply and by lessening the demand. The balance between oxygen demand and oxygen supply to the heart is, therefore, a fundamental physiological principle which explains the mechanism of action of these agents.

The final section covers the **therapy of heart disease**, including congestive heart failure, hypertension, ischemic heart disease and arrhythmias. In this rapidly changing area only the principles can be outlined; details of drug doses, trade names,[1] side-effects and pharmacokinetics are given in *Drugs for the Heart* (ed. LH Opie), American Edition, Grune & Stratton, Orlando, New York and London, 1984, and in *Drugs and the Heart* (by LH Opie) published by *The Lancet*, 1980.

In summary, the physiology and metabolism of the heart are best understood when closely integrated with an understanding of pharmacological agents and the pathophysiology of heart disease.

L. H. Opie
May 1984

---

[1]To the best of the author's knowledge, generic names have been used for all drugs. If any trade name has inadvertently been used the manufacturer is asked to correspond with the author so that it may be corrected in further editions.

Contents

III Pharmacology: Drug Action

IV Heart Disease:
Pathophysiology and Pharmacological Therapy

Introduction

Richard J. Bing

Evolution of science, like biological evolution, develops by a zigzag course of trial and error; the errors are soon forgotten though they serve as stepping-stones to new progress. The factors which determine both scientific progress and scientific error are dependent on the ability of the brain to be analytical, curious, critical, observant and imaginative. These are constant factors—qualities of the human brain which have evolved together with other properties of mind and body. There are, on the other hand, variables which determine progress in the natural sciences. Techniques and the spirit of the period, together with the personality of the scientist, make up these variables. Endowed with these constants, and blessed or cursed by these variables, the human mind attempts to discover single stones in the mosaic of the biological system, or if graced with a flash of genius, it can visualize whole parts of nature's mosaic.

A glance into the early beginnings of cardiac physiology and metabolism is not amiss, because we find that the pioneers wrestled with the same ideas that occupy us today, and that an astonishing amount of scientific truth is contained in early publications. Much of this important work, dating from the 1870s to 1920, was summarized in a remarkable fashion by Tigerstedt in 1923, in a volume on the physiology of the circulation.[1] Tigerstedt himself was an outstanding investigator, to whom we owe the discovery of renin. One section of his remarkable book deals with the "chemical conditions for cardiac action". In Chapter 33 he discusses the importance of inorganic substances for cardiac activity and subsequently that of organic material. He cites the literature of 40 years preceding this work in a comprehensive and critical fashion. Names that occur frequently in this review are those of Ludwig, Langendorff, Kronecker, Howell, Martin, Greene, Gaskell, Bowditch, Clark, Loewi, Locke and particularly of Ringer. Among those who contributed greatly to our understanding of the importance of organic material for cardiac function, he

[1]Tigerstedt RA (1923). Die Physiologie des Kreislaufes, Vol I, 2nd ed, pp 245–305, W. DeGruyter, Berlin and Wien.

mentions among others Starling, Evans and Clark. This book contains a wealth of information, for example: the Langendorff perfusion method was first introduced in 1890 by Martin and Applegarth of Johns Hopkins in Baltimore; Langendorff had no knowledge of this work when he described his perfusion method in 1895. Particularly fascinating is the story of the discovery of the role of calcium ions. It is interesting that Ringer was first misled by the use of sodium chloride enriched tapwater which contained, without his knowledge, not only calcium chloride but also potassium chloride which antagonized the calcium effect. A year later Ringer discovered that the arrested heart could be made to beat again by the addition of calcium chloride (see Fig. 1-4). He concluded in 1883 that calcium is absolutely essential for maintenance of cardiac contraction. Thus Ringer established that calcium increased the force of contraction and prolonged systole. Yet excess calcium could result in contracture of the heart and could diminish the duration of diastole.

What followed subsequently is remarkably well summarized in the first chapter of this book.

Other chapters of note are those on the cellular basis of contractility, protein synthesis, myocardial mechanics and hypertrophy, and the calcium cycle of the heart. Such landmarks concisely and clearly summarize our present knowledge. What distinguishes this book from the early publication by Tigerstedt is testimony to the major advances in the basic sciences, their influence on cardiac physiology and metabolism, and their application by cardiologists in daily clinical practice. This book also attests to the widespread permeation of physiology by metabolic studies, and to the development of cardiac pharmacology and therapy from these two basic disciplines. While in the late nineteenth and early twentieth century, knowledge of the function and nutrition of the heart was relatively limited, the present volume reflects advances in physical and biological chemistry, molecular biology, electron microscopy, electrophysiology and myocardial mechanics. In bringing together these basic disciplines into a volume which can be assimilated by clinical cardiologists and medical students, the present work achieves a milestone.

Acknowledgements

My interest in fundamental cardiology was awakened by one of the giants of cardiology, Sir John McMichael, formerly Professor of Medicine at the Royal Postgraduate Medical School, Hammersmith Hospital, London, and kept alive by Professor Jack Shillingford; this was followed by years of happy contact with Richard Bing, the "father of cardiac metabolism". To them my profound gratitude for their interest, guidance and training.

To my consultants, my appreciation is especially deep-felt. They have both contributed excellent chapters. Professor Winifred Nayler helped considerably with the early evolution of the plans. Professor Wieland Gevers has critically evaluated the biochemical content of the book; he has helped it to grow over many years by numerous discussions concerning the general planning and development. To him I owe more than I can state, because he imparted enthusiasm and scientific friendship.

Many other colleagues have also provided the stimulus, ideas and inspiration which I hope the present volume will reflect. The published proceedings of meetings which I have been privileged to attend bear testimony to the ways in which the organizers have advanced cardiology. Examples are Oliver's *Effect of Acute Ischaemia on Myocardial Function* (1972); Moret and Fejfar's *Metabolism of the Hypoxic and Ischaemic Heart* (1972); Maseri's *Myocardial Blood Flow in Man* (1972); Wildenthal's *Regulation of Cardiac Metabolism* (1976); Riecker, Weber and Goodwin's *Myocardial Failure* (1977); Hearse and de Leiris' *Enzymes in Cardiology* (1979); Winbury and Abiko's *Ischemic Myocardium and Antianginal Drugs* (1979); Gross' *Modulation of Sympathetic Tone in the Treatment of Cardiovascular Disease* (1979); Gerlach and Kübler's *Catecholamines and the Heart* (1981); Riemersma and Oliver's *Catecholamines in the Non-ischaemic and Ischaemic Myocardium* (1982); Ferrari's *Myocardial Ischemia and Lipid Metabolism* (1984); and *Regulation of Cardiac Function* (1984) edited by Abe, Ito, Tada and myself. It would also be appropriate to mention all those authors who contributed to *Calcium Antagonists and Cardiovascular Disease* (1984) and *Drugs for the Heart* (1984), both edited by myself. In each case, I learned much from the individual contributions and even more from the combined opinions.

Other valuable publications have been Katz's excellent *Physiology of the Heart* and the series on *Recent Advances in Function and Structure of the Heart* (now *Advances in Myocardiology*), edited by Dhalla and Rona, which reflects the activities of the International Society for Heart Research whom I have been privileged to serve in various capacities for ten years. One of the first meetings of that Society was published as *Calcium and the Heart* with Peter Harris and myself as co-editors (1971). Among the major authors was Fleckenstein, who presented his new discoveries on the calcium antagonist agents—in the days when clinicians were only just beginning to use beta-adrenergic blockers and when calcium antagonists were strictly for laboratory enthusiasts. Today's theory is tomorrow's practice.

Although this book was started in Italy in 1978 while on sabbatical leave with Professor A. Maseri, and largely completed in subsequent vacations, it could not have been finalized without study leave granted by the Heads of my Department, Dr S. J. Saunders (now Principal of the University of Cape Town) and Professor S. Benatar.

Jean Wicks gave years of splendid secretarial assistance, with a unique combination of devotion to duty and typing skills; I cannot thank her enough. The final typing was undertaken superbly by June Chambers. The artwork of Jeanne Walker and Jean Powell is in a superlative class of its own.

Members of the Ischaemic Heart Disease Research Unit, including Owen Bricknell, Francis Thandroyen, Cecilia Muller and Victor Claasen contributed significantly as did senior medical students of the University of Cape Town. Sections of the book were criticized by Dr Mark Noble, Midhurst Research Institute, London, England; Dr A. Lochner, University of Stellenbosch, South Africa; Dr W. Clusin, Cardiology, Stanford University, California; Professor W. Beck, Head of the Cardiac Clinic, Groote Schuur Hospital; and Dr T. Mabin, Cardiologist, Cape Town. Antiarrhythmic drugs were discussed with Dr B. Singh, Los Angeles, Professor E. Carmeliet, Leuven, Belgium, and Dr K. Courtney, Palo Alto, California. The advice of these and many other colleagues is gratefully acknowledged. I also owe much to the Medical Research Council of South Africa for creating the Ischaemic Heart Disease Research Unit and the Chris Barnard Fund for critical additional support.

It is my hope that this book will reflect the exciting blend of physiology, metabolism and pharmacology resulting from the continuing output of new facts and ideas in the midst of which we find ourselves. I believe that such an approach can be applied fruitfully to the principles of assessment and therapy of cardiac disease, thereby working towards the ultimate aim of helping mankind to achieve optimal health.

L. H. Opie

To Carol

who won a scholarship to Italy, thereby making possible our sabbatical stay in Pisa, Italy, where this book was born; it matured in Cape Town, nourished by her harmonious and beautiful garden.

I Physiology

Physiology and Metabolism
as the Basis of
Cardiac Function

No understanding of the circulatory reactions of the body is possible unless we start first
with the fundamental properties of the heart muscle itself, and then find out how these are
modified, protected and controlled under the influence of the mechanisms — nervous, chemical
and mechanical — which under normal conditions play on the heart and blood vessels

Starling (1920)

The heart is a restless organ, in a constant state of mechanical and metabolic flux. Its physiology is the study of the function of the normal organ, including its cellular organization and contractile activity. Metabolism, a term derived from the Greek word *change*, includes the conversion of oxygen and other foods into cell energy in the form of adenosine triphosphate (ATP). This book will emphasize three concepts. First, the physiology of the heart is increasingly based on an understanding of cellular function, especially when considering the role of calcium ions in the contractile cycle and the nature of the pumps and channels which control the movements of calcium, sodium and potassium ions into and out of the cell as well as within the confines of the cell membranes. Secondly, the major purpose of the metabolism of the heart is to provide sufficient energy in the form of ATP to balance the requirements of the mechanical function. When the energy supply is inadequate for the demand, then the metabolic changes are first those of ischemia (too little blood flow) and eventually those of infarction (cell death);

such an imbalance especially happens when the oxygen supply is limited by coronary artery disease. Energy is also required to keep in operation those pumps which regulate the concentrations of ions in the cell; abnormal distributions of ions occur when the cell dies or when irregularities of the heart rhythm such as ischemic ventricular arrhythmias develop. Thirdly, the heart is in the center of the circulation. When the mechanical load on the heart is sustained, the heart cells grow in size by the process of hypertrophy. Heart failure goes with a sustained overload or when the energy supply is severely diminished as in myocardial infarction. Important adjustments occur in the circulation so that there is an increased stimulation of the sympathetic nervous system as well as of certain hormones (renin–angiotensin system), the net result of these processes being to increase the load against which the heart works.

Clinicians can now modify the contractile activity of the heart as well as those receptors, pumps and channels responsible for normal function. Another category of drugs act on the circulation to relieve the failing heart by unloading. The myocardial oxygen balance can be favorably improved by agents reducing the heart rate (beta-adrenergic blocking agents), improving the blood supply (calcium-antagonist agents) or by reducing the load on the heart (nitrates). Antiarrhythmic agents act chiefly on diseased sodium and calcium channels to exert their beneficial effect.

Modern cardiology relies heavily on therapeutic manipulation of the physiology and metabolism of the heart. This current situation, where basic science and clinical practice are being integrated for the benefit of the patient, originated in simpler ideas which have gradually been built up over the centuries.

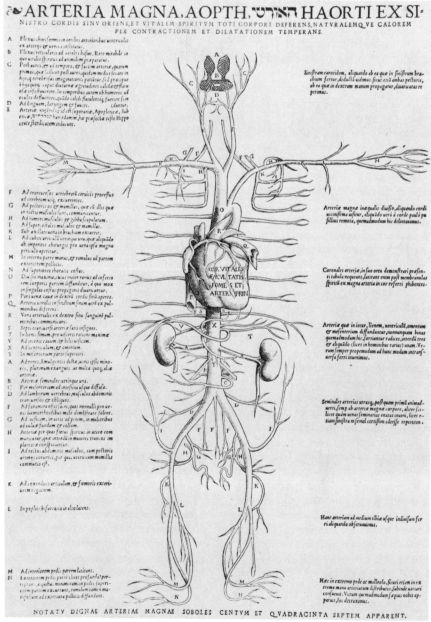

Fig. 1-1 The heart at the center of the circulation, as drawn by Vesalius (1514–1564) in his *Tabulae Anatomicae* (see Boyadjian, 1980).

From Pre-history to Harvey

The existence of the heart was well-known to the Greeks who gave it the name *kardia*, still surviving in words such as "cardiac", "tachycardia" and "bradycardia". Aristotle thought that the heart was the seat of the soul and the center of man. The Romans modified *kardia* to *cor*, the latter word still surviving in "cordial greetings" and in "cor pulmonale". The old Teutonic word *herton* is also derived from cor and gives us "heart" via the medieval English *heorte*.

Galen (about 200 AD), the "father of experimental physiology", knew that the heart set the blood in motion; he discovered that arteries contained blood and not air. Yet he wrote that pores in the septum allowed blood to flow from right to left ventricle, where the "vital spirit" is formed by the mixture of blood and air which reaches the ventricles from the lungs. Such was Galen's authority that his views on the circulation became dogma, dispelled only by the careful anatomical dissections of the Flemish anatomist, Vesalius (1514–1564), who became Professor of Anatomy at Padua in Italy and clearly showed that there were no pores in the ventricular septum. Not even the careful and beautiful anatomical drawings of the immortal Leonardo da Vinci (1452–1519) were entirely free from the erroneous pores.

The critical point that the circulations of the left and right heart were separate, was not grasped until Servetus (1511–1553) wrote:

> The connection between the cavities of the heart is not established through the median partition of the heart; a wonderful track conducts the blood, which flows in a long detour from the right of the heart to the lung and becomes red; at the moment of relaxation it reaches the left cavity of the heart.

Servetus hid this brilliant passage in a book of theology in which he criticized the Trinity, thereby falling foul of the Calvinist rulers of Geneva who burnt him at the stake. In 1571, an Italian, Cesalpino, clearly defined the pulmonary circulation and described the function of valves:

> Special membranes at the openings of the vessels prevent blood flowing back so that there is perpetual movement of the blood from the vena cava through the heart and lungs into the aorta.

Yet it was not till Harvey (1578–1657) that the pumping function of the heart and the circulation of the blood was scientifically established, to begin the modern era of cardiology. His *Anatomical Treatise on the Motion of the Heart and Blood in Animals* appeared in 1628 and is probably the most important single volume in the history of cardiology. Born in England and trained in Padua before returning to St Bartholomew's Hospital in London, he must have been influenced by Vesalius' masterly drawing of the circulation (Fig. 1-1). Thus it is to Harvey—and his predecessors—that we owe our knowledge of the heart as a mechanical pump.

Clinical Cardiology Develops

Five more recent discoveries helped to lay the foundations for modern clinical cardiology: that of digitalis by the botanist Withering in 1785; that of the stethoscope by Laennec, whose masterpiece on *Disease of the Chest and Mediate Auscultation* was translated into English in 1827; that of nitrates by Lauder Brunton in Edinburgh in 1867; that of chest x-rays by Röntgen in 1895; and that of electrocardiography by Einthoven in the Netherlands in 1903. Armed with digitalis for heart failure, nitrates for angina pectoris, a stethoscope and an electrocardiogram, early physicians such as Sir Thomas Lewis (Fig. 1-2) were able to cope reasonably well with the diagnosis and therapy of valvular and ischemic heart disease. Two more events were required for the "pumps and pressures" approach to flower fully; the description of the cardiac cycle by Wiggers (1934), who showed in detail all the critical events governing the circulation of blood through the heart, and the discovery of cardiac catheterization by Cournand in 1944.

Thus it was that those two great clinical cardiologists —Paul Wood at the National Heart Hospital, London, and the Bostonian Paul White—could write their classic books (Wood: *Diseases of the Heart and Circulation*, 1950; White; *Heart Disease*, first edition 1921, last edition in 1951) with great clinical accuracy and skill but scarcely a thought to the fundamental requirement of the heart to maintain its oxygen and energy metabolism, or to the role of contractility. These great clinicians were, however, aware of the anatomy of the conduction system which had been well-studied by the early 1900s.

Conduction System

The classical cardiac anatomists—Purkinje, His, Tawara, Kent—stained and studied the conduction

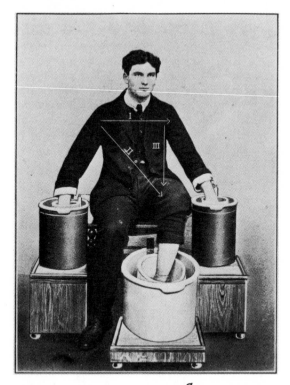

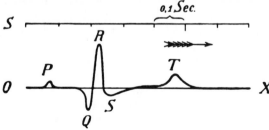

Fig. 1-2 Einthoven's electrocardiogram. The apparatus used to obtain an electrocardiogram in 1913 is taken from the book of Sir Thomas Lewis, *Clinical Electrocardiography*. The ionic currents underlying the electrocardiogram are discussed in Chapter 5.

system (Fig. 1-3). Purkinje (1845) worked in Prague and it was his description of the conducting cells which led to the realization that there were at least two populations of cells in the ventricular myocardium — the contractile and the conducting. The critical role of the atrioventricular node in receiving and transmitting the cardiac impulses was described by His (1893), Tawara (1906) and Keith and Flack (1908). Of these, the name of His is firmly linked with the bundle conducting the impulse from the atrioventricular node

to the bundle branches (all being composed of Purkinje fibers), while Kent (1914) is associated with the anatomical tract bypassing the atrioventricular node in patients with the Wolff–Parkinson–White (1931) syndrome (see page 63).

Classical Cardiac Physiology

In the meantime a more dynamic view was developing so that the heart came to be seen not just as a pump but as a sensitive organ responding to the needs of the body during exercise, rest, health and disease, by carefully regulating the rate and force of cardiac contraction. Some of the fundamental studies on the oxygen metabolism and contractile behavior, destined to become current concepts, were being carried out on isolated heart or heart–lung preparations.

Calcium and contractility

Perhaps the study with the greatest long-term repercussions was that of Sidney Ringer, Professor of Medicine at University College in London, to whom we can trace the current interest in calcium and therefore calcium-channel antagonists. Just over 100 years ago in 1883, he described the effects of deprivation of external calcium.

> When the circulating fluid is composed of saline solution, the ventricle grows weaker and weaker and contractility ceases. Calcium bicarbonate, or calcium chloride in physiological doses, or even in smaller quantities than are in the blood, restore good contractions . . . Calcium salts are necessary for the proper contraction of the heart   Ringer (1883)

Less well-known is that he emphasized the need for the "correct proportions" between calcium and potassium, without which the ventricle would be thrown into a state of tetanus or (as he called it) "persistent spasm". Thus Ringer defined two salient facts: the heart needs calcium for contraction, but calcium can have harmful effects if allowed to act in an unopposed way.

Since then generations of medical students have struggled with frog hearts and black drums to repeat Ringer's work; a particularly elegant trace was that obtained by a second-year student at the London Hospital in 1941 — the student's name was Shillingford, and he was later to become a leader in

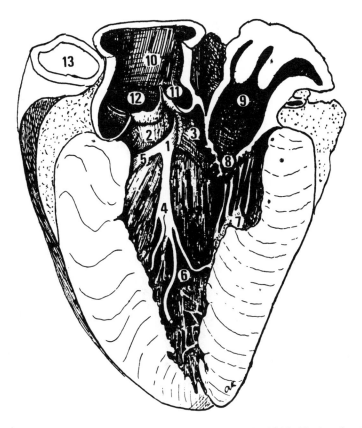

Fig. 1-3   The conducting system of the heart, as seen by Keith and Flack in 1906. The bundle of His (1) originates in the atrioventricular node (not shown) and divides into the left bundle branch (4) and right bundle branch (5) respectively, running down the left and right sides of the ventricular septum to become smaller branches (6) below the endocardial surface of the ventricles. This figure is also useful to trace the flow of flood, which is received into the left atrium (9) from the lungs, and leaves via the mitral valves (8) into the left ventricular cavity (between thick walls). The mitral valves are tethered to the left ventricle by the chordae tendinae (7). The left ventricle empties into the aorta (10) through the aortic valves. Reproduced with permission from The Lancet.

British cardiology at the Hammersmith Hospital and Royal Postgraduate Medical School in London (Fig. 1-4). Today the phenomena of calcium overload and calcium-induced contracture of the heart are held to be the basis of severe myocardial damage. Ringer's model of perfusion, in which calcium-free solution was followed by calcium-induced hypercontraction, may be the basis of the "calcium paradox". In the latter event, re-introduction of calcium ions after calcium-free perfusion causes massive damage.

Oxygen and fuels

Many of the early studies, like those of Ringer, were conducted on the frog heart which was much better

able to withstand the effects of oxygen-lack than was the mammalian heart. When deprived of oxygen, the frog-heart gradually ceased to beat, whereas the mammalian heart failed much sooner, within minutes. Based on the early work on frog skeletal muscle by Fletcher and Hopkins (1907), the theory arose that lactic acid "accumulates in the heart and produces paralysis fairly rapidly" (Clark et al., 1932). These theories proved viable and have been given fresh impetus by the recent findings that acidosis and lactate inhibit key enzymes of glycolysis. The source of the lactate was from glucose, by what is now called anaerobic glycolysis, which helps to protect the heart against oxygen-lack by provision of energy in the absence of oxygen.

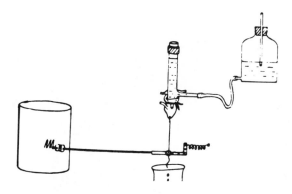

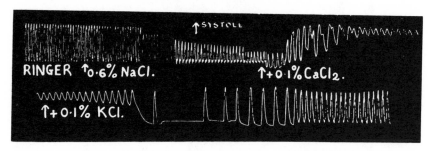

Fig. 1-4 Ringer's basic experiment on the perfused frog heart, showing the essential requirement for calcium ions for cardiac contraction (as recorded by Shillingford in 1940; reproduced with permission).

To study the uptake of glucose and other fuels by the mammalian heart, Langendorff in 1895 devised an isolated heart system which is still widely used. The provision of an adequate oxygen supply was critical. Equally important was maintenance of the correct ionic and pH conditions of the perfusion field—a condition not adequately met until Krebs and Henseleit (1932) described in detail the ionic composition of the mammalian blood; their bicarbonate buffer is now standard for heart perfusion systems.

These early workers correctly surmised what was later to be more clearly defined—that glucose could only make a minor contribution to the energy requirements of the heart unless insulin was added. The other carbohydrate fuel of significance was lactate; when lactate uptake was high, as in exercise, glucose uptake was low and vice versa. Glycogen was correctly classified as a reserve fuel for emergency situations. In the absence of glucose it was suspected that fats could account for about 90 percent of the oxygen uptake of the heart, but the poor lipid methodology then available limited more detailed conclusions.

The idea that all carbohydrate fuels—glucose, lactate and glycogen—had much in common in their metabolic history and constituted a common pabulum was put forth by Evans et al. (1935) who concluded that:

> Our work adds to the already large mass of evidence that the heart does not derive the whole of its energy from the oxidation of carbohydrates.

Later the classic studies of Bing (1954) proved that these principles also applied to the human heart.

Anaerobic glycolysis in hypoxia

Evans also made another fundamental observation on the dog heart–lung preparation: during hypoxia, the glucose uptake of the heart was increased, while lactate was produced instead of being taken up. This stimulation of glycolysis by hypoxia, reminiscent of what Pasteur had found in micro-organisms, is still called the Pasteur effect. The mechanism of the effect was unravelled years later by two American physiologists, Morgan and Neely, presently working in Hershey, Pennsylvania, who described the steps at which hypoxia accelerates glycolysis such as glucose uptake and the activity of the key enzyme, phosphofructokinase. Recently Neely has clarified the mechanism of inhibition of glycolysis during severe ischemia, a process which limits the potential benefit of the energy made by anaerobic glycolysis. Even today, the myocardial production of lactate is regarded as an excellent sign of myocardial ischemia (see Fig. 11-14), and is still used as a test of true metabolic myocardial ischemia in patients in whom the cause of an angina-like chest pain is doubtful.

Mechanics and Metabolism

Starling's "Law of the Heart"

It was Starling who first studied in detail the mechanical performance of the isolated mammalian heart and matched mechanics to metabolism. His fundamental observations were that:

> Within wide limits, the output of the heart is independent of arterial resistance and of temperature; up to a certain point, the output of the heart is proportional to the venous inflow. When this point is exceeded, the venous pressure rises and edema of the lungs supervenes.

The basic adaptation of the heart to an increased venous pressure was seen as an increased heart volume, and

> Within physiological limits, the larger the volume of the heart, the greater the energy of its contraction and the amount of chemical change at each contraction.

The latter conclusion was reached in Starling's fundamental lecture on the "Law of the Heart", given at Cambridge in 1915. He was aware of the longitudinal fibrils constituting muscle, and proposed that "lengthening the muscle increases the extent of the active surface" — very similar to the modern concept of cross-bridge interaction. He also gave an early view on molecular mechanisms in heart failure, proposing that the "concentration of active molecules becomes less" which leads to the modern view of abnormalities of the calcium cycle (shown in the Frontispiece).

Frank and isovolumic contraction

Whereas Starling stressed the role of the initial length of the muscle fiber and of the venous return, it was his German predecessor Frank (1895) who clearly emphasized that ventricular muscle could contract isovolumically. Also studying an isolated heart system (Fig. 1-5), Frank showed that when filled with different volumes, the heart could contract with varying tension even though there was no change in volume during

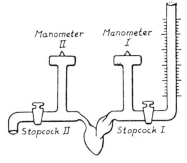

Fig. 1-5 Frank's much simplified isolated heart system. By turning off stopcocks I and II, he could make the system virtually isovolumic. By altering stopcock I, he could cause the isovolumic heart to contract at different critical tensions.

contraction — a situation corresponding to isometric contraction of skeletal muscle with unchanged muscle length but with different initial afterloads. By an ingenious yet simple system of valves and manometers, he could show a "family of isometric curves" (Fig. 1-6) with increasing initial tension (with the volume always remaining constant). This situation is in some ways a model of increasing the afterload on the ventricle, which increases the ventricular pressure generated during the isovolumic phase of the cardiac contraction cycle.

To recapitulate: Starling emphasized the role of the venous return in producing "maximal dilatation of the heart in the period of diastole", whereas Frank emphasized that increasing ventricular volume increased isovolumic systolic pressure generation. Today their names are frequently linked to describe the **Frank–Starling law of the heart** which relates initial heart volume to stroke volume and to the development of intraventricular pressure. If the initial volume is increased by increased venous filling, the usual term is the Starling law. If the emphasis is on the increased wall tension generated by an increased afterload, the

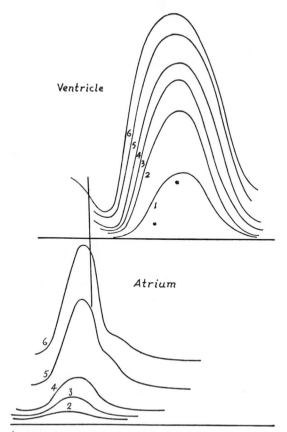

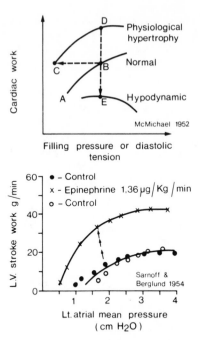

Fig. 1-6 Frank's family of isometric (isovolumic) curves. Each curve was obtained by a greater initial filling of the left ventricle by an increased left atrial filling pressure. Then valves were shut to produce isovolumic conditions (Fig. 1-7). Curve 6 has a greater velocity of shortening and hence the initial fiber length (volume of ventricle) can influence contractility. This effect of fiber length on contractility has recently been rediscovered.

best term is the Frank law. Frank also showed that altering the initial heart volume could alter contractility (Chapter 13), thus paving the way for the modern doubts about the validity of the distinction between the effects of the initial volume (or fiber length) and changes in contractility (independent of initial length).

Contractility

Neither Starling nor Frank used the term contractility, yet both helped to describe it. Starling called it "the tone" of the heart. The pioneering work of the great Harvard physiologist, Cannon (Cannon and de la Paz,

Fig. 1-7 The concept of the "family of Starling curves" and the therapeutic application of inotropic agents to the Starling Law. Note (i) decreased stroke volume for a given filling pressure in the failing heart; (ii) increased stroke volume for a given filling pressure with inotropic agents. From the original graphs of McMichael (Brit Med J 2: 525–529, 1952) and Sarnoff and Berglund (Circulation 9: 706–718, 1954). With permission from the British Medical Journal, Circulation and the American Heart Association.

1911) had already led to the concept that epinephrine was discharged in "fight or flight". According to Starling, the secretion of epinephrine during exercise could both increase coronary flow and "the energy available at each contraction". The central nervous system was seen as the mechanism which "reined and controlled" the heart to such an extent that dilatation—the basic control mechanism of the isolated heart—was no longer evident. Sarnoff and Berglund (1954) showed that the Starling curve is fundamentally altered by the contractility of the heart. There is a "family of Starling curves" each reflecting a different inotropic state of the heart (Fig. 1-7). McMichael (1952) put these curves into clinical context by showing how the failing human heart operated on a "lower Starling curve". An agent with a "positive inotropic effect" puts the heart onto a more favorable and higher Starling curve. Incidentally, we have a

German pharmacologist, Engelmann (1900), to thank for the immortal phrase "positive inotropic".

Frank also did not define contractility, but his data clearly show the concept. Increasing the initial fiber length (heart volume) was one mechanism for an increased contractility. Theoretically, a true increase in contractility can be achieved independently of an increased fiber length. Many workers have been challenged by the problem of defining true contractility. Sonnenblick (Sonnenblick and Downing, 1962) defined the phenomenon: "changing contractility induced by an inotropic intervention is characterized by a change in the rate of force development (dP/dt) from any initial muscle length". He also studied isotonic (i.e. unloaded) papillary muscle preparations, and postulated that the theoretical maximal rate of shortening was an index of contractility which he termed V_{max}. Later this concept came to be much criticized when it became apparent that the initial length of the preparation could also determine contractility. Nonetheless, the concept of contractility, independent of external determinants of muscle performance, remains viable.

Conversely, when the inotropic state (i.e. contractility) is constant, then "ventricular performance . . . is the product of two largely independent variables, the preload (establishing initial muscle length) and the afterload" (Sonnenblick and Downing, 1962). Like Frank (1895), Sonnenblick saw the afterload largely in terms of arterial blood pressure.

V_{max} and P_o in molecular terms

In an important joint symposium of the International Society of Cardiology and the World Health Organization in Geneva in 1971, Sonnenblick and Katz debated the meaning of contractility in molecular terms. Sonnenblick and Brutsaert (1971) summarized the then prevailing concepts of contractility:

> The velocity of shortening is inversely related to the load carried. When the load is increased till no shortening can occur, maximum isometric force (P_o) is manifest, while when the load is reduced, velocity increases. With the extrapolation to zero load, velocity is maximum and is termed V_{max}. This inverse force–velocity relation may be expressed as a displaced hyperbola. According to current theories, P_o represents the number of contractile sites activated, while V_{max} reflects the maximim rate of turnover of one contractile site independent of the number activated and of time [see Fig. 13-9].

At the same meeting, Katz related V_{max} to the rate at which myosin heads broke down ATP (myosin ATPase activity) while changes in P_o were explained by corresponding changes in the amount of calcium ions delivered to the contractile proteins in systole. Katz (1972) found "serious discrepancies" between the biochemical and biophysical postulates: "Variations in the amount of calcium delivered to the contractile proteins should modify P_o but be without effect on V_{max}". Yet Sonnenblick clearly showed that V_{max} was calcium-dependent: "A model of contraction based on the binding of calcium to troponin alone cannot explain these findings".

This discrepancy may now be explained by the proposed modulatory role of calcium ions in helping to regulate myosin–actin interaction. It now seems as if calcium ions can regulate all aspects of contractility — the number of cross-bridges interacting (P_o), the velocity of shortening (V_{max}), and hence, the maximal rate of pressure development (max dP/dt). Also the rate at which calcium is taken up by the sarcoplasmic reticulum can regulate the maximal rate of relaxation. The two major biochemical regulators of contractility (and hence of the myocardial oxygen uptake) are calcium ions and the sensitivity of the contractile proteins to calcium.

Myocardial Oxygen Balance

Catecholamines and oxygen uptake

Catecholamine stimulation is a major cause of an increased myocardial oxygen uptake, as Evans found in 1917. He could not explain all the increase of oxygen uptake achieved by a large dose of epinephrine as the result of increased heart work or heart rate, and introduced the idea of "oxygen-wastage" — a concept controversial even today. Two possible explanations are (i) that mechanical performance can in reality explain the increased oxygen uptake or (ii) that catecholamines stimulate myocardial lipid metabolism with a true metabolic "oxygen-wastage".

Beta-adrenoceptors and their antagonists

Years after Evans came the basic idea of Alquist (1948) that catecholamines stimulated alpha- or beta-adrenoceptors, defined by a rank order of cardiovascular reaction to infused catecholamines of various structures (Chapter 6). It is the beta-receptors which are concerned with enhanced contractility and heart rate. It was this idea of Alquist which subsequently inspired Black, working at Imperial Chemical Industries in England, to synthesize a new group of compounds antagonizing the beta-adrenergic receptor — usually now known as the beta-adrenergic blockers. Thereby Black achieved a new and fundamental therapy for angina pectoris.

> He wondered if there might be a chain of events in which stress induced by exercise or by emotion resulted in augmented sympathetic activity with increased noradrenaline release which would stimulate the heart with a resultant increase in the myocardial oxygen demand. If the supply of oxygen was inadequate, ischemia would occur with anginal pain.
>
> Shanks (1976)

In 1958 Black said that:

> I was able to argue that seeking to reduce myocardial oxygen demand by selective blockade of the cardiac actions of catecholamines would not be an exercise in wishful thinking.

Soon thereafter Black's group was to synthesize propranolol, still the standard beta-adrenergic antagonist ("beta-blocker") in the therapy of angina. His concepts were the basis of the idea that therapeutic improvement of the balance between the myocardial oxygen uptake and supply could fundamentally alter the severity of myocardial ischemia (Fig. 1-8).

Myocardial infarct size

A further development of the concept of "oxygen balance" is the direct result of the work of Braunwald and his group. Maroko *et al.* (1971) made the fundamental proposal that the size of the zone suffering infarction (cell death) after coronary artery occlusion was not fixed but dependent on the myocardial oxygen demand. Factors such as beta-adrenergic stimulation which increased the oxygen uptake could increase "infarct size" which they measured by histologic changes and the extent of depletion of the myocardial enzyme, creatine kinase.

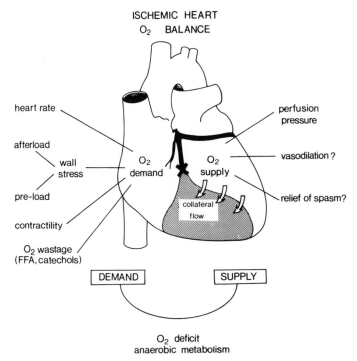

Fig. 1-8 The hypothesis that the oxygen supply to ischemic myocardial cells is a balance of the supply versus demand. When the demand is increased, as in exercise, angina of effort may be precipitated. When the supply is decreased, as in angina caused by coronary artery spasm, angina at rest may be precipitated. Beta-adrenergic blockers decrease the oxygen demand and calcium antagonists increase the oxygen supply. Modified from Opie (1980), with permission.

This enzyme, also called creatine phosphokinase, interconverts ATP and creatine phosphate. The ultimate "infarct size" could be predicted by the severity of acute ischemia at 15 minutes after coronary occlusion indirectly measured by the extent and severity of the epicardial ST segment elevation. Although these concepts have been subject to much scrutiny and criticism, the idea that excess catechol-amine activity acts harmfully in acute myocardial infarction in man is gaining ground, as is the possible beneficial effect of beta-adrenergic blockers when appropriately given.

Molecular effects of catecholamines

Many of the effects of catecholamines can now be explained in terms of the "second messenger" concept of the Nobel prize-winning team, Robinson, Sutherland and Rall. Beta-adrenergic catecholamines, by occupying the beta-receptor, stimulate adenylate cyclase to form the second messenger, cyclic AMP.

The latter in turn carries further messages by adding a phosphate group to critical cellular proteins, which then become activated to carry out the function finally desired. This is the chain of events thought to explain the enhanced rate of calcium ion entry into the cell with the positive inotropic effect, and the enhanced rate of relaxation in diastole. It is reversal of this chain of events that can explain the therapeutic benefit of beta-adrenergic blocking agents in angina pectoris.

Calcium

Whereas the beta-adrenergic blockers improve angina pectoris by decreasing the demand side of the oxygen balance, a new category of drugs can fundamentally influence calcium metabolism and improve the supply side of the equation, causing vasodilation. These drugs are thought to act predominantly on the slow calcium channel.

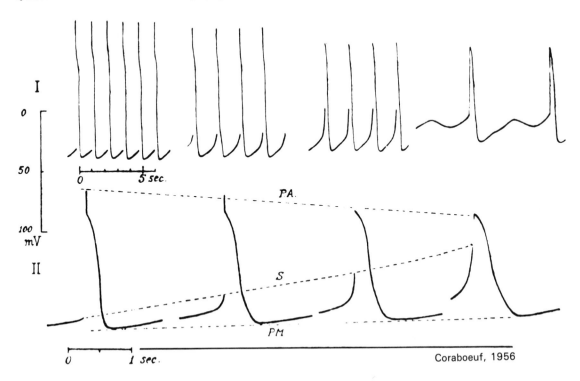

Fig. 1-9 In these experiments an increasing dose of quinidine progressively blocked the fast phase of the action potential (fast sodium channel) to uncover the slow calcium channel which is triggered by a higher threshold voltage. PA = peak potential; PM = resting membrane potential; S = threshold. Reproduced with permission.

Slow calcium channel

The existence of a fast component to the cardiac action potential had long been recognized both by analogy with the Hodgkin–Huxley model for nervous tissue, and by direct measurement using the voltage-clamp technique (Weidmann, 1955). Credit for the first suggestion of the slow channel possibly (but not certainly) goes to Coraboeuf (1957) who observed the development of a slowly rising action potential when the fast channel was markedly inhibited by very high concentrations of the antiarrhythmic agent quinidine (Fig. 1-9). Vaughan Williams (1958) independently found the same phenomenon and specifically recognized that more than one current could contribute to the formation of the cardiac action potential. The explanation for the slowly rising phase of the action potential is now known to be a calcium current, directly proven by voltage-clamp techniques. This current flows through the calcium channel which is largely though not entirely specific for calcium ions, justifying the name of "slow calcium channel". It is on this channel that the calcium-antagonist agents act.

Calcium-channel antagonists

The prototype calcium antagonist, verapamil, had been empirically used as an anti-anginal agent in Germany early in the 1960s. By 1968 a clear distinction could be made between the mode of action of verapamil and beta-adrenergic blockers (Nayler et al., 1968). It was left to Fleckenstein to clarify the fundamental qualities of these new agents. In a classic paper delivered to a selected audience of no more than fifty at a Satellite Symposium to the World Congress of Cardiology in London in 1970, Fleckenstein (1971) emphasized the properties of a

> new group of extremely potent calcium-antagonists which can inhibit excitation-contraction coupling in a highly specific way, probably by blocking special calcium channels.

He also described the properties of "the most potent agent" Bayer 1040, or nifedipine as it is now known. For the first time an excess of intracellular calcium was seen as a harmful pathogenic phenomenon. Calcium overload of the myocardium could be induced by high doses of the beta-agonist isoproterenol, and prevented by verapamil or nifedipine. The proposed mechanism was that an excess of calcium led to excitation–contraction "over-coupling" with excess breakdown of high-energy phosphate compounds. Today an excess influx of calcium is thought by many workers to be a lethal event in ischemic injury, and calcium-antagonists may protect the ischemic myocardium by several complex mechanisms. For example, calcium-antagonists have an even more powerful effect on vascular smooth muscle than on contractile myocardium, so that coronary vasodilation may increase the myocardial blood supply while peripheral vasodilatation lessens the afterload and decreases the work of the heart. Thus beta-adrenergic blockers and calcium-channel antagonists are able to alter, in different ways, myocardial calcium metabolism; in addition, calcium antagonists have a major effect on vascular smooth muscle.

Digitalis compounds

Myocardial calcium metabolism can also be therapeutically influenced by other drugs and procedures. As far back as 1917, Loewi thought that digitalis exerts its positive inotropic effect by a mechanism depending on calcium (Loewi, 1917). Subsequent studies over the years by Schwartz and his colleagues, and many others, have shown how digitalis inhibits the sodium–potassium pump of the sarcolemma, thereby indirectly enhancing the intracellular calcium ion concentration of the heart cell (see Chapter 4).

Load Reduction

In congestive heart failure, the current principles of therapy are also based on a consideration of the myocardial oxygen balance. Reduction of the preload (for example, by nitrates or diuretic therapy), makes use of the Starling principle; by reducing the volume of the over-distended ventricle, the oxygen demand lessens and contractile activity improves. Reduction of the afterload by arterial vasodilators such as nitroprusside, hydralazine or nifedipine makes use of the Frank principle, by reducing the afterload and thereby lessening the heart volume and the initial tension on the myocardial fibers. Combined venous and arterial vasodilators such as prazosin change both preload and overload. Inotropic agents such as digitalis allow a greater stroke volume at the same filling pressure and afterload, thereby moving the failing

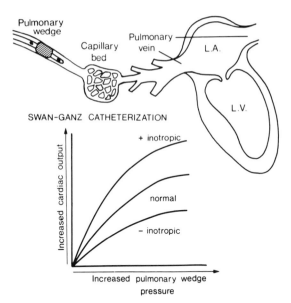

Fig. 1-10 By means of a Swan–Ganz catheter, the concepts of Starling, Frank and McMichael can be applied to the management of patients with myocardial failure as in acute myocardial infarction.

heart from one ventricular function curve to a more favorable one so as to allow a bigger stroke volume for the same filling pressure. The measurements required to test these hypotheses at the bedside can now be made (Fig. 1-10).

Summary

Myocardial cellular metabolism is fundamental to an understanding of the physiological function of the contraction cycle of the heart, and to the mode of action of modern therapeutic agents such as beta-adrenergic blockers, calcium-channel antagonists and load-reducing agents.

References

Alquist RP (1948). A study of the adrenotropic receptors. Am J Physiol 153: 586–600.

Bing RJ (1954). The metabolism of the heart. Harvey Lecture Series 50: pp 27–70, Academic Press, London, Orlando and New York.

Black JW (1958). In: Ahlquist and the development of beta-adrenoceptor antagonists. Postgrad Med J (1976), 52 (Suppl 4): 11–13.

Boyadjian, N (1980). The Heart. Its History, Its Symbolism, Its Iconography and Its Diseases, Esco Books, Antwerp, Belgium.

Cannon, WB, de la Paz D (1911). Emotional stimulation of adrenal secretion. Am J Physiol 28: 64–70.

Clark AJ, Gaddie R, Stewart CP (1932). The anaerobic activity of the isolated frog's heart. J Physiol 75: 321–331.

Coraboeuf, E, Boistel, J, Distel, R (1956). L'action de la quinidine sur l'activité électrique élémentaire du tissu conducteur du coeur de chien. C.R. Acad Sci (Paris) 242: 1225–1228.

Einthoven W (1903). Die galvanometriche Registrirung des menschlichen Elektrokardiogramms, zugleich eine Beurtheilung der Anwendung des Capillar-Electrometers in der Physiologie. Pflügers Arch Physiol 99: 472–480.

Engelmann Th W (1900). Uber die Wirkungen der Nerven auf das Herz. Arch Anat Physiol Leipzig S, 315–361.

Evans CL (1917). The mechanism of cardiac acceleration by warmth and by adrenaline. J Physiol (London) 51: 91–104.

Evans CL, Grande F, Hsu FY (1935). The glucose and lactate consumption of the dog's heart. Qtly J Exper Physiol 24: 347–364.

Fleckenstein A (1971). Specific inhibitors and promoters of calcium action in the excitation-contraction coupling of heart muscle and their role in the prevention or production of myocardial lesions. In: Calcium and the Heart, Eds. P Harris, LH Opie, pp 135–188, Academic Press, New York, London and Orlando.

Fletcher WM, Hopkins FG (1907). The oxidative intra-muscular removal of lactic acid. J Physiol 35: 247.

Frank O (1895). Zur Dynamik des Herzmuskels. Zeitschrift für Biologie 32: 370–447. Translated in Am Heart J (1958) 58: 282–317, 467–478.

Katz AM (1972). The force-velocity curve. A biochemist's point of view. Cardiology 57: 2–10.

Keith A, Flack, M (1906). The auricular ventricular bundle of the human heart. Lancet ii: 359–364.

Kent AFS (1914). Observations on the auricular–ventricular junction of the mammalian heart. Qtly J Exper Physiol 7: 193–195.

Kent S (1893). Researches on the structure and function of the mammalian heart. J Physiol 14: 233–254.

Krebs HA, Henseleit K (1932). Untersuchungen uber die Harnstoffbildung im Tierkorper. Hoppe-Seylers Zeitschrift Physiologie Chemie 210: 33–66.

Langendorff O (1895). Untersuchungen am uberlebender Saugethierherzen. Pflügers Arch Physiol 61: 291–332.

Loewi O (1917). Uber den Zusammenhong zwisohel digitalis-und calcium wirkung. Naunyn Schmiedebergs Arch Exper Pathol Pharmakol 82: 131–158.

Maroko PR, Kjekshus JK, Sobel BE, Watanabe T, Covell JW, Ross J Jr, Braunwald E (1971). Factors influencing size following experimental coronary artery occlusions. Circulation 43: 67–82.

McMichael J (1952). Dynamics of heart failure. Brit Med J ii: 525–529.

Nayler WG, McInnes I, Swann JB, Price JM, Carson V, Race D, Lowe TE (1968). Some effects of isoptin (Iproveratril) on the cardiovascular system. J Pharm Exper Therap 161: 83–96.

Opie LH (1980). Drugs and the Heart. Lancet, London.

Ringer S (1883). A further contribution regarding the influence of different constituents of the blood on the contraction of the heart. J Physiol 4: 29–42.

Sarnoff SJ, Berglund E (1954). Ventricular function. I. Starling's law of the heart studied by means of simultaneous right and left ventricular function curves in the dog. Circulation 9: 706–718.

Shanks RG (1976). The properties of beta-adrenoceptor antagonists. Postgrad Med J 52: 14–20.

Sonnenblick EH (1962). Force–velocity relationships in mammalian heart muscle. Am J Physiol 202: 931–939.

Sonnenblick EH, Brutsaert DL (1972). Vmax: its relation to contractility of heart muscle. Cardiology 57: 11–15.

Sonnenblick EH, Downing SE (1962). Afterload as a primary determinant of ventricular performance. Am J Physiol 204: 604–610.

Starling EH (1920). In: Starling on the Heart. Eds CB Chapman, JH Mitchell, pp 148–165, Dawsons, London, 1965.

Vaughan Williams EM (1958). The mode of action of quinidine on isolated rabbit atria interpreted from intracellular potentials. Brit J Pharm 13: 276–287.

Weidmann S (1955). The effect of the cardiac membrane potential on the rapid availability of the sodium-carrying system. J Physiol 127: 213–224.

White PD (1931) Heart Disease, Macmillan, New York.

Wiggers CJ (1934). Physiology in Health and Disease, p 568, Lea and Febiger, Philadelphia.

Wolff L, Parkinson J, White PD (1930). Bundle branch block with short P–R interval in healthy young people prone to paroxysmal tachycardia. Am Heart J 5: 685–704.

Wood P (1950). Diseases of the Heart and Circulation, Eyre and Spottiswoode, London.

2 Heart Cells and Organelles

W. Nayler, W. Gevers and L. H. Opie

Prior to Harvey, the true function of the heart was unknown. However, when in 1628 Harvey wrote "the blood is driven round a circuit with an increasing sort of movement; this is an activity or function of the heart which it carries out by virtue of its own pulsation", he was not only describing the circulation; he was also drawing attention to the heart's ability to provide the mechanical force necessary to sustain the circulatory flow. It was Ringer who showed that calcium ions are required for normal contractile activity (see Fig. 1-4). His work led to the modern concept that calcium ion fluxes into and within the myocardial cell explain most aspects of the contractile behavior of the heart. To understand this proposal requires a prior knowledge of the organization, structure and function of the myocardial cell (Table 2-1).

General Organization

Most of the heart is made up of **muscle cells** (also known as **cardiocytes** or **myocytes**). The remainder consists of pacemaker and conducting tissues (which are concerned with the generation and propagation of the heart's electrical activity), blood vessels and an extracellular space that is occupied mainly, but not exclusively, by viscous molecules called the proteoglycans which are soaked with interstitial fluid. A small amount of collagen is also present to provide a fibrous support, thereby keeping the various other tissues in their correct anatomical situations.

Cardiocytes

The individual muscle cells that account for more than half of the heart's weight are roughly cylindrical in shape (Fig. 2-1). Those in the atrium are quite small being less than 10 microns (μm) in diameter and about 20 μm in length. Relative to the atrial cells, the ventricular myocytes are large measuring about 10–25 μm in diameter and 50–100 μm in length (Table 2-2). When examined under the light microscope, the atrial and ventricular muscle cells have cross striations and are branched. Each cell is bounded by a complex membrane, the **sarcolemma**, and is filled with "rod-like" bundles of **myofibrils**: these are the contractile elements (Fig. 2-2). The sarcolemma invaginates to form an extensive tubular network (T-tubules) which extends the extracellular space into the interior of the cell. The nucleus, which contains almost all of the cell's genetic information, is centrally located; some myocytes have several nuclei. Interspersed between the myofibrils and immediately beneath the sarcolemma are the **mitochondria**, the main function of which is to generate the energy in the form of adenosine triphosphate (ATP) needed to maintain the heart's function and viability.

Pacemaker and conducting tissues

The electrical activity of the heart starts in specialized cells known as "pacemaker cells". These are located in the sinoatrial (= sinus) node. The node lies close to the junction of the superior vena cava and the right

Table 2-1

Composition and function of rat ventricular heart cell

Organelle	Percent of cell volume	Function
Myofibril	About 50%[1]	Interaction of thick and thin filaments during contraction cycle
Mitochondria	16% in neonate[1] 33% in adult[1]	Provide ATP chiefly for contraction
T-system	1%[2]	Transmission of electrical signal from sarcolemma to cell interior
Sarcoplasmic reticulum	33% in neonate[1] 2% in adult[1]	Takes up and releases Ca^{2+} during contraction cycle
Terminal cisternae	0.33% in adult[2]	? site of calcium storage and release[3]
Rest of network	Rest of volume	? site of calcium uptake *en route* to cisternae
Sarcolemma	Very low	Control of ionic gradients. Channels for ions (action potential). Maintenance of cell integrity. Receptors for drugs and hormones
Nucleus	5%	Protein synthesis
Lysosomes	Very low	Intracellular digestion and proteolysis
Sarcoplasm (= cytoplasm) (+ nuclei + other structures)	12%[2]	Provides cytosol in which rise and fall of ionized calcium occurs; contains other ions and small molecules

[a]Includes glycogen; see Reference 1.
[1]David et al. (1979). J Molec Cell Cardiol 11: 631.
[2]Page and McCallister (1973). Am J Cardiol 31: 172.
[3]Page and Surdyk-Droske (1979). Circ Res 45: 260.
Modified from Page and McCallister (1973).

Table 2-2

Micro-anatomy of heart cells

	Ventricular myocyte[1,2]	Atrial myocyte[1,3]	Purkinje cells[1,4]
Shape	Long and narrow	Elliptical	Long and broad
Length, μm	50–100	About 20	150–200
Diameter, μm	10–25	5–6	35–40
T-tubules	Plentiful	Rare or none	Absent
Intercalated disc	Prominent end-to-end transmission	Side-to-side as well as end-to-end transmission	Very prominent; abundant gap functions. Fast end-to-end transmission
General appearance	Mitochondria and sarcomeres very abundant. Rectangular, branching bundles with little interstitial collagen	Bundles of atrial tissue separated by wide areas of collagen	Fewer sarcomeres, more glycogen

[1]Legato (1973). The Myocardial Cell for the Clinical Cardiologist.
[2]Laks et al. (1967). Circ Res 21: 671.
[3]McNutt and Fawcett (1969). J Cell Biol 42: 46.
[4]Sommer (1982). J Molec Cell Cardiol 14 Suppl 3: 77.

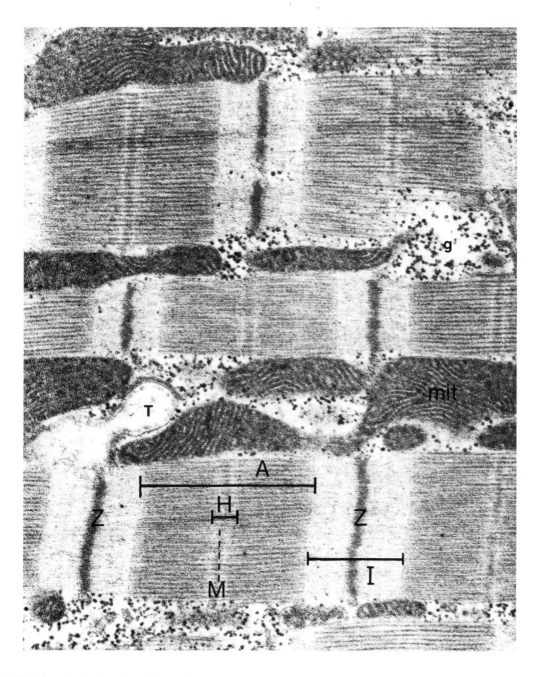

Fig. 2.1 Longitudinal section of rat papillary muscle showing regular arrays of myofibrils, divided into sarcomeres. Note the presence of numerous mitochondria (mit) sandwiched between the myofibrils, and the presence of T-tubules (T) which penetrate into the muscle at the level of the Z-bands. This two-dimensional picture should not disguise the fact that the Z-line is really a "Z-disc", as is the M-line. For description of A, I and H zones, see text. M = M-band; g = glycogen granules. × 32 000. By courtesy of Dr J Moravec, Paris.

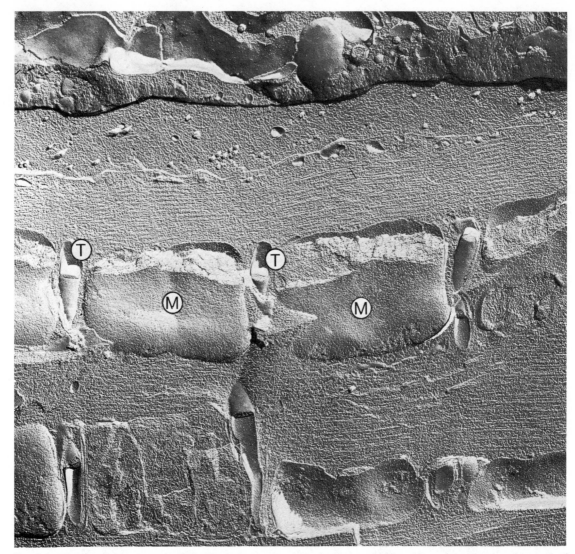

Fig. 2-2 The extensive network of the T-tubular system lying between mitochondria and penetrating the rows of sarcomeres at the Z-lines, delineated by a freeze-fracture micrograph. The lumen of the T-tubules is continuous with the extracellular space and brings the extracellular fluid into the ventricular myocyte. M = mitochondria; T = T-tubule; × 31 580. By courtesy of Dr Scales (1981), with permission.

atrium, and some of its cells spontaneously generate electrical activity. Hence the term "pacemaker". Certain substances, including the sympathetic neurotransmitter substance norepinephrine (noradrenaline), increase pacemaker activity; others, including the parasympathetic transmitter substance, acetyl choline, slow it down.

The electrical activity which is generated in the pacemaker cells of the sinoatrial node rapidly spreads throughout the atrium to reach the **atrioventricular node** which consists of fibers that have an unusually slow rate of propagation. Malfunction of this node can lead to heart block. Correct functioning, however, ensures that the delay between excitation of the atria and that of the ventricles is sufficient to allow time for the atria to empty and the ventricles to fill. The impulse is now distributed to the surface of the two ventricles by way of another set of specialized conducting fibers. The cells in this conducting pathway were first dissected out and described by the Czech physiologist, Purkinje. These Purkinje cells are located in a specialized conducting system starting off as the "bundle of His" and splitting into bundle branches.

Purkinje cells are unusually large, being 35–40 μm in diameter and about 150–200 μm long. This makes them about three times wider than the ventricular muscle cells and about eight times wider than the cells of the atrium. The individual Purkinje cells are packed tightly together, with each cell abutting closely against its neighbor. This tight packing, together with the relatively few connections between the Purkinje cells and the absence of T-tubules, minimizes the resistance to longitudinal conduction, because the diameter effectively available for conduction is that of the entire bundle rather than that of an individual Purkinje cell (Sommer, 1982). The rate of longitudinal conduction is also enhanced by the frequency of the junctions spanning the interrelated discs (gap-junctions).

The ability of the Purkinje cells to conduct electrical impulses so quickly enables the numerous cells of the ventricles to be excited almost synchronously, so as to eject blood into the aorta at pressure rather than simply moving it between different parts of the ventricular cavities—as may happen, for example, during very rapid ventricular arrhythmias.

Extracellular space

About 40 percent of the heart is not occupied by myocytes or pacemaker and conducting tissues. This extracellular space contains blood vessels (the coronary vasculature), interstitial fluid, some collagen and ground substances which consist mainly of proteoglycans. The latter are very large, aggregated molecules (formerly called mucopolysaccharides) in which long carbohydrate chains (bearing negative sulphate and carbohydrate charges) are attached to a protein "core"; this molecular structure helps to hold the ground substance together.

Blood vessels

A little over half of the extracellular space is occupied by the coronary vasculature. The capillaries lie close to the surface of the cells and come into contact with about one-third of the total cell surface. This large area of surface contact must mean that the intervening diffusion pathways are relatively short to facilitate the supply of substrates and oxygen for metabolism and the removal of any metabolic waste products.

Extracellular fluid

That half of the extracellular space in the heart not occupied by coronary vessels is filled with interstitial fluid, some of it entering into the interior of the cell by the T-tubular system. The ionic composition of the extracellular fluid differs markedly from that found within the cells, for the intracellular fluid (or **cytosol** as it is now called) is rich in potassium and low in sodium, whereas the reverse is true for the interstitial fluid that bathes the cells. The maintenance of the ionic gradients that result from this distribution of ions between the inside and outside of the cells depends upon a number of factors. The high-energy phosphate compound, ATP (Chapter 11), is required for the various pumps that drive the ions against their respective concentration gradients. An example of such a pump is the sodium–potassium pump that moves potassium into and sodium out of the cells. This pump is also called the sodium, potassium ATPase (Na^+/K^+-ATPase), or more simply the sodium pump. It is inhibited by the cardiac glycosides, including ouabain and digoxin.

Also contributing to the ability of cell membranes to maintain ionic gradients is the correct orientation of their phospholipids and proteins. This orientation is lost when cells are exposed to detergents or to certain naturally occurring toxins. The membranes then become much more permeable and ions move along their concentration gradients; the cells become overloaded with sodium and calcium and lose potassium, just as when an ischemic episode precipitates a decline in the tissue levels of ATP.

Collagen and elastic fibers

The small number of collagen fibers that are present in the extracellular space lie close to the surface of the myocytes, forming a supporting "framework" or "tissue skeleton". Small microfibrils and even smaller microthreads extend from the surface of the cells to the "tissue skeleton", as well as from cell to cell. Some of these microfibrils and filaments are collagenous, others are carbohydrate–protein complexes. These fine fibrils and filaments probably limit the amount by which the heart can be dilated by volume overload. Elastic fibers are found in close approximation to collagenous tissues, for example around the collagen "skeleton", on the surface of capillaries and around the myocytes. The two components of the elastic fiber are a glycoprotein which forms a microfilament about 11 nm in diameter, and the amorphous *elastin* component (Sato et al., 1983). The whole elastic fiber has properties similar to that of polymeric rubber. The elastic fibers account for a part of the elasticity of the myocardium; however, the major part lies in the cross-bridges so that the myocardium becomes less elastic as cross-bridges interact during systole. In the blood vessels of the heart, a protein called **fibronectin** lies in the subendothelial layers. When the endothelium is damaged as in atheromatous lesions, fibronectin may contribute to the connective tissue reaction (Effron and Harrison, 1983).

Sarcolemma and Glycocalyx

Most mammalian cells have a complex cell surface and cardiac muscle cells are no exception. The whole of the complex surface structure that surrounds each muscle cell can be subdivided into three layers, from the periphery inwards (Fig. 2-3). First, the glycocalyx can be split into (i) an outer coating or external lamina

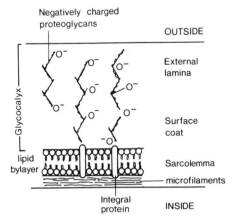

Fig. 2-3 The glycocalyx can be split into the external lamina (upper layer) and the surface coat (adherent to the sarcolemma) by means of a calcium-free perfusion (Frank et al., 1982). Upon reperfusion with a normal calcium medium, excess calcium ions enter the ventricular myocyte. Therefore it is proposed that the glycocalyx helps to protect heart cells against the much higher external calcium ion concentration.

which is about 30 nm wide and (ii) an inner coating about 20 nm thick, known as the surface coat (1 nm = 1 mm × 10⁻⁹ = 10 Ångstrom units). Secondly, immediately adjacent to the surface coat there is the true plasmalemma consisting of the lipid bilayer with its associated proteins. Thirdly, just beneath the plasmalemma there is a thin, mat-like layer of fine microfilaments which provides structural support. The term **sarcolemma** sometimes includes all three layers; more frequently it is a synonym for the "unit" plasma membrane or plasmalemma which encloses the cardiac muscle cell (McNutt and Fawcett, 1974). The structural and dynamic roles assigned to the glycocalyx and plasmalemma warrant further discussion.

The glycocalyx

The two outermost layers of the cell surface, the external lamina and the surface coat, together constitute the glycocalyx, which literally means "sweet husk". Synonyms for the glycocalyx include basement membrane, basal lamina, surface coat and boundary layer. Chemically it is composed of polysaccharides which may be associated with lipids (glycolipids) or with proteins (glycoproteins). Sialic acid residues are found at the ends of short branched carbohydrate chains attached to proteins. Calcium can be displaced from superficial binding sites by adding certain di- and trivalent cations, such as manganese and **lanthanum**. When Langer (1978) noted that the amount of calcium that could be displaced was proportional to the tension generated during contraction, he concluded that during excitation some of this calcium is displaced from the binding sites into the cell to activate contraction. He first thought that sialic acid (= neuraminic acid) in the glycocalyx constitutes the binding site; his recent data show that the binding is to the phospholipids of the outer layer of the sarcolemmal bilayer (Langer, 1984).

The major function of the glycocalyx is to provide an ionic trap to ensure that the external surface of the sarcolemma has a reasonably constant ionic environment. Under certain conditions the glycocalyx peels away from the underlying sarcolemma (Fig. 2-3). This happens, for example, when calcium is re-introduced to the heart after a short perfusion period with solutions containing less calcium than 50 μmol/L (micromoles per liter; instead of the millimolar amounts that are usually present). The end result is the loss of an effective ionic barrier at the periphery of the cell, so much so that when the calcium is added back it "floods" into the cells causing massive damage. Zimmerman et al. (1967) called this the **calcium paradox**.

The sarcolemma or plasmalemma

The sarcolemma, which lies immediately below and adjacent to the surface coat of the external lamina, is a bilayered structure. As in almost all other mammalian cells it contains phospholipids. The molecules of phospholipids are arranged so that their **hydrophilic (water-loving), phosphate-containing heads extend outwards, whilst their hydrophobic** (water-repelling) fatty acid tails are directed inwards towards the center of the membrane (molecules with these properties are called **amphiphiles**). The lipids provide the structural framework of the plasmalemma into which proteins are also inserted.

Two types of proteins are associated with the plasmalemma. First, the **intrinsic** or **integral proteins** are tightly associated and released only when the sarcolemma is damaged. These integral proteins are held in the plasmalemma by the side-chains of hydrophobic amino acids which interact with the lipid tails in the center of the membranes. Hydrophilic regions of the proteins project into the surrounding water on the inner or outer surface of the plasmalemma. **Transport proteins**, such as the sodium pump, are integral proteins which penetrate through the entire bilayer, bridging its innermost and outermost layers. Other integral proteins are involved in the formation of specialized "channels" which selectively transport certain ions into or out of the interior of the cell, often in a controlled, or "gated" manner.

Secondly, the **extrinsic** or **peripheral proteins** are rather loosely held to the inner surface of the plasmalemma by charge interactions with the lipid polar heads. Such extrinsic proteins merge into various cytoplasmic structures which attach to the plasmalemma, such as the sarcoplasmic reticulum and the actin-containing filaments at the intercalated discs.

Entry of ions through voltage-activated channels in the sarcolemma

Whilst the sarcolemma is normally relatively impermeable to ions, this condition changes when the cells are electrically excited. Then ion-selective channels that are embedded in the plasmalemma open to specific ions. There are sodium channels which are highly specific for the rapid entry of sodium ions, while the calcium channels are predominantly, but not exclusively, selective for the slow entry of calcium ions. Potassium channels allow an outward potassium current as the action potential ends. The passage of these ions does not happen in a haphazard fashion, but in a well-defined pattern which will be described in Chapter 4.

Intercalated discs

When the ends of neighboring cells make contact with one another, the sarcolemma becomes highly specialized forming the intercalated disc (Fig. 2-4). The major part of the intercalated disc is the **fascia adherens**, where the actin filaments insert themselves (*fascia* is Latin for band—the adherent band; the Greek *desmo* means bound, so that the alternative name is **belt desmosome**). **Spot desmosomes**, on the other hand, are localized micro-areas, about 5 percent of the surface of the disc, where thin filaments link cell-to-cell (Hüttner, 1980).

Thus the fascia adherens and spot desmosomes link contractile proteins from the ends of one cell to another. Another small part of the disc (perhaps 5 percent) has microchannels which allow communication of the cytosol of one cell with that of the next—the **nexus** junctions or **gap** junctions (*nexus* is Latin for "bond"). Here the space between the opposing surface of the adjacent cells (Fig. 2-5) is reduced to only 1 or 2 nm, and fine filaments appear within it, as if to connect the facing membranes of the opposing cells. Probably these gap junctions transport small molecules and ions from cell to cell, and also act as low-resistance electrical pathways. The depolarizing current therefore spreads directly from cell to cell, explaining the heart's capacity to function as a syncytium though anatomically it consists of discrete cells.

The transverse tubular system

This system involves (Fig. 2-2) the invagination of the sarcolemma to provide a series of hollow tubules that penetrate inwards, usually at the level of a Z-line (the latter are the regularly spaced electron-dense bands that are responsible for conferring the cross striation

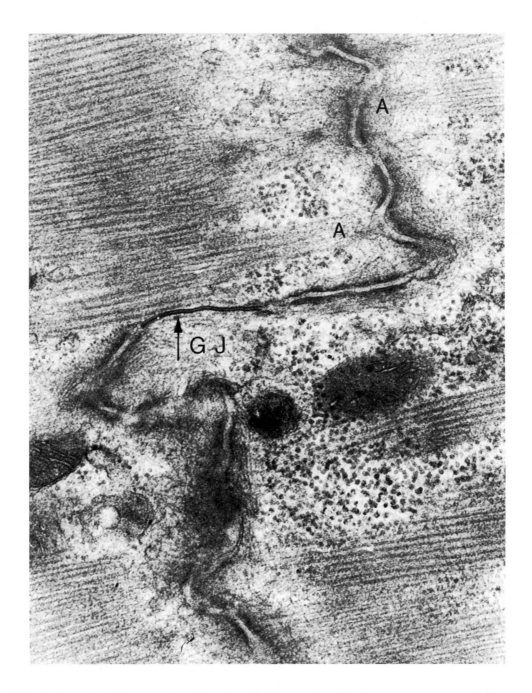

Fig. 2-4 The intercalated disc connection adjacent ventricular myocytes. The disc serves to anchor actin filaments, to bind cells to each other, and to communicate between cells. A = actin filaments inserting into fascia adherens; GJ = gap junction (see also Fig. 2-5). × 43 000. By courtesy of Dr J Moravec, Paris.

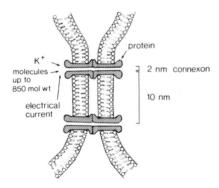

protein

K⁺ molecules → up to 850 mol wt

2 nm connexon

10 nm

electrical current

Fig. 2-5 Diagrammatic representation of the **gap** or **nexus junction**, where the distance between the adjacent cells is reduced to only 1 or 2 nm. (One nanometer (nm) is one thousandth of a millionth part of a meter.) Note the proposed connexons or microchannels which allow end-to-end communication between cells and are particularly prominent in Purkinje fibers.

Table 2-3

Membrane areas of ventricular cells (μm^2 membrane area/μm^3 cell volume).

	Area/volume
External sarcolemma	0.3
External sarcolemma plus T-tubules	0.4[a]
Sarcoplasmic reticulum	1.2
Mitochondrial cristae	11

[a]Other workers estimate that the T-tubules increase the area/volume ratio by several times.
From Page and McCallister (1973). Am J Cardiol 31: 172, with permission.

the fibers requires a correspondingly more prominent T-system.

Intracellular Organelles: Myofibrils

Almost half of each cardiac muscle cell is occupied by the contractile proteins. The remaining intracellular space contains the mitochondria, one or more nuclei, the sarcoplasmic reticulum (a specialized lace-like network of tubules that sequesters and releases calcium), the lysosomes (which are like small "bags" of degradative proteins), glycogen granules, a Golgi network and intracellular fluid (often referred to as the cytosol or sarcoplasm).

Micro-anatomy of myofibrils

Cardiac muscle resembles skeletal muscle in that its contractile proteins form longitudinally orientated, rod-like structures. These are the **myofibrils** (Frontispiece). Each myofibril is assembled from a large number of small filaments — the **myofilaments**.

The first recorded description of myofibrils was probably made by Felix Fontana in 1787. When dissecting skeletal muscle he noted the presence of "fleshy threads . . . solid cylinders equal to each other and very perceptibly marked at equal distances". In 1840 Bowman actually measured the distance between adjacent striations and reported it as being one thousandth of an inch — a measurement which agrees fairly closely with that obtained from electron-micrographs (2.2 μm for resting muscle).

Even under the light microscope, the myofibrils can be seen to contain bands of differing birefringence

pattern on the myofibrils). Initially, it was thought that the T-tubules ran in only one plane — at right angles to the main axis of the myofibrils. More recent studies have shown that they branch and ramify in all directions to interconnect. Usually only a single T-tubule is seen at the level of each Z-band. Occasionally they are paired. Probably the easiest way of tracing their course is to add an electron-dense marker substance (such as horse-radish peroxidase) that does not penetrate the sarcolemma (Fig. 2-6).

The important features of the **T-tubules** are as follows:

(a) their lumen is an extension of the extracellular space and contains modified interstitial fluid;

(b) in cardiac myocytes the lumen of the T-tubules at the surface of the cell is about 250 nm wide; this makes them ten times wider than their skeletal muscle counterparts. The existence of these very wide T-tubules in ventricular myocytes may ensure that an adequate supply of oxygen and nutrients is available to satisfy the needs of the mitochondria. Other possible advantages include the rapid removal by diffusion of metabolic waste products and a rapid and adequate supply of calcium for the contractile cycle; and

(c) since the T-tubules are extensions of and have the same ultrastructure as the cell surface, they increase the surface area of the cell, at least by 30 percent (Table 2-3) and possibly much more, thereby facilitating the spread of the excitatory stimulus. This function is not nearly as important in cardiac as in some types of skeletal muscle, where the much larger diameter of

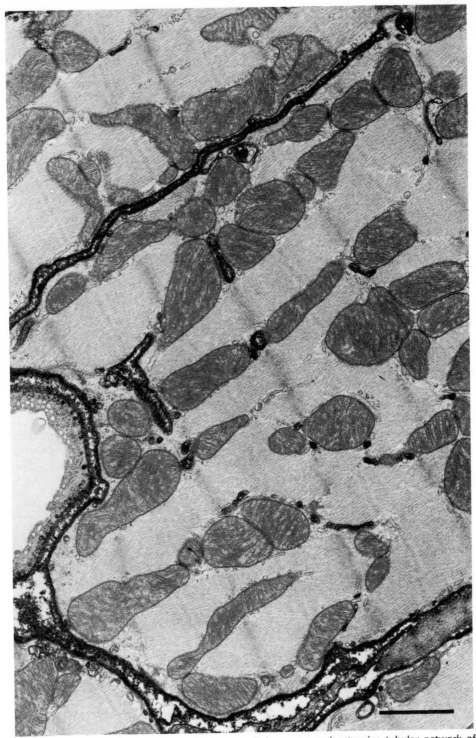

Fig. 2-6 Cardiac muscle cells from rat heart, with extracellular space and extensive tubular network of T-system delineated by the marker horse-radish peroxidase. × 20 000. By courtesy of Hüttner (1980) and Elsevier/North Holland Biomedical Press.

(light-scattering properties). For more than a century, the bands with the strongest birefringence have been designated as A (anisotropic) bands whilst those that are more weakly birefringent have become known as I (isotropic) bands. Each I-band is bissected by a dense staining band—the Z-disc (or line). The segment between two successive Z-lines is called a **sarcomere** and this is the fundamental unit of muscle function. Each sarcomere (Frontispiece and Fig. 2-1) consists of thick myosin filaments and thin filaments containing several different proteins including actin (which accounts for 60 percent of the thin filaments), troponin and tropomyosin. Myosin and actin are usually classed together as contractile proteins, whilst troponin and tropomyosin are known as regulatory proteins. This is because the actual physical process of contraction involves a displacement of filamentous actin along the myosin-containing thick filaments, while troponin and tropomyosin simply regulate the phenomenon (Chapter 8).

In the centre of each A-band there is a relatively clear zone known as the **H-zone** (from the German word *helle* meaning clear). Here only myosin is present, because the overlapping of the thin and thick filaments falls short of this region. Each H-zone contains a central dark region, the **M-line**, which contains M-line proteins that extend across the filaments as if to hold them in register.

The thick and thin filaments of the A- and I-bands overlap for part of their length, and the spacing between them is such that they can slide past each other without restriction. It is this sliding motion which is responsible for the shortening process of contraction. The force for the sliding movement comes from "rowing" movements of many cross-bridges which project from the myosin filaments and attach to the thin filaments, energy being provided by hydrolysis of adenosine triphosphate (ATP).

The Sarcoplasmic Reticulum

The sarcoplasmic reticulum consists of a network of tubules that are less than one thousandth of a millimeter in diameter (Scales, 1981). These wrap around the myofilaments and spread across Z-lines, extending from one sarcomere to the next. They anastamose and divide in all directions (Fig. 2-7) forming a lace-like network. The sarcoplasmic reticulum is entirely intracellular, and occupies about 2% percent of each ventricular myocyte (Table 2-1).

The total surface area exceeds that of the combined sarcolemma and T-tubules, at least in the rat myocardium. The main function of the sarcoplasmic reticulum is to regulate the intracellular movements of calcium ions, so that (i) calcium is released in response to the calcium entering the cell by the slow channel (or in direct response to depolarization); and (ii) calcium is retrieved from the myofilaments to decrease the cytosolic calcium ion concentration to facilitate relaxation.

When lying in close opposition to the sarcolemma or T-tubules, the tubules of the sarcoplasmic reticulum expand into bulbous swellings, still hollow, which lie along the inner surface of the sarcolemma or are wrapped around the T-tubules. These expanded areas of the sarcoplasmic reticulum have several names— **subsarcolemmal cisternae** (Latin for baskets), or caveolae (small caves) or the junctional component. Sometimes the cisternae occur in pairs (**diads**) lying astride the T-tubule, the whole having the appearance of **triads**. The close physical contact between the cisternae and the sarcolemma is made even more intimate by the development of small **electron-dense feet** found at coupling sites. Speculatively, the feet may reduce the distance between the opposing surfaces of the plasma membrane (or T-tubule) and the sarcoplasmic reticulum to help facilitate the spread of electrical activity from sarcolemma to reticulum.

A second part of the sarcoplasmic reticulum consists of ramifying tubules. At the start of diastole, a calcium pump thought to be located on the tubules of the sarcoplasmic reticulum, rapidly transfers enough calcium from the cytosol to the interior of these tubules. Calcium is thought to be released from the cisternae and taken up by the tubules of the sarcoplasmic reticulum, along which the calcium ions presumably flow along to the cisternae, again ready to be released. (Note that the longitudinal tubules of the sarcoplasmic reticulum and the T-tubules have completely different functions.)

By regulating the supply of calcium ions to the myofilaments, the sarcoplasmic reticulum determines precisely how much calcium is available for interaction with the regulatory proteins of the contractile mechanism.

Mitochondria

Mitochondria occupy a large proportion (see Table 2-1) of each myocyte. Located beneath the sarcolemma

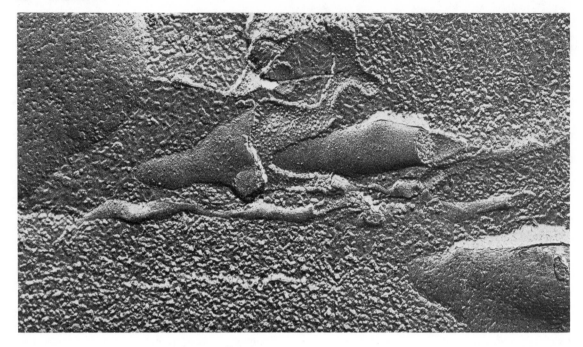

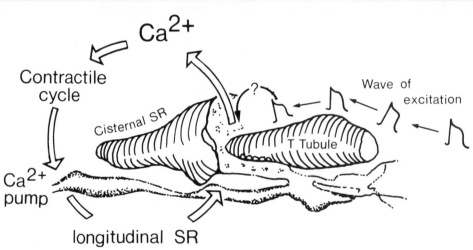

Fig. 2-7   Release of calcium from the cisternal or junctional component of the sarcoplasmic reticulum is rapid — in the heart it is potentiated by entry of calcium from the T-tubule, around which the cisternal sarcoplasmic reticulum is wrapped. The rapid release of calcium may be caused by collapse of a proton gradient established by the calcium pump (Shoshan et al., 1981) but this is controversial. Alternatively, the wave of depolarization may directly discharge the calcium ions. The freeze-fracture electron micrograph is taken from Scales (1981) with permission from the author and Academic Press. × 86 400.

they are wedged in between the myofibrils, presumably so that the chief source of energy supply is close to the chief site of energy utilization. Phase-contrast cinephotomicrography of cells in culture shows the overall shape of mitochondria is in constant flux. "Mitochondria may branch, fuse and focally enlarge or constrict" (McNutt and Fawcett, 1974). In fixed cardiac tissue the mitochondrial shape is pleomorphic, although elongated to fit between the myofilaments. Mitochondria may be in communication with each other through end-to-end connections (Bakeeva et al., 1983). Branching and formation of thin side-arms may

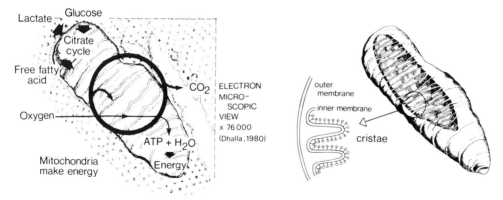

Fig. 2-8 The traditional "cocoon" mitochondrion is shown here. In reality mitochondria are in constant flux and may communicate with each other. The left part of the figure shows the fundamental role of mitochondria in the production of ATP. The right part stresses the transport function of the inner mitochondrial membrane, which separates the cell into two major compartments, the cytoplasm and the mitochondrial matrix. The electron microscopic view is drawn with permission from Dhalla et al. (1980). In: Drug-induced Heart Disease, Ed. Bristow MR, p 41, Elsevier/North Holland, Amsterdam.

either reflect formation of new mitochondria or the way in which constantly changing mitochondria are "snapped" in different shapes at the stage of fixation.

Mitochondria are often described as the "power-houses" of the cell, producing the energy (as ATP) that the cells need to survive and function (Fig. 2-8). Much of the "machinery" that is responsible for producing this energy is located on the inner multifolded membrane of the cristae, which occupy a vast membrane area when compared with other cell membranes (Table 2-3). The enzymes located here produce carbon dioxide and hydrogen atoms by the Krebs or citrate cycle. The energy that is released during the transfer of these hydrogen atoms to oxygen is harnessed for the synthesis of ATP: hence the term **oxidative phosphorylation** (see page 140).

Besides generation of ATP cardiac mitochondria have another important role, the accumulation of calcium (Carafoli and Crompton, 1978). A "back-ground" uptake helps to prevent the level of calcium in the cytosol from becoming too high in conditions of calcium overload. Thereafter, the mitochondria must again release such calcium to prevent the damage to mitochondria that comes from excess sustained accumulation of calcium. Mitochondria that are isolated from heart muscle that has been made ischemic for an hour or more and then reperfused, are overloaded with calcium and hence produce ATP at a very slow rate.

The Nucleus

Cardiac myocytes usually contain only one nucleus, although binucleate and multinucleate cells are also found (see Chapter 16). Nuclei are usually located near the center of the cell and account for about 5 percent of the cell's volume. Apart from the small amount of DNA that is found in the matrix of the mitochondria, all of the genetic information that is needed for each myocyte to maintain and repair its structure is contained in its nucleus or nuclei. Each nucleus is surrounded by an envelope formed by two membranes that are each about 10 nm thick. The envelope is perforated at frequent intervals and the pores are believed to be responsible for the selective passage of material into and out of the nucleus.

The major role of the nucleus is to control the systems that are responsible for tissue maintenance and repair. The genetic information that is required for this process is stored as sequences of bases in deoxyribonucleic acid (DNA). The actual process of protein synthesis (Chapter 3) takes place in the cytosol on very small particles called **ribosomes**, some of which are attached to the sarcoplasmic reticulum embedded in the cytosol. There must be a system which allows the coding information stored in the genes to be transferred to the amino acid assembly sites on the ribosomes. This function of information-transfer is performed by a special form of ribonucleic acid called messenger RNA (mRNA) which leaves the nucleus through the nuclear pores, carrying within it the required coding sequence. mRNA is bound to ribosomes free in the cytosol or attached to a net-like system known as the **endoplasmic reticulum**. These bound ribosomes are lined up on the outside of the endoplasmic reticulum giving a "rough" appearance. (Note the major distinction between the endoplasmic and the sarcoplasmic reticulum.) Hence mRNA molecules originating in the nucleus "alert" the ribosomes to the particular amino acid sequences that are required. Another form of RNA, known as transfer RNA, or tRNA, supplies the required amino acids in activated form to the ribosomes where the amino acids are joined in the sequences dictated by messenger RNAs. Once assembled, the proteins fold, associate with others and are distributed throughout the cell.

Golgi network

The Golgi apparatus, situated at the poles of the nucleus, is functionally associated with the endoplasmic reticulum. It is concerned with the processing and completion of those proteins due for secretion from cells or for incorporation into lysosomes or membranes of the cell.

Lysosomes and Peroxisomes

The cytosol contains numerous membrane-bounded sacs that are filled with enzymes. Some of these sacs are the **lysosomes**, discovered by de Duve. Lysosomes are spherical, membrane-bound organelles found mainly in the perinuclear region of cardiac myocytes, but more widely distributed in other cell types. Their interiors are more acid than the surrounding myoplasm and contain, in free or membrane-bound form, a very large number of different hydrolytic (digestive) enzymes which work best at pH values between 3 and 6. Cathepsins attack proteins and co-operate to produce total degradation to the level of free amino acids, which diffuse back into the cytosol. They are often regarded as "clearing houses" for unwanted intracellular substances, but probably also participate in the handling of some internalized nutrients such as cholesterol.

Susceptible proteins can be brought into contact with cathepsins within lysosomes by autophagy or they may be taken up in tiny droplets of cytoplasm engulfed in lysosomal membranes (micropinocytosis). Alternatively, lysosomal enzymes may leak into the cytosol under certain conditions, but the evidence for this is weak. Normally the pH of the cytosol is neutral, which excludes active proteolysis by cathepsin.

Peroxisomes are also membrane-bounded sacs but they contain enzymes that are responsible for producing and degrading peroxides — hence the name, peroxisomes. An accumulation of peroxides can lead to excess production of free radicals which in turn can damage cell membranes.

Receptors

Receptors are specialized sites in the cell membrane, chiefly the sarcolemma, which "receive" stimuli from circulating drugs or hormones. For example, the heart rate and contractility can be increased by stimulation of the autonomic sympathetic nervous system, which releases the catecholamine norepinephrine from nerve terminals to act as a neurotransmitter on the sarcolemmal beta-adrenergic receptors (or beta-adrenoceptors). Receptors have a particular molecular structure which can "recognize" and selectively interact with an agent such as norepinephrine, which is called an agonist. Receptors also interact with antagonist agents which can "fit in" the receptor site to "block" it from the agonist. Thus beta-adrenergic blocking agents can compete with catecholamine molecules for the beta-adrenoceptor, and by competitive inhibition can minimize the increase of heart rate or contractility resulting from sympathetic activity.

Receptors link the activity of the autonomic nervous system to the function of the heart. The beta-agonist catecholamine (or first messenger) interacts with the sarcolemmal beta-adrenoceptor (Chapter 6), which initiates a biochemical signal to "tell" a specialized part of the inner lipid layer, adenylate cyclase, to form the second messenger which is the compound cyclic adenosine monophosphate or cyclic AMP. The latter carries out the intracellular physiological effects of catecholamines by further biochemical signals which "tell" the pacemaker cells to increase the heart rate and myofibers to increase their contractility.

Microsomes

The term **microsome** includes a variety of subcellular organelles, which sediment together on centrifugation of myocardial homogenates. Mitochondria, being heavier, are excluded. The microsomal fraction, containing ribosomes, lysosomes and endoplasmic as well as sarcoplasmic reticulum, is a biochemical rather than an anatomical entity.

Summary

When considered in terms of the heart's capacity to function as a pump, the biochemical functions of the various intracellular organelles can be subdivided as follows:

(a) Firstly, there are the organelles that are responsible for maintaining ionic homeostasis. The sarcolemma, with its sodium pump, its calcium–sodium exchanger and its calcium pump would belong here. This group also includes the sarcoplasmic reticulum (by virtue of its ability to sequester and release calcium) and the mitochondria (because of their ability to provide a "background" regulation for calcium).

(b) As a second group, there are organelles which are responsible for the processes involved in control of calcium. This group includes the glycocalyx (a protective ionic trap), the sarcolemma (with its ion-selective channels), and the sarcoplasmic reticulum—which provides an intracellular store from which calcium is released to cause contraction and into which calcium is pumped back to cause relaxation.

(c) A third group includes the contractile and regulatory proteins such as actin, myosin, tropomyosin and the various troponins.

(d) The fourth group comprises the mitochondria which are concerned primarily with providing the energy (as ATP) that is needed for the functioning of the other organelles.

(e) Fifthly, there must be provision for tissue maintenance and repair—this is the role of the nucleus, the endoplasmic reticulum and the cyto-plasmic ribosomes.

(f) Finally, the function of the heart must be linked to the requirements of the body as a whole; this is accomplished by the autonomic nervous system which releases neurotransmitters to interact with receptors situated on the plasmalemma. Such receptors receive the signals and convert them to intracellular second messengers which appropriately regulate the physio-logical functions of the heart.

References

Bakeeva LE, Chentsov YS, Skulachev VP (1983). Intermitochondrial contacts in myocardiocytes. J Molec Cell Cardiol 15: 413–420.

Bowman W (1980). On the minute structure and movements of voluntary muscle. Trans Roy Soc London, Series B, 130: 457–501.

Carafoli E, Crompton M (1978). The regulation of intracellular calcium. In: Current Topics in Membrane and Transport. Eds. F Bonner, A Kleinzeller, Vol 10 pp 151–216, Academic Press, New York, London and Orlando.

Effron MK, Harrison DC (1983). Fibronectin: cardiovascular aspects of a ubiquitous glycoprotein. Am J Cardiol 52: 206–208.

Fontana F (1787). Treatise on the venom of the viper; on the American Poisons and on the Cherry Laurel and some other vegetable poisons. (J Skinner, trans.), Vol 2, London.

Frank JS, Rich TL, Beydler S, Kreman M (1982). Calcium depletion in rabbit myocardium. Circ Res 51: 117–130.

Huttner I (1980). The sarcolemma. In: Drug-induced Heart Disease. Ed. MR Bristow, pp 3–37, Elsevier/North Holland Biomedical Press, Amsterdam.

Isenberg G, Klockner U (1980). Glycocalyx is not required for slow inward current in rat heart myocytes. Nature 284: 358–360.

Langer GA (1978). The structure and function of the myocardial cell surface. Am J Physiol 235: H461–H468.

Langer GA (1984). Calcium at the sarcolemma. J Molec Cell Cardiol 16: 147–153.

McNutt, NS, Fawcett DW (1974). Myocardial ultrastructure. In: The Mammalian Myocardium. Eds. GA Langer, AJ Brady, pp 1–49, Wiley, New York.

Page E, McCallister LP (1973). A quantitative electron microscopic description of heart muscle cells: application to normal, hypertrophied and thyroxin-stimulated hearts. Am J Cardiol 31: 172–181.

Sato S, Ashraf M, Millard RW, Fujiwara H, Schwartz A (1983). Connective tissue changes in early ischemia of porcine myocardium: an ultrastructural study. J Molec Cell Cardiol 15: 261–275.

Scales DJ (1981). Aspects of the mammalian cardiac sarcotubular system revealed by freeze fracture electronmicroscopy. J Molec Cell Cardiol 13: 373–380.

Shoshan V, McLennan DH, Wood DS (1981). A proton gradient controls a calcium-release channel in sarcoplasmic reticulum. Proc Nat Acad Sci USA 78: 4828–4832.

Sommer JR (1982). Ultrastructural considerations concerning cardiac muscle. J Molec Cell Cardiol 14 Suppl 3: 77–83.

Zimmerman ANE, Daems W, Hulsmann WC, Snijder J, Wisse E, Durrer D (1967). Morphological changes of heart muscle caused by successive perfusion with calcium-free and calcium-containing solutions (calcium paradox). Cardiovasc Res 1: 201–209.

Synthesis and Turnover of Cardiac Proteins

W. Gevers

A striking feature of the proteins making up about one-sixth of the wet mass of the heart is the ceaseless synthesis and degradation, assembly into functional structures and disassembly that they undergo in the steady state. The precise concentration of proteins and organelles at any time in a cardiac cell is a result of these opposing processes. The cellular heterogeneity of the heart requires that different proteins must be made and degraded in a variety of cell types at different rates. Non-contractile cells outnumber the power-producing muscle cells in the mature heart, whilst making up less than 30 percent of the cardiac volume because of their considerably smaller average size (Fig. 3-1).

Polypeptide chains

Proteins consist of one or more linear amino acid polymers called polypeptide chains, each species of which has a defined sequence in which the constituent amino acid residues (up to 20) occur. The chains may be linked covalently (strong chemical bonds) or non-covalently (multiple weak forces) to non-polypeptide components such as iron-containing heme groups, metal ions or carbohydrates. The physical properties of the "backbone" peptide bonds and of the many different side chains (which vary in size, charge and hydrophobicity) ensure that polypeptide chains, as they are synthesized, fold spontaneously in a sequential and ordered manner. They eventually attain a size,

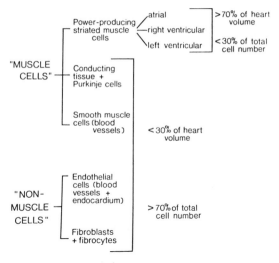

Fig. 3-1 Cells of the heart.

shape and surface topography which is quite distinctive and unique for each species of protein. Many proteins have some flexibility in their shape, and reversible conformational changes are one of the hallmarks of protein function, for example, contractile proteins and membrane pumps. Proteins show highly complex surfaces (specific as regards shape and the position of reactive chemical groups) to each other and to all the other proteins in their environment. This leads to spontaneous and specific aggregation and assembly, creating the structures and organelles in the cells of the heart.

Types of cardiac proteins

The major proteins are found in the myofibrils, and function in contraction. Myofibrils contain about 50 percent of total cardiac protein, and are made up of the proteins myosin, actin, tropomyosin, troponin, actinins, C-protein, M-line proteins and other minor species. Myosins and actins are also present at much lower concentrations in non-muscle cells (actin predominating) and contribute to the total complement of cardiac proteins. The second major group of proteins lies in the mitochondria, which make up more than one-third of the cardiac muscle cell volume. The third most plentiful group is found in the cytoplasm and comprises enzymes concerned with glycogen metabolism, glycolysis, phosphate transfers and fatty acid utilization.

Nucleoproteins are prevalent in the nucleus and also occur as ribosomal particles in the cytoplasm. Membrane proteins, apart from those in mitochondrial membranes, are present in the sarcoplasmic reticulum, nuclear membranes and in the specialized and unspecialized parts of cell surface membranes. Finally, extracellular proteins in the heart include collagen (about 4 percent of the total protein), other glyco-proteins such as fibronectin (Chapter 2), as well as proteoglycans and elastin in the walls of the arteries and other blood vessels.

Cardiac proteins are a relatively small part of the total muscle protein mass of the body. As such, they help to fulfil the general muscular role of nitrogen and energy reserve, and this may be one of the reasons for the existence of protein degradation mechanisms which are stepped up when an athlete hangs up his running shoes, during prolonged starvation or in the course of disease states.

Synthesis and degradation

The characteristic protein composition (phenotype) of individual cells reflects a balance between synthesis and degradation (Fig. 3-2). The great majority of cardiac proteins are not present in free solution but are organized into multi-molecular assemblies, which may be large and complex (organelles) or smaller and designed for a single function. Such assemblies are at once stable and evanescent, because they depend for their organization on multiple weak (non-covalent) interactions. Many of the proteins serve both as structural components and as specific functional units.

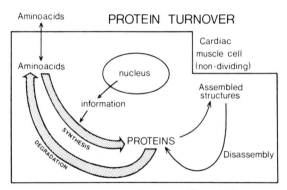

Fig. 3-2 Protein turnover in the heart. Note the important role of the nucleus in providing the information for the continuous ''replacement'' of proteins degraded in the cells.

Protein formation in the heart (Fig. 3-3) is not simply a question of polymerizing amino acids on ribosomes, but also of a large variety of post-synthetic modifications and events which are necessary for the formation of functioning proteins. A striking feature of intracellular protein degradation is the absence of repair mechanisms which could reverse the damage done by one or more ''cuts'' inflicted by a proteinase on a polypeptide chain. In general, any protein which has sustained even a single ''cut'' is rapidly degraded to its component amino acids, so that no intermediates accumulate.

One function of protein turnover seems to be selectivity, or the continued ability to select the most appropriate member(s) of a family of related proteins for use in particular physiological situations (see below). The action of thyroid hormones on rabbit hearts appears to be a good example of a large-scale substitution in cardiac muscle cells of one type of myosin for another. This could not happen without continuous turnover of the protein population, which in the case of myosin heavy chains operates with a half-life of 5–6 days.

Amino Acids

Amino acids are low molecular weight substances taken up from the plasma by the heart or formed within heart cells from intermediates of glycolysis or the Krebs cycle. Their principal function is to be incorporated into and excised from proteins in the ceaseless process of cardiac protein turnover. The branched-chain amino acids, leucine, isoleucine and

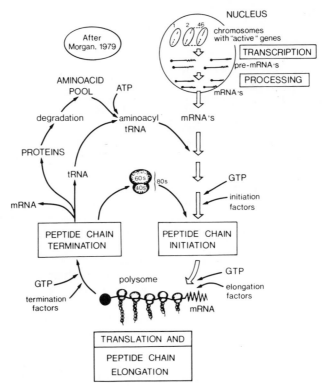

Fig. 3-3 Pathways for polypeptide and protein synthesis and turnover in heart. Modified from Morgan et al. (1979), with permission.

valine can be oxidized by the heart as physiologically trivial substrates when the normal flow of glycolysis is inhibited in starvation or severe diabetes, when such amino acids are oxidized more freely. These amino acids also exert effects on protein metabolism which entail the simultaneous enhancement of protein synthesis and inhibition of protein degradation. The inward transport of amino acids into heart cells is unlikely to be a rate-determining step in protein synthesis, because there usually is an adequate intracellular supply in the form of amino acids derived from protein breakdown (Fig. 3-4).

Protein Synthesis in the Heart

There is an important distinction between the two nucleic acids involved in protein synthesis (Fig. 3-5). Both are chains of many nucleotide base units ("polynucleotides"; for structure of nucleotides see Chapter 11); by far the larger is deoxyribonucleic acid or DNA, which may contain millions of base units.

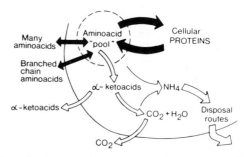

Fig. 3-4 Amino acids are taken up into an intracellular "pool" for use in protein biosynthesis. They also arise from protein turnover and may leave heart cells unchanged or in the alpha-ketoacid form; some of them are oxidized to CO_2.

The smaller, with anything from 120 to 50 000 base units, is ribonucleic acid or RNA, differing only by the presence of an extra oxygen atom on the sugar residues.

Molecules of DNA constitute the master file of genetic information carefully reproduced in successive generations of cells, whereas molecules of RNA are used as working copies and as tools for making proteins. These differences in function are reflected in the life-span of the molecules; the cell does not intentionally destroy DNA, whereas it constantly degrades and remakes RNA as a necessary part of its adjustment to changing circumstances.

McGilvery (1979)

It is the DNA molecules which have the well-known regular double-helical structure. When DNA forms, the RNA which conveys its genetic signal to the ribosomes (sites of protein assembly), then part of the DNA molecule, is unfolded so that one of the strands of the helix is used as a template ("blue-print") on which messenger RNA (mRNA) is newly synthesized from many molecules of the appropriate nucleoside triphosphates (Fig. 3-5). The nucleoside concerned may be either adenosine (A) or cytidine (C) or guanosine (G) or uridine (U). That these are the four nucleoside triphosphates involved in the synthesis of mRNA may seem confusing when considering the four nucleosides which constitute the "4-letter language" of the DNA molecule: they are A, T, C and G, standing for adenosine, thymidine, cytidine and guanosine. However, uridine differs from thymidine only in the absence of a methyl group and it forms the same type of hydrogen bonds. Thus DNA and RNA speak the same 4-letter language.

An enzyme, **RNA polymerase**, incorporates the correct nucleosides into the growing mRNA molecule, whilst shedding two of the phosphate units (as pyrophosphate = PP_i). Thus each nucleoside is incorporated in the precise sequence dictated by the genetic code.

Healthy muscle cells do not divide in mature hearts, yet the genes coding for proteins are continuously active within the chromosomes of the nucleus as DNA templates for the synthesis of RNA copies or transcripts. The genes thus expressed are scattered on the 46 chromosomes and represent a small fraction of the total coded information present. The RNA copies are chemically modified and shortened (edited) to form mRNAs which emerge from the cell nucleus and are used to dictate the sequences of proteins being synthesized on cytoplasmic ribosomes; the latter may be free (the majority in heart cells) or bound to internal cellular membranes. Most individual mRNAs, their coded information written in triplets of succeeding bases called codons, are simultaneously bound and translated by several ribosomes, forming **polysomes**. To these polysomes are brought activated amino acids, bound to a type of RNA concerned with the transfer process and therefore called transfer RNA (tRNA). In the ribosomes, the nascent polypeptide chains fold spontaneously as they are lengthened, until they are released from the ribosomal factories when complete as molecules with a defined shape and size. The translation of linear sequence information from the 4-letter language of nucleic acids (DNA strands or RNA strands), to the 20-letter language of proteins is

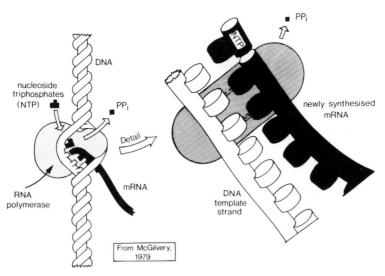

Fig. 3-5 Synthesis of new mRNA (pre-messenger variety) on the DNA template. Modified from McGilvery (1979), with permission.

extraordinarily error-free. (The protein language has 20 letters because 20 amino acids are involved.)

The rate at which new proteins of various kinds are synthesized in the cytoplasm, is mainly a function of (i) the differential availability of genes for transcription; (ii) processing and presentation of mRNA to ribosomes; (iii) the initiation of new peptide chains and (iv) the ability of the ribosomal apparatus to synthesize polypeptides.

Genes

The definition of a gene is constantly changing as modern knowledge of mammalian chromosomes expands. The gene for a given protein is that part of the total DNA present in a cell which is required ultimately to provide the sequence information for a particular polypeptide chain. In diploid cells the 22 autosomal chromosomes, present in duplicate, provide at least two identical or near-identical copies (alleles) of every gene functioning in this way. Additional non-allelic copies, which may be identical (amplified genes), near-identical, or greatly modified by mutations (homologous genes), are frequently found in clusters which have arisen as a result of serial gene duplications and mutations during the evolution of the species. These **gene families** provide the basis for the occurrence of isoproteins in the tissues of the body. Such isoproteins are separately encoded species of proteins with a particular function, which are closely similar but may differ in respect to some physiological properties. Different tissues characteristically express their own variants of proteins (**isoproteins**) especially in the case of enzymes (**isoenzymes**); these closely related molecular variants have properties which suit local conditions.

Messenger RNA

One of the crucial areas of control in protein biosynthesis is the very first step, namely the copying of the DNA gene sequence (Fig. 3-3) as a "photo-negative" to become part of the mRNA being formed (Brown, 1981). Because the mRNA ultimately exported from the nucleus is modified from that originally formed, the latter is termed **pre-mRNA**. The molecular mechanics dictate that the copying of DNA on to pre-mRNA is the negative–positive type used in photography and not the positive–positive type used

in auditory transmission. RNA synthesis or transcription is initiated only when the coded product protein is actually required. The majority of genes (>95 percent) are not active but **repressed**. The tremendous "packing ratio" achieved in condensing about 2 meters of linear DNA into a tiny nucleus about 10 μm wide, implies that many of the constraints imposed on RNA transcription in differentiated cells may be purely physically determined (Kornberg and Klug, 1981).

The enzymes capable of synthesizing RNA from DNA templates are called RNA **polymerases** (DNA-dependent RNA polymerases or reverse transcript-ases). These enzymes add the "correct" nucleoside at each step, so that the base of the nucleoside is the complement of the corresponding base in the exposed strand of the DNA template. Perhaps 6–10 of the base pairs in the double helix of the DNA become exposed at a time, with the polymerase advancing from base to base to incorporate the appropriate complementary nucleoside base into the progressively growing mRNA chain.

The number of molecules of each nucleoside used, and the order in which they are added, is precisely dictated by the sequence of complementary bases in the DNA template strand. Destruction of the product pyrophosphate from ATP or GTP or UTP or CTP makes biosynthesis irreversible. As the ribonucleotide residues are added, the enzyme moves along the double helix to the next DNA template. The process is repeated until a sequence signal says "stop" so that RNA is not made indefinitely and transcription stops. Then a different enzyme uses ATP to construct a long run (usually 100–200) of adenine residues, giving the linear pre-mRNA its characteristic **poly A "tail"**. Certain proteins immediately become tightly associated with this "tail" (Revel and Groner, 1978).

These highly intricate enzymatic reactions and associations convert pre-mRNA molecules into mRNA-containing ribonucleoprotein complexes (mRNP) which can transfer the complex genetic message out of the nucleus probably leaving via the nuclear pores.

Transfer RNA

For mRNA to convey the genetic message to the site of protein synthesis requires: (i) ribosomal subunits which will combine to provide a suitable site for the formation of polypeptide chains; and (ii) the arrival of activated amino acids at the ribosomal sites. Transfer RNA is concerned with intracellular collection of amino acids and transfer to the ribosomes. ATP-requiring enzymatic reactions fulfil the double purpose of "activating" the amino acids so that they can be polymerized, and coupling them to the tRNA molecules (Fig. 3-5). A separate enzyme (**aminoacyl tRNA synthetase**) is present for the transfer of each amino acid to tRNA, but the number of tRNAs is greater than 20 because the 4-letter triplet code requires about 60 different anticodons and as many tRNA molecules.

In structure, all tRNA molecules are very similar, consisting of a double helix of two RNA molecules, bent at about a right angle to form an L-shape. There are about 70–80 nucleotides in the molecule, rather rigidly held together by a great number of hydrogen bonds. At the one end of the "L", tRNA carries the activated amino acid required for protein synthesis; at the other end is the anticodon site which will link up with the codon of mRNA. By responding to the genetic information in the mRNA codon and synthesizing the polypeptide chain, the relatively simple tRNA molecule can convert the 4-letter genetic language into the 20-letter protein language (Quigley and Rich, 1976).

Ribosomes

The actual machinery for the formation of peptide bonds required for protein synthesis lies not in the mRNA molecules but in the ribosomes (Fig. 3-6). These are particles composed of many different molecules of proteins, some of which are enzymes required for formation of peptide chains and some of which help to determine the structure and shape of the ribosomal particle. Ribosomal particles are distinguished by having different sedimentation characteristics (due to their different size). The functioning ribosome 80s unit is formed when the 40s ribosomal subunit is combined with the 60s unit. Many such "whole units" bind to the same mRNA chain to form a polysome (Fig. 3-3) to which activated amino acids are transported by many transfer RNA molecules.

> The complete ribosome is in effect a sleeve that passes over the messenger RNA, the transfer RNA's, and the growing peptide chain to effect their contact with the protein factors in the ribosome necessary for the translational process   McGilvery (1979)

As each amino acid is added to the growing polypeptide chain, the ribosome moves along the

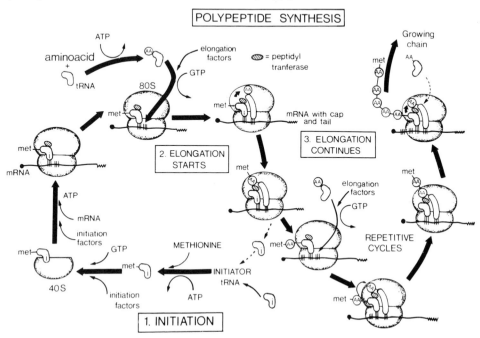

Fig. 3-6 Details of polypeptide synthesis. Note role of initiation and elongation factors. i = initiator mRNA; AA = amino acid.

mRNA molecule. Now molecules of tRNA come in, carrying appropriate amino acids to the site of synthesis of the peptide chain; there the tRNAs are bound to the mRNA with the anticodon of the tRNA linking to the codon of the mRNA.

The most effective way to control the rate of overall protein synthesis by a population of ribosomes is to make the step of initiation rate-limiting, thus avoiding a build-up of intermediates or of half-completed polypeptide chains (Hunt, 1980). At least seven **initiation factors** (all proteins called eiFs) are directly involved in getting protein synthesis going and there are also participating ribosomal proteins, placed at strategic points on the ribosomal surface, as well as mRNA-associated proteins. In addition, GTP and ATP are hydrolyzed (Fig. 3-6).

In this completed ribosomal unit, the anticodon of tRNA is apposed to the codon of mRNA to form a short segment of a double helix. This **codon–anticodon** pairing creates a site where the genetic information, originally in the DNA molecule, can be transferred to the nascent (= being born, Latin) protein as the appropriate amino acids are brought in by various tRNAs.

The first molecule of tRNA to bind to the small ribosomal subunit has something special about it and is called an **initiator tRNA**; it conveys the amino acid methionine, so is also called a methionyl-tRNA; the synthesis of all peptides starts with methionine. One particular codon of the mRNA recognizes the anticodon of the initiator transfer RNA, so that the methionine group is "ready" to be transferred to the next amino acid arriving with the next tRNA.

The binding of the initiator tRNA molecule also sets in process the formation of the "whole" ribosomal unit, to which the next tRNA can bind; this next tRNA will be selected because its anticodon binds to the next codon on the mRNA molecule. At this stage there are two tRNA molecules bound to mRNA (two anticodon sites on two codon sites), and the first two amino acids are ready to be joined to form the first peptide bond. Thus all is ready for elongation (Fig. 3-6).

Polypeptide chain elongation and termination

The 80s ribosomal initiation complexes are one of the requirements for polypeptide chain elongation, the others being GTP and a heterogeneous population of amino acyl tRNAs. The catalysts of the reaction are two important cytoplasmic proteins, the **elongation factors** (EF-1 and EF-2), and an enzyme which is an integral part of the larger ribosomal subunit (**peptidyl transferase**) (Clark, 1980). These proteins bind the molecule of the initiator tRNA (carrying the activated methionine) to a site on the ribosomal surface, which in turn allows the binding of the second tRNA bearing the appropriate amino acid to a second site on the ribosomal surface. As soon as the first peptide bond is formed by transferring the methionine chain to the amino acid of the second tRNA molecule, then the "empty" initiator tRNA molecule leaves the ribosomal complex. Its vacant site is occupied by the second tRNA molecule, bearing the first peptide linkage (methionine plus another amino acid), which forsakes its first binding site. The mRNA chain can now move along through the ribosomal "sleeve", till the next codon is in place to attract the anticodon of the next (now the third) tRNA—which will bear the next appropriate amino acid—required for that particular polypeptide. So the whole elongation cycle can go on and on, churning out the peptide bonds and rapidly forming the polypeptide chain, until there is a signal for **termination**. The appearance of a special termination codon in the mRNA sequence, for which there is no tRNA, causes the binding of GTP and a termination factor. As a result, the polypeptide is liberated, tRNA is released and the ribosomal subunits separate, ready for use in the biosynthesis of other proteins.

There is no evidence for the regulation of protein synthesis at the level of chain termination; any such control would be late in the day and highly uneconomical. The release of ribosomal subunits by the termination event completes the ribosomal cycle (Fig. 3-6) and sets the stage for further initiation.

Post-translational Assembly of Proteins

Most nascent polypeptide chains begin to fold as soon as they have reached a length sufficient to be clear of the ribosomal "sewing machine". The structure assumed is determined by multiple, weak chemical interactions between the polypeptide backbone chains themselves (secondary structure) or between side-chains which may be charged. Side-chains may also form hydrogen bonds with other appropriate groups, or they may have a hydrophobic character. Such intermolecular forces guide the growing molecule through a series of conformational changes, until the complete molecule assumes a specific "native" shape (tertiary structure) with a definite limit to its flexibility.

Each completed native protein becomes concentrated within the cellular compartment or organelle where it normally functions. This may entail remaining in the cytoplasm, either as an organized structure associated specifically with other proteins and components (myofibrils, glycogen particles), or free in solution, where loosely organized complexes of proteins are prevalent as in the glycolytic pathway. Some proteins migrate through membrane barriers to become associated more or less exclusively with structures such as mitochondrial inner membranes, the mitochondrial matrix, or chromatin within the nucleus.

Mitochondrial Protein Synthesis

A considerable fraction of newly produced cardiac proteins are taken up by the mitochondria, most of them becoming components of the thick and functionally important inner membrane, which is extensively convoluted and therefore has a vast surface area. A lesser amount of mitochondrial protein is synthesized on site. Mitochondrial protein synthesis would be expected to have some sort of reciprocal control relationship with cytoplasmic ribosomes, since growth of cardiac cells is always accompanied by enhanced protein synthesis both in the cytoplasm and in the mitochondria. Various schemes have been put forward to account for the co-ordination of the "import" and "on site" production lines in mitochondria.

Protein Secretion

In all cardiac cells, a significant part of the total protein production is either secreted into membrane-bound intracellular organelles (such as lysosomes) or to the cell exterior. In the case of muscle cells which are not striated, such as fibroblasts and smooth muscle cells, secretion to the exterior is a major pathway of protein flux. Collagen, elastin, proteoglycans and glycoproteins are produced in large quantities by the specialized processes of intracellular protein secretion followed by extrusion (**exocytosis**).

Extensive post-translational modifications are characteristic of this group of proteins, including the addition of carbohydrate side-chains (glycosylation), hydroxylation, oxidation and subsequent cross-linking

of side-chain groups, as well as **limited proteolysis** or protein processing. Membrane proteins are probably produced partly by a modified secretion mechanism or by uptake of polypeptides into existing membranes (Davies and Tai, 1980).

Such maturational changes are well illustrated by the formation of the **collagen fibers** in the heart which join with fibronectin, elastin and proteoglycan to form the extracellular matrix of arterial or arteriolar walls (see page 20), the modified "micronet" of similar composition which surrounds every cardiac cell, basement membranes for endothelia of cardiac vessels and the more obvious macroscopic connective tissue in the valves and cardiac ring of the heart.

Protein Degradation in the Heart

The concentration of a given protein in the heart will, at any given time, be a function not only of the rate of the synthetic processes already described, but also of the rate of degradation; both can be varied independently. General features of protein degradation have become apparent from studies of various systems, which have pointed to the existence of at least two major pathways (Ballard, 1977). During **basal proteolysis**, native proteins are continuously removed from their individual cellular pools by enzymes breaking down protein—the **proteinases**. Such removal occurs at random within the population, so that molecules do not have a fixed life-span. The process of degradation is complete to the amino acid level. The rate of degradation is different for different proteins. Some physical properties of proteins appear to be associated with rapid rates of basal turnover. These include a large size of individual polypeptide chains, the prevalence of large numbers of acidic groups on the surfaces of proteins and the presence of carbohydrate side-chains. Proteins which are rendered more susceptible to physical denaturation by the removal of prosthetic groups or substrates, by replacement of natural residues by analogs or after mutant substitutions, are degraded more readily than their "normal" counterparts.

Secondly, during **accelerated proteolysis**, hormonal stimulation of cellular proteolysis occurs with much less or no discrimination, and is compatible with a bulk destruction mechanism. Areas of the cell become sequestered in membrane envelopes (segresomes) by a process known as **autophagy**. The **segresomes** undergo fusion with lysosomes and complete destruction of proteins, with other macromolecules, then occurs in the secondary lysosomes so formed, by the action of lysosomal proteases (Chapter 2). Now degradation is complete to the level of amino acids.

Possible rate-limiting steps

Cardiac muscle contains a variety of other proteinases which may function in the breakdown of proteins. These proteinases have pH optima in the neutral or mildly alkaline range. Some of these are constituents of mast cells and the cellular location of others is in doubt. Some proteins are more susceptible than others to digestion by proteinases. Thus the susceptibility of proteins not assembled into organelles, large complexes or oligomers is much greater than that of proteins which are organized into such protected and functioning entities. Disassembly of protein structures is, therefore, a crucial step in the initiation and promotion of protein degradation. Proteolytic "nicking" is probably not the rate-determining step in the degradation of individual proteins; more important are reversible conformational or state changes which predispose proteins to cleavages in exposed regions. One consequence of "nicking" is the opening up of the compact protein structure and the exposure of normally internal hydrophobic groupings. This may lead to membrane binding (e.g. to lysosomal membranes), which would tend to destabilize the native conformation further, and would expose susceptible bonds to the action of cellular proteinases. Fragments thus created would be candidates for lysosomal uptake; alternatively, the non-lysosomal "neutral protease" battery may suffice to degrade the polypeptic chains completely.

Turnover of extracellular molecules

Turnover of extracellular molecules such as collagen, fibronectin and proteoglycans occurs normally in the heart. Contributing to this may be (i) cell-derived tissue collagenases and other proteinases present in latent form and proteolytically activated by cellular release of key enzymes; (ii) serum-derived proteinase cascades (e.g. the fibronolysis or kallikrein systems); or (iii) the production of proteinases by infiltrating phagocytes. These processes play a part in growth or remodelling.

Physiological control

Although a large number of metabolic signals have been identified which exert significant effects on the synthesis or degradation of proteins in isolated heart preparations (Fig.3-7), there is no certainty that such factors normally operate with the exception of the work load which determines the rate at which protein turnover is "set" and the size of the organ by an unknown mechanism (Chapter 16).

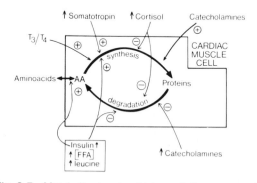

Fig. 3-7 Metabolic signals which can influence rate of protein synthesis or degradation in the heart. The exact physiological role of these factors is still not known, nor is it clear which signals are involved in the enhanced protein synthesis occurring during a hemodynamic load (Chapter 15). T_3/T_4 = thyroid hormones; AA = intracellular amino acids; FFA = concentration of circulating free fatty acids.

Summary

The heart contains many cell types; mechanical work is done by cardiocytes which do not divide but are capable of continuous protein synthesis and degradation. The steps in protein synthesis are: (i) the formation of mRNA molecules on the "template" of the DNA in the genes of the nucleus; (ii) binding of the mRNA to ribosomes which initiates protein synthesis in the presence of various initiation factors; (iii) for such synthesis to proceed, a supply of activated amino acids combined with tRNA (aminoacyl-tRNA) is needed; (iv) various aminoacyl-tRNAs arriving successively, are acted on repetitively by a ribosomal enzyme system to incorporate the amino acids into the growing polypeptide chain; the aminoacyl-tRNAs are selected by their ability to bind to the mRNA code words; and (v) completion of chain growth when the appropriate termination code word appears in the mRNA on the ribosome. Regulation of protein synthesis is exerted mainly, but not exclusively, at two levels: (i) RNA synthesis in the nucleus; and (ii) protein synthesis in the cytoplasm. The complex processes of synthesis and degradation are finely balanced and do not interfere with function despite their occurrence at a rate which means that most of the cardiac protein is replaced every 7–14 days.

The workload influences the rate at which the protein turnover mechanism is "set" and, therefore, the size of the organ as a whole.

References

Ballard FJ (1977). Intracellular protein degradation. Essays Biochem 13: 1–37.

Brown DD (1981). Gene expression in eukaryotes. Science 211: 667–674.

Clark BRC (1980). The elongation step of protein biosynthesis. Trends Biochem Sci 5: 207–210.

Davis BD, Tai PC (1980). The mechanism of protein secretion across membranes. Nature 283: 433–437.

Gevers W (1984). Protein metabolism. J Molec Cell Cardiol 16: 1–32. [This article contains a systematic set of references to matters alluded to in this chapter.]

Hunt T (1980). The initiation of protein synthesis. Trends Biochem Sci 5: 178–181.

Kornberg RD, Klug A (1981). The nucleosome. Sci Am 244 (2): 52–64.

McGilvery RW (1979). Biochemistry. A Functional Approach, p 298, Holt-Saunders, Philadelphia.

Morgan HE, Rannels DE, McKee EE (1979). Protein metabolism of the heart. In: Handbook of Physiology: Circulation. Ed. R Berne, pp 845–871, American Physiol Soc, Washington.

Quigley GJ, Rich A (1976). Structural domains of transfer RNA molecules. Science 194: 796–806.

Revel M, Groner Y (1978). Post-transcriptional and translational controls of gene expression in eukaryotes. Ann Rev Biochem 47: 1079–1126.

New References

Morkin E (1984). Hormonal effects on cardiac performance. In: Physiology and Pathophysiology of the Heart. Ed. N Sperelakis, pp 593–603, Nijhoff, Boston.

4 | Pumps, Channels and Currents

A common concept of the sarcolemmal membrane is that of a semipermeable sac, holding vital subcellular organelles including enzymes and other macromolecules such as the contractile apparatus. On irreversible cell damage, as in infarction, this membrane ruptures to liberate diagnostic enzymes into the circulation and a general breakdown of cellular structure follows. This simplified version makes no allowance for the molecular heterogeneity of the cell membrane nor for its vitality—innumerable different molecules and assemblies, such as receptors, participate in the structure of the membrane, while a constant flux of ions passes in and out through carefully regulated "channels", "pumps" or exchange mechanisms. Above all, the membrane maintains its essential function of maintaining vast gradients of ions, enzymes and subcellular organelles between the intracellular and extracellular environments. The structure of the normal sarcolemma should be recalled at this point.

Lipid Bilayer

The pattern of most cell membranes is that of a lipid bilayer, providing both the structural framework and maintaining the permeability barriers. Another way of viewing the membrane is as a trilaminar unit, the three layers being the two outer zones with the polar hydrocarbon heads, and the inner layers being the hydrocarbon tails pointing towards each other. This "fluid mosaic" structural model supposes that the polar hydrocarbon tails are not fixed but "fluid", and that the lipid molecules can move laterally to exchange places by "lateral diffusion"; rarely can the lipid molecules of one layer change with those of the other.

Besides the movement of lipid molecules, biosynthesis and biodegradation occur continuously, some of the membrane being renewed with a half-life of only hours or days.

As the wave of electrical excitation speeds throughout the ventricular myocardium, the sarcolemma becomes highly permeable to a number of ions by the opening of "channels" which allow ions to flow across the sarcolemma. Such ionic movements occur in a characteristic sequence—first sodium, then calcium and then potassium—determining the typical shape of the ventricular action potential. The distribution of ions across the sarcolemma, when there is no excitation during diastole, must be examined to understand the normal electrical properties of the ventricular cells.

Resting Membrane Potential

In the normal resting myocardial cell, there is a difference in the electric charges within and without the sarcolemma, which can be metered by insertion of a very fine tipped micro-electrode. The charges inside and outside the cell are different so that the **resting membrane potential** is about -85 mV (millivolts) less inside the cell. During the passage of the electrical wave, this "polarity" of charges existing across the sarcolemma is lost. The cell now becomes depolarized; the juxtaposition of depolarized and polarized sarcolemma allows current to flow inwards to the polarized negative part of the cell, opening the sodium and other channels by the process of **voltage-activation**. The voltage is the electrical force moving the current.

Generation of resting membrane potential

Hypothetically, a "resting" cell could have equal concentrations of the principal charge-bearing ions (Na^+, K^+, Cl^-) on either side of the sarcolemma, and a low concentration of anions associated with intracellular proteins on the inside. The activity of the sodium pump transfers potassium ions inwards; as they accumulate on the inner surface they start moving back to the outer surface, sarcolemma being highly permeable to potassium ions (the **conductance** to K^+ is high). Similarly, sodium ions pumped out of the cell accumulate on the outer surface of the sarcolemma and will tend to diffuse inwards (Fig. 4-1); the latter process is much slower than the outward diffusion of potassium ions because the sarcolemma is about 50 times less permeable to sodium than to potassium (low Na^+ conductance across resting membrane).

A simple example assumes that the sodium pump is neutral, exchanging Na^+ and K^+ equally. As an example, let 400 000 Na^+ and K^+ ions be pumped per msec per unit area (Woodbury, 1963). Suppose that of the 400 000 K^+ ions pumped inwards only 200 K^+ ions will diffuse outwards in contrast to 4 Na^+ ions (conductance differences) with a charge difference of 196 negative ions on the inside to cause the electrical potential which can be calculated by the **Nernst equation**

$$E_m = 61.5 \log K_i/K_0$$

If the external potassium is 4 mM and the internal value 140 mM, the calculated **equilibrium potential** (= **reversal** potential) is −95 mV; 80mM is a better value for the "active" intracellular K^+ concentration so that the calculated potential is −80 mV. Allowing for the electrogenic component of the sodium pump (about −10 mV), the total of −90 mV is not far from the measured value. Thus many workers think of the resting potential as being generated solely by potassium ions, but other ions also contribute during depolarization, when the permeability of each ion must

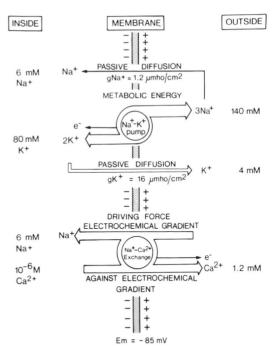

Fig. 4-1 Role of sodium pump (Na^+−K^+ pump), Na^+−Ca^{2+} exchange and passive diffusion in maintaining ion gradients across sarcolemmal membrane. The intracellular concentrations are those "free to act", i.e. the activities (see Table 4-1). For conductances during action potential see Fig. 4-5.

be considered. These complexities are better taken care of by the more evolved **Goldman field equation** (Goldman, 1943).

It requires emphasis that only a fraction of the total cell K^+ ions are involved in the generation of the resting membrane potential.

Intracellular Concentrations and Activities

In the idealized, simplified cell just described, it is assumed that intracellular ions are distributed uniformly throughout the cell. In reality, the apparent concentration of an ion in the heart cell must be distinguished from its activity (Table 4-1).

To measure the concentration of an ion in the myocardium requires a ventricular biopsy. The limits of the extracellular space must be defined to allow correction for those ions outside the cell. The central elements of the T-system are in direct communication with the exterior of the cells, and should contain high

Table 4-1

Intracellular and extracellular concentrations of ions in normal heart

Ion	Extracellular concentration		Apparent ventricular content (mmol/kg wet wt)	Intracellular concentration ionized in cytosol (mM)	References
	Total (mM)	Ionized (mM)			
Na^+	140	140	40	About 6	1, 5
K^+	4	4	70	About 80	1, 5
Mg^{2+}	1.20	0.60	8	About 0.6	2
Ca^{2+}	2.50	1.25	0.6	0.0003–0.001	3
Cl^-	140	140	35	About 30	4

[1]Dalby et al. (1981). Cardiovasc Res 15: 588.
[2]Page and Polimeni (1972). J Physiol 224: 221.
[3]Jennings and Shen (1972). Myocardiology 1: 639.
[4]Spector (1956). Handbook of Biological Data, p 71, Saunders, Philadelphia.
[5]Values refer to activities. See Lee and Fozzard (1975). J Gen Physiol 65: 695.

concentrations of sodium ions. Yet extracellular markers, such as insulin or radioactive sulfur, do not completely penetrate to those seemingly sequestered intracellular sites. The exact extracellular ion concentration is therefore very difficult to determine. Hence of more importance is the **activity** of the ion — the actual concentration that is in a free state in cytosolic water. Measurements of the activities of sodium and potassium by special micro-electrodes (Cohen et al., 1982) show that only a part of the cellular value of each ion is active, so that the gradient across the sarcolemma for both sodium and potassium is about 20-fold (Table 4-1). For calcium, the intracellular ionized concentration in diastole is very low, about 10 000 times below the extracellular value. For other ions, only estimates are available. Most of the magnesium seems to be bound to or contained in various cellular organelles (mitochondria), or associated with ATP and other nucleotides; only a fraction is free and ionized.

Sodium–Potassium Pump

The sodium–potassium pump shunts sodium out of the cell and potassium into the cell against the electrochemical gradients; although commonly called the sodium pump, more accurate names are the sodium–potassium pump or the Na^+/K^+-ATPase. The enzyme is activated by internal sodium and/or external potassium and uses energy in the form of ATP complexed to magnesium.

$$3 (Na^+) \text{ in} \longrightarrow 3 (Na^+) \text{ out}$$
$$2 (K^+) \text{ out} \longrightarrow 2 (K^+) \text{ in}$$
$$MgATP^{2-} + H_2O \longrightarrow MgADP^{1-} + P_i^{2-} + H^+$$

One ATP molecule is used per transport cycle, which adequately covers the energy requirements. One positive charge leaves the cell for each 3 sodium ions exported so that the pump is electrogenic, tending to make the inside of the cell negatively charged; hence another name is the **electrogenic sodium pump**. The pump probably contributes about -10 mV to the resting membrane potential. The sodium pump indirectly extrudes calcium ions from the cell by removing those internal sodium ions which have entered as calcium ions leave. Because the influx of calcium ions via the calcium channel is very rapid and the flux through the sodium pump very much slower,

Table 4-2

Density of channels, pumps and receptors in sarcolemmal membrane

	Per μm^2 of sarcolemma
Sodium pump	About 400
Sodium channel	16
Calcium channel	0.1
Beta-adrenergic receptor	2
Muscarinic receptor	6
Nitrendipine binding sites	1

Data from Reuter, 1984; Colvin et al., 1983.

there is a much larger number of sodium pumps per unit surface of the sarcolemma than of calcium channels (Table 4-2).

Properties of the sodium pump

The sodium–potassium pump is asymmetrically situated in the sarcolemma so that sodium-activation sites are located on the internal surface and most of the potassium activation sites on the external surface (Fig. 4-2). The exact location of this pump in the sarcolemma depends on the membrane model favored. According to the fluid mosaic model, the lipid bilayer is interspersed with globular proteins, some of which penetrate all the way through the membrane. The sodium–potassium pump is presumably one of these

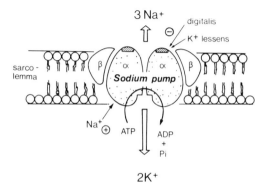

Fig. 4-2 Schematic representation of the sodium pump, which is thought to consist of two alpha-subunits, each of molecular weight about 100 000, and of two surrounding beta-subunits of molecular weight about 45 000. The ionic channel is located in the alpha-domain which also has: (i) the external digitalis binding site; (ii) the external potassium binding site; (iii) the internal sodium binding site; and (iv) the ATP hydrolysis site. For simplicity, these sites are shown on only one of the alpha-subunits. Note that potassium binds to two external sites to inhibit the binding of digitalis to the pump. Modified from Schwartz and Adams (1980), with permission.

proteins. When K^+ binds to the outside or Na^+ to the inside surface, then the enzyme undergoes a change in configuration. This molecular change is transmitted via the neighboring cell membrane to other subunits of the sodium pump which also change their molecular properties to the "active" form. Thus the pump is activated, ATP broken down and Na^+ exchanged for

K^+. ATP binds to the enzyme to form a phosphory-lated intermediate which breaks down to provide the energy required.

Digitalis compounds bind to the outer part of one subunit of the pump, which is the digitalis receptor site (see Fig. 20-3). The sensitivity of various species to the inotropic effect of digitalis is similar to the avidity with which the sodium pump concerned binds with digitalis glycosides. How these events link to increased contractility is not known, but the ultimate signal is an increased intracellular calcium ion concentration.

Vanadium is a trace metal which potently inhibits the sodium pump with a positive inotropic effect (Scholz et al., 1980) like digitalis; trace amounts present in the myocardium could theoretically act as a physiological regulator of the pump.

One theory for the **ischemic loss of potassium** is that accumulated fatty acid intermediates inhibit the pump; another theory is that the loss of potassium (and the later gain of sodium) is caused by lack of ATP for the sodium pump. Yet potassium starts to leak even when the total ATP is more than adequate for the activity of the pump. Furthermore very early loss of potassium cannot involve the sodium pump because there is no net gain of sodium. In contrast, in digitalis toxicity the marked loss of cellular potassium is clearly related to excessive inhibition of the pump.

Calcium Pumps

Calcium pumps also require energy to transport calcium ions against the large concentration gradients that exist between the relatively low calcium ion concentrations in the cytosol and the much higher values in the sarcoplasmic reticulum or the extra-cellular space. The sarcoplasmic reticulum needs so much pumping activity to take up the calcium ions from the cytosol that the membrane of the sarco-plasmic reticulum has been described as a "battery of pumps". This pump is "switched on" by a membrane protein called phospholamban which requires a phosphate group for its maximal activity. Such phosphorylation is achieved either by (i) the effect of catecholamine stimulation or (ii) an increased cytosolic calcium ion concentration, acting by combination with the calcium modulator compound, calmodulin (for details, see Chapter 7). Therefore the systolic rise of calcium ions will stimulate the uptake of calcium into the sarcoplasmic reticulum to help initiate diastole.

Catecholamine stimulation will accelerate the uptake of calcium ions into the sarcoplasmic reticulum to shorten diastole and to accelerate relaxation so that the heart can fill better. Another calcium pump, in the sarcolemma, responds to similar stimuli but is far less important than that in the sarcoplasmic reticulum. Usually calcium ions leave the myocardial cell by an exchange with sodium (see later).

Sodium Channel

The normal negative resting membrane potential of atrial and ventricular cells is abruptly lost when the sodium channels open to increase the conductance for sodium and to allow the rapid influx of sodium ions. Differentiation between the fast channel and the slow channel of the action potential was first achieved by electrophysiologists using toxic doses of quinidine which markedly inhibited the fast channel to uncover the slow channel (see Fig. 1-9), whose permeability for calcium is about 100 times that for sodium (Reuter and Scholz, 1977). Hence a practical classification is into the fast sodium channel and the slow calcium channel (Table 4-3).

Model for sodium channel

A good working hypothesis is that there are several "gates" which open to "activate" the channel (the "m" gates or activation gates (Fig. 4-3). Sodium ions rapidly enter the cell when the activation gates are opened by a voltage stimulus (**voltage-activation**); the gates close with full depolarization. There are other gates, the **inactivation-gates** ("h" gates), which when closed render the channel inactive. It is thought that Class I antiarrhythmic agents such as lidocaine and quinidine preferentially bind to sodium channels in the inactivated state (for details, see Chapter 23). Hence, the affinity of such drugs for the sodium channel of partially depolarized cells is greater than for that of normal cells (Hondeghem and Katzung, 1977), so that abnormal heart rhythms may be inhibited while normal rhythm is maintained.

Pharmacological dissection

Studies with **tetrodotoxin** (TTX) tell us that the sodium channel is selectively inhibited by the binding of this poison to an external membrane site. The number of

Table 4-3

Contrasting properties of fast and slow channels

Property	Fast action potential	Slow action potential
Ion specificity	Sodium	Calcium
Inhibitors	TTX,[a] lidocaine quinidine	Ca^{2+}-antagonists *l*- more than *d*-verapamil
Physiologic occurrence	Atrial, Purkinje and ventricular tissue	Nodal and vascular tissue; as component of normal atrial, Purkinje or ventricular action potential
Effect of beta-adrenergic receptor stimulation	No effect	Enhances Ca^{2+} entry by "opening" channels
Threshold of activation	-60 to -70 mV	-30 to -40 mV
Resting membrane potential	-80 to -90 mV	-40 to -70 mV
Overshoot	$+20$ to $+35$ mV	0 to $+15$ mV
Maximal rate of depolarization (phase 0)	100–1000 V/sec	1–10 V/sec
Type of conduction	Fast	Slow
Role in arrhythmias	Tachyarrythmias; ectopic activity; possibly in ischemia as "slow" fast responses	Slow conduction predisposes to re-entry; possible additional role in "slow response", and in ventricular fibrillation

[a]TTX = tetrodotoxin.
Electrophysiological data from Singh et al. (1980).
See also Fig. 23-8.

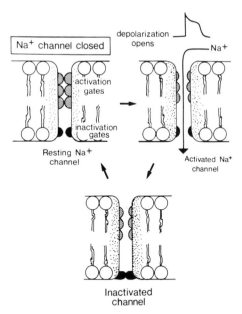

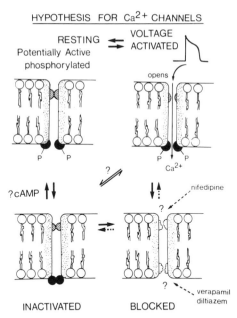

HYPOTHESIS FOR Ca^{2+} CHANNELS

Fig. 4-3 Hypothetical model of the sodium channel. The three activation gates (m-gates) open upon activation, whereas the single inactivation gate (h-gate) closes in the inactivated state. Each of the above arrows is reversible; the sequence shown is thought to occur during the normal cardiac cycle. These gates are based on the Hodgkin–Huxley model (Hauswrith and Singh, 1979). For another model see Fig. 23-9. The rate of activation the sodium current is rather slow, and that of inactivation rather rapid, suggesting that the rather slow decay of the current (Fig. 23-11) depends on the slow kinetics of activation (Aldrich et al., 1983).

Fig. 4-4 Provisional "thought-diagram" of calcium channel modified from Sperelakis (1984) and Bean et al. (1984). Note the proposed role for phosphorylation of calcium channel in changing inoperative channels to operative channels. Operative channels can go through the same cycle as shown in Fig. 4-3, and change from the resting to the activated and then to the inactivated and back to the resting state. The proposal is that catecholamine beta-adrenergic stimulation acts by its second messenger cyclic AMP (cAMP) to transfer charged phosphate groups (P) from ATP to the calcium channel so that there is a molecular change which allows a greater probability of the channels opening during depolarization (Bean et al., 1984). For details of calcium antagonist drugs see Chapter 19.

molecules of TTX which bind to the surface is an indirect measure of the density of the sodium channels (about 100/μm^2). The alkaloid neurotoxin **aconitine,** which "forces" the sodium channel open and is used experimentally to produce tachyarrhythmias, is closely related. This model shows that the fast sodium channel must be involved in certain arrhythmias, especially those firing at a fast rate and requiring rapid opening and closure of the sodium channel.

Calcium Channel

Although the calcium ion concentration outside the heart cell is very much higher than inside, the concentration gradient is effectively maintained because the sarcolemma is virtually impermeable to

calcium. Calcium enters the myocardial cell chiefly through a very strictly controlled calcium channel, by the process of voltage-activated "opening" of the channel (Fig. 4-4). When the fast sodium channel is inactivated either by voltage clamping or by an abnormally high extracellular potassium concentration, then calcium fails to enter the cell and the contractile force decreases rapidly. It is the "opening" of the sodium channel that changes the voltage to bring it into the range which "opens" the calcium channel. The amount of calcium entering with each wave of depolarization is very small when compared with the total cellular content of calcium. The very rapid intracellular turnover and release of calcium all make it difficult to measure accurately calcium ion movements. Nevertheless, it is probably the entry of calcium through the slow channel which is the critical event in triggering the intracellular calcium cycle. Some calcium may also enter through a reversal of the sodium–calcium exchange system (Fig. 4-1).

The calcium channel has an increasing probability of opening in bursts as the trans-sarcolemmal voltage becomes more positive than -40 mV until further depolarization decreases the driving force with less opening (Reuter, 1984). To obtain such data, the voltage is fixed across a small patch of a single cardiac cell in culture (**patch clamp**) and the flow of current measured. There are many more sodium than calcium channels (Table 4-2), explaining the greater amplitude of the sodium current.

Important properties of the calcium channel are its inhibition by calcium antagonists such as verapamil, its stereospecificity (*l*-verapamil inhibits much more than *d*-verapamil), its "opening" facilitated by catecholamine beta-agonist stimulation, and its insensitivity to the specific inhibitor of the sodium channel (TTX).

Model for calcium channel

One model for the calcium channel (Fig. 4-4) proposes that the channel has two external sites which bind chiefly calcium but also some sodium (Schneider and Sperelakis, 1975). According to the model, the channel is normally "opened" by depolarization to the threshold potential which converts the slow channel to the active state by opening a "gate". Calcium ions flow in (rather slowly though when compared with sodium) until an unknown signal shuts the gate to inactivate the channel. There is also thought to be another gate, located on the "inner mouth" of the channel, which can be "closed" by verapamil so that the normal voltage stimulus no longer opens the channel, and the channel is blocked.

Catecholamine beta-adrenergic stimulation, on the other hand, can hypothetically alter the electrical charges around the inner mouth of the channel so the time the channel remains open is increased and more calcium ions flow in during the normal voltage-activation; alternatively, beta-stimulation may bring into activity channels which were previously inactive (Fig. 4-4). The mechanism is thought to involve the second messenger, cyclic AMP, which promotes the transfer of a phosphate group from ATP to the channel, thereby altering the charges and inducing a change in the molecular conformation of the channel (Sperelakis, 1984; Bean et al., 1984).

Potassium Channels

Whereas potassium ions are brought into heart cells by the activity of the sodium pump, they leave the cells spontaneously by virtue of the high permeability of the sarcolemma to potassium (Fig. 4-1). There is a "background" outward potassium current (I_{k1}) and other potassium currents which are involved in shaping the action potential (Table 4-4). The voltage-invoked decrease in potassium conductance (Fig. 4-5) is called **inward-going rectification.** As the membrane current becomes more negative at the start of repolarization, the potassium current again starts to flow to help terminate the action potential plateau by **delayed rectification** (Fig. 4-5). To achieve such rectification, there is another predominantly potassium current, called I_x, which is both time and voltage-dependent, so that it is induced a certain time after the onset of depolarization and at a certain voltage. Noble called this **current I_x** because he wished to emphasize the possible contributions of components other than potassium; another name is simply I_k. I_x has also been separated into a fast (I_{x1}) and a slow component (I_{x2}) but these differences are not of practical importance. A third potassium current has been described—I_{k2}. Originally it was thought that I_{k2} contributed to delayed rectification and that its characteristics also contributed to spontaneous diastolic depolarization in the sinus node and in Purkinje fibers. More recently it has become clear that I_{k2} is in fact identical (at least in the sinus node and in Purkinje fibers) with a new inward pacemaker current I_f which is more fully evaluated in Chapter 5. So it seems as if I_{k2} should now be eliminated from the electrophysiological terminology.

The outward-going potassium currents which help to terminate the action potential plateau might be triggered by the inward calcium current. Yet the fact that the highly specific calcium channel blocker nisoldipine blocks I_{si} but does not reduce I_x is a strong argument against the suggestion that I_x is a calcium-activated current (Kass, 1982). Rather, I_x is voltage-activated and therefore indirectly the result of the sodium and calcium ion movements occurring early in the action potential (Fig. 4-7).

In contrast to the sodium channel, pharmacological

Table 4-4

Currents associated with cardiac action potential (see Brown, 1982)

Current	Abbreviation	Qualities
Fast inward sodium current	I_{Na}	Abolished by tetrodotoxin; inhibited by Class I antiarrhythmic agents
Slow inward calcium current	I_{si}	Important for plateau phase of cardiac action potential; involved in excitation-contraction coupling; inhibited by "calcium-antagonist" agents
Outward voltage- and time-dependent potassium current	I_x or I_k	Slow outward predominantly potassium current helps to terminate action potential plateau by delayed rectification; **voltage-dependent** so that it increases as the membrane potential returns towards normal ("regenerative"); **time-dependent** so that it increases with time after the start of I_{Na}
		Subdivisions of I_x
		Early rapid component (I_{xi}); major component of delayed rectification in Purkinje fibers
		Slow late component (I_{x2})
Background potassium current	I_{k1}	Background outward current occurring throughout the cardiac cycle that lessens during depolarization so that outward currents do not inhibit inward currents. Also called inward rectification current
Diastolic pacemaker current in Purkinje fibers	$I_{k2} = I_f$	Diastolic outward current whose decay was thought to cause spontaneous firing in Purkinje or nodal cells. Now known to be identical to inward current I_f
	I_f	Inward "funny" sodium and potassium current may be responsible for initial phase of spontaneous depolarization in Purkinje tissue. Replaces I_{k2}
Transient outward current	I_{to}	Transient outward early potassium current, previously called the chloride current

dissection has not helped elucidate the nature of the potassium channels. **4-Aminopyridine** is a specific inhibitor of the potassium channel but the nature of the block is very complex (Meves and Pichon, 1977). The classical inhibitor of potassium conductance is **tetraethylammonium** (TEA) which not only blocks the potassium channel but in the high doses required (20–40 mM) also blocks the sodium channel.

Magnesium and its Channel

Magnesium is an important constituent of the cytosol and is essential for numerous enzymatic reactions (including the sodium pump, myosin ATPase, oxidative phosphorylation and various enzymes of glycolysis). The vital functions of ATP and other adenine nucleotides are carried out in the ionized form chelated with magnesium. The total magnesium in the cell is about 43 μmol/g wet weight with a calculated overall intracellular concentration of 17 mM (Page and Polimeni, 1972). Of this, about 10 mM should be related to adenine nucleotides and a small proportion is bound to mitochondria (12 percent of total) and myofibrils (2 percent of total).

Recently ionized magnesium has been measured by the formation of a magnesium complex with aequorin blue and found to be 3.0–3.5 mM in the squid axon. The free intracellular magnesium concentration in the heart can be measured by an ion-selective micro-electrode and is about 3.0 mM in ventricular muscle (Hess et al., 1982). This value is of more than academic interest. If true (and there are many technical problems), it is thought to be too high for the process of calcium-induced calcium release from the sarcoplasmic reticulum which operates at 0.3 mM magnesium or less.

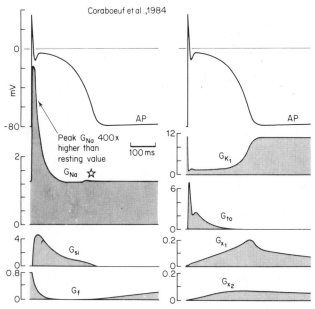

Fig. 4-5 Computed Purkinje fiber action potential (AP in mV) and ionic conductances per unit of membrane surface (G_{Na}, G_{si} etc. . . . in 10^{-4} S/cm^2). G_{Na}: sum of rapid sodium conductance and background sodium conductance. The initial peak of conductance (arrow) reaches 11×10^{-2} S/cm^2, i.e. about 400 times that shown here. This large magnification has been chosen to visualize the G_{Na} "window" which occurs as a small hump (star) on the background sodium conductance. G_{si} = slow conductance giving rise to the slow inward current. G_f = new pacemaker conductance replacing G_{K2}; the corresponding pacemaker current is carried by both sodium and potassium ions. G_{K1} = background K conductance exhibiting strong anomalous (inward going) rectification, i.e. decreasing during depolarization. G_{to} = conductance giving rise to the transient outward potassium current. G_{x1} and G_{x2} = delayed potassium conductances (A. Coulombe, unpublished). Figure and data kindly provided by Professor E. Coraboeuf, Paris. For comparison with Fig. 4-1, 1 Sieman = 1 mho.

A Magnesium channel?

It is usually thought that magnesium ions are also carried inwards by the slow channel of the action potential. Spah and Fleckenstein (1979) recently proposed the existence of a third inward channel (in addition to the sodium and calcium channels) which preferentially carries magnesium. The beta-adrenergic catecholamines stimulate the calcium channel but in-

hibit the proposed magnesium channel. The speed of the proposed magnesium channel is in between that of the sodium and calcium channels. The proposed magnesium channel is not thought to contribute to electrogenesis, but it may serve as a source of intracellular magnesium. It is not clear whether all magnesium transport into the cell takes place by this proposed third channel, or whether there is also a pump.

Chloride

Throughout this chapter the emphasis has been on movements of positively charged cations. In general, the distribution of chloride ions follows that of its dominant partner which is sodium (Table 4-1). It is generally accepted that there is an inward chloride current early during depolarization which contributes to repolarization; it was even proposed that a chloride current could play a pacemaking role in the sinus node. Recent evidence is that the "chloride current" is in fact an early transient outward (I_{to}) potassium current, evoked by the inward movement of calcium, and responsible for the initial notch on the action potential of Purkinje fibers (Coraboeuf and Carmeliet, 1982).

Ventricular Action Potential

The characteristic appearance of the ventricular action potential can now be interpreted in terms of opening and closing of sodium, calcium and potassium channels with the resultant flow of currents (Fig. 4-6). The resting potential of -70 to -90 mV is largely the result of the unequal distribution of potassium ions across the sarcolemma. The rapid phase of depolarization of the action potential (phase 0) is the result of opening of the sodium channels to allow the rapid influx of sodium which depolarizes the cell. The wave of depolarization changes the resting potential to less negative values which "open" the sodium channel activation gates at -60 to -70 mV and then almost immediately start to close the "inactivation" gates. Sodium conductance increases, as does the flow of the inward current I_{Na}, to peak rapidly within 1 msec and then rapidly falls off (Bosteels and Carmeliet, 1972). The "flash" of inward sodium movement, carrying positive charges, continues to depolarize the cell to reach 0 mV with a small overshoot.

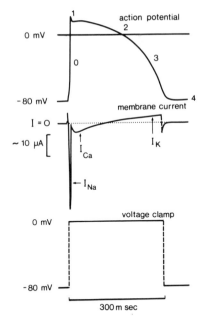

Fig. 4-6 Schematic drawing of a ventricular cardiac action potential (top) of total membrane current flowing (middle) and of a voltage-clamp step from a holding potential of −80 mV to 0 mV (bottom). When the voltage across the heart membrane is artificially fixed by the voltage-clamp technique, the change in current required to keep the voltage constant reflects the change in membrane conductance for various ions. If the voltage is changed in a step-like fashion (voltage-step) then the patterns of the current required to keep the voltage fixed despite the changes in conduction for the various ions, allows a diagram of the currents to be constructed and triggered by a depolarizing clamp to a level more positive than −60 to −90 mV. When the voltage-step rises to above −40 to −30 mV, the slow inward largely calcium current (I_{si}) is activated. When the calcium current dies, the outward potassium current I_k is left to rectify the electrical charge changes caused by the previous currents, i.e. it is the rectifying current. For phases of action potential (0–4) see text. Taken from Reuter (1984), with permission.

Conductance vs current

The maximal conductance measures the permeability of the membrane to an ion when all the channels are fully open; for values across resting membrane, see Fig. 4-1. The actual rate of current flow is not the same as the conductance. Taking sodium as an example

$$I_{Na} = gNa(V_m − V_{Na})$$

where I_{Na} = sodium current; gNa = sodium conductance; V_m = voltage across the membrane; and V_{Na} = sodium equilibrium or reversal potential. The latter is +40 mV for sodium. As depolarization drops the voltage across the membrane (V_m), I_{Na} decreases to become very low.

Phase 1-4

In the meantime the much slower calcium channel has already been opened at the time when the depolarization process reached −30 to −40 mV. As the sodium current fades away, it is replaced by the slow inward calcium current, I_{si}, which forms the plateau. Thus, from the peak depolarization, the overshoot is lost (phase 1) (see I_{to} above) to form the relatively flat plateau (phase 2), which merges into the phase of rapid repolarization (phase 3). In atrial and ventricular cells the resting membrane potential is regained and remains stable throughout diastole, so that these cells cannot fire spontaneously. So also for normal Purkinje cells. In injured Purkinje cells and in the sinus and atrioventricular nodes, spontaneous diastolic depolarization can occur (phase 4) by complex mechanisms to be described in Chapter 5.

The factors leading to **repolarization** are poorly understood (Fig. 4-7). A good possibility is that the voltage changes associated with depolarization invoke

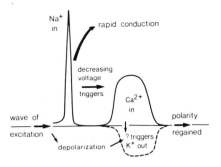

Fig. 4-7 Proposal for the sequential triggering of currents. The inward fast sodium current responds to the wave of depolarization; the inward slow calcium current to a greater degree of depolarization; and the outward potassium current responds probably to the voltage change or less probably to the calcium current. The potassium current helps to "rectify" the depolarizing effects of the inward sodium and calcium channels.

the delayed rectifier (I_x) potassium currents which terminate the action potential (Kass, 1982). Additionally, or alternatively, the calcium gate is "shut" by the build-up of intracellular calcium ions. A third and currently less favored possibility is that the calcium current "switches on" the rectifying potassium current (Bassingthwaite et al., 1976). During phase 3 the voltage required to "open" the sodium current is again passed "on the way down", so that a short "window" sodium current flows again (for conductances, see Fig. 4-5) to help maintain the **action potential duration**.

Once the action potential is over, the resting membrane is restored and maintained. In contrast to this picture is the situation in nodal tissue (see Fig. 5-1) where the resting membrane potential is much less negative and where spontaneous diastolic depolarization takes place to initiate the whole cardiac cycle.

The wave of conduction is self-propagated, because depolarization sets up a current between the site of depolarization and the adjacent sarcolemma (the potential difference would exceed 70–90 mV because of the overshoot to about 10 mV during depolarization). Thus the cardiac impulse can travel very rapidly over the ventricular syncytium to cause an opening of sodium and calcium channels virtually simultaneously throughout the ventricular myocardium, so that co-ordinated contraction results.

Calcium Exit from the Cell

Although only relatively small amounts of sodium and calcium ions enter by the fast and slow channels respectively, over a period the cytosol would potentially gain substantial amounts of these ions. The exit mechanism for sodium is the sodium pump while the chief exit for calcium is the sodium–calcium exchange mechanism (Fig. 4-1).

Sodium–calcium exchange

Evidence for the sodium–calcium exchange is no longer in doubt — probably three sodium ions are exchanged with one calcium (Pitts, 1979) — thereby revising the original proposals of Reuter (1974) and showing that the exchanger generates an electrical current with a gain of intracellular positive charge. (Note that this effect opposes that of the electrogenic

sodium pump.) The exchanger responds to low concentrations of calcium ions, similar to those found within the cell, and transports these ions very effectively. Calcium ions can also leave the heart cell by the ATP-requiring calcium pump, although the maximal rate of the sodium–calcium-exchanger is about 30 times higher than that of the pump. Carafoli (1982) proposes that it is the exchanger which operates during systole when the cytosolic calcium ion concentration rises to 10^{-5} M, whereas the calcium pump probably functions in diastole to help keep the cytosolic calcium ion concentration low.

Influence of internal sodium on calcium

An interesting prediction was made by Reuter (1974) concerning the effects of increasing the internal sodium concentration. His sodium–calcium exchange scheme can be simplified to the following equation:

$$(Ca^{2+})_i/(Ca^{2+})_o = (Na^+)_i^2/(Na^+)_o^2$$

where i = inside the cell and o = outside. With the recent knowledge that the exchange is 3 sodium ions per calcium ion, the equation becomes:

$$(Ca^{2+})_i/(Ca^{2+})_o = (Na^+)_i^3/(Na^+)_o^3$$

If internal sodium ions are increased in concentration by inhibition of the sodium pump by digitalis, then only a very small increase will dramatically increase the internal free calcium ion concentration to enhance contractility.

Overall Rates of Ion Flux

Sodium flux

To recapitulate — ions are in a constant state of flux across the sarcolemma. The resting membrane is relatively impermeable to sodium but becomes highly permeable with the opening of the sodium "gate" which is induced by depolarization. Such sodium must eventually be returned to the extracellular space. Most of this flux of sodium across the sarcolemma is linked to the activity of the sodium–potassium pump; another component is not linked to potassium, but to calcium.

The sodium–calcium exchange system depends on the existence of a sodium gradient from without to within the cell (sodium enters as calcium leaves), and the activity of the sodium pump is required to eject the sodium ions thus accumulated (Pitts, 1979). Thus, in the end, exchange of sodium for either potassium or calcium is linked to active transport of sodium by the sodium–potassium pump.

Potassium flux

The intracellular potassium ion activity is about 80 mM with an intracellular–extracellular ratio of about 20 (Table 4-1). Hence energy must be expended in keeping potassium within the cell. Unlike sodium flux, the flux of potassium is fixed over a wide range of heart rates. The reason for this constancy of potassium exchange may be the backward outward current I_{k1} (Table 4-3), which is "turned off" sufficiently to cancel the increased outward flux of potassium during the phase of rapid repolarization.

Calcium flux

The rate of calcium influx can be estimated indirectly by labelling myocardial pools with ^{45}Ca, measuring the rate of washout and presuming that the rate of influx and efflux are in balance.

The amount of calcium influx is 0.4×10^{-9} mol/g wet wt/sec in the resting state, and $1.5–8.7 \times 10^{-9}$ mol/g/beat are required for activation of the contractile process (Langer, 1974). Voltage-clamp studies also show that Ca^{2+} entry during the action potential is only one-fifth of that needed for full activation (Kaufmann et al., 1974). Such arguments lead to the proposal that small amounts of "activator" calcium entering by the calcium channel during the plateau phase of the action potential can release much more calcium from a superficial site by the process of "calcium-induced calcium release" (see Fig. 2-6).

Magnesium flux

The very slow rate of exchange of magnesium suggests that (i) magnesium is not involved in beat-to-beat regulation of contraction; (ii) magnesium will be lost only gradually from ischemic cells; and (iii) little energy is spent on magnesium transport.

Manganese flux

Little is known of manganese. Presumably it is important in the heart, as in other cells, in the control of oxidative phosphorylation. The trace amount of manganese in the circulation may enter heart cells by calcium channels (Hunter et al., 1981).

Energy for Ion Fluxes

Whenever an ion is transported against a concentration gradient, energy is required. To estimate how much ATP is expended on maintenance of ionic gradients is not easy and requires a number of assumptions. It is simplest to take the case of potassium ion flux which is independent of the heart rate.

The transport of 0.7 µmol K^+/g/min (Table 4-5) requires 0.35 µmol ATP/g/min or about 4 µL O_2/g/min. This contrasts with the oxygen uptake of the human heart in basal conditions of about 100 µL/g/min. Thus very roughly up to 4 percent of the energy needs of the heart might be expended on potassium movements by the sodium–potassium pump. Higher estimates, up to 20 percent, are obtained when based on sodium influx (Table 4-5). Only about 2 percent of the total ATP production is required for sodium entry by the fast sodium channel.

Energy for calcium flux

Estimates suggest that the entry and exit of calcium ions across the sarcolemma requires relatively little energy—perhaps up to 10 percent of the myocardial oxygen uptake (Table 4-5). Quite different is the situation with intracellular calcium ion movements. Calcium uptake by the sarcoplasmic reticulum in diastole requires 1 mol of ATP for 2 mol of calcium and calcium can be concentrated by 1000–5000 times. A significant percentage of the total oxygen uptake (up to 20 percent) of the heart is required for calcium movements associated with relaxation.

Summary

The myocardial cell takes up potassium and ejects sodium ions to produce the resting negative membrane potential. This is achieved by the sodium–potassium (Na^+/K^+-ATPase) or sodium pump, which probably

Table 4-5

Estimated ATP requirements for ion fluxes and phases of cardiac action potential

Ion	K+-arrested heart (μmol/g wet wt/min)	Effect of increasing beating rate		
		75 beats/min (μmol/min)	150 beats/min (μmol/min)	330 beats/min (μmol/min)
Total sodium flux[a]	up to 0.1	3.1	6.2	13.6
Fast channel[b] (I_{Na})	—	0.4	0.8	1.7
Potassium flux[c]	included in above	included in above	included in above	included in above
Calcium flux				
(a) slow channel[d] (I_{si})	—	0.1–0.5	0.2–1.0	0.4–2.2
(b) contractile Ca^{2+} flux				
(1) for 50% tension[e]	—	about 1.2	about 2.4	—
(2) for peak tension[f]	—	—	—	about 30
Total ATP needed[g]	10	23	41	152
Percentage breakdown				
Na^+ flux	up to 1%	15%	15%	9%
I_{Na}	—	2%	2%	1%
I_{si}	—	0.4–2.2%	0.5–2.4%	0.3–1.5%
Average internal Ca^{2+} flux	—	5%	6%	—
Peak internal Ca^{2+} flux	—	—	—	20%

[a]Calculated from steady state flux of 0.2–0.3 μmol/g/min and from the measured flux of 4.2 μmol/g/min at 80 beats/min (Langer, 1974).

[b]Calculated using the flux of 14 pmol/cm^2 per impulse, and assuming that this flux requires energy via the sodium pump.

[c]Assuming that all K^+ fluxes are covered by sodium pump.

[d]Net Ca^{2+} influx per impulse is 1.5 nmol/g and assuming that the sarcolemma calcium pump is required to eject this calcium influx; pump needs 1 ATP for each Ca^{2+}. Alternatively, 3 Na^+ exchange for 1 Ca^{2+}, and 1 ATP is needed for 3 Na^+ movements via sodium pump.

[e]Derived from data of Marban et al. (1980), assuming that all such Ca^{2+} flux is taken up by the Ca^{2+} pump of the SR which requires 1 ATP for 2 Ca^{2+}.

[f]Derived from data of Marban et al. (1980).

[g]Data for non-beating K^+-arrested perfused rat heart from Opie et al. (1971); for 75 and 100 beats/min from basal O_2 uptake of dog heart in situ of 104 μL/g/min and from working rat heart data of Opie et al. (1971); and peak O_2 uptake from rat hearts working against an aortic column height of 120 cm H_2O, at an atrial filling pressure of 25 cm H_2O, paced at 330 beats/min, and perfused with glucose 11 mM, lactate 10 mM and insulin 2 u/l (unpublished data of Noakes and Opie). In every case a P/O ratio of 3 was assumed.

stretches across the cell membrane; its outer side binds potassium and digitalis glycosides, whereas its inner site binds sodium and uses ATP. The ratio of molecules involved is 3 Na^+ : 2 K^+ : 1 ATP. From 4 to 20 percent of myocardial ATP production could be used for this pump. Depolarization of an adjacent cell causes a current to flow which "opens" the voltage-activated "gates" of the sodium channel to allow the very rapid entry of positively charged sodium ions (phase 0 of the action potential). As the cell loses its polarity, the calcium channel "opens" because it is activated by a less negative voltage than the sodium channel. Inflow of calcium ions and outflow of potassium ions cause the action potential plateau (phase 2). Potassium ions leave the cell both as a background current (because the sarcolemma is highly permeable to K^+) and more rapidly during the re-polarization phase of the action potential as the rectifying current which helps to terminate the action potential plateau (phase 3), so that the resting potential is regained (phase 4). This description applies to contractile myocardial cells and conducting Purkinje fibers, not to spontaneously firing nodal tissue (see Chapter 5).

References

Aldrich RW, Corey DP, Stevens CF (1983). A reinterpretation of mammalian sodium channel gating based on single channel recording. Nature 306: 436–441.

Bassingthwaite JB, Fry CH, McGuigan JAS (1976). Relationship between internal calcium and outward current in mammalian ventricular muscle: a mechanism for the control of the action potential duration? J Physiol 262: 15–37.

Bean BP, Nowycky MC, Tsien RW (1984). Beta-adrenergic modulation of calcium channel in frog ventricular heart cells. Nature 307: 371–375.

Bosteels S, Carmeliet EE (1972). Estimation of intracellular Na concentration and transmembrane Na flux in cardiac Purkinje fibers. Pflügers Arch 336: 352–359.

Brown HF (1982). Electrophysiology of the sinoatrial node. Physiol Rev 62: 505–530.

Carafoli E (1982). Transport of calcium across the inner membrane of mitochondria. In: Membrane Transport of Calcium. Ed. E Carafoli, pp 109–139, Academic Press, London, Orlando and New York.

Cohen CJ, Fozzard HA, Sheu SS (1982). Increase in intracellular sodium ion activity during stimulation in mammalian cardiac muscle. Circ Res 50: 651–662.

Colvin RA, Ashavaid TF, Katz AM, Herbette LG (1983). Estimation of receptor densities in canine cardiac sarcolemmal vesicles. Circulation 68 Suppl III (Abstract): 399.

Coraboeuf E, Carmeliet E (1982). Existence of two transient outward currents in sheep cardiac Purkinje fibers. Pflügers Arch 392: 352–359.

Coraboeuf E, Deroubaix E, Hoerter J (1976). Control of ionic permeabilities in normal and ischemic heart. Circ Res 38, Suppl 1: 92–98.

Goldman DE (1943). Potential impedance and rectification in membranes. J Gen Physiol 27: 37–60.

Hauswrith O, Singh BN (1979). Ionic mechanisms in heart muscle in relation to the genesis and the pharmacological control of cardiac arrhythmias. Pharm Rev 30: 5–63.

Hess P, Metzger P, Weingart R (1982). Free magnesium in sheep, ferret and frog striated muscle at rest measured with ion-selective micro-electrodes. J Physiol 333: 173–188.

Hondeghem L, Katzung BG (1977). Time- and voltage-dependent interactions of antiarrhythmic drugs with cardiac sodium channels. Biochimica Biophysica Acta 472: 373–398.

Hunter DR, Haworth RA, Berkoff HA (1981). Cellular manganese uptake by the isolated perfused rat heart: a probe for the sarcolemma calcium channel. J Molec Cell Cardiol 13: 823–832.

Kass RS (1982). Nisoldipine: A new, more selective calcium current blocker in cardiac Purkinje fibers. J Pharm Exp Therap 223: 446–456.

Kaufmann R, Bayer R, Furniss T, Krause H, Tritthart H (1974). Calcium-movement controlling cardiac contractility. II. Analog computation of cardiac excitation-contraction coupling on the basis of calcium kinetics in a multi-compartment model. J Molec Cell Cardiol 6: 543–559.

Langer GA (1974). Ionic movements and the control of contraction. In: The Mammalian Myocardium. Eds. GA Langer, AJ Brady, pp 193–217, Wiley, New York.

Marban E, Rink TJ, Tsien RW, Tsien RY (1980). Free calcium in heart muscle at rest and during contraction measured with Ca^{2+}-sensitive micro-electrodes. Nature 297: 845–850.

Meves H, Pichon Y (1977). The effect of internal and external 4-aminopyridine on the potassium currents in intracellularly perfused squid giant axons. J Physiol 268: 511–532.

Opie LH, Owen P and Mansford KRL (1971). Effects of heart work on glycolysis and adenine nucleotides in the perfused heart of normal and diabetic rats. Biochem J 124: 475–490.

Page E, Polimeni PI (1972). Magnesium exchange in rat ventricle. J Physiol 224: 121–139.

Pitts BJR (1979). Stoichiometry of sodium–calcium exchange in cardiac sarcolemmal vesicles. Coupling to the sodium pump. J Biol Chem 254: 6232–6235.

Reuter H (1974). Exchange of calcium ions in the mammalian myocardium. Circ Res 34: 599–605.

Reuter H (1984). Electrophysiology of calcium channels in the heart. In: Calcium-Antagonists and Cardiovascular Disease, Ed. LH Opie, pp 43–51, Raven Press, New York.

Reuter H, Scholz H (1977). The regulation of the calcium conductance of cardiac muscle by adrenaline. J Physiol 264: 49–62.

Schneider JA, Sperelakis N (1975). Slow Ca^{2+} and Na^+ responses induced by isoproterenol and methylxanthines in isolated perfused guinea pig hearts exposed to elevated K^+. J Molec Cell Cardiol 7: 249–273.

Scholz H, Hackbarth I, Schmitz W, Wetzel E (1980). Effect of vanadate on myocardial force of contraction. Basic Res Cardiol 75: 418–422.

Schwartz A, Adams RH (1980). Studies on the digitalis receptor. Circ Res 46: 154–160.

Singh BN, Collett JT, Chew CYC (1980). New perspectives in the pharmacologic therapy of cardiac arrhythmias. Prog Cardiovasc Dis 22: 243–301.

Spah F, Fleckenstein A (1979). Evidence of a new, preferentially Mg-carrying, transport system besides the fast Na and slow Ca channels in the excited myocardial sarcolemmal membrane. J Molec Cell Cardiol 11: 1109–1127.

Sperelakis N (1984). Properties of calcium-dependent slow action potentials, and their possible role in arrhythmias. In: Calcium-Antagonists and Cardiovascular Diseases, Ed. LH Opie, pp 277–291, Raven Press, New York.

Woodbury JW (1963). Interrelationships between ion transport mechanisms and excitatory events. Fed Proc 22: 31–35.

The cardiac action potential is not uniform throughout the heart, but is modified to suit the requirements of impulse generation in the sinus node, rapid conduction through the atria, "filtration" and delay in the atrioventricular node, followed by another phase of rapid conduction in the His bundle and bundle branches, which finally leads to excitation–contracting coupling in the ventricular myocyte (Fig. 5-1). The initiator of these events is in the automatic behavior of the sinus node which generates the cardiac impulse.

Sinoatrial Node Automaticity

Structure of the sinoatrial node

Anatomically, the human sinus node (= sinoatrial or SA node) is spindle-shaped and measures 20 × 3 × 1 mm (Harriman et al., 1980). It contains clusters of

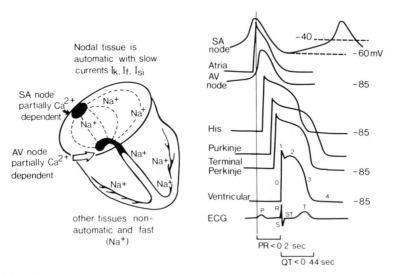

Fig. 5-1 Nodal tissue is automatic. The sinoatrial (SA) node has three depolarizing currents. The slow upstroke is largely calcium-dependent. In other tissues such as atrial muscle, Purkinje fibers and ventricular muscle, the impulse travels very rapidly because the initial phase of depolarization is much faster and sodium-dependent. The patterns of the cardiac action potential in different sites are modified from Singer et al. (1981) Prog Cardiovasc Dis 24: 97, with permission.

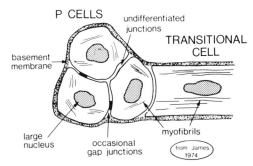

Fig. 5-2 The heart beat originates in the P (pacemaker) cells of the sinus node. Note very low content of myofibrils. Transitional T cells are closer to normal myocardial cells in histology. From James (1974), with permission.

cells, poor in contractile filaments, where the automatic activity mostly resides in the **pacemaker**, or **P, cells** (Fig. 5-2). Such primary pacemaker cells are also called B cells, in contrast to **transitional** A cells which lie near the periphery of the node (Brown, 1982). Each cluster of P cells is enveloped by a basement membrane and junctions between P cells are largely undifferentiated. P cells connect with each other by simple apposition of plasma membranes at a constant distance, so they have well-conducted electrical activity although there are only a few gap junctions (which are the sites of communication between ordinary myocardial cells). The co-ordination is good enough for the transmembrane potential to change almost simultaneously in all P cells in one cluster. In contrast, different clusters of cells are probably not well coupled because the upstrokes of the action potentials from adjacent recording sites in the canine node are not synchronous. Functionally, the site of predominant discharge can move as the dominant autonomic tone changes from sympathetic to parasympathetic or vice versa. Such nervous innervation is more dense in the sinus than in the atrioventricular node, so that autonomic variations normally govern the activity of the pacemaker (sinoatrial node) rather than that of the "filter" (atrioventricular node).

Decaying potassium currents

In sinoatrial tissue there is spontaneous diastolic depolarization in phase 4 of the action potential, so the threshold of the cell is reached to fire the node at about $-40\,\text{mV}$ (Fig. 5-1). A high intracellular

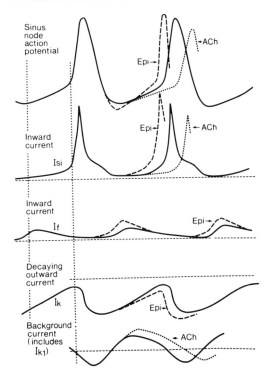

Fig. 5-3 Tentative proposals for currents in the sinus node. The activity of the slow inward current I_{si} probably coincides with the overall pattern of the depolarization. The recently described inward pacemaker current I_f is thought to occur simultaneously with the phase of spontaneous diastolic depolarization and to fire the I_{si}. The outward potassium current is responsible in part for the decay of the action potential, but is not nearly so important as in Purkinje fibers. I_{k2} is not shown and has properties similar to I_f according to one hypothesis. Epi = epinephrine effects; ACh = acetyl choline effects.

potassium concentration is responsible for the resting membrane potential of ventricular cells (Chapter 4). Here it would be logical to suppose that increased potassium loss from the nodal cell in diastole explains the progressive loss of the resting potential which results in spontaneous depolarization. In ventricular muscle, the various **potassium currents** associated with the ventricular action potential include a constant "background" outward potassium current, K_1, which helps to maintain the resting membrane potential (Fig. 5-3). Isolated Purkinje fibers are frequently studied as a model of tissue that can spontaneously depolarize, being easier to work with than the sinus node itself. Voltage-clamp studies on such fibers have shown that there is a second potassium current, K_2, which is quite distinct from those outward currents that determine the plateau phase of the action potential. The current K_2 was long thought to be the pacemaker current, causing depolarization in spontaneously firing Purkinje cells by producing an outward-flowing current which progressively decreased, until a separate constant inward current eventually took over to fire the Purkinje fibers. A similar sequence was thought to occur in the sinoatrial node. The nature of the constant inward current was not so well understood, but thought to be carried by sodium and other ions. As will be seen, this concept of the decaying potassium current as the pacemaker in Purkinje fibers now needs revision, although still partially valid for the sinoatrial node.

Slow inward nodal current

In nodal tissue, the slow inward calcium current (I_{si}) explains the distinctive, slowly rising depolarization phase. When normal ventricular muscle has the fast phase eliminated by tetrodotoxin (TTX) or by a sodium-free and calcium-rich perfusion solution, the nature of the resultant slow current resembles that found in nodal tissue. The inward current in nodal tissue is blocked by lowering the external calcium ion concentration to zero or by the calcium antagonist agent verapamil. Verapamil depresses the sinus pacemaker so as to increase the cycle time for spontaneous firing; this effect is opposed by beta-adrenergic receptor agonists which are thought to "open" calcium channels to enhance I_{si} (see Fig. 4-6).

The slow calcium channel is not the only channel of importance in the sinus node. Rather, the modern view (Brown, 1982) is that the spontaneous firing of nodal tissue is not wholly dependent on one current. The decay of the potassium current plays a major role in depolarization, with the slow inward current governing the action potential itself. In addition, a new current now to be described plays a variable and probably minor role.

Voltage-clamp technique

A new inward pacing current has been identified by the **voltage-clamp technique** (Fig. 4-6). The voltage across the membrane is artificially fixed and the ionic movements which result from the voltage chosen are then balanced by an artificial current, required to keep the voltage constant or clamped. Any changes in the current must reflect changes in the conductance of the membrane for specific ions. It is these changes in the

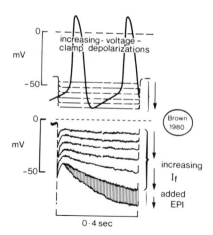

Fig. 5-4 Application of hyperpolarizing voltage clamps to pacemaker tissue. The initial "holding" potential is −42 mV, and progressively increasing voltage-clamp steps have been superimposed on the spontaneous pacemaker activity. The bottom panel shows the records of the current required to balance the hyperpolarizing clamps (units = nanoamps). Note the progressively increased current that flows as the voltage-clamp becomes more and more negative. This current flows despite the added presence of both a calcium antagonist (D-600) and the sodium channel blocker, tetrodotoxin. This current is the I_f current. From Brown and DiFrancesco (1980), with permission.

current flow which measure the **conductance** for any specific ions at the voltage chosen. In the case of heart tissue, there are major technical problems involved because of the smallness of heart cells and because of the difficulty of achieving a uniform transmembrane potential (Fozzard and Beeler, 1975). The technique cannot designate the ions which carry the currents. Thus the additional use of inhibitors (TTX, calcium antagonists) is required, or else the ion concerned is left out of the bath. Local anesthetic agents such as cocaine will inhibit the rapid phase of fast current change, so that at any given clamp potential there is a less rapid rate of change of current I_{Na}. In these ways the fast channel has been identified as that carrying the sodium current and the slow channel as that carrying the calcium current.

Inward current, I_f

Once voltage-clamp techniques could be adapted to the sinus node, two currents were found, the first being the slow inward current, and the second being an outward time-dependent potassium current. Of greater interest was the discovery of a third current, an inward current activated during hyperpolarizing clamps. (Hyperpolarizing clamps are those in which the voltage clamp is increased in progressively more negative steps—see Fig. 5-4.) Because of its "funny" properties, the new current is called I_f. The range of activation of this current (-65 to -55 mV) overlaps but does not fully coincide with the normal diastolic voltage range of the spontaneously beating sinus node (Brown and DiFrancesco, 1980), so that I_f may only be fully operative when the sinus node is hyperpolarized by adrenergic stimulation or in Purkinje fibers when partially depolarized. Other workers have studied the inward current activated during hyperpolarization and called it I_h; it is probably the same current I_f which plays little role in the normal action potential, rather being involved in the generation of the pacemaker activity. Probably both sodium (Maylie et al., 1981) and potassium (DiFrancesco, 1981) ions are responsible for carrying this new pacemaker current. In Purkinje fibers, the range in which I_f operates is less negative than the normal resting membrane potential (-85 mV). In injured, partially depolarized Purkinje fibers, I_f is probably the pacemaker current (Chapter 22).

Safety factors

In the sinoatrial node, the existence of three pacemaking currents (I_k, I_{si} and I_f) gives a "safety factor" so that inhibition of any one current still leaves two others to carry on the vital depolarizing function. Additional protection is given by the metabolic pattern of the sinus node, which depends more on glycolysis than does the rest of the myocardium, the general rule being that tissue with a high population of mitochondria is more dependent on fatty acids for its energy, whereas more primitive tissue depends more on glycolysis. Dependence on glycolysis explains why the sinus node can recover even after prolonged hypoxia, especially in the presence of glucose (Fig. 5-5).

The internal time clock

How does the "internal time clock" of the sinus node "know" to undergo regular diastolic depolarization at a regular interval and thereby satisfactorily to regulate our hearts and lives? The explanation for the

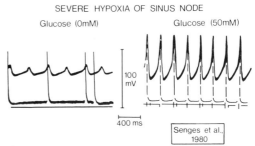

SEVERE HYPOXIA OF SINUS NODE

Glucose (0mM)   Glucose (50mM)

100 mV

400 ms

Senges et al.,
1980

Fig. 5-5 Effect of deprivation of glucose on sinus node. Note the irregular, low currents in the hypoxic preparation on the left. After the introduction of glucose, there are now high-amplitude frequent contractions on the right despite persisting hypoxia. Nodal tissue and conducting tissue is more dependent on glycolysis than is normal myocardium. From Senges et al. (1980), with permission.

pacemaker current underlying automaticity in the sinoatrial node has swung away from the idea that the outward decaying potassium current is the only factor to emphasize the additional role of inward currents such as I_f and I_{si}. As yet these descriptions have not led to any clarity about the cyclical nature of the repetitive spontaneous depolarizations of the sinus node.

Pollack (1977) has postulated an obligatory role for catecholamines in the cyclical pacemaking changes of the sinus node, as shown by the abundance of adrenergic nerve terminals, the high content of norepinephrine, and the arrest of the node when catecholamines are depleted by high doses of reserpine or when synthesis of catecholamines is inhibited by alpha-methyl tyrosine. The basis of Pollack's hypothesis rests on three assumptions: the first that the pacemaker current is carried by calcium ions; the second that the external catecholamines cause calcium influx into pacemaker cells; and the third that calcium influx causes catecholamines efflux. Hence "the elements of a regeneration feedback loop are at hand" (Pollack, 1977). The first assumption is not correct in view of the role of the inward current I_f and decaying potassium current in the pacemaker cells. The second assumption is probably valid. The third assumption depends on extrapolation from the neuromuscular junction. Evidently, the cause of the repetitive spontaneous firing of the sinus node which is essential for the pumping action of the heart, and hence for human and animal life, is still not known.

Autonomic Control of Heart Rate

Sympathetic stimulation of sinoatrial node

Sympathetic stimulation increases the heart rate, hence tachycardia is characteristic of emotional excitement or exercise. Beta-adrenergic stimulation may act on all three pacemaker currents. While the exact mechanism whereby beta-stimulation acts is still unresolved, it is clear that the previously held view that it only enhances the potassium-carrying outward current does not really make sense, because a larger potassium current will take longer to decay and should, therefore, lead to a prolonged interval between the action potentials (Brown et al., 1975). Whatever the cellular mechanism, the effect of beta-adrenergic stimulation plays a major role in causing the tachycardia of exercise to increase the cardiac output (Chapter 14).

Vagal stimulation and acetylcholine

Whereas beta-adrenergic catecholamine stimulation increases the spontaneous rate of firing of the sinus node, vagal stimulation decreases the rate. Acetyl choline, the "messenger" of vagal stimulation, reduced the amplitude, rate of rise and duration of the action potential of the sinus node. During physiological vagal stimulation, the sinus node does not arrest; rather, only parts of the sinus node respond to acetylcholine and pacemaker function shifts to those cells which fire albeit at a slower rate. Traditionally acetyl choline "opens" additional potassium channels, so that the outward potassium current flow should be enhanced. Presumably this change inhibits the pacemaker current, I_f. Acetyl choline also inhibits sinoatrial conduction, but again the mechanism is not clear (Woods et al., 1981).

Intrinsic heart rate

The intrinsic heart rate is uncovered when autonomic control is removed by combined sympathetic beta-adrenergic and parasympathetic vagal blockade (Jose, 1966). In controls, the intrinsic rate can be up to 50 percent higher than the resting rate, showing that normally vagal inhibition is more powerful than adrenergic stimulation. In heart failure, the resting rate is increased and the intrinsic rate rises less after autonomic blockade; the effect of the parasympathetic system is blunted (Eckberg et al., 1971). Normally, with exercise, the heart rate increases as parasympathetic tone is withdrawn and sympathetic tone increases. In heart failure, the limited ability of the heart rate to rise means that the cardiac output cannot increase to the levels required for adequate muscle perfusion, so that fatigue sets in.

Positive and Negative Chronotropic Agents

The major pharmacological agents increasing the heart rate (positive chronotropic effect) are the beta-adrenergic receptor agonists; the major agents slowing the heart are the beta-adrenergic receptor blockers or antagonists (Tables 5-1 and 5-2). The cellular sites of action of these agents are described under the autonomic nervous system (Chapter 17). Although the calcium antagonists slow the rate of isolated heart preparations, they also cause peripheral vasodilation which normally gives a reflex tachycardia to return the sinus rate to normal. An alternative explanation is that the other sites of action of calcium antagonists (AV node for verapamil and diltiazem, muscular smooth muscle for nifedipine) are more sensitive than the sinoatrial node to the drug concerned. Digitalis decreases heart rate by vagal stimulation and it may also have a direct inhibitory effect. An important point is that therapeutic concentrations of these agents do not totally obliterate sinus node pacemaking (unless there is pre-existing disease of the node—sick sinus syndrome). The basement membrane enveloping the clusters of P cells seals off the pacemaker sites from the drug concentrated in the interstitial fluid. Of the agents which decrease heart rate, it is only the beta-blockers which have thus far been used therapeutically to slow the sinus node.

Table 5-1

Positively chronotropic agents

Agent	Presumed mechanism
Beta-adrenergic receptor agonists	Formation of second messenger
Phosphodiesterase inhibitors	Formation of second messenger
Atropine	Binding to muscarinic cholinergic receptor
Quinidine, disopyramide	Atropine-like

For cellular sites of action see Chapters 6 and 17.

Table 5-2

Negatively chronotropic agents

Agent	Presumed mechanism
Beta-adrenergic receptor antagonists	Inhibition of formation of adrenergic second messenger
Ca²⁺-antagonists (high dose)	Inhibition of slow inward current
Acetylcholine	? inhibition of release of norepinephrine
Vagal stimulation	**Release of acetylcholine** ? inhibition of release of norepinephrine
Digitalis	Vagal stimulation
Alinidine¹ (a clonidine derivative)	?? inhibition of chloride current
Adenosine	Inhibition of adenylate cyclase
Reserpine	Depletion of catecholamines
Alpha-methyl tyrosine	Inhibition of catecholamine synthesis

For cellular sites of action see Chapters 6 and 17.
¹Harron et al. (1981). Lancet i: 351.

Propagation of Impulse

Once the impulse has formed in the sinus node it spreads very rapidly throughout the atrium to reach the atrioventricular node (Fig. 5-6). In atrial tissue, a new sort of action potential is dominated by a fast sodium channel. When the electrical impulse arrives at the sarcolemma it "opens" the sodium gate, which in turn opens the calcium gate. Sodium and calcium ions enter causing a zone of positive changes within the cell while potassium ions leave to cause a zone of negative changes. Positive ions will be attracted to the negative zone on the outside of the sarcolemma and negative ions to the inner side where the sodium and calcium ions are. Thus the surrounding sarcolemma will tend to lose its polarity and this in turn will open more surrounding sodium channels. A self-perpetuating process occurs so that the impulse very readily spreads throughout the sarcolemma of a single heart cell.

Conduction between cells is explained as follows. There is an efflux of potassium ions during depolarization into that narrow part of the extracellular space found between the intercalated discs separating

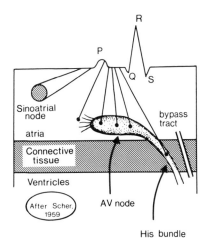

Fig. 5-6 Components of the conduction system and their contribution to the PR interval of the electrocardiogram. Modified from Scher et al. (1959), with permission.

the cells, so that a local micro-accumulation of potassium ions depolarizes the intercalated disc of the next cell (Sperelakis, 1979). A further mechanism for intercellular conduction is the existence of the low-resistance **gap** or **nexus junctions** between cells (see Fig. 2-4). Each gap junction is thought to be composed of protein-lined channels (connexons) which penetrate the lipid bilayer of two adjacent cells. The central pore is about 2 nm (20 Ångstrom) in diameter. The result is that potassium and other small molecules (mol. wt up to about 850) can pass from cell to cell by the gap junctions as can, presumably, the electrical current (for critical analysis, see Sperelakis, 1979).

Atrial Conduction

From the origin of the heart beat in the specialized cells of the sinus node to the contraction of the ventricular myofibril is a big gap. That gap is bridged first by the rapid conduction of the electrical impulse through the atria, so as to fire the atrioventricular (AV) node which in turn sends another impulse down the specialized bundle of His and Purkinje fibers. The terminal branches (arborization of the Purkinje system) spread the impulse throughout the ventricles, eventually travelling along the sarcolemma of the myocytes whence the process of excitation–contraction coupling links the cell surface and its invaginations to the contractile system.

Are there specialized conducting fibers carrying the

impulse through the atria from the sinus to the atrioventricular node? Three **internodal tracts** have been thought to serve as pathways that preferentially conduct the cardiac impulse through the atria. Histologically, they consist of cells somewhat similar to those of the Purkinje system. Physiologically, these cells are highly resistant to an increased extracellular potassium concentration, a property which resembles that of the sinus node. Recently the pattern of atrial activation has been studied and displayed in the form of isochrones (Scher and Spah, 1979). **Isochrones** look like weather charts and display wavy lines which link sites of simultaneous excitation. The pattern of movement of isochrones shows how the impulse spreads. Such studies show that from the functional point of view there are no narrow specialized atrial tracts. Rather, the entire atrial septum functions as a conduction system to take waves from the sinus to the atrioventricular node. According to this view, those atrial cells with specialized functional properties (resistance to high potassium, spontaneous diastolic depolarization) are not necessarily found in the three internodal tracts.

Atrioventricular Node

Atrial impulses cannot travel directly to the ventricles because of separating connecting tissue. Hence the impulse is "collected" in the atrioventricular node (Fig. 5-6) which is located in the right atrium just above the origin of the tricuspid valve; when this node is stimulated, it sends off the impulse along the bundle of His through the connective tissue separating atria and ventricles. The depolarization of ventricular cells starts about 80 msec after the impulse leaves atrial tissue (Scher and Spah, 1979); this is the time taken for the impulse to traverse the atrioventricular node, His bundle and bundle branches. Electrocardiographically, this interval corresponds to the **PR interval** (beginning of P to beginning of R wave, normal upper limit 0.20 sec, Fig. 5-6), most of which reflects conduction from the sinus to the atrioventricular node. The benefit of this delay is that the atrial booster contraction (page 168) occurring with the P wave has time to empty into the ventricle before ventricular contraction starts.

The AV node may be divided into three regions— atrionodal (AN), nodal (N) and nodal-His (NH), on the basis of striking differences in the shape of the action potential rather than on anatomical grounds

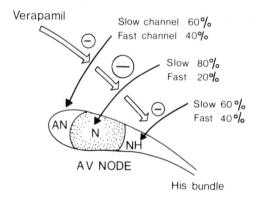

Fig. 5-7 Contributions of slow (Ca^{2+}) and fast (Na^+) channels to the three parts of the atrioventricular node; the atrionodal zone (AN), middle zone of "true" nodal cells (N) and the nodal-His (NH) zone.

(Fig. 5-7). The blood supply to the atrioventricular node is usually from the right coronary artery, which explains the association between atrioventricular block and posterior myocardial infarction (reflexes are another factor, see below). Most of the cells of the atrioventricular node are slender traditional cells, similar to the T cells of the sinus node; these are a few simple rounded cells identical to P cells of the sinus node; and at the margin of the node are ordinary working myocardial cells. As the atrioventricular node forms the His bundle and conduction system, the cells become more linearly arranged (Fig. 5-8).

Autonomic control

The space just behind the atrioventricular node (**retronodal space**) is richly supplied with autonomic nerves. Here adrenergic nerves deliver sympathetic stimuli to the atrioventricular node and cholinergic nerves deliver vagal stimuli. An interesting characteristic of autonomic control is that the inhibitory effects of the vagus on the sinus node become more pronounced as the sympathetic tone increases. In contrast, in the atrioventricular node it seems that the effects of vagal stimulation are independent of the prevailing sympathetic tone (Levy and Martin, 1979). Receptors in the nodal area are thought to convey different stimuli for the reflex vagal symptoms associated with posterior myocardial infarction— bradycardia, AV conduction delay, nausea and sweating.

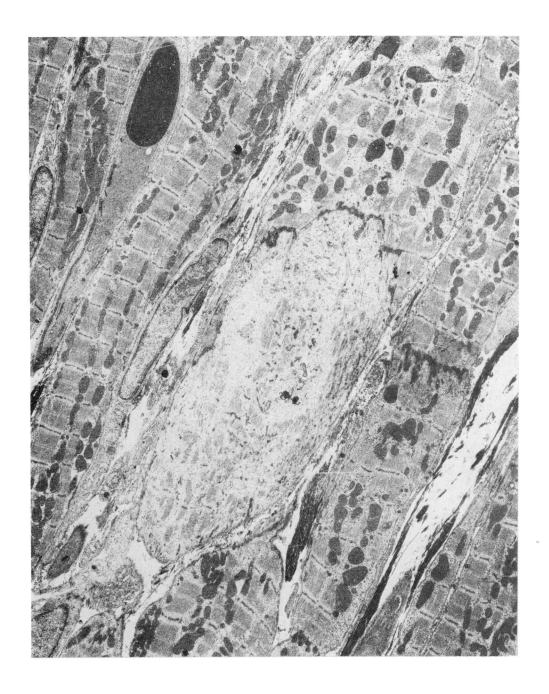

Fig. 5-8 Ventricular portion of the conduction system of rat heart. Note (i) the central Purkinje cells with relatively clear cytoplasm and only a few myofibrils; and (ii) above and to the right of the Purkinje cells, several transitional cells more closely resembling contracting myocytes. × 4500. By courtesy of Dr J Moravec, Paris.

Electrophysiological properties

Many of the electrophysiological properties of the atrioventricular node closely resemble those of the sinus node; in particular, there is a spontaneous slow diastolic depolarization, a slow upstroke and a low amplitude type of action potential found in the AV junctional cells. The spontaneous diastolic depolarization is less prominent in the junctional cells of the atrioventricular node than in the sinus node so that the AV node acts largely to regulate conduction from atria to ventricles, rather than to act as a subsidiary pacemaker, except in pathological circumstances such as complete heart block. The atrioventricular node functions as a sorting box or filter so that the number and order of the supraventricular impulses can be controlled.

The rate of conduction from the atria to the ventricles is largely dependent on the slow channel of the atrioventricular node and hence is inhibited by verapamil or diltiazem (Fig. 5-7); a small sodium-dependent component may explain why sometimes the Class I (sodium-channel blocking) antiarrhythmic agents of the quinidine group can depress atrioventricular conduction. The contribution of the slow channel to the action potential of nodal tissue is most in the N (nodal) zone of the AV node, where automaticity is absent and where the upstroke of the action potential rises most slowly. In contrast, automaticity is found in the AN (atrionodal or upper part) and NH (nodal-His) regions, where verapamil is least active (Wit and Cranefield, 1974).

Metabolism

Both adenosine and severe hypoxia depress atrioventricular conduction (Belardinelli et al., 1980). Adenosine is a breakdown product of ATP normally concerned with coronary vasodilation. Adenosine also inhibits the slow calcium channel, which would explain its inhibitory effect on the atrioventricular node and its potential use in supraventricular tachycardia effect (similar to verapamil, see Fig. 23-4). If adenosine were carried to the atrioventricular node cells from other acutely ischemic cells it could be a cause of transient atrioventricular conduction disturbances in acute infarction. An interesting prediction has been made: methylxanthines, which prevent adenosine from interacting with its cell receptor, could be useful therapeutically in combating atrioventricular heart block in some patients with acute myocardial infarction.

AV nodal disease

When the AV node is damaged by disease such as ischemia or myocarditis, then the conduction of the impulse can become abnormally slow so that AV nodal block occurs. This is classically recognized on the electrocardiogram as a prolonged PR interval and called **first-degree heart block** (Fig. 5-9). Any of the drugs inhibiting the AV node can also cause first-degree block—digitalis, verapamil, diltiazem, beta-adrenergic blockade. In the case of digitalis poisoning, one risk is total inhibition of the AV node and, by quite another effect of digitalis, increased ventricular automaticity which frequently occurs at the AV junction in the His bundle. Thus a pacemaker takes over to form a **junctional escape rhythm** (less correctly called a **nodal** rhythm).

When the conduction between the atria and ventricles is severely inhibited, usually as a result of disease of AV node and His bundle, then the P-wave intermittently fails in its efforts to reach the ventricles (**second-degree heart block**) or there is a total block between atria and ventricles (third-degree or **complete heart block**). In the latter instance, ventricular asystole occurs and death is inevitable unless a subsidiary ventricular pacemaker takes over. Such an **idioventricular rhythm** usually arises in the His bundle or upper Purkinje fibers and fires at a much lower spontaneous rate than the sinus node. When there is the sudden development of complete heart block, the idioventricular rhythm may take some time to develop; during the period of asystole, cerebral ischemia and syncope develops (Stokes–Adams attack).

Drugs acting on the AV node

Conduction through the atrioventricular node needs to be reduced in many supraventricular arrhythmias (page 331). Physiologically, carotid sinus massage may be successful by reflexly enhancing vagal tone. Pharmacologically, slow channel blockade by verapamil or diltiazem may be very effective; alternatively, beta-adrenergic blockade or digitalis compounds may be used (Table 5-3). Conversely, when conduction through the node must be accelerated,

Table 5-3

Agents or procedures acting on the atrioventricular node

Effect	Agent or procedure	Proposed mechanism
Physiological inhibition	Carotid sinus massage, breath-holding	Vagal stimulation
Pharmacological inhibition	Verapamil	Inhibition of slow calcium current
	Diltiazem	
	Beta-adrenergic blockade	Inhibition of beta-adrenergic effects
	Digitalis	Enhanced vagal effect
	Adenosine	Inhibition of slow calcium channel
	Amiodarone	? calcium current inhibition
Pharmacological stimulation	Beta-adrenergic agonists	Increased formation of second messenger
	Atropine	Decreased vagal effect; competition with acetyl choline at muscarinic receptors
Mixed pharmacological effects	Quinidine	Decreased vagal effect versus direct inhibition
	Disopyramide	

For cellular sites of action see Chapters 6 and 17.

as in some patients with myocardial infarction and serious block of atrioventricular conduction, then atropine (see Fig. 17-3) is used.

Bypass tract

Sometimes the presence of the atrioventricular node is bypassed by an additional conduction pathway. The classic example is the bundle of Kent, a strand of cardiac muscle crossing the fibrous barrier between atria and ventricles (Fig. 5-6).

> It is now clear that there are several types of accessory atrioventricular conduction pathways, that these are about 1 mm in diameter and approximately 5–10 mm in length and that they occur around the entire atrioventricular ring   Scher and Spah (1979)

Conduction along these pathways bypasses the slower atrioventricular node to give the shortened PR interval (less than 0.12 sec) and abnormal **delta wave** with widened QRS (more than 0.10 sec) which together characterize the **Wolff–Parkinson–White syndrome**.

His Bundle and its Branches. Purkinje Fibers

The bundle of His, which divides into left and right bundles, runs from the atrioventricular node. It penetrates the connecting tissue dividing atria and ventricles and is the only muscular connection between these chambers. The cells found in the common bundle

and bundle branches are the characteristic Purkinje cells which much more closely resemble (Fig. 5-8) embryonic muscle than normal working myocardium. The analogy with embryonic cells should imply slow conduction of the electrical impulse whereas in reality the conduction velocity is 200 cm/sec in contrast to that in the sinus node P cells of 5 cm/sec. There are specific membrane characteristics to accelerate conduction — possibly the numerous end-to-end rather than side-to-side connections (James and Sherf, 1971).

Purkinje fibers have the potential for spontaneous diastolic depolarization at a much slower rate than nodal tissue, but the threshold for firing is also lower in keeping with the very active fast sodium channel. Two factors keep Purkinje fibers from firing. First, the rate of spontaneous firing is very slow, being only about 30/min. Secondly, the Purkinje pacemaker current, I_f, operates at a voltage range less negative than that of normal Purkinje fibers, so that only partially depolarized Purkinje fibers can fire rapidly. The sinus node normally suppresses the automaticity of the Purkinje fibers, except in cases of complete heart block (for electrocardiographic pattern, see Fig. 5-9).

The His bundle divided into the two bundle branches — the **left bundle branch** is distributed to the left ventricle to give early activation of the septum and the areas of the papillary muscles. The left bundle divides into anterior and posterior fascicles, which when damaged as by ischemia, cause respectively **left anterior hemiblock** or **left posterior hemiblock**. Anatomically, the basis for such a strict division is less

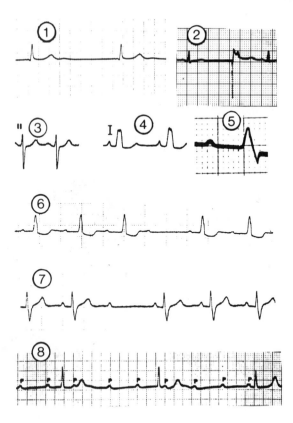

Fig. 5-9
1. Sinus bradycardia, 36/min.
2. Same + demand atrial pacing.
3. Left anterior hemiblock.
4. Left bundle branch block.
5. First-degree AV block.
6. Second-degree Wenkebach block.
7. Second-degree Mobitz block.
8. Third-degree ''complete heart block''.
By permission of D Dubin (1974). Rapid interpretation of EKG's, Cover Publishing Co, Tampa, Florida (traces 5 and 8) and FL Meijler et al. (1975). Electrocardiography for intensive care units, Excerpta Medica, Amsterdam (traces 3, 4, 6, 7).

clear. When both fascicles are blocked the pattern of left bundle branch block emerges (Fig.5-9). The **right bundle branch** continues from the His bundle down the interventricular septum to start branching at the apex of the right ventricle.

Terminal branches of the left and right bundles form an extensive lacy network of **Purkinje fibers** on the endocardial layer of the ventricles which penetrate only the inner third of the ventricular wall. From these terminal arborizations the impulse must be conducted through the ventricular wall by ordinary myocardial contractile cells.

The blood supply of the bundle of His is from both left anterior and posterior descending coronary arteries so that ischemic damage is unusual. On the other hand, the bundle branches reach the ventricles where coronary artery disease can cause ischemia of the bundles.

Sick Sinus Syndrome

In the sick sinus syndrome, the sinoatrial node intermittently and progressively fails to fire. There may be associated episodes of tachycardia or periods of sinus arrest. This disease characteristically occurs in the older age group, frequently as a result of coronary artery disease or idiopathic fibrosis. In one type, the diagnosis is electrocardiographically evident because the associated episodes of tachycardia give the characteristic **bradycardia–tachycardia syndrome**. In other cases overdrive pacing may be required to show delayed recovery of the sinoatrial node at the end of pacing.

Overdrive Suppression

Overdrive suppression or **post-pacing inhibition** is the phenomenon whereby pacemaker activity is slow to resume when an induced tachycardia is terminated. The mechanism of overdrive suppression is usually studied in isolated Purkinje fibers rather than in the sinus node. After overdrive induced by tachycardia, the slope of diastolic depolarization is decreased and the threshold voltage is more positive, and hence it is more difficult to initiate the action potential. A proposed mechanism is that the high heart rate causes repetitive entry of sodium ions with each action potential (Courtney and Sokolove, 1979); the sodium pump is stimulated and the electrogenic outward current increases so that the net inward pacemaker current is less. Recent measurements with an ion-selective micro-electrode favor this view (Cohen et al., 1982).

A secondary mechanism is by an accumulation of calcium ions (Musso and Vassalle, 1982), also to be expected because of repetitive entry of calcium during the action potential; such calcium ions can increase the conductance of potassium so that more potassium ions flow outwards to promote hyperpolarization.

His Bundle Electrogram

In the conventional electrocardiogram, conduction between the sinoatrial node and the ventricles is readily monitored by the PR interval (Fig. 5-9). To separate conduction abnormalities in the AV node from those in the His bundle and bundle branches requires the invasive placing of a catheter with three electrodes at its tip near to the tricuspid valve to record the His bundle electrogram (Fig. 5-10). Another catheter is introduced high into the right atrium, to be positioned near the sinoatrial node; this catheter has two stimulating and two recording electrodes. A third catheter goes into the right ventricle. Other electrodes may be placed low in the right atrium or in the coronary sinus. The **PA interval** is from the earliest P wave recorded to the atrial depolarization taken from the His bundle electrogram (Fig. 5-11). The **AH**

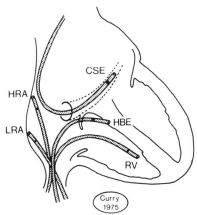

Fig. 5-10 Some catheter electrode positions used for intracardiac recording. HRA = high right atrium. LRA = lower right atrium; HBE = His bundle electrogram; RV = right ventricle; CSE = coronary sinus electrogram (for indirect monitoring of left atrial and left ventricular sites). With permission from Curry PUL (1975). In: Cardiac Arrhythmias. Ed. DM Krikler, JF Goodwin, p 48, Saunders, London.

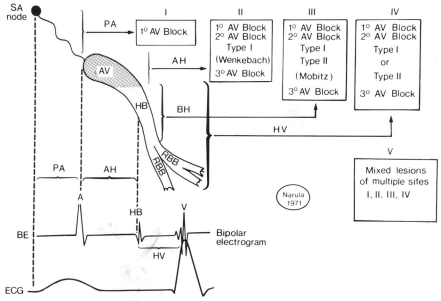

Fig. 5-11 The atrioventricular conduction system illustrating the different varieties of AV block that occur as a result of lesions in the conduction system. In the lower left-hand corner are recordings taken from the bipolar electrogram from the area of the His bundle. The PA (P wave to atrial depolarization), AH (atrial depolarization to His depolarization) and HV (His to ventricular depolarization) intervals are outlined. They are compared with the PR interval of the normal electrocardiogram (L2, bottom trace). Recordings such as this allow clear localization of the site of conduction block and of the effect of antiarrhythmic drugs on conduction. SAN = sinoatrial node; AVN = atrioventricular node; BH = Bundle of His; LB = left bundle branch; RB = right bundle branch. Modified from Narula et al. (1971). Am J Med 50: 146, with permission.

interval is from the A point to the start of His depolarization, which gives the conduction time through the AV node. The **HV interval** is from the H point to the earliest component of ventricular contraction and gives the conduction time through the His bundle and Purkinje system. Accordingly, conduction delay can be localized. Slowing of conduction induced by antiarrhythmic drugs can be defined.

In cases of suspected abnormalities of AV nodal conduction (Chapter 23), including those involving the bypass tract, a tachycardia may be provoked by an appropriately introduced atrial or ventricular ectopic beat, the direction of the conduction determined, and the effect of various antiarrhythmic drugs shown. This procedure is called programmed electrical stimulation (Chapter 23).

Summary

The spontaneous heart rate is chiefly governed by the rate of diastolic depolarization of the pacemaker (P) cells of the sinus node, the mechanism of which is still ill-understood. There are three pacemaker currents: the decaying potassium current, the slow inward current, and the newly described inward current I_f. These currents respond to beta-adrenergic or cholinergic stimulation to raise or lower the heart rate. Such changes occur especially in response to exercise and allow for changes in the cardiac output to be independent of the venous filling pressure. The rate of sinus firing can be slowed by beta-adrenergic blockers. Temporary suppression of the sinus node pacemaker by overdrive is a useful test for the sick sinus syndrome.

The electrical impulse travels from the sinus node to the atrioventricular node through the atrial septum. In the atrioventricular node some cells similar to the P cells of the sinus are found, with the majority resembling the transitional cells. Conduction through the atrioventricular node is normally slow but can be very rapid when a circus tachycardia passes through the atrioventricular node. Only rarely is there evidence of the ability of the His–Purkinje system to fire spontaneously, as in the condition of complete heart block. Conduction through the His bundle and down the bundle branches to the ventricular endocardium is by Purkinje cells, which is some ways are primitive and resistant to hypoxia, and in other ways are highly specialized with a very rapid rate of conduction. The

cardiac impulse has now arrived at the sarcolemma of the ventricular myocyte; the next step is depolarization of the sarcolemma, "opening" of the calcium channels, and triggering of contraction by calcium ions.

References

Belardinelli L, Belloni FL, Rubio R, Berne RM (1980). Atrioventricular conduction disturbances during hypoxia. Possible role of adenosine in rabbit and guinea pig heart. Circ Res 47: 684–691.

Brown H (1982). Electrophysiology of the sinoatrial node. Physiol Rev 62: 505–530.

Brown H, DiFrancesco D (1980). Voltage-clamp investigation of membrane currents underlying pacemaker activity in rabbit sino-atrial node. J Physiol 308: 331–351.

Brown HF, McNaughton PA, Noble D, Noble SJ (1975). Adrenergic control of pacemaker currents. Phil Trans Roy Soc London 270: 527–537.

Cohen CJ, Fozzard HA, Shen SS (1982). Increase in intracellular sodium ion activity during stimulation in mammalian cardiac muscle. Circ Res 50: 651–662.

Courtney KR, Sokolove PG (1979). Importance of electrogenic sodium pump in normal and overdriven sinoatrial pacemaker. J Molec Cell Cardiol 11: 787–794.

DiFrancesco D (1981). The pacemaker current 'i(K₂)' in Purkinje fibres is carried by sodium and potassium. J Physiol 308: 32P–33P.

Eckberg DL, Drabinsky M, Braunwald E (1971). Defective cardiac parasympathetic control in patients with heart disease. N Engl J Med 285: 877–883.

Fozzard HA, Beeler GW (1975). The voltage clamp and cardiac electrophysiology. Circ Res 37: 403–413.

Harriman RJ, Hoffman BF, Naylor RE (1980). Electrical activity from the sinus node region in conscious dogs. Circ Res 47: 775–791.

James TN (1974). Selective experimental chelation of calcium in the sinus node. J Molec Cell Cardiol 6: 493–504.

James TN, Sherf L (1971). Fine structure of the His bundle. Circulation 44: 9–28.

Jedeikin LA (1964). Regional distribution of glycogen and phosphorylase in the ventricles of the heart. Circ Res 14: 202–211.

Jose AD (1966). Effect of combined sympathetic and parasympathetic blockade on heart rate and cardiac function in man. Am J Cardiol 18: 476–478.

Levy MN, Martin PJ (1979). Neural control of the heart. In: Handbook of Physiology. Sect 2, Vol. 1, The Heart, pp 581–620, Am Physiol Soc, Bethesda, Maryland.

Maylie J, Morad M, Weiss J (1981). A study of pacemaker potential in rabbit sinoatrial node: Measurement of potassium activity under voltage-clamp conditions. J Physiol 311: 161–178.

Musso E, Vassalle M (1982). The role of calcium in overdrive suppression of canine cardiac Purkinje fibers. Circ Res 51: 167–180.

Narula OS, Scherlag BJ, Samet P, Javier RP (1971). Atrioventricular block: localization and classification by His bundle recordings. Am J Med 50: 146–165.

Pollack GH (1977). Cardiac pacemaking: an obligatory role of catecholamines. Science 196: 731–738.

Scher AM, Spah MS (1979). Cardiac depolarization and repolarization and the electrocardiogram. In: Handbook of Physiology, Vol 1, The Cardiovascular System. Ed. RM Berne, pp 357–392, Am Physiol Soc, Bethesda.

Scher AM, Rodriquez MI, Liikane J, Young AC (1959). The mechanism of atrioventricular conduction. Circ Res 7: 54–61.

Senges J, Brachman J, Pelzer D, Kramer B, Kubler W (1980). Combined effects of glucose and hypoxia on cardiac automaticity and conduction. J Molec Cell Cardiol 12: 311–323.

Sperelakis N (1979). Propagation mechanisms in heart. Ann Rev Physiol 41: 441–457.

Wit AL, Cranefield PF (1974). Effect of verapamil on the sinoatrial and atrioventricular nodes of the rabbit and the mechanism by which it arrests re-entrant atrioventricular nodal tachycardia. Circ Res 35: 413–425.

Woods WT, Urthaler F, James TN (1981). Electrical activity in canine sinus node cells during arrest produced by acetylcholine. J Molec Cell Cardiol 13: 349–357.

New References

Favale S, Di Biase M, Rizzo U, Belardinelli L, Rizzon P (1985). Effect of adenosine and adenosine-5′-triphosphate on atrioventricular conduction in patients. J Am Coll Cardiol 5: 1212–1219.

Irisawa H, Noma A (1984). Pacemaker currents in mammalian nodal cells. J Molec Cell Cardiol 16: 777–781.

6 | Receptors, Adrenergic Effects and Cyclic AMP

Properties of Receptors

In 1905, Langley made the fundamental proposal that agents acting at the nerve-endings did not directly interact with the cells concerned; rather, "receptive substances" mediated the cellular response. The term "receptor" was used by Ehrlich in 1913 to designate the hypothetical specific chemical groupings of the cell which reacted with chemotherapeutic drugs. It is this concept of receptors (Table 6-1) which is fundamental to modern cardiovascular pharmacology.

Definition of receptor

A good definition of "receptor" is that of Kahn (1976):

> There is general agreement that the term "receptor" refers to a molecule (or molecular complex) which is capable of recognizing and selectively interacting with the hormone or neurotransmitter, and which, after binding it, is capable of generating some signal that initiates the chain of events leading to the biological response.

The biological response is generated by a functionally separate unit, the **effector** (Fig. 6-1). Generally, the receptor is a specialized part of the external layer of the sarcolemma, sometimes extending through the sarcolemma, whereas the effector is a specialized part of the internal layer; communication between the two

is called **coupling**. Structurally, many receptors appear to be integral membrane proteins which require strong detergents to break the hydrophobic bonds holding them to the membrane. Sometimes, as in the case of thyroid hormone, the receptors are located within the cell so that the hormone has to cross the sarcolemma to reach the receptor. For a typical hormone such as a catecholamine:

$$R + H \longrightarrow RH$$
$$RH + effector \longrightarrow RH - E$$
$$RH - E \longrightarrow biological\ effect$$

Receptors for drugs

In the case of drugs, the hormone-receptor theory applies within certain limits (Ariens and Beld, 1977). First, the active drug must be released from the form in which it is administered; next, the active drug must be absorbed into the bloodstream when all the factors governing its concentration become important — liver metabolism, protein-binding, water or lipid solubility, as well as rates and routes of secretion. All these processes are part of the study of **pharmocokinetics**. The interaction of the drug with the molecular sites of action on the tissues (the receptors) then leads to a stimulus which in turn produces the desired pharmacological effect. Sometimes drug receptors are active sites on enzymes as in the case of digitalis (Chapter 20). Sometimes another well-defined receptor molecule is involved as in the case of the beta-

Table 6-1

Classification of cardiac receptors, including vascular and myocardial sites

Broad types and agonists	Sub-types	Comments
1. Classical neurotransmitters		
Adrenergic	alpha	Chiefly vascular
	beta-1	Chiefly myocardial (? coronary vascular)
	beta-2	Chiefly vascular, also nodal
Cholinergic	muscarinic	Vascular, myocardial and nodal
2. Adrenergic-related receptors		
Histamine	H_1	Chiefly vascular
	H_2	Chiefly myocardial
Thyroid	—	Additional intracellular receptor
Glucagon	—	Bypasses beta-1 receptor
Dopamine[1]	Multiple	Significance of subtypes controversial
3. Vascular receptors (other than adrenergic-cholinergic)		
Adenosine[2]	R	Requires ribose, activates adenylate cyclase; vascular and myocardial
Serotonin	—	May vasoconstrict
Thromboxane[3]	—	Vascular. Helps regulate Ca^{2+} influx
Prostacyclin[4]	—	Vasodilates
Purinergic[5]	P_1	Adenosine-sensitive, vascular and atrial
	P_2	ATP-sensitive, vascular
Peptidergic[6]	—	Vascular
4. Enzymes		
Digitalis[7]	?	Sodium–potassium pump
5. Other hormonal receptors		
Insulin	—	—
Steroid	—	—

[1]Woodruff (1982). Trends Pharm Sci 3: 4.

[2]Londos and Wolff (1977). Proc Nat Acad Sci USA 74: 5482.

[3]Smith and Lefer (1981). Am J Physiol H493.

[4]Dusting and Vane (1980). Circ Res Suppl 1: 183.

[5]Burnstock and Meghji (1981). Brit J Pharmacol 73: 879.

[6]Weihe et al. (1981). J Molec Cell Cardiol 13: 331.

[7]Schwartz and Adams (1980). Circ Res Suppl 1: 154.

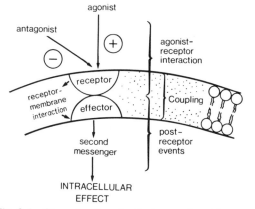

Fig. 6-1 General pattern for the interaction of hormone or other agonist with membrane-bound receptor.

adrenergic receptor. Isolation of receptors is now possible, especially when they are separated from adjacent macromolecules by polar groups which cleave upon isolation. For many drugs the receptors are as yet ill-defined and possibly rather non-specific. Thus the term "receptor" is not always as specific as might be imagined.

Receptor models

Initial models stressed the close molecular fit with a "lock-and-key" pattern, where the **agonist** molecule is the "key" and the receptor molecule the "lock". The key turns the lock to produce an intercellular effect, mediated by a second messenger. The current

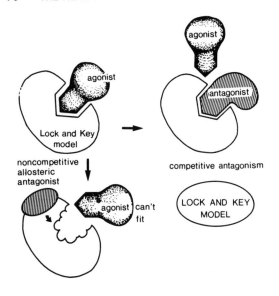

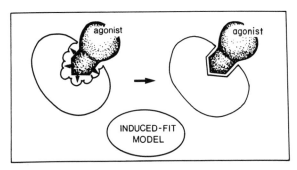

Fig. 6-2 Agonist–receptor models largely have their origins in the concepts of substrate–enzyme interactions.

working model for the effects of polypeptide hormones and catecholamines (Fig. 6-2) is as follows:

hormone → receptor → effector → second messenger

A second "**induced-fit**" model has been evolved for the effects of hormones such as the glucocorticoids (De Meyts and Rousseau, 1980). The agonist steroid molecule combines with the receptor, altering its molecular configuration; the combination exerts an intracellular effect such as influencing the rate of synthesis of messenger RNA (Chapter 3) by the nuclei.

Antagonists may act in one of two ways. An allosteric antagonist interacts with another spatially different site to induce the inactive state. During competitive inhibition, there is a steric interaction whereby both agonist and antagonist compete for that site. In a second model there are two sites on the

receptor. The agonist molecule is bound to the receptor at the **binding site**, while stimulation of the receptor takes place at a second **active site**. Antagonists could act to prevent the interaction of the agonist with the active site or the binding site or both. The two-site model can explain the phenomenon of **partial agonism**. A partial agonist stimulates the active site yet prevents access of other agonists by combining with the binding site. Thus both beta-adrenergic inhibition and beta-adrenergic stimulation can simultaneously be achieved, for example by the compound pindolol.

The interaction between receptor sites and antagonists may be reversible or irreversible. **Reversible** agonists and antagonists compete for the same receptor site, and the degree of effectiveness of each depends on the concentration at the receptor site. **Irreversible** agonists and antagonists bind irreversibly and no amount of increased concentration of an agonist can overcome the blockade of the receptor site by the antagonist. Fortunately the effect of most physiological and pharmacological agonists is reversible, so that **receptor binding** agents can displace physiological agonists with irreversible inhibition.

Drugs and hormones seldom only stimulate or block one receptor. The explanation may be either that there are molecular similarities between receptor sites, or that agonist molecules lack complete molecular specificity for various receptors. The interaction of only a very limited part of the molecular structure of agonist and receptor seems to determine the "fit" and the subsequent interaction.

Receptor kinetics and ligands

Initially kinetics were considered only in terms of the **occupancy theory** whereby the intensity of the pharmacological effect is proportional to the number of receptors occupied by the drug. Thus

$$R + D \rightleftharpoons RD \rightarrow \text{effect}$$

where R is the concentration of free receptors, D the concentration of free molecules of the drug, RD the concentration of the drug–receptor complex, and the latter gives a proportional effect. Maximal effect will require maximal occupancy.

The allosteric theory allows for completely different kinetics because the response can rapidly change as the molecular structure of the receptor is altered by the agonist. This gives rise to the idea of a **critical concentration** of agonist (or antagonist) which induces the maximal change in receptor structure; below or above this concentration the effects are either very slight or maximal. Therefore, the allosteric theory can allow for an (almost) all-or-none response to an agonist.

Ligands are highly radioactive agonists or specific hormones which bind to the receptor. Lefkowitz (1979) has defined the criteria required to show that the binding of a particular ligand to the cell membrane is not merely a non-specific phenomenon but is specific to the physiologic or pharmacologic receptor:

> These criteria generally include that the binding phenomenon should be saturable, that is, to a finite, usually small number of sites; ligand binding should have high affinity consonant with the known high affinity for that particular drug or hormone's action; the kinetics of binding should be appropriate to the kinetics of drug action; and, most importantly, the detailed specificity of binding should be identical in all respects to the specificity inferred from physiologic experiments.

The use of radiolabeled beta-agonists have shown that each ventricular cell has hundreds of receptor sites or even more (the value can be calculated from Tables 2-2 and 4-2). These sites have the characteristics of beta-adrenergic receptors, including stereo-specificity for beta-agonists and beta-antagonists, the absence of reaction with alpha-antagonists, and firm binding of labeled agonists and antagonists.

The **dissociation constant**, K_D, is defined from the concentration of antagonist or agonist required to displace a radioligand from a receptor, being approximately half the concentration required for a maximal effect. The correct formula is:

$$K_D = 1/2 \, (L) \, . \, (1 - f_L)$$

where $1/2 \, (L)$ is half the concentration of the labeled ligand and f_L is the fractional degree of saturation of the labeled ligand in the absence of competing ligand (Maguire et al., 1977). Thus the K_D for the beta-adrenergic receptor of the antagonist propranolol is about 10^{-8} M (Fig. 6-3).

Receptor effects and dose–response curves

The classical way of relating the concentration of a drug or hormone to its effect, is by a dose–response curve (Fig. 6-4). The dose causing 50 percent of the maximal effect is known as the ED_{50} (ED = effective dose). When the effect is inhibition, the concentration of the

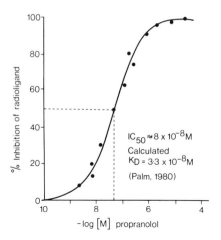

Fig. 6-3 Kinetics of the interaction of propranolol with beta-receptor as defined by radioligand binding. From Palm (1980). In: Advances in Beta-blocker Therapy, Eds H Roskamm, K-H Graefe, pp 3–15, Excerpta Medica, Amsterdam, with permission.

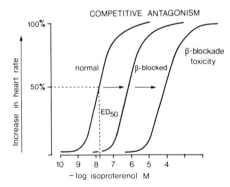

Fig. 6-4 Pattern of competitive antagonism between the beta-adrenergic agonist, isoproterenol, and a beta-adrenergic receptor antagonist, propranolol. These estimates are based on (i) a "high" plasma catecholamine concentration of 10^{-9} M; (ii) a K_D for propranolol of 10^{-8} M (see Fig. 6-3) which might need an agonist concentration of 10^{-7} M to be displaced from the beta-adrenergic receptor; and (iii) the much higher doses of propranolol required for toxicity. Thus beta blockade moves the ED_{50} to the right.

agent causing 50 percent of the maximal inhibition is the IC_{50} (IC = inhibitory concentration). Determination of the ED_{50} or IC_{50} can show whether a drug or hormone is very active in producing its effect (low ED_{50} or IC_{50}) or not so active (high ED_{50} or IC_{50}). When a low concentration of a drug initiates a marked response, it has "high **intrinsic activity**"

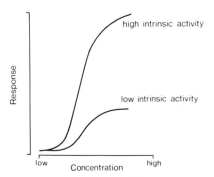

Fig. 6-5 Variations in intrinsic activity of agonist molecules.

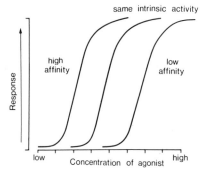

Fig. 6-6 Agonists with different affinities for the receptor, but with the same intrinsic activity, have the same ultimate effects but at different concentrations.

because the drug is assumed to bind to its receptor in such a way that a maximal signal is elicited (Fig. 6-5). Another drug with a "low intrinsic activity" will elicit little or no response even at a high concentration. The **affinity** of the agonist and receptor molecules for each other may be explained by the molecular "fit". Perfect compatibility (lock and key) explains a high affinity. An agonist molecule that is not very active (low intrinsic activity) can still bind to the receptor with high affinity, thereby separating these two qualities (Fig. 6-6).

Thus the receptor concept allows understanding of two important characteristics of drug–tissue interaction—high **affinity** and marked **specificity**. High affinity explains why a low concentration of a drug can be so effective; marked specificity explains why only a small change in molecular structure can decisively change the properties of that drug.

Knowing the K_D for a particular antagonist of a receptor can be useful in distinguishing non-specific

from specific effects. Specific effects are those mediated only by the interaction with the receptor; non-specific effects are those mediated by additional properties and usually at a higher concentration. A practical example is in the assessment of the anti-arrhythmic properties of beta-adrenergic blocking agents against reperfusion arrhythmias (Thandroyen et al., 1983). In the case of propranolol, half of the concentration (ED_{50}) required to abolish reperfusion arrhythmias in an isolated rat heart is about 10^{-6} M. Yet the KD_{50} of propranolol is 10^{-8} M from ligand studies. Therefore the antiarrhythmic effect of propranolol in this preparation is not due to a specific agonist–receptor interaction but probably resides in another non-specific "membrane" effect.

Regulation of receptors

Not all the factors governing the chain of events between agonist and tissue response (Table 6-2) are well understood. Among the most difficult to understand is the way in which receptor numbers and activity can change. The number of receptors per unit area of the sarcolemma (the **receptor density**) is not fixed, but can rise or fall in response to certain physiologic or pathophysiologic circumstances; these changes are called **up-regulation** and **down-regulation**. The hormones or drugs that cause up- and down-regulation can be divided into those that help regulate the concentration of their own receptors by the process of **homologous receptor regulation**, whereas **heterologous receptor regulation** is by non-specific agents. An example of heterologous regulation is the increase in beta-adrenergic receptors caused by experimental hyperthyroidism (Lefkowitz, 1979). An example of homologous regulation is the process whereby high concentrations of beta-adrenergic catecholamines "down-regulate" the number of receptors, so that there is a decrease in tissue responsiveness. Chronic high-level exposure to such catecholamines leads to a marked decrease in tissue responsiveness by the process of **desensitization** or **tachyphylaxis**.

It must not be assumed that an altered number of receptors automatically leads to a corresponding alteration in the activity of the system. Not all receptors are always in use; those present but out of use are **spare receptors**. Variations in the proportions of spare receptors mean that even with an unchanged total number of receptors, the response to a given

Table 6-2

Comparative cardiovascular effects of alpha- and beta-adrenergic receptor stimulation

	Alpha-mediated	Beta-mediated
Electrophysio-logical effects	±	+ + Conduction ↑ Pacemaker ↑ HR ↑
Myocardial mechanics	±	+ + Contractility SV ↑ CO ↑
Myocardial metabolism	± ? glycolysis	+ + O₂ uptake ↑ ATP ↓
Coronary arterioles	+ + constriction	+ direct dilation + + + indirect dilation (metabolic)
Peripheral arterioles	+ + + constriction PVR ↑ BP ↑	+ dilation

HR = heart rate; SV = stroke volume; CO = cardiac output; PVR = peripheral vascular resistance; BP = blood pressure.

concentration of agonist can vary. What makes receptors spare or fully used is not known.

Changes in receptor affinity

Even if the receptor density and proportion of spare receptors were fixed, the activity of the receptor can be altered by molecular changes which regulate the affinity for the agonist. This concept is only now being explored. For example, beta-agonist catecholamines induce or stabilize a "high affinity" form of the beta-adrenergic receptor, which is specific for agonists and binds antagonists rather weakly (Lefkowitz and Hoffman, 1980).

Beta-adrenergic Receptors

The critical experiments of Ahlquist (1948) distinguished the function of alpha- from beta-adrenergic receptors of the heart; he proposed that the major effect of alpha-adrenergic receptor stimulation was on the blood vessels to cause vasoconstriction, while beta-adrenergic receptor stimulation caused inotropic and vasodilatory responses. This pattern of effects is largely still valid, but has been refined by further knowledge, and especially by the description of the cardiac beta-1 and the non-cardiac beta-2-adrenergic receptors. Similarly alpha-adrenergic receptors are now divided into two classes, the alpha-1 postsynaptic and alpha-2 presynaptic receptors. Cholinergic receptors mediate the function of the vagal nerve, which in general have a function opposing that of the adrenergic receptors. Of all these receptors, the best understood is the beta-adrenergic receptor which is of great clinical importance because of the widespread use of beta-adrenergic receptor blocking drugs in cardiovascular diseases.

Beta-1- and beta-2-adrenergic receptors

Cardiac receptors are chiefly the beta-1-adrenergic receptor subtype, while most other receptors are beta-2 (Lands et al., 1967). The introduction of relatively **cardioselective beta-adrenergic blocking agents**, acting chiefly on the heart, supports this functional classification of beta-adrenergic receptors. Even stronger evidence for the existence of different receptors rests on recent molecular and immunological studies (Venter, 1981) which allow an exact differentiation of the distribution of beta-adrenergic receptor subtypes, varying from 100 percent beta-1-adrenergic receptors in the dog ventricle to 100 percent beta-2-adrenergic receptors in the liver. In man, there is a substantial population of beta-2 receptors in the atria (Robberecht et al., 1983), with perhaps about 15 percent beta-2 receptors in the left ventricle (Stiles et al., 1983). The major clinical significance in the different distribution of beta-adrenergic receptor subtypes lies in the concentration of beta-1-adrenergic receptors in the ventricular myocardium and beta-2-adrenergic receptors in the lungs. It must be emphasized that the beta-1- and beta-2-adrenergic receptors still have some molecular similarity despite their major differences, so that beta-2-adrenergic stimulants or beta-1-blockers are only relatively selective and at high concentrations selectivity is lost. Molecular proof of receptor subtypes is still awaited.

Beta-1-adrenergic **receptor density** varies throughout the heart, and the sinus node has about 7–8 times more receptors than has the surrounding atrial muscle or atrioventricular node. The next highest concentration of receptors is found in the ventricles. It seems likely that differences in beta-adrenergic receptor density are one factor determining the magnitude of the tissue response to adrenergic beta-stimulation. Differences in receptor density could explain why the sinus node and the ventricles are the major sites for beta-1 effects.

It has also been postulated that the beta-1-adrenergic receptors can be further subdivided into inotropic and chronotropic receptors, to explain why some beta-1-agonist agents such as dobutamine have a more marked inotropic than chronotropic effect. An alternate proposal rests on the recent finding that both beta-1- and beta-2-adrenergic receptors are found in the myocardium. The ventricles contain chiefly beta-1-adrenergic receptors, whereas the sinus nodal tissue contains both subtypes (Hedberg et al., 1980). Hence beta-2-stimulants also cause tachycardia, whereas beta-1-agonists such as dobutamine may have an apparently dominant inotropic selectivity.

Adenylate cyclase

The molecular beta-adrenergic receptor is only part of a complex which translates the stimulus of the first messenger, the beta-agonist, to the second messenger, usually cyclic AMP (Fig. 6-7). Situated on the outer surface of the sarcolemma, the beta-adrenergic receptor couples to adenylate (= adenyl) cyclase. The beta-adrenergic receptor site is highly stereospecific (Wrenn and Haber, 1979) and the "best-fit" among catecholamines is obtained with isoproterenol, rather than with the naturally occurring catecholamines, norepinephrine and epinephrine.

To transmit the message from the receptor, on the outer surface of the sarcolemma to adenylate cyclase on the inner surface, requires the presence of a protein which binds GTP (guanosine triphosphate)-binding protein (Rodbell, 1980). The latter protein faces the cytoplasm in part so as to gain access to cytosolic

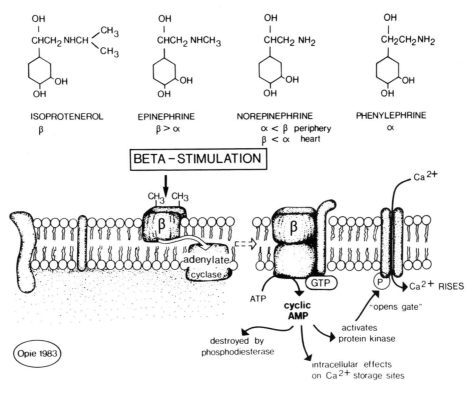

Fig. 6-7 Hypothetical interaction of beta-adrenergic receptor with beta-stimulants to interact with adenylate cyclase by proposed "lateral fluidity" of sarcolemmal lipids. In the presence of guanosine triphosphate (GTP), ATP is converted to the second messenger, cyclic AMP. There is competitive antagonism of beta-agonist stimulation by the non-selective beta-antagonist, propranolol, or the beta-1-selective agents such as atenolol and metoprolol.

guanosine triphosphate and is bound to the guanyl nucleotide-binding subunit of the receptor complex. Both the beta-agonist and **guanosine triphosphate** are required for full activity of adenylate cyclase (Fig. 6-8).

Rodbell (1980) proposes that the beta-adrenergic receptor basically inhibits adenylate cyclase by preventing a GTP-binding protein from reacting with GTP. Beta-stimulation releases the constraint by occupation of the receptor, which allows the GTP-binding protein (Gs) to interact in the required stimulatory manner with adenylate cyclase. This requirement for GTP is shared by the glucagon receptors which couple to adenylate cyclase in a generally similar way. Another GTP-binding protein (Gi) is responsible for the inhibition of adenylate cyclase. The ratio between the stimulating protein, Gs, and the inhibitory protein, Gi, may be an important signal switching adenylate cyclase on and off (Gilman, 1984).

The exact link between occupation of the beta-adrenergic receptor and the activation of adenylate cyclase is still not clear. Possibly there are changes in the physical properties of the cardiac lipid bilayer. For example, phospholipid methylation caused by beta-stimulation is thought to increase membrane fluidity to allow a lateral movement of the beta-agonist adrenergic receptor complex, so that it interacts more readily with adenylate cyclase and thus increases "coupling" (Fig. 6-1).

Lefkowitz and others (1981) have studied the nature of the **receptor binding sites** with radioligands. The binding sites are many, up to a thousand or two per cell, and share the **potency order** of the beta-adrenergic receptor (isoproterenol > epinephrine > norepinephrine) as well as the stereospecificity (*l*-isomer ≫ *d*-isomer); by definition the binding sites also interact with beta-adrenergic antagonists because it is with the aid of radiolabeled beta-adrenergic antagonists that they are identified. Beta-antagonist agents limit the degree of binding of the beta-agonist to the receptor site by competitive antagonism. In the case of agents such as propranolol with additional membrane-stabilizing properties, the latter effect is associated with non-specific binding sites.

Alpha-adrenergic Receptors

Alpha-adrenergic receptors may help mediate the influx of calcium in cardiac and especially in vascular smooth muscle. Identification of the alpha-adrenergic

receptor and its properties lags behind knowledge of the beta-adrenergic receptor (Table 6-2). Pharmacologically, an alpha-adrenergic receptor mediates the response in which the agonist potencies are: norepinephrine > epinephrine > isoproterenol; the antagonist properties are mediated by phentolamine and phenoxybenzamine at low concentrations. Subdivisions of the alpha-adrenergic receptor are complex. The basic division is into presynaptic alpha-2-adrenergic receptors (inhibited by yohimbine) and the postsynaptic alpha-1-adrenergic receptor (inhibited by prazosin). An important but continuing recent advance is that alpha-2 postsynaptic vascular receptors have been described which have their vasoconstrictive effects inhibited by calcium antagonists (Van Meel et al., 1981). Such alpha-2 vascular receptors (see Fig. 18-3) may be predominantly in the inner layer of the vascular wall and are not innervated according to the concept of Langer and Shepperson (1982), in contrast to the innervated alpha-1 receptors found in the outer vascular wall. In the heart, the myocardial receptors are almost exclusively alpha-1 in type (U'Prichard and Snyder, 1979) and their stimulation usually causes a modest inotropic effect by increased trans-sarcolemmal calcium influx (Scholz and Bruckner, 1982). In a minority of studies alpha-stimulation is reported to have negative inotropic effects; here the mechanism appears to be a reduction of the cyclic AMP levels (Watanabe et al., 1977).

An interesting recent hypothesis is that alpha-adrenergic receptors are involved in the production of arrhythmias during myocardial ischemia; the basic observation is that the density of alpha-adrenergic receptor in the myocardium increases soon after the onset of ischemia (Corr et al., 1981).

Cholinergic Receptors

According to the classical point of view, there are two types of cholinergic receptors: the nicotinic receptors at the autonomic ganglia and the muscarinic receptors at the effector tissue. Thus it is the **muscarinic** receptor which is specifically associated with the activity of the vagal nerve endings and has as its characteristics the production of a negative inotropic response and inhibition by atropine. The **nicotinic** receptor by definition responds to nicotine and is inhibited by ganglionic-blocking agents such as hexomethanium. This differentiation between the nicotinic ganglionic receptor sites and the tissue muscarinic sites is broadly correct, although some nicotinic receptors have also been found at the nerve endings.

The major effects of vagal stimulation on the heart are well-known—bradycardia and a negative inotropic effect. Thus there are opposing effects of cholinergic and of adrenergic stimulation on the heart. The chief function of muscarinic cholinergic receptors is seen as the modulation of the effects of sympathetic stimulation, either by modifying the rate of release of transmitter, or by lessening the degree of formation of cyclic AMP in response to the transmitter (Fig. 6-8), or by forming another second messenger (cyclic GMP) within the cell to oppose the effects of cyclic AMP (see page 84). The major pharmacological agents acting on the muscarinic receptors include those which inhibit cholinesterases to promote the action of acetylcholine, and those which inhibit acetylcholine.

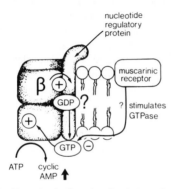

Fig. 6-8 Hypothetical molecular interaction between myocardial muscarinic and beta-receptors. According to this hypothetical scheme, acetylcholine stimulates the muscarinic receptor to allow breakdown of GTP thus inhibiting adenylate cyclase. The production of cyclic AMP falls. GDP = guanosine diphosphate; GTP = guanosine triphosphate.

Physiological Catecholamine Effects

"Turn-off" of inotropic response

An interesting aspect of the catecholamine-induced inotropic response is that it passes off rapidly, within minutes, even though the catecholamine stimulation is maintained. One reason for this effect is that the tissue level of cyclic AMP rises much more initially than later. When cyclic AMP rises in the myocardial cell, the enhanced cytosolic calcium concentration activates calmodulin which in turn enhances the

activity of phosphodiesterase, so that the rate of cyclic AMP breakdown is increased (see Chapter 7). Another factor is that prolonged stimulation of the beta-adrenergic receptor leads to desensitization, probably by down-grading of the population of active receptors. These phenomena are of chemical importance because the administration of beta-agonist agents may initially achieve a good positive inotropic response which then tails off, whereafter an increasingly higher dose is required for a sustained inotropic effect as the receptor density falls (Colucci et al., 1981).

Chronotropic effect

Besides an increased rate of contraction and relaxation characteristic of the positive inotropic effect, the beating rate of the heart also increases during catecholamine stimulation. This is the positive chronotropic effect which results from the stimulation of the pacemaker (Chapter 5).

Dromotropic effect

Not only does beta-stimulation cause the positive inotropic and chronotropic effects, but the impulse is conducted more rapidly down the atrioventricular node, His bundle and Purkinje fibers. This is called the positive dromotropic effect. Conduction velocity through the atrioventricular node is enhanced, probably as a result of stimulation of calcium ion entry into atrioventricular nodal cells. Clinically, the result is shortening of the PR interval on the electrocardiogram and the AH interval on the His bundle electrogram is also shortened.

The Second and Third Messenger Concept

The basis of the second messenger concept is that the initial extracellular signal is the first messenger and is a hormone. The second messenger is formed at the cell surface or some other superficial site, and acts within the cell. The second messenger can cause amplification effects, for example in the case of the glycogenolysis cascade.

The classic first messenger is a catecholamine such as epinephrine, and the classical second messenger is cyclic AMP produced from ATP (Fig. 6-9). The original concept was that the adenylate cyclase

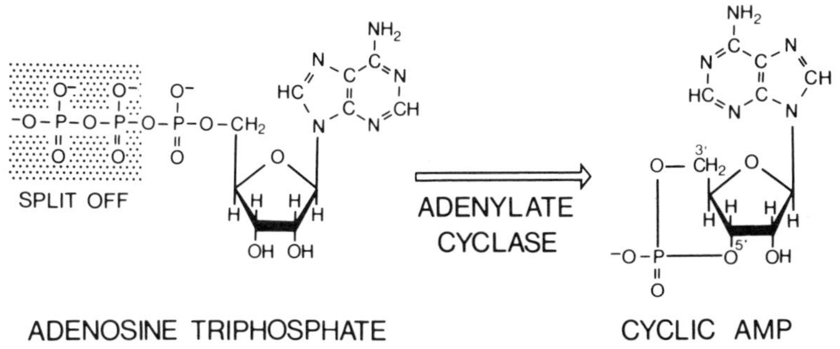

ADENOSINE TRIPHOSPHATE

CYCLIC AMP

Fig. 6-9 Cyclic AMP is formed from ATP by the activity of adenylate cyclase.

consisted of two subunits, namely the receptor unit which responded to the first messenger and the catalytic unit, which responded to the receptor unit and converted ATP to cyclic AMP. The general

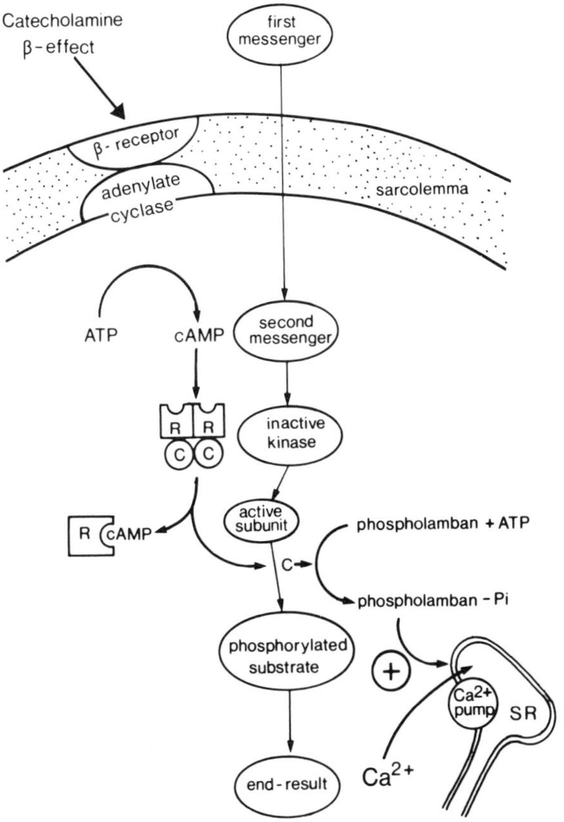

Fig. 6-10 In between the first messenger and the end-result lie a complex sequence of events. Thus catecholamine stimulation of adenylate cyclase eventually enhances calcium uptake by the sarcoplasmic reticulum (SR). Similar principles apply to other end-results.

hypothesis that cyclic AMP acts as a second messenger of catecholamines has gained wide acceptance, although it does not appear to explain all catecholamine effects.

Sometimes calcium seems to be the second messenger of beta-stimulation, especially in those experiments when an inotropic effect is achieved without a rise in cyclic AMP. Another idea is that calcium is the **third messenger** of beta-stimulation, brought into play by the intermediate effect of the protein kinases. Due to the numerous intermediate steps between cyclic AMP and calcium (Fig. 6-10), this idea of calcium as the third messenger is not too accurate—it is closer to being the fifth messenger. Another cyclic nucleotide, cyclic GMP, may act as a second messenger for some aspects of vagal activity.

All of these messenger chemicals are present in heart cells in minute concentrations. The cellular contents are: cyclic AMP about 10^{-10} M and cyclic GMP about 10^{-11} M. The real concentrations in the cytosol are somewhat higher, because 80 percent of the cell is water. A basic feature of the concept of cyclic AMP as second messenger is its very rapid turnover as a result of a constant dynamic balance between its formation by adenylate cyclase and removal by phosphodiesterase. In general, changes in the tissue content of cyclic AMP can be related to the inotropic effects of catecholamines (Table 6-3).

Adenylate cyclase

Adenylate cyclase is the only enzyme system producing cyclic AMP, and specifically requires low concentrations of ATP (and magnesium) as substrate. The concentration of cyclic AMP in the cell is about 1000

Table 6-3

Effects of elevated intracellular levels of cyclic AMP on the heart

Target	Effect
Sinus node	Accelerated discharge
AV node	Accelerated conduction
Purkinje fibers	Accelerated conduction
Normal action potential	Increased slow channel activity (increased Ca^{2+} entry)
Blocked action potential	Provocation of slow responses
Troponin I	Decreased sensitivity of ATPase to Ca^{2+}
Sarcoplasmic reticulum	Phosphorylation of phospholamban with increased activity of calcium pump
Sarcolemma	Phosphorylation of a protein with increased entry of calcium by the slow channel
Glycogen	Synthase kinase stimulated; glycogen synthase *b* formed; less glycogen synthesis. Phosphorylase kinase stimulated; increased conversion of phosphorylase *b* to *a*; increased glycogenolysis
Lipases	Stimulation of lipolysis with provision of energy

times lower than the overall cell content of ATP. Thus activity of adenylate cyclase is unlikely to be limited by decreases in the cell ATP level (even in ischemia or hypoxia), nor is the conversion of ATP to cyclic AMP by adenylate cyclase an important route of ATP utilization in the cell.

Adenylate cyclase is localized to the sarcolemmal membrane although an additional location on the sarcoplasmic reticulum cannot be excluded. A major problem in the study of adenylate cyclase is that it has not been isolated and purified because it is relatively stable and membrane bound.

Adenylate cyclase in broken cell preparations generally responds to the same hormones which are effective in the intact heart and this evidence is particularly good for catecholamine stimulation. One of the mysteries of adenylate cyclase is why sodium fluoride should stimulate the activity; that this stimulation occurs in fragmented preparations but not in whole-cell preparations supports the idea that adenylate cyclase is tightly linked to the cell membrane.

The simple and early hypothesis that adenylate cyclase is a component of the beta-receptor is increasingly attractive because the beta-agonists bind to that cellular fraction which also contains adenylate cyclase activity.

Are Beta-adrenergic Effects Mediated by Cyclic AMP?

Inotropic effect

The first and most obvious question is whether the level of cyclic AMP increases within the myoplasm whenever the catecholamines exert their inotropic response and at catecholamine concentrations which are physiologically relevant. When epinephrine is added to the isolated perfused working heart, cyclic AMP rises before the positive inotropic response (Fig. 6-11). Only a few studies have explored the dose–effect relationship between concentrations of catecholamines required to produce a rise in cyclic AMP and to increase contractile force. In one such study (Fig. 6-11) isoproterenol 10^{-8} M increased guinea-pig papillary muscle cyclic AMP from 0.58 to 0.88 nmol/g wet wt and contractile force rose. A lower concentration of isoproterenol (10^{-9} M) had no effect at all. Bearing in mind that the circulating catecholamine levels are about 10^{-10} M and rise no more than 10-fold to 10^{-9} M in various pathological states such as myocardial infarction, it is difficult to be sure that the concentrations of catecholamines used in animal studies have physiological relevance. This problem is

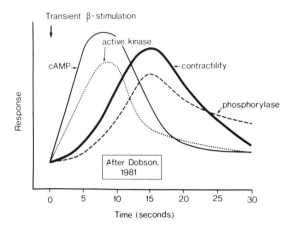

Fig. 6-11 After stimulation of the heart by a bolus injection of epinephrine at zero time, cyclic AMP rises before protein kinase is activated. Thereafter an index of contractility (dP/dt) rises and only later does phosphorylase rise. From Dobson (1981). In: Catecholamines and the Heart. Eds. W Delius, E Gerlach, H Grobecker, W Kubler, pp 128–141, Springer-Verlag, Berlin, with permission.

accentuated by the recent hypothesis that some beta-receptors are "innervated" and others are "hormonal" with the latter responding to circulating catecholamines (Bryan et al., 1981). Yet stimulation of the sympathetic nerves running to the dog heart causes a concomitant increase both in tissue cyclic AMP and in contractility (Pindok et al., 1981). All such data argue for an association between tissue cyclic AMP and the contractile response, but do not prove causality.

Relaxing effect

Catecholamine stimulation also has a relaxing effect on the heart besides the positively inotropic effect; there is a good agreement between the effects of catecholamines and those of dibutyryl cyclic AMP on cardiac relaxation. At a subcellular level, those agents enhancing relaxation are also those known to enhance the activity of the protein phospholamban situated in the sarcoplasmic reticulum (Chapter 7). Cyclic AMP enhances the uptake of calcium ions by the sarcoplasmic reticulum by phosphorylations thereby enhancing the rate of relaxation. For these reasons it is frequently possible to link cyclic AMP with positive inotropic and relaxant effects of catecholamines.

Chronotropic effects

There is a general correspondence between the chronotropic effects of those catecholamines which increase heart rate with those which increase cyclic AMP. A notable agent causing both effects is isoproterenol. An outstanding question relates to the physiological relevance of the concentrations of catecholamines used to obtain an inotropic effect. Isoproterenol in the physiologically "relevant" concentration of 10^{-10} M can increase the beating rate of the right atrial preparation by 30 percent but atrial cyclic AMP does not rise. Again, as in the case of contractility, this disturbing discrepancy could perhaps be explained by the recent postulate that beta-adrenergic receptors respond chiefly to neurally released and not to circulating catecholamines so that experiments with added catecholamines are not really "relevant". Alternatively, cyclic AMP could have risen locally in those cells concerned with the initiation of the heart beat.

Factors other than cyclic AMP

There is more involved in these responses to adrenergic stimulation than changes in the overall tissue levels of cyclic AMP. When catecholamines are bound covalently to glass beads, which severely limits the amount of contact of the catecholamines with the cell surface, then maximum contraction of cat papillary muscles can be achieved without a measurable change in tissue cyclic AMP concentrations (Venter et al., 1975). One explanation for this puzzling phenomenon is that there is very localized but intense stimulation of the receptors, resulting in elevation of cyclic AMP only at points of contact with the glass beads, and that the cyclic AMP then mediates calcium-responses which spread the inotropic effect throughout the muscle fibers. This may be an example of beta-agonism acting through only a very small percentage of receptors, according to the **spare receptor** concept. A second possible explanation is that calcium ions are acting as the second messenger. Thirdly, at any given level of cyclic AMP, it is the degree of stimulation of various protein kinases by cyclic AMP which is of ultimate importance. Theoretically, changes in the activity of specific protein kinases (Fig. 6-12) could occur in response to very small localized changes in compartmentalized cyclic AMP.

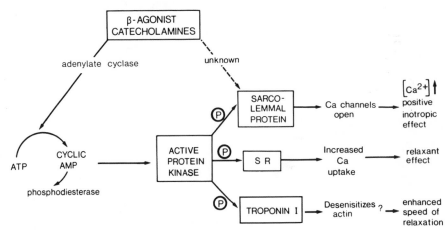

Fig. 6-12   The major intracellular effects of beta-agonist catecholamines is by formation of cyclic AMP which in turn increases the activity of protein kinases which phosphorylate various proteins, including enzymes (Chapter 12). SR = sarcoplasmic reticulum.

Cyclic AMP Removal by Phosphodiesterase

Cyclic AMP is broken down by the enzyme phospho-diesterase, whose activity is increased when calmodulin is activated by calcium ions. There is a self-regulating mechanism at work:

beta-agonist → adenylate cyclase → cyclic AMP → increased cytosolic (Ca^{2+}) → increased activity of phosphodiesterase → reduction of cyclic AMP level.

Inhibition of phosphodiesterase by methylxanthines

The inhibition of the activity of phosphodiesterase by methylxanthines is probably the basis of their best-known therapeutic effect, that of bronchodilation as in bronchial asthma. In the heart an infusion of aminophyllin causes a sustained and prolonged elevation of tissue cyclic AMP, which contrasts with the short-lived elevation after beta-agonist stimulation. The differences could be explained by the effect of calcium ions which activate phosphodiesterase during beta-agonist stimulation, whereas during an amino-phyllin infusion, the dominant effect is inhibition of phosphodiesterase.

Additional modes of action not directly involving cyclic AMP are also likely. Methylxanthines inhibit the uptake of calcium by the sarcoplasmic reticulum so that the development of peak tension is delayed and

relaxation is prolonged. This action of methyl-xanthines on the sarcoplasmic reticulum is termed the **calcium-sequestration blocking effect** and can be overcome by the local anesthetic procaine or by a high heart rate. There are further complex effects which increase the rate of release of calcium from the sarcoplasmic reticulum, and impair accumulation of calcium by mitochondria, which further increases the cytosolic calcium ion concentration. This explains why theophyllin has a positive inotropic effect at concentrations which are not strong enough to inhibit phosphodiesterase.

Methylxanthines are commonly regarded as coronary vasodilators because they inhibit phosphodiesterase in smooth muscle to cause a vasodilation mediated by cyclic AMP. They also have an opposing effect because they inhibit the vasodilation caused by adenosine, by preventing the interaction of adenosine with its receptors. Thus the actions of methylxanthines are not related solely to an accumulation of intra-cellular cyclic AMP, but also to an action on calcium ion movements and on the coronary vasculature.

If methylxanthines have such powerful and multiple effects on myocardial cyclic AMP and calcium ion movements, besides inhibiting the formation of adenosine, then the obvious question is why theo-phyllin is standard therapy in bronchial asthma with only occasional serious side-effects on the heart. The probable answer is that most of the myocardial effects, including that in reducing the threshold to ventricular fibrillation, and the effects on adenosine, have been found at about millimolar concentrations (10^{-3} M), whereas therapeutic levels in man are much lower, being 10–20 μg/mL, i.e. 0.6–1.1 × 10^{-4} M.

Papaverine

Although papaverine is a more powerful inhibitor of phosphodiesterase than the methylxanthine group, it does not always have a positive inotropic effect because of many ancillary properties including verapamil-like and quinidine-like effects. Papaverine is also a powerful coronary vasodilator, apparently acting independently of inhibition of phosphodiesterase and possibly by its verapamil-like effect.

Cyclic AMP and phosphodiesterase: summary

In general, factors inhibiting phosphodiesterase activity increase tissue cyclic AMP and enhance contractility. The data support but do not prove the hypothesis that cyclic AMP mediates the positive inotropic effect sometimes found with these agents. A major problem is that the regulation of phosphodiesterase activity is poorly understood, although the identification of calmodulin as a regulator is a distinct advance. Phosphodiesterase inhibitors also have effects besides those on cyclic AMP, for example on intracellular movements of calcium ions.

Protein Kinases

At a subcellular level most, if not all, of the effects of cyclic AMP are ultimately mediated by protein kinases which phosphorylate various important proteins and enzymes (Fig. 6-12). Each protein kinase is composed of two subunits: regulatory (R) and catalytic (C). Cyclic AMP binds to the R subunit to liberate the C subunit (Fig. 6-10). The inactive kinase, composed of both R and C subunits, is split by cyclic AMP so that active kinase (C) forms:

$$(R_2 + C_2) + cAMP \rightarrow 2\ RcAMP + 2C$$

The ratio of the inactive protein kinase to the active form is called the **protein kinase activity ratio**. The activity ratio rises in direct relation to the rise of intracellular cyclic AMP level during stimulation by a variety of agents increasing cyclic AMP, such as epinephrine, glucagon and phosphodiesterase

inhibition. The activated kinase in turn acts as the trigger for a variety of physiological effects, because it "switches on" or "switches off" several different enzymes concerned with the regulation of calcium ion movements and the breakdown of glycogen and lipid. The protein kinase activated by the cyclic AMP sometimes achieves this aim by phosphorylating a second kinase, which in turn responds by a change in molecular structure to become active (or inactive) and ultimately to achieve a particular physiological function. There are at least eight phosphorylations mediated by the active form of the cyclic AMP-dependent protein kinase. **Phosphorylation**—the donation of a phosphate group to the enzyme concerned—is therefore a fundamental metabolic "switch" which can function as a "cascade" to produce extensive amplification of a signal.

> Phosphorylation of proteins has become recognized as a major mechanism of cellular control. It constitutes the only well-documented mode of action of cyclic AMP in metazoan cells.   Will et al. (1979)

At a molecular level, the basic action of the cyclic AMP-dependent protein kinase is to catalyze the transfer of the terminal phosphate of ATP to serine and threonine residues of the protein substrates, leading to a modification of the properties of the proteins concerned. This then leads to further key reactions.

The protein kinase activated by cyclic AMP, with its many diverse intracellular substrates, occurs in different cells in two forms with different but similar regulator subunits; the type called "protein kinase II" predominates in cardiac cells. The aim of much current work is to determine the order of phosphorylation of the various proteins that occur in response to a given cyclic AMP "signal" within heart cells, as this "pecking" order determines the order of the ultimate physiological response. Clearly the concentrations of the respective substrate proteins and their affinities for the protein kinase, as well as their locations in the cell, will be prime determinants of this "pecking" order.

Cyclic AMP is not the only agent causing critical intracellular phosphorylations. Some phosphorylations such as that of phospholamban can be promoted either by cyclic AMP or calmodulin bound to Ca^{2+}. Phosphorylations such as those catalyzed by kinase acting on myosin light chains are mediated only by calmodulin. Hence one critical phosphorylation set in motion by cyclic AMP, such as that of a protein associated with the calcium channel, could lead to an increase in the intracellular free calcium ion concentration, which would in turn activate calmodulin to **cause yet other phosphorylations such as that of the myosin light chains and phospholamban.**

Dephosphorylations

If phosphorylation of various critical cellular proteins by kinases is so important in the regulation of heart cell function, then it follows that the **phosphoprotein phosphatase** enzymes catalyzing the breakdown of the phosphorylated proteins are equally important in regulation. (This idea will be met in the regulation of glycogen synthesis and glycogen breakdown.) A specific phosphatase is known to convert inactive pyruvate dehydrogenase to the active form, while another dephosphorylates the P light chain of myosin. Most of the phosphoprotein phosphatases concerned with the cardiac contraction cycle are not well studied, nor is much known about their regulation.

Organelles Influenced by Cyclic AMP

Sarcolemma

Of the many functions of cyclic AMP, that exerted on calcium influx into the heart cell is of prime importance. The fundamental observation was made by Fleckenstein's group in 1961 who found that in fibers inhibited by a high potassium medium, a new type of action potential without the preceding sodium-spike could be elicited by the addition of epinephrine (Engstfeld et al., 1961). This action potential had a slow upstroke. It was also provoked by the use of caffeine. It was presumed that cyclic AMP had promoted this slowly rising type of action; decisive evidence for the role of cyclic AMP has since been established by the introduction of cyclic AMP by micro-iontophoresis into heart cells. The molecular mechanism of the action on cyclic AMP in promoting calcium entry during the slow response is not yet fully established, but appears to involve phosphorylation of a sarcolemmal protein (Fig. 4-4).

Thus a possible sequence of events is:

beta-stimulation → stimulation of adenylate cyclase
→ formation of cyclic AMP → protein
phosphorylation → increased entry of calcium
by the slow channel → inotropic effect.

Sarcoplasmic reticulum

The phosphoprotein of the sarcoplasmic reticulum which is phosphorylated in the presence of a cyclic AMP-dependent protein kinase is called phospholamban (Chapter 7). If the phosphorylation of phospholamban is prevented by digestion with trypsin, then the cyclic AMP-dependent protein kinase is unable to stimulate calcium uptake. So it seems that phospholamban controls the activity of the calcium pump of the sarcoplasmic reticulum. To reverse the effect of cyclic AMP on phospholamban requires a subsequent dephosphorylation (phosphatase) reaction which is not well-understood.

Contractile proteins

Cyclic AMP also mediates the phosphorylation of the inhibitory subunit of troponin (troponin-I). Originally this phosphorylation was thought in some way to facilitate the inotropic effect of epinephrine; now it appears that the phosphorylation of troponin-I decreases the sensitivity of the actomyosin ATPase to calcium, thereby tending to decrease the inotropic response. It has been proposed that this is a built-in "braking mechanism" so that the other stimulatory effects of catecholamines are modulated to prevent "excess" cardiac contraction upon catecholamine stimulation.

Cytosol

Cyclic AMP is able to meet the needs for increased myocardial energy during an inotropic response by the rapid activation of glycogenolysis. Additionally, the breakdown of high-energy phosphate compounds stimulates glycolysis and the increased formation of $NADH_2$ stimulates oxidative phosphorylation. Whether stimulation of lipolysis can occur rapidly enough to be of energetic significance is not known.

Other Agents Stimulating Formation of Cyclic AMP

An additional way of trying to resolve the relation between catecholamines, cyclic AMP and contractility is to ask whether or not those agents, other than beta-agonists, that also increase cyclic AMP, increase contractility as well (Table 6-4).

Table 6-4

Pharmacologically active agents which alter myocardial levels of cyclic AMP and contractile activity of the heart

Agent	Mechanism	Effect on cyclic nucleotide	Effect on contractile activity
Epinephrine } Norepinephrine }	Stimulate adenylate cyclase via beta-receptor	cyclic AMP ↑	↑
Glucagon } Histamine }	Stimulate adenylate cyclase via non-beta-receptor	cyclic AMP ↑	↑
Forskolin	"Directly stimulates" adenylate cyclase e	cyclic AMP ↑	↑
Beta-adrenergic blocking agents	Antagonize effects of beta-stimulating catecholamines	cyclic AMP ↓	↓
Adenosine	Inhibits adenylate cyclase	cyclic AMP ↓	↓
Papaverine	Inhibits phosphodiesterase	cyclic AMP ↑	↑ in presence of isoproterenol

Glucagon

Glucagon has positive inotropic and chronotropic effects, whereas the chronotropic effect was inhibited by propranolol. The inotropic effect bypasses the beta-receptor (Fig. 6-13) so that glucagon is used in the therapy of overdoses of beta-blocking agents.

Histamine

Histamine has a positive chronotropic and inotropic effect, mediated by H_2-receptors in the ventricles. The inotropic effect is potentiated by theophyllin; histamine stimulates the formation of cyclic AMP by adenylate cyclase derived from guinea-pig heart, and the effect is not blocked by propranolol but by H_2-blockers. As in the case of glucagon, a receptor site coupled to adenylate cyclase but not involving the beta-adrenergic site has been postulated (Fig. 6-13). This histamine receptor site is blocked by the H_2-blocking agent, burimamide. In man, there is good evidence linking the activity of the cardiac histamine H_2-receptors to stimulation of adenylate cyclase and to inotropic effects (Bristow et al., 1982).

Thyroid

Thyroid hormone can also activate adenylate cyclase independently of the beta-adrenergic receptor. A membrane-bound thyroid receptor is by no means the only receptor involved in the explanation of thyroid effects; the basic site of thyroid action is probably the

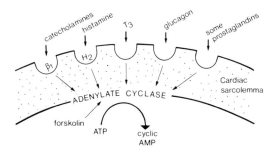

Fig. 6-13 The histamine H_2-receptor is one of several receptors, in addition to the beta-adrenergic receptor, which promotes the formation of cyclic AMP by cardiac adenylate cyclase.

nuclear receptor for triiodothyronine which stimulates the formation of a diversity of messenger RNA complexes in the presence of this hormone. Formation of cyclic AMP is not likely to be the sole or even the chief effect of thyroid hormone on the heart.

Adenosine

Adenosine inhibits myocardial adenylate cyclase which would explain negative inotropic and negative chronotropic effects. In addition, adenosine also directly inhibits calcium ion entry by the slow channel. Hence inhibition of the formation of cyclic AMP could explain some but not all of the negative inotropic effects of adenosine.

Forskolin

Cardiac adenylate cyclase responds directly to stimulation by forskolin, a diterpene isolated from the roots of *Coleus forskohlii*. Even a low concentration of forskolin increases the formation of cyclic AMP (Seamon et al., 1981) and has a positive inotropic effect. It is now being tested as a possible therapeutic agent in experimental heart failure.

Cyclic GMP and Vagal Effects

Cyclic GMP is present in the myocardium at about one-hundredth the level of cyclic AMP. The structure of cyclic GMP is very similar to that of cyclic AMP except that guanine replaces adenine. Many of the effects of cyclic GMP on various other tissues are the opposite of those of cyclic AMP which has led to the influential "yin–yang" hypothesis. While cyclic GMP undergoes opposite changes to those of cyclic AMP during the frog cardiac cycle (next section), the general function of cyclic GMP in the mammalian heart is still obscure. Cholinergic stimulation is frequently suspected of acting on guanyl cyclase in a manner similar to beta-agonists acting on adenylate cyclase. In some experiments acetyl choline can increase the

cyclic GMP content of the heart while leaving the content of cyclic AMP unchanged (Fig. 6-14). The beauty of this argument is destroyed by marked dissociations between cyclic GMP and contractility when sodium nitroprusside elevates cyclic GMP (with no effect on contractility) and when low concentrations **of acetylcholine depress contractility (with no effect on cyclic GMP). The best explanation for the vagal** effects is that acetyl choline, liberated by vagal stimulation, decreases the formation of cyclic AMP by acting on muscarinic receptors both at a pre-junctional and postjunctional level. Any effect of vagal stimulation in increasing cyclic GMP seems not to be fundamental but rather an additional secondary inhibitory mechanism which can only be detected in selected experimental circumstances. The "yin–yang" contrasting effects of sympathetic and parasympathetic stimulation can be adequately explained without invoking cyclic GMP which remains "a nucleotide in search of a function" (Brooker, 1977).

Cyclic Variations in Cardiac Cycle

In a classic study, Wollenberger's group showed that there were cyclical variations of the overall cardiac contents of cyclic AMP in the cardiac cycle of the frog

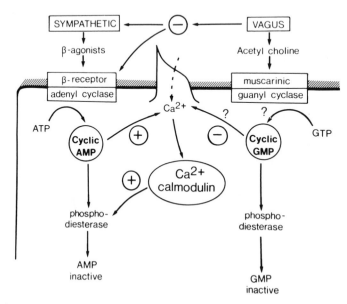

Fig. 6-14 Interaction between parasympathetic and sympathetic systems at a cellular level may involve two opposing cyclic nucleotides, cyclic AMP and cyclic GMP. Many effects of vagal stimulation could best be explained by the inhibitory effect on the formation of cyclic AMP (Chapter 7).

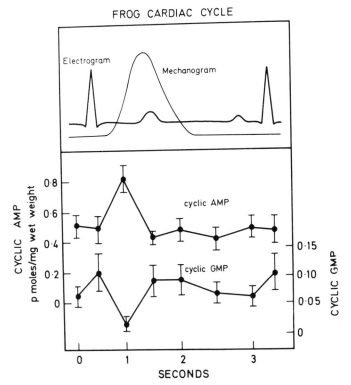

FROG CARDIAC CYCLE

Fig. 6-15 Cyclic changes in cyclic AMP and cyclic GMP found in the frog cardiac cycle (from Wollenberger et al. (1973) with permission). Similar cyclic AMP changes have now also been found in the mammalian heart.

(Fig. 6-15). There was a brief peak of increase of cyclic AMP occurring between the Q and the T wave of the electrocardiogram, but before the peak of mechanical activity. At the time when cyclic AMP peaked, cyclic GMP levels reached a nadir. These fascinating changes are difficult to explain; in the case of cyclic AMP they have now been confirmed for the mammalian heart (Wikman-Coffelt et al., 1983). Hypothetically, increased cyclic AMP in early systole could help "open" calcium channels to increase the cytosolic calcium concentration.

Pathological Effects of Cyclic AMP

Ventricular arrhythmias can be caused by catecholamine stimulation and the mechanism may in part involve formation of excess cyclic AMP (Chapter 27). Three possible mechanisms are: (i) the provocation of delayed after-depolarizations; (ii) in depolarized cells, the formation of calcium-dependent slow responses may also be important; or (iii) cyclic AMP

might stimulate intracellular lipolysis, to produce lysophospholipids with detergent and arrhythmogenic properties.

Myocardial necrosis can be caused by large doses of beta-adrenergic agonists such as isoproterenol. Similar necrosis can also be found after the administration of dibutyryl cyclic AMP, especially in the presence of additional phosphodiesterase inhibition. Possible mechanisms might include calcium overload and activation of cardiac lipases with resultant "oxygen wastage".

Summary

Receptors no longer remain a concept. Some, such as the beta-adrenergic receptor, have been well characterized at a molecular level; the existence of others is still only postulated. Agonist agents such as beta-adrenergic agents interact with the receptor at two sites—the binding site and the active site where stimulation takes place. There then follows a change in the molecular structure of the receptor, so that a further effector molecule is stimulated to release the "second messenger", such as cyclic AMP, for the beta-agonist. Antagonist agents such as beta-blockers compete with beta-agonists for the same binding site. Most binding of agonist and antagonists to the receptor is reversible so that any given physiological effect is transient. Similarly, the action of pharmacological blocking agents is not permanent. Ligand binding studies show that the density of receptors can be increased (up-regulation) or decreased (down-regulation) and that many hormones regulate the density of their own receptors.

At present, the probable sequence of events describing the inotropic effect of catecholamines is:

catecholamine stimulation → beta-receptor → molecular changes → catalytic subunit of adenylate cyclase → formation of cyclic AMP from ATP → activation of protein kinase(s) → phosphorylation of a sarcolemmal protein → increased entry of calcium ion through the cell membrane → calcium-induced calcium release → rise of intracellular free calcium ion concentration → inotropic effect → increased uptake of calcium by the sarcoplasmic reticulum **(phosphorylation of phospholamban by cAMP and by calcium-calmodulin).**

Discrepancies between total cyclic AMP and actions of catecholamines may be ascribed to an imperfect understanding of the molecular effects of cyclic AMP, and to a lack of full knowledge of the control of cyclic AMP-dependent protein kinases. Calcium ions sometimes act as the co-messenger or third messenger of catecholamine beta-stimulation. Many effects of vagal stimulation, mediated by acetyl choline, can be explained by inhibition of the formation of cyclic AMP.

References

Ahlquist RP (1948). A study of the adrenotropic receptors. Am J Physiol 153: 586–600.

Ariens EJ, Beld AJ (1977). The receptor concept in evolution. Biochem Pharmacol 26: 913–918.

Bristow MR, Cubbicciotti R, Ginsburg R, Stinson EB, Johnson C (1982). Histamine-mediated adenylate cyclase stimulation in human myocardium. Mol Pharmacol 21: 671–679.

Brooker G (1977). Dissociation of cyclic GMP from the negative inotropic action of carbachol in guinea-pig atria. J Cycl Nucleotide Res 3: 407–413.

Bryan LJ, Cole JJ, O'Donnell SR, Wanstall JC (1981). A study designed to explore the hypothesis that beta-1 adrenoceptors are "innervated" receptors and beta-2 adrenoceptors are "hormonal" receptors. J Pharm Exp Therap 216: 395–400.

Colucci WS, Alexander RW, Williams GH, Rude RE, Holman BL, Konstam MA, Wynne J, Mudge GH, Braunwald E (1981). Decreased lymphocyte beta-adrenergic-receptor density in patients with heart failure and tolerance to the beta-adrenergic agonist pirbuterol. New Engl J Med 305: 185–190.

Corr PB, Shayman JA, Kramer JB, Kipnis RJ (1981). Increased alpha-adrenergic receptors in ischemic cat myocardium. J. Clin Invest 67: 1232–1236.

De Meyts P, Rousseau GG (1980). Receptor concepts: a century of evolution. Circ Res 46, Suppl 1: 3–9.

Engstfeld G, Antoni H, Fleckenstein A (1961). Die Restitution der Erregungsfortleitung ünd Kontraktionskraft des K⁺-gelahmten Frosch- und Saugtiermyokards durch Adrenalin. Pflügers Arch Physiol 273: 145–163.

Ehrlich P (1913). Chemotherapeutics: scientific principles, methods and results. Lancet ii: 445–450.

Gilman AG (1984). Guanine nucleotide-binding regulatory proteins and dual control of adenylate cyclase. J Clin Invest 73: 1–4.

Hedberg A, Minneman KP, Molinoff PB (1980). Differential distribution of beta-1 and beta-2 adrenergic receptors in cat and guinea-pig heart. J Pharm Exp Therap 212: 503–508.

Kahn CR (1976). Membrane receptors for hormones and neurotransmitters. J Cell Biol 70: 261–286.

Lands AM, Arnold A, McAuliff JP, Ludvena FP, Brown RG Jr (1967). Differentiation of receptor systems activated by sympathomimetic amines. Nature 214: 597–598. 597–598.

Langer SZ, Shepperson NB (1982). Prejunctional modulation of noradrenaline release by alpha₂-adrenoceptors: physiological and pharmacological implications in the cardiovascular system. J Cardiovasc Pharmacol 4: S35–S40.

Langley JN (1905). On the reactions of cells and of nerve-endings to certain poisons, chiefly as regards the reaction of striated muscle to nicotine and to curare. J Physiol (London) 33: 374–413.

Lefkowitz RJ (1979). Direct binding studies of adrenergic receptors: biochemical, physiologic and clinical implications. Ann Int Med 91: 450–458.

Lefkowitz RJ, Hoffman BB (1980). Adrenergic receptors. Adv Cycl Nucleotide Res 12: 37–47.

Lefkowitz RJ, Delean A, Hoffman BB, Stadel JR, Kent R, Michel T, Limbird L (1981). Molecular pharmacology of adenylate cyclase — coupled alpha- and beta-adrenergic receptors. Adv Cycl Nucleotide Res 14: 145–161.

Maguire ME, Ross EM, Gilman AG (1977). Beta-adrenergic receptor: ligand binding properties and interaction with adenyl cyclase. Adv Cycl Nucleotide Res 8: 1–83.

Pindok MT, Sukowski E, Glaviano VV (1981). Cardiac cyclic nucleotides and norepinephrine during neural sympathetic stimulation. Am J Physiol 240: H630–H635.

Robberecht P, Delhaye M, Taton G, De Neef P, Waelbroeck M, De Smet JM, Leclerc JL, Chatelain P, Christophe J (1983). The human heart beta-adrenergic receptors. Mol Pharmacol 24: 169–173.

Rodbell M (1980). The role of hormone receptors and GTP-regulatory proteins in membrane transduction. Nature 284: 17–22.

Scholz H, Bruckner R (1982). Effects of beta- and alpha-adrenoceptor stimulating agents on mechanical activity, electrophysiological parameters and cyclic nucleotide levels in the heart. In: Advances in Studies on Heart Metabolism. Ed. CR Caldarera and P Harris, CLUEB, Bologna.

Seamon KB, Padgett W, Daly JW (1981). Forskolin: unique diterpene activator of adenylate cyclase in membranes and intact cells. Proc Nat Acad Sci USA 78: 3363–3367.

Stiles GL, Taylor S, Lefkowitz RJ (1983). Human cardiac beta-adrenergic receptors: subtype heterogeneity delineated by direct radioligand binding. Life Sci 33: 467–473.

Thandroyen FT, Worthington MG, Higginson LM, Opie LH (1983). The effect of alpha- and beta-adrenoceptor antagonist agents on reperfusion ventricular fibrillation and metabolic status in isolated perfused rat heart. J Am Coll Cardiol 1: 1056–1066.

U'Prichard DC, Snyder SH (1979). Distinct alpha-nor-adrenergic receptors differentiated by binding and physiological relationships. Life Sci 24: 79–88.

Van Meel JCA, de Jonge A, Kalkman HO, Wilfert B, Timmermans P, van Zwieten RA (1981). Vascular smooth muscle contraction initiated by postsynaptic alpha-2-adrenoceptor activation is induced by an influx of extracellular calcium. Europ J Pharm 69: 205–208.

Venter JC (1981). Beta-adrenoceptors, adenylate cyclase, and the adrenergic control of cardiac contractility. In: Adrenoceptors and Catecholamine Action. Vol. 1. Ed. G Kunos, pp 213–245, Wiley, New York.

Venter JC, Ross J Jr, Kaplan NO (1975). Lack of detectable change in cyclic AMP during the cardiac inotropic response to isoproterenol immobilized on glass beads. Proc Nat Acad Sci USA 72: 824–828.

Walsh DA, Clippinger MS, Sivaramakrishnan S, McCullough TE (1979). Cyclic adenosine monophosphate dependent and independent phosphorylation of sarcolemma membrane proteins in perfused rat heart. Biochemistry 18: 871–877.

Watanabe AM, Hathaway DR, Besch HR, Farmer BB, Harris RA (1977). Alpha-adrenergic reduction of cyclic adenosine monophosphate concentrations in rat myocardium. Circ Res 40: 596–602.

Wikman-Coffelt J, Sievers R, Coffelt RJ, Parmley WW (1983). Oscillations in cAMP with the cardiac cycle. Biochem Biophys Res Comm 111: 450–455.

Will H, Misselwitz HJ, Levchenko TS, Wollenberger A (1979). Some characteristics of low molecular weight phosphoprotein constituents of cardiac sarcoplasmic reticulum and sarcolemma. In: Advances in Pharmacology and Therapeutics. Vol. 3. Ed. JC Stoclet, Pergamon Press, Oxford.

Wollenberger A, Babskii EB, Krause EG, Genz S, Blohn D, Bogdanova EV (1973). Cyclic changes in levels of cyclic AMP and cyclic GMP in frog myocardium during the cardiac cycle. Biochem Biophys Res Comm 55: 446–452.

Wrenn S, Haber E (1979). An antibody specific for the propranolol binding site of cardiac muscle. J Biol Chem 254: 6577–6582.

New References

Brown MS, Anderson GW, Goldstein JL (1983). Recycling receptors: The round-trip itinerary of migrant membrane proteins. Cell 32: 663–667.

Bruckner R, Mugge A, Scholz A (1985). Existence and functional role of alpha$_1$-adrenoceptors in the mammalian heart. J Molec Cell Cardiol 17: 639–645.

Dobson JG, Schrader J (1984). Role of extracellular and intracellular adenosine in the attenuation of catecholamine evoked responses in guinea pig heart. J Molec Cell Cardiol 16: 813–822.

Homcy CJ, Graham RM (1985). Molecular characterization of adrenergic receptors. Circ Res 56: 635–650.

Limas CJ, Limas C (1984). Rapid recovery of cardiac beta-adrenergic receptors after isoproterenol-induced "down"-regulation. Circ Res 55: 524–531.

Linden J, Hollen CE, Patel A (1985). The mechanism by which adenosine and cholinergic agents reduce contractility in rat myocardium. Circ Res 56: 728–735.

7 Calcium Fluxes

L. H. Opie, W. Nayler and W. Gevers

After propagation of the cardiac impulse from the pacemaker cells of the sinus node to the ventricular cells, the next event of critical importance is the voltage-induced increased "opening" of the calcium channels of contractile cells, followed by a series of intracellular movements of calcium ions leading to myocardial contraction and relaxation. This chapter will concentrate on the calcium ion fluxes which link the wave of excitation to contraction by the process of **excitation–contraction coupling**, followed by the uptake of calcium ions into the sarcoplasmic reticulum which is associated with the relaxation phase. The next chapters will explain the contractile mechanism and the role of the beta-adrenergic receptor and its second messenger, cyclic AMP, in the control of cellular calcium and the inotropic state.

Calcium Ion Movements

The overall pattern of calcium ion movement associated with the contraction cycle may be summarized as follows. Only small amounts of calcium actually enter and leave the cell with each cardiac cycle, so that the majority of calcium ion movements are from the calcium stores to the cytosol and back again (Fig. 7-1). The sarcolemma maintains a vast gradient of calcium ion concentration from the extracellular value of about 1 mM (10^{-3} M) to intracellular values which fluctuate between about 10^{-7} M in diastole and 10^{-5} M in systole (Fig. 7-2). The major intracellular calcium store is probably in the sarcoplasmic reticulum. It is from here that relatively large amounts

of calcium ions are liberated by the small, but varying, amounts of calcium entering the cell during depolarization according to the theory of "calcium-induced calcium release" (Fabiato, 1983). Another less established theory is that calcium is released from some other superficial store, possibly from the calcium bound to the phospholipids of the sarcolemma (Langer, 1974). As intracellular calcium is released, its concentration in the cytosol rises to interact with troponin C so that the interaction of actin and myosin is facilitated and contraction takes place. The rise of cytosolic calcium comes to an end as the wave of excitation passes, so that no more calcium is released and the cytosolic calcium is rapidly taken up by the calcium pump of the sarcoplasmic reticulum; a lesser amount is pumped out of the cell.

To balance the small amount of calcium entering the heart cell with each depolarization, calcium ions can leave by one of two processes (Table 7-1). First, calcium ions leaving can be exchanged for sodium ions entering, and secondly an ATP-consuming calcium pump can transfer calcium back into the extracellular space, against a concentration gradient. In addition, cytosolic calcium may be taken up into the mitochondria. Mitochondria are rich in calcium and are thought to be a major site of storage for these ions. The exchange of calcium from cytosol to the mitochondria is not susceptible to those many drugs acting on the calcium uptake of the sarcoplasmic reticulum (catecholamines, beta-adrenergic blockers, methylxanthines), nor to the calcium channel antagonist drugs. Probably the mitochondrial calcium stores **are only indirectly related to the contraction–**

CALCIUM FLUXES IN HEART CELL

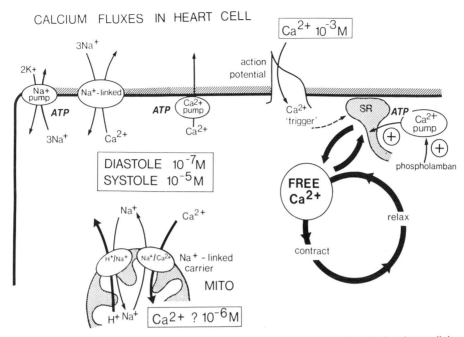

Fig. 7-1 Calcium fluxes in the myocardium. Note the much higher extracellular (10^{-3} M) than intracellular value, and a hypothetical mitochondrial value of about 10^{-6} M. The mitochondria could act as a "buffer" against excessive changes in the free cytosolic calcium concentration. SR = sarcoplasmic reticulum; MITO = mitochondria.

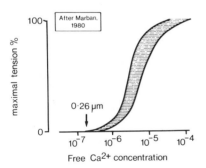

Fig. 7-2 Relation of free ionized calcium concentration to tension development in heart. The resting diastolic value is about $0.26\,\mu$mol, rising to 10^{-5} M with maximal tension development. For details see Marban et al. (1980). For criticism of techniques used see Langer (1982).

Table 7-1

Mechanisms for lowering cytosolic Ca^{2+} concentration in myocardial cells

	% of total uptake
Sarcoplasmic reticulum	88
Sarcolemma	
1. Na^+–Ca^{2+} exchange	5
2. Ca^{2+}-pump	1
Mitochondria	6

Relative contribution at 1 μM Ca^{2+} and 1–3 mM Mg^{2+}
From Carafoli (1982). Membrane Transport of Calcium, p 134, Academic Press, London, Orlando and New York, with permission.

relaxation cycle, by being one of the slower sites of calcium exchange and hence a potential "second-line" regulator.

Such calcium ion fluxes govern the contraction–relaxation cycle of the contractile cardiac cells. A critical site of regulation is calcium ion entry by the calcium channel.

Calcium Influx

The opening of the slow calcium channels by a voltage stimulus during the depolarization phase of the action potential has already been described (Chapter 4); these are the **depolarization-operated channels**. Non-electrical factors also regulate slow channel activity. The interaction of a beta-adrenergic agonist with its receptor can help to increase either the number of calcium channels that can operate or the duration that a given number stay in the open state (see Fig. 4-4). In vascular smooth muscle such **receptor-operated channels** are thought to be a different population from the voltage or depolarization-operated channels (Chapter 18). In heart muscle, it seems more probable that beta-adrenergic stimulation acts via its receptor on the same channels that depolarization acts on, because no amount of catecholamine stimulation will open the calcium channels in the absence of an accompanying voltage stimulus.

The calcium antagonist drugs (Chapter 19) have as their major action the inhibition of the channels allowing calcium ions into either nodal or vascular cells. Differences in the membrane binding sites for various calcium antagonists may in part explain the clinical differences between verapamil and diltiazem (active on nodal tissue besides vascular smooth muscle), and nifedipine (chief site of action: vascular smooth muscle). Other investigators suggest that the different antagonist agents bind with different affinities to more than one population of calcium channels.

Other routes for calcium ion influx

Besides the highly controlled entry of calcium ions by the calcium channel, there are two other possible routes. First, calcium can flow into the cells by a non-specific process. Despite the relative impermeability of the resting sarcolemma to calcium ions, such a "downhill" transport of calcium ions is possible because of the vast concentration gradient from without to within the cell. Secondly, calcium ions can theoretically enter the cytosol by a reversal of the pumps and exchange mechanisms used for calcium efflux. Although the magnitude of these processes has not been defined, it is still sometimes proposed that calcium ions entering independently of the calcium channel could help to activate contraction.

Calcium Ion Efflux

The major route for calcium ion efflux from the heart cell is the sarcolemmal **sodium–calcium exchange** mechanism (Chapter 4), which is designed to eject calcium ions whenever the cytosolic calcium ion concentration exceeds a certain critical value, probably

reached in systole (Carafoli, 1984). The activity of the exchanger is presumably regulated by mechanisms which activate calcium ion efflux following the intracellular surge of the calcium ion concentration occurring in systole.

The **sarcolemmal calcium pump** is a back-up calcium ejection system which uses ATP and pumps calcium ions outwards (Fig. 7-3). The chief function of the calcium pump may be as follows. The pump is just active enough in diastole to respond to the low cytosolic calcium ion concentration normally found in diastole (0.3×10^{-6} M; Marban et al., 1980), thereby maintaining the diastolic cytosolic calcium concentration. During systole or during catecholamine stimulation the pump is "switched on" to function more actively, but it is not fast enough to cope with all the calcium ions, so the much more active sodium–calcium exchange system is brought into action to eject more calcium.

A second energy-requiring calcium pump may be concerned with calcium ion entry (Dhalla et al., 1981); yet it is difficult to understand why any considerable amount of ATP should be used to admit calcium ions down a favorable concentration gradient.

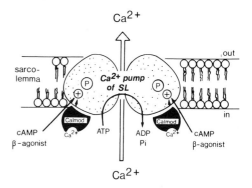

Fig. 7-3 Model of the calcium pump of the sarcolemma. Note that the major route for efflux of calcium ions is by the sodium–calcium mechanism (Fig. 4-1). The calcium pump probably plays a supportive role.

Role of Sarcoplasmic Reticulum

Most of the fall of the calcium ion concentration in the cytosol at the start of diastole is not by efflux from the cell, but by uptake into the sarcoplasmic reticulum. It is only the small amount of calcium entering the cell during each depolarization that needs to be ejected to avoid calcium overload. It is the much larger fraction of calcium released from the sarcoplasmic reticulum that must be returned to its site of origin in preparation for release in the next cardiac cycle.

Calcium accumulation

Studies in which fragments of the reticulum have been isolated (as tiny vesicles called microsomes) indicate that the calcium-accumulating activity of the sarcoplasmic reticulum requires ATP. Such true uptake of calcium must be distinguished from non-specific binding which occurs more quickly but has much less physiological significance (Fig. 7-4). Once it was realized that the calcium-accumulating activity of the sarcoplasmic reticulum depended upon ATP, there was little doubt that an endogenous calcium pump had to be present. This ATP-requiring enzyme, now isolated and characterized, is the major protein component of the reticulum (Fig. 7-5). It has a molecular weight of about 105 000 and is distributed asymmetrically across the membrane (Tada and Katz, 1982) in such a way that part of it actually protrudes into the cytosol. Probably it consists of dimers of a single polypeptide, but there may be a relatively low molecular weight (about 6000) proteolipid co-factor. For each mole of ATP that is hydrolyzed by this enzyme two calcium ions are accumulated within the reticulum, so that calcium is taken up from the vicinity of the myofibrils. This calcium-pumping ATPase of the sarcoplasmic reticulum differs in many ways from that of the sarcolemma, despite their common capacity to pump calcium.

Calcium accumulation and relaxation

An important but as yet unresolved question is whether or not the reticulum can accumulate calcium ions fast enough to account for relaxation. The average time for relaxation in mammalian heart muscle is about 200 msec, during which time the sarcoplasmic reticulum can accumulate as much as 100 mol calcium/kg ventricle (Schwartz, 1971). Since only 2 mol calcium/kg muscle are needed to elicit a strong contraction (Solaro et al., 1974), it seems likely that the calcium-accumulating activity of the reticulum is more than adequate to cause relaxation. Whether or not calcium can be taken up fast enough to account for the rate of relaxation is a different, unsolved issue (Blayney, 1983).

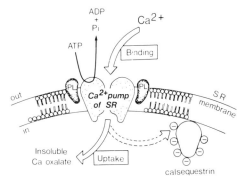

Fig. 7-4 Calcium transport in isolated vesicles of the sarcoplasmic reticulum. The addition of oxalate permits continuing accumulation of pumped calcium as the insoluble oxalate in the interior of the vesicles. Calsequestrin and other highly negatively charged proteins are present in the sarcoplasmic reticulum (SR) to provide what is the physiological equivalent to oxalate.

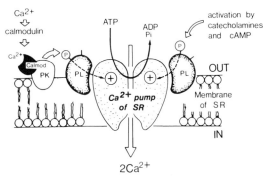

Fig. 7-5 Calcium is taken up into the sarcoplasmic reticulum by a calcium pump whose activity is regulated by phospholamban (PL). The calcium-dependent ATPase pumps two calcium ions inwards and splits one molecule of ATP to ADP and inorganic phosphate (P_i) in the process. The rate of pumping, especially at low cytosolic calcium concentrations, is enhanced by phosphorylation (P) of the associated phospholamban molecule. There are two such activating phosphorylations, at distinct sites, and their effects are additive: one is activated by catecholamines via cyclic AMP, and the other is dependent on the binding of activated calmodulin to an enzyme of the sarcoplasmic reticulum called protein kinase (PK, see Chapter 8).

Phosphorylation and calcium accumulation

The activity of the calcium pump of the sarcoplasmic reticulum is subject to complex regulation, as befits the requirement for fine regulation of the rate of relaxation. The major signal regulating the calcium pump is **phospholamban**, which means "phosphate receptor" (Tada and Katz, 1982). Agents that increase the ability of adenylate cyclase to form cyclic AMP and to enhance the cytosolic calcium concentration, such as the beta-adrenergic agonists isoproterenol, epinephrine and norepinephrine, should all enhance sequestration of calcium (Lindemann et al., 1983) and abbreviate systole. The ultimate mechanism is the same — the transfer of a phosphate group from ATP to phospholamban, so as to increase the activity of the pump (Fig. 7-5).

Phospholamban is a dimer or oligomer (mol. wt 22 000) consisting of two to four polypeptide chains and is an integral part of the proteins of the membrane of the sarcoplasmic reticulum (Tada and Inui, 1983). Most is embedded in the membrane, a small part being exposed to the cytosol. Upon phosphorylation, phospholamban undergoes a profound molecular change which in turn alters the conformation of the calcium pump to increase the uptake of calcium into the sarcoplasmic reticulum. Phospholamban can be phosphorylated in two different ways at two different sites (Walsh et al., 1980). Both systems respond physiologically to beta-adrenergic stimulation which increases both the intracellular level of cyclic AMP and the intracellular calcium concentration (Chapter 8). In pathological circumstances, as in early ischemia, when calcium overload of the cytosol may threaten the cell, then the existence of a system requiring only calcium to "switch" it on may be a protective mechanism. The calcium-accumulating activity of the sarcoplasmic reticulum is depressed in congestive heart failure, which may in part explain the depressed contractile state. Drugs such as catecholamines enhance the intake of calcium (Table 7-2), while others, such as methylxanthines (caffeine, amino-phylline) are inhibitory. This effect of the methyl-xanthines is quite distinct from their ability to inhibit the enzyme (phosphodiesterase) which breaks down cyclic AMP (see Chapter 8), thereby increasing cyclic AMP and the activity of phospholamban. The experimental agent **ryanodine** inhibits chiefly the release of calcium by the sarcoplasmic reticulum (Wier et al., 1983) without altering cyclic AMP levels.

Calcium-induced calcium release

In steady-state conditions that amount of calcium that is taken up and accumulated by the sarcoplasmic

Table 7-2

Effect of drugs on sarcoplasmic reticulum

Substance	Ca^{2+} accumulation	Ca^{2+} release
Catecholamines	+	Indirectly increased by enhanced slow inward current
Low-dose caffeine	Delayed[1]	Nil
High-dose caffeine (5–10 mM)	No effect	Enhanced[2]
Local anesthetics (procaine)	No effect	Inhibit[2]
Ca^{2+}-antagonists	No effect	No direct effect
Ryanodine	No effect	Inhibits

[1]Calcium sequestration blocking effect, Weber (1968). J Gen Physiol 52: 760.
[2]Hunter et al. (1982). Circ Res 51: 363.

reticulum is released again during the next beat. Despite the importance of this release process, comparatively little is known about the signal which triggers it. There are at least two possibilities: (i) the depolarizing signal at the cell surface may spread directly to the sarcoplasmic reticulum and cause the release of stored calcium ions, perhaps by collapsing a proton gradient across the membrane of the sarcoplasmic reticulum. Alternatively, (ii) the calcium that enters during the plateau phase of the action potential may act as the trigger for release, by the process of "calcium-triggered calcium release" (Fabiato, 1982, 1983).

Which of these two possibilities is correct is still being vigorously debated. Radiolabeled calcium has been used to show the existence of an intracellular pool of calcium in the heart which has the characteristic features expected of calcium located in the sarco-plasmic reticulum, being released by high concen-trations of caffeine or by external calcium, while being retained by the local anesthetic procaine, which inhibits the release from the sarcoplasmic reticulum (Hunter et al., 1982). Such data suggest that it is calcium in the sarcoplasmic reticulum that is involved in the calcium-induced calcium release. Another way of looking at the problem is by chemically "skinning" muscle fibers to remove the lipid bilayer of the sarcolemma. Addition of calcium to "skinned" cells can now react with the sarcoplasmic reticulum to release calcium. Such release is a graded effect, being greater when the sarcoplasmic reticulum is pre-loaded with calcium, or when the concentration of "triggering" calcium is greater (Fabiato, 1982). It follows that beta-adrenergic stimulation by preloading the sarcoplasmic reticulum with more calcium will indirectly enhance the subsequent calcium-triggered release of calcium. Because beta-adrenergic stimulation "opens" more calcium channels to increase internal calcium which triggers the release of yet more calcium from the sarcoplasmic reticulum, both the contraction and relaxation phases of the contractile cycle (Chapter 8) will be stimulated.

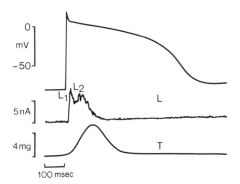

Fig. 7-6 The aequorin signal associated with the action potential (top panel) of Purkinje fibers is shown in the middle panel (L = luminescence). The aequorin signal is activated by an increase in the cytosolic calcium ion concentration and consists of two components. The first component L_1 is probably calcium entry by the slow channel, and the second component (L_2) is probably calcium-induced calcium release from the sarcoplasmic reticulum. The bottom panel shows how tension increases in response to the rise of calcium. Verapamil decreases both the light signals (Morgan et al., 1983) probably by inhibiting calcium ion entry which then decreases the amount of calcium release from the sarcoplasmic reticulum. From Wier and Isenberg (1982). Pflügers Arch 392: 284, with permission.

Direct evidence favoring the theory of calcium-induced calcium release has been obtained by monitoring intracellular calcium ion concentrations by aequorin, which emits a light-sensitive signal in the presence of calcium. The aequorin signal shows two peaks in Purkinje fibers—the first is closely related to the slow inward current. The second peak does not require depolarization and is probably the phenomenon of calcium-induced calcium release (Fig. 7-6).

Uptake vs release of calcium by sarcoplasmic reticulum

How does the sarcoplasmic reticulum "know" when to take up calcium from the cytoplasm, and when to release it? One theory is that the capacity to take up calcium is there throughout the cardiac cycle, but that when the wave of depolarization reaches the sarcoplasmic reticulum via the T-tubules (see Fig. 2-7) there is a temporary release of calcium to exceed the potential rate of uptake. This theory fails to explain why the release of calcium is graded in response to an increasing external calcium ion concentration. Fabiato (1983) explains the cyclical uptake and release of calcium by the sarcoplasmic reticulum as follows. He proposes that there are two different stimuli to the sarcoplasmic reticulum: the rate of rise of the calcium ion concentration in the cytoplasm, and the absolute value thereof. While the calcium ion concentration rises rapidly soon after "opening" of the calcium channel (Fig. 7-6), the sarcoplasmic reticulum responds by releasing more calcium. Then, when the rate of rise of calcium slows down as the absolute concentration of the calcium rises, the uptake mechanism is activated and the release mechanism shut off. Thus the sarcoplasmic reticulum responds sensitively and oppositely to the rate of rise and the absolute concentration of calcium. This hypothesis requires that the internal calcium ion concentration should fluctuate, as indirectly suggested by measurements with aequorin (Fig. 7-6; Wier et al., 1983).

Calmodulin

The previous sections have described how a rise in the cytosolic calcium concentration promotes the activity of at least three processes which remove calcium from the cytosol: the uptake of calcium by the sarcoplasmic reticulum, the extrusion of calcium through the sarcolemmal calcium pump, and the activity of the sodium–calcium exchanger. Hence it is not too fanciful to suppose that calcium ions self-regulate their concentration in the cytosol—an important concept, because when self-regulation fails, calcium overload ensues and lethal cellular damage can follow. The calcium regulator protein, calmodulin, is thought to play a critical role as the intracellular calcium sensor (Gevers, 1981; Fig. 7-7).

Calmodulin is a small but ubiquitously distributed protein consisting of a single polypeptide chain with

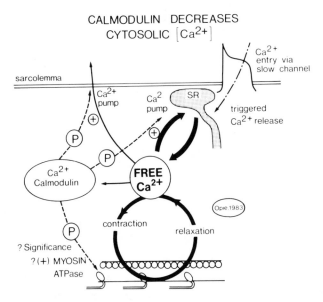

CALMODULIN DECREASES
CYTOSOLIC $[Ca^{2+}]$

Fig. 7-7 Calmodulin probably plays an important role in the self-regulation of calcium ions, whereby a rise of cytosolic calcium increases calmodulin activity to enhance those processes which in turn decrease the cytosolic level. Calmodulin is activated when calcium ions displace magnesium ions from three of the four divalent ion binding domains. Calcium–calmodulin exerts its functions by combining with enzymes, thereby regulating their activity. For example, by increasing the activity of a protein kinase, calcium–calmodulin can phosphorylate the sarcoplasmic reticulum to increase the uptake of calcium (LePeuch et al., 1980).

a molecular weight of 16 700 (Cheung, 1980) and a high affinity for calcium. It has four calcium-binding domains within its structure, with varying dissociation constants which lie neatly between the diastolic calcium ion concentration of 10^{-7} M and the systolic value of 10^{-5} M. When calcium is absent the four binding sites are occupied by magnesium ions. It is thought that the rise in free calcium which accompanies excitation–contraction coupling, displaces all the magnesium from three sites, but only a small fraction of magnesium from the fourth site. Thus the active form is Ca_3Mg_1—calmodulin (Walsh et al., 1980). However, this view may be a simplification (Lee et al., 1980). As calcium binds, the molecular form of calmodulin changes and it becomes able to combine with certain enzymes. For example, calcium–calmodulin stimulates the activity of the calcium pumps of both the sarcoplasmic reticulum and of the sarcolemma, thereby acting as a general calcium sensor.

Drug action and calmodulin

The effects of calmodulin are specifically inhibited by the phenothiazine compounds. For example, 1 mol calmodulin binds 2 mol trifluoperazine with a dissociation constant of 10^{-6} M to become inactive (Levin and Weiss, 1977). This effect may explain the antipsychotic properties of the phenothiazines such as chlorpromazine. Normally calmodulin stimulates the phosphodiesterase of the brain, thereby reducing cyclic AMP levels. Phenothiazines may reverse this effect to increase cyclic AMP levels, thereby having the same ultimate effect as other antipsychotic agents which increase cerebral release of catecholamines. In the case of the heart and vascular tissue, an effect of calcium antagonists on calmodulin has been proposed but not confirmed.

Excitation–Contraction Coupling

The sequential release of calcium ions and subsequent uptake into the sarcoplasmic reticulum are therefore regulated by (i) the amount of calcium entering the calcium channels, which in turn regulate the amount of calcium released by the sarcoplasmic reticulum, and (ii) the rate of uptake of calcium ions by the calcium pump of sarcoplasmic reticulum. To prove that the postulated rise and fall of cytosolic calcium is directly linked to myocardial contraction and relaxation requires demonstration that (i) the calcium ion concentration rises and falls just prior to contraction and relaxation, and (ii) that the extent of the rise of calcium can be related to the force of subsequent contraction. Direct evidence of these postulates has now been obtained through measurement of the aequorin signal in contracting papillary muscle (Fig. 7-8).

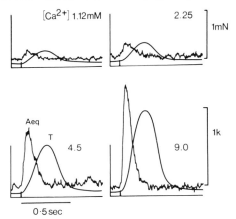

Fig. 7-8 Influence of extracellular calcium ion concentration on the aequorin (Aeq) signals for intracellular calcium and on isometric tension development (T) of papillary muscle. The calcium concentrations are given in the individual panels (mN). The symbol k denotes thousands of photon counts per second, and is a reflection of the calcium ion concentration which activates the aequorin signal. The contractile activity is shown as the smooth continuous line. From Morgan et al. (1983), with permission. The exact relation in time between the intracellular free calcium and contractile force needs further study.

Internal Calcium and Slow Inward Current

Internal calcium may be a "key intracellular messenger" (Marban and Tsien, 1982) in controlling inward currents. On incomplete evidence, a provisional scheme is as follows. Internal calcium may either enhance or inhibit the slow inward current, I_{si}. During modest increases of internal calcium, as found during digitalis therapy, a positive feedback loop promotes the flow of I_{si}; this effect is quite different from the stimulation of I_{si} resulting from beta-adrenergic stimulation and acting via cyclic AMP (see Fig. 6-7). During pathological rises of internal calcium it would be much more logical to have a negative rather than positive feedback system, so that the high internal calcium could inhibit calcium entry and limit calcium overload (see next section). Preliminary evidence supports this concept (Marban and Tsien, 1982). Therefore there should be an intriguing "switch-over" mechanism, yet to be discovered, to allow a rising internal calcium to stimulate and then to inhibit the slow inward current. During ischemia, when internal calcium also rises, calcium-induced calcium currents may help produce arrhythmias (see next section).

Calcium Overload

An important concept in cardiac pathology is that of calcium overload, first emphasized by Fleckenstein (1971, 1984). He described how experimental myocardial necrosis occurred in response to high doses of catecholamines, with a greatly increased uptake of calcium by the myocardium; the whole process was inhibited by calcium-channel antagonists such as verapamil and nifedipine (Fig. 7-8). It is thought that cytosolic calcium overload may occur in response to myocardial ischemia (the evidence is not clear), reperfusion and excess catecholamine stimulation. Fleckenstein (1971) proposed that calcium overload could damage myocardial cells by excessive splitting of ATP as a result of the increased activity of the contractile mechanism in response to calcium (Fig. 7-9). Now it is known that calcium overload can occur even while the myocardial levels of ATP are normal (Horak and Opie, 1983) so that other mechanisms may also be involved: (i) as the mitochondria tend to buffer the cytosolic calcium, they become overloaded with calcium and "waste" ATP in the process, thereby demanding more oxygen and extending the severity of ischemia; (ii) calcium may stimulate the phospholipase enzymes which break down cell membranes (see Fig. 10-20); and (iii) calcium overload may cause the development of ischemic contracture.

Internal calcium in ischemia

A new concept is that there is a role for calcium overload in the genesis of early arrhythmias of myocardial infarction (Clusin et al., 1984). The action potential duration shortens early in myocardial ischemia; the mechanism may be the inhibition of glycolysis that occurs in severe ischemia (Chapter 22). Such glycolytic inhibition will also, it is proposed,

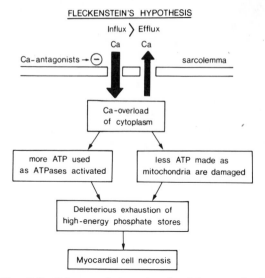

FLECKENSTEIN'S HYPOTHESIS

Fig. 7-9 Scheme of the role of calcium overload of cytoplasm in the development of myocardial cell necrosis. See Fleckenstein (1984); reproduced with permission.

decrease the uptake of calcium by the sarcoplasmic reticulum by lessening the amount of ATP available for that purpose (Bricknell et al., 1981). Thus, in ischemia two events will occur simultaneously: decreased uptake of calcium by the sarcoplasmic reticulum and a shortened action potential duration. As less calcium is taken up by the sarcoplasmic reticulum, it accumulates in the cytosol to increase the resting diastolic tension (ischemic contracture) and there is also less calcium available for release by the wave of excitation (decreased calcium-triggered calcium release). As the cytosolic calcium ion concentration increases it should diminish the slow inward current, thereby further decreasing the action potential duration and increasing the risk of arrhythmias (Chapter 22).

Calcium overload may also provoke arrhythmias by inducing a diastolic inward current to cause **delayed after-depolarizations**. These may, in turn, trigger automatic activity. Such mechanisms are thought to be of major importance in the arrhythmias of **digitalis toxicity**, which causes calcium overload by severe inhibition of the sodium pump. Intracellular sodium thus accumulates and the sodium–calcium exchange mechanism becomes inhibited.

Summary

Cardiac contraction and relaxation is explained by a calcium cycle. During depolarization, a small amount of calcium enters the heart cell and is thought to trigger the release of more calcium from the sarcoplasmic reticulum by the process of calcium-induced calcium release. The cytosolic calcium rises and contraction occurs. At the same time the increased concentration of cytoplasmic calcium activates the calcium-modulator protein, calmodulin, which in turn hastens the efflux of calcium ions from the cell by (i) "switching on" the uptake of calcium into the sarcoplasmic reticulum; and (ii) the pump ejecting calcium from the cell. The major route for calcium ion entry into the cardiac cell is by the slow calcium channel, which is triggered as the sodium channel opens and the cell depolarizes to a certain critical value. The probability of the calcium channel being open can be increased by catecholamine stimulation, acting via the second messenger cyclic AMP. Beta-adrenergic catecholamine stimulation and other agents with a positive inotropic effect also increase the cytosolic calcium concentration. Both entry and exit of calcium ions into and from the cytosol are promoted by adrenergic stimulation, yet there must be a small net gain of calcium to permit the positive inotropic effect. Enhanced relaxation during adrenergic stimulation is mediated by enhanced uptake of calcium ions into the sarcoplasmic reticulum, as cyclic AMP "switches on" the regulator protein phospholamban. When the control mechanisms regulating the cytosolic calcium concentration fail, calcium overload may develop, with pathological effects such as enhanced necrosis, shortening of the action potential duration and the emergence of delayed after-depolarizations.

References

Blayney L (1983). Cardiac sarcoplasmic reticulum. In: Cardiac Metabolism. Ed AJ Drake-Holland, MIM Noble, pp 19–47, John Wiley, Chichester.

Bricknell OL, Daries PS, Opie LH (1981). A relationship between adenosine triphosphate, glycolysis and ischaemic contracture in the isolated rat heart. J Molec Cell Cardiol 13: 941–945.

Carafoli E (1984). How calcium crosses cell membranes. In: Calcium Antagonists and Cardiovascular Disease. Ed LH Opie, pp 29–41, Raven Press, New York.

Cheung WY (1980). Calmodulin plays a pivotal role in cellular regulation. Science 207: 19–27.

Clusin WT, Buchbinder M, Bristow MR, Harrison DC (1984). Evidence for a role of calcium in the genesis of early ischemic cardiac arrhythmias. In: Calcium Antagonists and Cardiovascular Disease. Ed LH Opie, pp 293–302, Raven Press, New York.

Dhalla NS, Anand-Srivastava MB, Tuana BS, Khandelwal RR (1981). Solubilization of a calcium-dependent adenosine triphosphatase from rat heart sarcolemma. J Molec Cell Cardiol 13: 413–423.

Fabiato A (1982). Calcium release in skinned cardiac cells: variations with species, tissues and development. Fed Proc 41: 2238–2244.

Fabiato A (1983). Calcium-induced release of calcium from the cardiac sarcoplasmic reticulum. Am J Physiol 245: C1–C4.

Fleckenstein A (1971). Specific inhibitors and promoters of calcium action in the excitation–contraction coupling of heart muscle and their role in the prevention or production of myocardial lesions. In: Calcium and the Heart. Eds P Harris, LH Opie, pp 135–188, Academic Press, London, Orlando and New York.

Fleckenstein A (1984). Calcium antagonism: history and prospects for a multifaceted pharmacodynamic principle. In: Calcium Antagonists and Cardiovascular Disease. Ed LH Opie, pp 9–28, Raven Press, New York.

Gevers W (1981). Calcium: the managing director. SA Med J 59: 406–408.

Horak AR, Opie LH (1983). Energy metabolism of the heart in catecholamine-induced myocardial injury. In: Advances in Myocardiology, Vol 4, Ed E Chazov, V Saks, G Rona, pp 23–43, Plenum Press, New York.

Hunter DR, Haworth RA, Berkoff HA (1982). Cellular calcium turnover in perfused rat heart. Circ Res 51: 363–370.

Langer GA (1982). Sodium–calcium exchange in the heart. Ann Rev Physiol 44: 335–349.

Langer GA (1984). Calcium at the sarcolemma. J Molec Cell Cardiol 16: 147–153.

Lee CB, Crouch TH, Richman PG (1980). Calmodulin. Ann Rev Biochem 49: 489–515.

LePeuch CJ, Guilleux JC, Demaille JG (1980). Phospholamban phosphorylation in the perfused rat heart is not solely dependent on beta-adrenergic stimulation. FEBS Letters 114: 165–168.

Levin RM, Weiss B (1977). Binding of trifluoperazine to the calcium-dependent activator of cyclic nucleotide phosphodiesterase. Molec Pharm 13: 690–697.

Lindemann JP, Jones LR, Hathaway DR, Henry BG, Watanabe AM (1983). Beta-adrenergic stimulation of phospholamban phosphorylation and Ca^{2+}-ATPase

activity in guinea-pig ventricles. J Biol Chem 258: 464–471.

Marban and Tsien (1982). Enhancement of calcium current during digitalis inotropy in mammalian heart: positive feedback regulation by intracellular calcium? J Physiol (London) 329: 589–614.

Marban E, Rink TJ, Tsien RW, Tsien RY (1980). Free calcium in heart muscle at rest and during contraction measured with Ca^{2+}-sensitive microelectrodes. Nature 286: 845–850.

Morgan JP, Wier WG, Hess P, Blinks JR (1983). Influence of Ca^{2+}-channel blocking agents on calcium transients and tension development in isolated mammalian heart muscle. Circ Res 52: Suppl 1, 47–52.

Schwartz A (1971). Calcium and the sarcoplasmic reticulum. In: Calcium and the Heart, Eds P Harris, LH Opie, pp 66–90, Academic Press, London, Orlando and New York.

Solaro RJ, Wiese RM, Shiner JS, Briggs FN (1979). Calcium requirements for cardiac myofibrillar activation. Circ Res 34: 525–530.

Tada M, Inui M (1983). Regulation of calcium transport by the ATPase–phospholamban system. J Molec Cell Cardiol 15: 565–575.

Tada M, Katz AM (1982). Phosphorylation of the sarcoplasmic reticulum and sarcolemma. Ann Rev Physiol 44: 401–423.

Walsh MP, LePeuch CJ, Vallet B, Cavadore JC, Demaille JG (1980). Cardiac calmodulin and its role in the regulation of metabolism and contraction. J Molec Cell Cardiol 12: 1091–1101.

Wier WG, Kort AA, Stern MD, Lakatta EG, Marban E (1983). Cellular calcium fluctuations in mammalian heart: direct evidence from noise analysis of aequorin signals in Purkinje fibers. Proc Nat Acad Sci 80: 7367–7371.

New References

Carafoli E (1985). The homeostasis of calcium in heart cells. J Molec Cell Cardiol 17: 203–212.

Clusin WT (1985). Do caffeine and metabolic inhibitors increase free calcium in the heart? Interpretation of conflicting intracellular calcium measurements. J Molec Cell Cardiol 17: 213–220.

Fabiato A (1985). Calcium-induced release of calcium from the sarcoplasmic reticulum. J Gen Physiol 85: 189–320.

Valdeolmillos M, Eisner DA (1985). The effects of ryanodine on calcium-overloaded sheep cardiac Purkinje fibers. Circ Res 56: 452–456.

The Mechanism of
Myocardial Contraction

W. Gevers

The essential components of the heart's "contractile machinery" are those proteins concerned primarily with contraction (actin and myosin) and those whose function is regulatory (troponin and tropomyosin). By far the greater percentage of myofibrillar protein is that concerned with contraction, with about 10 percent concerned with its regulation and another 10 percent concerned with maintenance of the structure of the myofibril (Table 8-1). In living muscle, no matter how correctly these proteins are orientated, contraction will not occur unless ATP and calcium are also present.

Table 8-1

The proteins of myofibrils.

Function	Location	% of myofibrillar protein	Molecular weight
Contractile			
Myosin	Thick filaments	55–60	500,000
Actin	Thin filaments	20	43,000
Regulatory			
Tropomyosin	Thin filaments	5	70,000
Troponin-I	Thin filaments		
Troponin-C	Thin filaments	7	86,000
Troponin-T	Thin filaments		
Structural			
C-protein	Thick filaments		
alpha-actinin	Thick filaments and Z-lines		
beta-actinin	Thin filaments	8–13	40,000–750,000
M-line proteins	M-lines		
Other proteins	Various		

There are about 7 actins : 2 myosins : 1 tropomyosin : 1 troponin in the myofibrils, but their different molecular weights account for the different picture given by the percentage contribution each makes to the total myofibrillar mass (third column). These data are partly from Perry (1979).

Molecular Events Associated with Myocardial Contraction

The involvement of the myosin heads

The transformation of chemical energy into mechanical work involves a series of reactions which center around the splitting of ATP by hydrolysis. The term hydrolysis describes a reaction in which a compound is split by the addition of water ("lysis by water"). In the case of muscle, the enzyme that is involved is an integral part of the myosin molecule—hence the enzyme is known as the **myosin ATPase**. For this function the important part of ATP is the terminal pyrophosphate (P–O–P) linkage. It is customary to refer to this as a "high-energy bond"

(a concept that was introduced by Fritz Lipmann in 1941) because when the bond is split off, useful energy is "released". Thus in general terms, all the energy needed to support muscle extraction is obtained by splitting the terminal phosphate bond in ATP, as follows:

$$ATP + H_2O \longrightarrow ADP + P_i + H^+ + energy$$

where ADP is adenosine diphosphate and P_i is inorganic phosphate. A little more than 30 kJ (kilojoules) of energy are released for each mole (500 g) of ATP that is hydrolyzed (or split off).

The heart contains about 3 mg ATP/g fresh weight or about 5 μmol/g or 5 × 10^{-6} mol/g of ATP. Together with the roughly threefold greater pool of creatine phosphate, this represents an energy

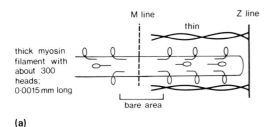

(a)

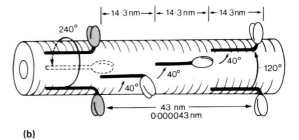

(b)

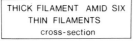

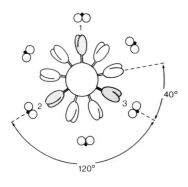

(c)

Fig. 8-1 Proposed scheme of thick and thin filaments (a), with myosin "heads" coming off at right angles to the "body". The thickness of the thick filament is only relative, since the length to width proportion is approximately 100 : 1. The heads emerge in groups of three and shift their positions by 40° in succession (b). Thus nine rows of about 16 heads each are placed in a line on the surface of each arm of the bipolar filament. Note the position of the thick filament between six thin filaments (c). In the cross-sectional view, the shaded "heads" of myosin correspond to a group of three heads coming off at the same level (two of these three heads are shaded in part (b).

reserve sufficient for only 50–75 beats in an adult heart.

Micro-anatomy of contraction

To explain the contraction cycle requires first a brief recapitulation of the micro-anatomy of the contractile elements. The thick filament of myosin (about 1.5 μm long and 10–15 nm wide) is composed of about 300 individual myosin molecules, each very large and ending in a myosin head which is bilobed (Fig. 8-1). Half of these heads are orientated towards one end of the sarcomere and half to the other, leaving a bare area in the middle of the thick filament where the centrally placed disc of the M-line proteins holds the entire array of thick filaments in register within the sarcomere. The pattern in which myosin heads emerge from the body of the thick filaments is still controversial, but in a commonly accepted version the heads appear in groups of three, each group 14.3 nm from the next (Squire, 1981). This means that about 50 such sets occur on each ''half'' of a single thick filament. The sets are ''rotated'' with respect to each preceding one in a spiral fashion, so that every head emerges displaced at an angle of about 40° in relation to its predecessor. A head will accordingly reappear in the same ''line'' as another every 43 nm.

Thin filaments (about 1 μm long and only 5–7 nm wide) contain two helical chains of actin units, each carried on a backbone of tropomyosin, with troponin complexes placed at intervals of about 38 nm (Fig. 8-2). Troponin-C (for calcium) is that component to which calcium can bind to remove the inhibitory effect of troponin-I (I for inhibitor) on the interaction between actin and myosin heads. Troponin-T links the whole troponin complex to tropomyosin.

The bilobed head of each myosin molecule is connected to the thick filament by a rod-like ''stalk'' or ''neck'', which then merges into the remaining rod-like ''body'' of the molecule which is permanently built into the filament by side-to-side aggregation with its fellows (Fig. 8-3). These three domains of the molecule are thus joined by two flexible hinges which enable the head to reach out to the thin filaments even when the muscle shortens. This is necessary because sarcomeres ''swell'' when they shorten since the system has a constant volume; accordingly, the thick and thin filaments become separated from each other more and more during contraction and the myosin hinges enable the system to operate unchanged during these processes.

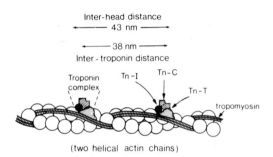

Fig. 8-2 Thin filament structure. The rope-like filament is essentially a double helix of two half-filaments each consisting of seven actins lying along a dimeric coiled tropomyosin molecule with one troponin complex attached to it. The filament depicted would look identical from the back. The structure of the members of the troponin is purely diagrammatic, especially in the case of troponin-C which is the molecule undergoing a change in its configuration in the presence of enough calcium ions, as will be shown in Fig. 8-4.

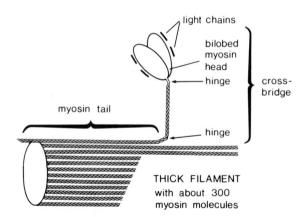

Fig. 8-3 The bilobed myosin head is at the end of the cross-bridge and projects from the thick filament. Each lobe of the head lies at the end of a long strand; two such strands are twisted together to form a long rigid helical structure, the tail of which is buried in the thick filament and held in tight apposition to the tails of other myosin molecules. The two hinges at either end of the ''neck'' of the cross-bridge allow (i) flexion–extension movements of the head on the neck (Fig. 8-4); and (ii) the cross-bridge to stretch across the increased gap between thick and thin filaments during contraction. Figure modified from Murphy RA (1983), with permission.

Cross-bridge Cycle

The best way to understand individual contraction cycles is to start in diastole when the sarcomeres are

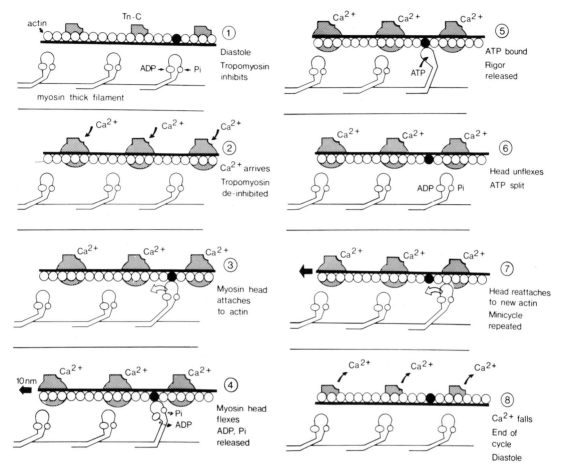

Fig. 8-4 (Steps 1–7). The cross-bridge cycle starts with relaxation in diastole, when tropomyosin (Tm) "blocks" the myosin heads from binding to actin. At the start of systole, calcium ions combine with troponin-C (Tn-C) to unblock the actin so that myosin heads can bind (Step 2) and then "flex" whereupon ADP and inorganic phosphate (P_i) are released (Step 3). The "rigor state" develops transiently (Step 4). ATP moves in to the same binding site on the myosin head, vacated by ADP, to "release" the myosin head (Step 5). After ATP has been split to ADP and P_i by the myosin ATPase, the head extends (Step 6) to rebind to another actin 2–4 units "downstream" (Step 7). Steps 1–7 are repeated until calcium ions leave at the start of diastole (Step 8).

in a state of relaxation. There is then no interaction between any of the myosin heads and the actin units of the thin filaments. The absence of actin–myosin interactions in the relaxed state centers around the properties of troponin and tropomyosin, which inhibits the potential interaction of myosin heads with actin units (Step 1, Fig. 8-4). In diastole, when the cytosolic calcium ion concentration falls, the loss of calcium from its binding sites on troponin-C is associated with a series of complex interactions among the proteins of the rope-like thin filament, which result in a shift in the relative positions of the filamentous molecules: tropomyosin

moves to a position that essentially blocks any interaction of actin units with myosin (Perry, 1979). The inhibition is only imposed on actin subunits in the immediate vicinity of the particular "unoccupied" troponin-C molecule; about 7 actins are thus controlled "at a distance" by the master-switch sited in the troponin complex.

When the concentration of calcium ions rises in the cytosol as a result of excitation, these ions bind to two (or more) specific sites on troponin-C so that the thin filaments revert to the conformation that permits interaction between the myosin heads and adjacent actin units. The myosin heads now attach to the actin or induce local conformation changes (Yanagida et al., 1984); at this stage the product of (prior) hydrolysis of ATP, in the form of ADP and inorganic phosphate, are bound to the head. The attachment to actin occurs at a preferred angle of about 90° (Step 2, Fig. 8-4).

The next step in the cross-bridge cycle is a concerted movement of the myosin head towards an angle of about 45°, with discharge first of the bound inorganic phosphate and then of bound ADP (Step 3). This (together with the action of other cross-bridges in the half sarcomere) performs the mechanical work of contraction by sliding the entire thin filaments over the thick filament, by a distance of about 10 nm (Huxley, 1969). The distance between the thick and thin filaments increases slightly (Fig. 8-3).

The state in which the flexed myosin head is bound to an actin at a preferred angle of 45° without any bound ADP or inorganic phosphate is the "rigor state" (Step 4). When ATP occupies this site there is a shape change in the myosin head which causes it to "loosen its grip" on the actin unit (Step 5). Hydrolysis of the bound ATP immediately follows, so that the head is returned to its unattached, 90° position, with bound ADP and inorganic phosphate (Step 6). In essence, the head is now in a position to bind a second time to an actin 2–4 units further along the thin filament than the one that has just participated in the cycle described (Step 7), provided that the nearest troponin-C still binds calcium ions. When the calcium concentration falls the thin filament is again "switched off" and relaxation occurs in that region of the sarcomere (Step 8).

During a single beat, tension develops by recruitment of more and more rapidly cycling cross-bridges as the cytosolic calcium concentration rises to a peak; relaxation begins when cross-bridge cycling activity diminishes in response to the removal of calcium from the thin filament sites where it acts. Since the cross-bridges cycle asynchronously, tension is maintained by those members of the population of cross-bridges which are attached at any given moment, while the rest are moving through the various detached phases of their individual cycles (Fig. 8-5).

Rate-limiting steps

The rate-limiting step in the slow hydrolysis of ATP by purified myosin is the release of bound inorganic

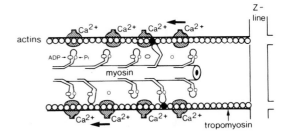

Fig. 8-5 Asynchronous nature of cross-bridge cycling during sarcomeric contraction. Many myosin heads are unattached, with bound ADP and P_i, because attachment is probably the rate-limiting step in each individual cross-bridge cycle at low afterloads. Those which are attached to actin units (●) either exert tension towards the center of the sarcomere or they are about to do so. For simplification only two thin filaments are shown and only one strand (actin–tropomyosin) of each; in addition, only two "lines" of heads emerging from a thick filament are shown (there are seven others). All actins are switched on because the Ca^{2+} occupancy of troponin-C is complete.

phosphate (P_i) during the following sequence (where M = myosin head):

$$M + ATP \longrightarrow M.ATP \longrightarrow M.ADP.P_i \xrightarrow{\text{slowest step}}$$
$$\longrightarrow M.ADP + P_i \longrightarrow M + ADP + P_i$$

When actin is available for interaction with myosin (which is essentially what happens during the cross-bridge cycle) the rate of ATP hydrolysis is greatly speeded up. In the following equation, A = actin, AM = actomyosin:

$$AM + ATP \longrightarrow M.ATP + A \longrightarrow M.ADP.P_i + A$$
$$\uparrow \qquad\qquad\qquad\qquad\qquad\qquad \searrow (1)$$
$$AM + ADP \longleftarrow AM.ADP + P_i \xrightarrow{(2)} AM.ADP.P_i$$

There is disagreement as to the rate-limiting step of the new sequence, which is thought to be reaction (2) by Taylor and co-workers (Lymn and Taylor, 1971), while Eisenberg and Greene (1980) favor reaction (1). Although the resolution of this controversy would appear to be relatively trivial, there are important implications arising from the correctness of one or the other view. Most of the molecules taking part in cyclical processes such as these normally find themselves "waiting" in anticipation in the molecular form just before the rate-limiting step. For reaction (1) this means that most of the myosin heads would be detached during very rapid shortening, while for reaction (2) the heads would predominantly be attached.

When one considers that cross-bridge action during muscle contraction is generally held to be asynchronous, i.e. the heads are all cycling independently of one another whenever calcium is present to "switch on" a local region of thin filament, then it becomes clear that enormous mechanical disadvantages will accrue from a situation where most cross-bridges are attached, some pulling in the manner depicted in Step 3 and others attached at either 90° (Steps 2 and 8) or 45°. This situation is analogous to the disastrous consequences of asynchrony in a rowing eight where all the rowers are at different stages of their strokes but most of the oars are in the water. A simple calculation, taking account of the number of cross-bridges on one-half of a thick filament which are in a straight line (about 15 or 16), shows that the model of Eisenberg and Greene (1980) has the attractive feature that the 5 percent (1 in 16) of the cross-bridges which they believe are actually attached at any given moment in the myofibrils, would represent one cross-bridge out of the set that can interact with a particular thin filament. The mechanical disadvantage is then virtually zero and we have a single explanation also for the fact that the most rapid shortening of the muscle occurs at zero load (V_{max} conditions). Addition of a load would immediately increase the number of attached cross-bridges (by an unknown mechanism) and slow down the rate of contraction.

Alternative Theories of Contraction*

Although the cross-bridge theory is almost universally accepted, it does not fit nor explain all the facts. In particular, length-dependent activation is difficult to understand. According to an alternative **electrostatic theory**, force generation is achieved by the thin filaments acting as dielectric rods suspended in electric fields between the cross-bridges which act as capacitors. The inequalities of the distribution of electrical charges are achieved by ATP hydrolysis. Length-dependent activation is explained by assuming that the tips of the thin filaments are at lower calcium concentrations during shorter sarcomere lengths, and at higher concentrations at longer lengths. Although this hypothesis is an interesting alternative, it is not presently widely espoused. (For further arguments, see Noble and Pollack, 1977.)

Another variant of the cross-bridge theory,

supported by studies with sophisticated x-ray diffraction techniques, is as follows. When seen end-on (Fig. 8-1) it is thought that the myosin heads can undergo radial movement during systole to lie in close apposition to the thin filaments. Although the myosin heads do move away from actin in diastole, this is a slow process. Some of the myosin heads remain close to the actin, without actually engaging in further cross-bridge cycling and without generating tension. The number of such quiescent "heads-in-waiting" increases during inotropic stimulation and such heads are "more ready" to engage in contraction. This theory is particularly good in explaining **paired stimulation** (page 171) when it is proposed that the myosin heads have not yet regained their diastolic state, so that the extra stimulus "catches" the heads closer to the actin.

Control of Contraction Cycle

The overall concept is thus that a single contraction of a heart cell involves a period of time (about 600 msec) during which the cytosolic calcium concentration rises to a peak (about 200 msec) and falls (about 400 msec). During this time calcium ions bind increasingly to troponin-C molecules all over the thin filaments, turning on an increasing total "length" of actin for interaction with any adjacent myosin heads. Thousands of mini-contractile cycles occur in ever-increasing numbers as long as the calcium concentration rises (systole). As soon as the calcium concentration begins to fall, however, increasing numbers of actins become unavailable to waiting myosin heads and the number of mini-contractile cycles per unit time diminishes, until ultimately the beat is over when the possibility of interactions has declined to near zero (diastole).

The peak difference in tension between systole and diastole that is reached during a beat is given by integration of the total number of cross-bridge cycles which occur from the beginning of systole up to the point where the calcium concentration reaches its peak (Table 8-2). The peak tension thus depends both on the initial sarcomeric length (see page 106) and on the amount of calcium released from the sarcoplasmic reticulum. Additional factors of importance are the affinity of troponin-C for calcium ions and the efficiency of the thin filament transduction process during calcium-induced "switch-on".

The maximum rate at which tension increases

---

*For conformational changes in cross-bridges, see Eisenberg and Hill (1985), Science 227: 999–1006.

Table 8-2

Proposed metabolic explanations for mechanical parameters of cardiac function

Mechanical parameter	Definition	Proposed explanation
V_{max}	Maximal rate of shortening at zero load	Proportional to maximum rate of actin-stimulated ATP hydrolysis by myosin species present (a) isoenzyme: V_1 V_2 V_3 and (b) P-light chain phosphorylation may enhance V_{max}. Also proportional to rate of Ca^{2+} release and diffusion to interior of myofibrils
P_o	Maximal tension at zero shortening rate	Related to number of cross-bridges attached
Peak tension increment (= peak force)	Difference between maximum systolic tension and minimum diastolic tension	Total number of cross-bridges attached since beginning of systole—a function of (a) initial sarcomere length and (b) total calcium released
dP/dt (i) (+) dP/dt_{max}	Maximal rate of pressure development in LV	Related to same factors as V_{max} above and to afterload through enhanced release of Ca^{2+} at greater initial sarcomere lengths. Also related to sensitivity of thin filaments to Ca^{2+} regulation, which is decreased by phosphorylation of Tn-I
(ii) (−) dP/dt_{max}	Maximal rate of fall of pressure in LV	Related to rate of Ca^{2+} removal by sarcoplasmic reticulum and to sensitivity of thin filaments to Ca^{2+} regulation, which is decreased by phosphorylation of troponin-I

$(+ dP/dt_{max})$ is a function of (i) the rate at which calcium is released from the sarcoplasmic reticulum and hence the rate of rise of the calcium concentration in the interior of the myofibrils, and especially (ii) the rate at which the myosin heads can break down ATP (Table 8-2). The latter quality is determined by the magnitude of the "turnover number" or catalytic efficiency of the particular type of myosin present in a given type of muscle (see below).

The maximum rate at which tension declines from the peak systolic level $(- dP/dt_{max})$ is a function of (i) the rate at which calcium is removed from the cytosol bathing the sarcomeres and also (ii) of the sensitivity of the thin filaments to calcium (Table 8-2). In relaxation, the opposite processes occur to those already discussed for tension increments.

Speed of contraction: determination of ATPase activity

It has long been held that the activity of the myosin ATPase is one of the fundamental points of control of the cardiac contraction cycle. The maximal possible activity of myosin ATPase has to date been considered

to be an intrinsic characteristic of the molecule concerned. According to the classic theory of Barany (1967), myosin from white muscle (fast twitch) has a higher ATPase activity and therefore catalyzes a more rapid breakdown of ATP. Myosin from red muscle, such as heart, has a lower ATPase activity, a slower rate of ATP breakdown and a slower rate of contraction. However, the ATPase activity of any given muscle type can vary, as is shown by the effect of thyrotoxicosis in increasing both cardiac myosin ATPase activity and the velocity of circumferential fiber shortening. This is caused by the re-emergence of an "embryonic" form of myosin (the so-called V_1 isoprotein coded by a different gene) in preference to the normal "adult" V_3 isoprotein. V_1 has an appreciably greater catalytic activity in hydrolyzing ATP than V_3, with an intermediate hybrid form, V_2, occupying an intermediate position (Samuel et al., 1983; see also Fig. 15-6).

Located on the myosin heads are **light chains** which in turn may gain a phosphate group under the influence of a kinase enzyme which "moves" (kinesis = movement) the phosphate from its donor molecule (ATP) to the light chain. This is an example of a **phosphorylation–dephosphorylation cycle** which can change some enzymes from inactive to active forms and back again, thereby switching them on and off. Phosphorylation of myosin light chains may increase the capacity of the myosin heads to split ATP, i.e. there is increased myosin ATPase activity, which may increase the maximal possible velocity of contraction at zero load (V_{max} of contraction). Since the kinase concerned is indirectly controlled by the concentration of calcium (see below), the cytosolic calcium concentration could be a factor determining the V_{max} of contraction (Fig. 8-6). This role of calcium (which is currently controversial) would be in addition to the more generally known role of this ion in regulating the number of cross-bridges which interact, and thereby controlling the maximum amount of isometric tension that can be developed (P_0, or the tension when there is no shortening of muscle).

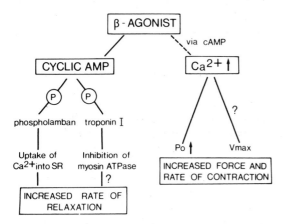

Fig. 8-6 Proposed links between beta-adrenergic agonist stimulation by catecholamines and changes in rates of relaxation and contraction of heart muscle. P = phosphorylation mediated by cyclic AMP (Fig. 6-4); P_0 and V_{max} are terms used in muscle mechanics (see Table 8-2 and Fig. 13-11).

Calcium and calmodulin

As its name implies, calmodulin is a substance which "modulates" (or conveys) the effects of calcium. It is a naturally occurring and remarkably widely distributed protein which binds up to four calcium ions with a high affinity and specificity. The binding of calcium causes conformational changes which confer biological activity on the molecule and activate some enzyme systems:

$$Ca^{2+}.calmodulin + inactive\ enzyme \longrightarrow$$
$$Ca^{2+}.calmodulin\ .\ active\ enzyme$$

One of the enzyme systems thus activated is **myosin light chain kinase**, which exists as an inactive protein at low calcium concentrations. This kinase probably becomes active when the cytosolic calcium ion concentration rises at the start of contraction. Increased calcium ion concentrations occur particularly after adrenergic stimulation or treatment with digitalis (Resink and Gevers, 1981). The activation of myosin light chain kinase is reversed when the phosphate group is removed by another enzyme, **myosin light chain phosphatase**, the control of which is not yet understood. Because only one of the two types of light chains on myosin heads are phosphorylated, these are called the P light chains.

Kopp and Barany (1979) found a positive correlation between the degree of myosin P light chain phosphorylation and active tension in perfused rat hearts, in the presence of a wide variety of agents increasing or decreasing cardiac contractility. Although one would expect that adrenergic stimulation would cause P light chains of myosin to become more highly phosphorylated, many groups have failed to detect such changes, while others have reported increases which never exceeded 0.5 phosphate per P light chain. Hence the true role of P light chain phosphorylation is still uncertain (England, 1984). Other explanations for the links between calcium and contractility include the idea that the calcium ion concentration at the contractile sites might change the physical properties of the sarcomere to allow a greater velocity of contraction (Ter Keurs, 1983).

Troponin-I

The troponin-I component of the troponin complex can also, like the myosin P light chains, gain a phosphate group. A different kinase is concerned which becomes active during adrenergic stimulation (cyclic AMP-dependent protein kinase). When this happens, higher concentrations of calcium are required to achieve the same degree of "switch on" of thin filaments. The physiological significance of this phosphorylation is likely to be that contraction can be "switched off" more rapidly when calcium falls at the start of diastole (increased relaxation rate).

Relaxation rate: another factor

Brutsaert et al. (1980) have described a mechanism whereby there is a "striking sensitivity of relaxation to the prevailing load". Thus an increased load increases the rate of relaxation although the molecular mechanisms involved are unknown. "**Active relaxation**", suggested by the occurrence of a negative early diastolic intraventricular pressure, could be explained by high rates of activity of the ATP-requiring calcium pump in the sarcoplasmic reticulum.

The Rigor State and Contracture

Hearts that are subjected to long periods of ischemia become stiff and non-compliant; this is called the **rigor state**. There appears to be a close association between its development and marked depletion of the tissue stores of ATP. If only small amounts of ATP are available the cross-bridges are frozen in the attached state and no active movement occurs, nor can the muscle be stretched under load—the rigor state.

> Rigor complexes can be formed in the laboratory by adding actin to myosin in the absence of ATP. The resultant complexes are extremely stable but can be dissociated by adding ATP.   Katz (1970)

In marked contrast to active tension development, the development of the rigor state does not require calcium and can occur in the absence of ATP. This condition should not be confused with that of **ischemic contracture**, although in both instances the sarcomeres do not return to their normal resting length. Contracture, which is often referred to as an increase in resting, or diastolic tension, may occur as a result of an increased cytosolic calcium concentration when:

(a) the myofibrils and the surrounding cytosol may have been swamped and therefore overloaded with calcium—as occurs, for example, when ischemic heart muscle is reperfused or anoxic heart muscle is reoxygenated;

(b) there is insufficient ATP produced by glycolysis to serve as substrate for the calcium-activated ATPase of the sarcoplasmic reticulum that is responsible for removing calcium from the cytosol (Bricknell et al., 1981). The **stone heart** is a dreaded complication of cardiac surgery which may be a combination of the rigor state (very low ATP) and of calcium overload.

Cardiac Ultrastructure and Starling's Law

According to the cross-bridge hypothesis the filaments in sarcomeres are anatomically so arranged that an optimal number of cross-bridges can form at optimal sarcomere lengths, usually held to be 2.0–2.2 μm. It is easy to argue that suboptimal overlap at short sarcomere lengths can impair the development of tension; it is less easy to understand why tension falls off in cardiac muscle when the fibers are supposedly overstretched. Whereas in skeletal muscle relaxation is truly a state of relaxation (so that the resting tension is close to zero), the heart has a very high resting tension. Resting **stiffness** may in part be attributed to the unique myocardial collagen network thought to counter the high systolic pressures normally developed in the ventricles (Borg and Caulfield, 1981). This low compliance means that a very small increase in cardiac muscle length will cause a large increase in tension development. This structural factor could explain why sarcomeres in chronically dilated hearts are just under 2.2 μm (Ross et al., 1971). Other explanations for the descending limb of the Starling curve (see Fig. 1-7) must be found. "Slippage" between myofibrils is suggested because the Z-lines lose their normal alignment at larger ventricular diastolic volumes, when more layers of the myocardium are uncovered.

Thus the relationship between cardiac ultrastructure and the contractile performance of the whole heart is by no means self-evident. The puzzled reader may be consoled by Katz ("It is not possible to provide a clear explanation for the Frank–Starling relationship in the intact heart"—Katz, 1977) and Sonnenblick ("In cardiac muscle, this decrease in force cannot be entirely explained by sarcomere elongation and a decrease in myofilament overlap"—Sonnenblick and Skelton, 1974). A better understanding of the contractile performance of the heart may now be achieved by thinking in molecular terms.

To explain the Frank–Starling relationship, length-dependent activation is now invoked—that is, an increased initial muscle length somehow makes more calcium available to the contractile proteins so that tension development increases. Possibly more calcium is available to interact with troponin-C; thus, the first action potential after a stretch releases more calcium from intracellular stores (Lab, 1982). More probably the cross-bridges are more sensitive to any given calcium ion concentration (Housmans *et al.*, 1983). Therefore, according to the current concepts, both the Frank–Starling law and an inotropic stimulus ultimately increase the contractile performance of the heart by increasing the availability of cytosolic calcium ions to the contractile apparatus.

Summary

The energy that is needed to sustain the contractile activity of the heart comes from the hydrolysis of ATP. The particular ATPase that is involved in contraction is located in the myosin head. In diastole the interaction between actin and myosin is suppressed because of an inhibitory effect exerted by troponin-I which forms part of the troponin complex. Other parts of the troponin complex include troponin-T (which binds the complex to tropomyosin) and troponin-C, which is a calcium receptor. When calcium is supplied to troponin-C during systole the inhibitory effect of troponin-I is overcome, and actin and myosin can then associate; thus the actin-induced increase of the myosin ATPase activity takes place.

The physical nature of the actin–myosin interaction involves steps in which the attached heads pull the thin filaments a very small distance towards the center of the sarcomeres in which they occur, before detaching and re-attaching further along the thin filament to repeat the cross-bridge cycle. During the detachment stage of one cross-bridge, tension is maintained by other cross-bridges which are attached during that time. During a single heart beat, tension develops by recruitment of more and more cross-bridge cycles as the cytosolic calcium concentration rises to a peak, to be followed by relaxation as the cross-bridge cycling activity diminishes in response to a falling calcium concentration.

References

Barany M (1967). ATPase activity of myosin correlated with speed of muscle shortening. J Gen Physiol 50: 197–218.

Borg TK, Caulfield JB (1981). The collagen matrix of the heart. Fed Proc 40: 2037–2041.

Bricknell OL, Daries PS, Opie LH (1981). A relationship between adenosine triphosphate, glycolysis and ischemic contracture in the isolated rat heart. J Molec Cell Cardiol 13: 941–945.

Brutsaert DL, Housmans PR, Goethals MA (1980). Dual control of relaxation: its role in venticular function in the mammalian heart. Circ Res 47: 637–652.

Eisenberg E, Greene LE (1980). The relation of muscle biochemistry to muscle physiology. Ann Rev Physiol 42: 293–309.

England PJ (1984). The significance of cardiac myosin light chain phosphorylation. J Molec Cell Cardiol 16: 591–595.

Housmans PR, Lee NKM, Blinks JR (1983). Active shortening retards the decline of the intracellular calcium transient in mammalian heart muscle. Science 221: 159–161.

Huxley HE (1969). The mechanism of muscular contraction. Science 164: 1356–1361.

Katz AM (1970). Contractile proteins of the heart. Physiol Rev 50: 63–158.

Katz AM (1977). Physiology of the Heart, pp 146, 152, 153. Raven Press, New York.

Kopp SJ, Barany M (1979). Phosphorylation of the 19 000-dalton light chain of myosin in perfused rat heart under the influence of negative and positive inotropic agents. J Biol Chem 254: 12007–12012.

Lab M (1982). Contraction–excitation feedback in myocardium. Circ Res 50: 757–766.

Lymn RW, Taylor EW (1971). Mechanism of adenosine triphosphate hydrolysis by actomyosin. Biochem 10: 4617–4624.

Murphy RA (1983). Contraction of muscle cells. In: Physiology. Eds RM Berne, MN Levy, pp 359–386. CV Mosby, St Louis.

Noble MIM, Pollack GH (1977). Controversies in cardiovascular research: molecular mechanisms of contraction. Circ Res 40: 333–342.

Perry SV (1979). The regulation of contractile activity in muscle. Biochem Soc Trans 7: 593–617.

Resink TJ, Gevers W (1981). Altered adenosine triphosphatase activities of natural actomyosin from rat hearts perfused with isoprenaline and ouabain. Cell Calcium 2: 105–123.

Ross J Jr, Sonnenblick EH, Taylor RR, Spotnitz HN, Covell JW (1971). Diastolic geometry and sarcomere length in the chronically dilated canine left ventricle. Circ Res 28: 49–61.

Samuel JL, Rappaport L, Mercadier JJ, Lompre AM, Sartore S, Triban C, Schiaffino S, Schwartz K (1983). Distribution of myosin isoenzymes within single cardiac cells: an immunohistochemical study. Circ Res 52: 200–209.

Sonnenblick FH, Skelton CL (1974). Reconsideration of the ultrastructural basis of cardiac length-tension relations. Circ Res 35: 517–526.

Squire JM (1981). The Structural Basis of Muscular Contraction, pp. 471–521, Plenum Press, New York.

Ter Keurs HED (1983). Calcium and contractility. In: Cardiac Metabolism. Ed. AJ Drake-Holland, MIM Noble, pp 73–99. John Wiley, England.

Yanagida T, Nakase M, Nishiyama K, Oosawa F (1984). Direct observation of single F-actin filaments in the presence of myosin. Nature 307: 58–60.

II | Energy Metabolism and Ventricular Function

Fuels

Knowledge of the fuels of the human heart started with the introduction of coronary sinus catheterization by Bing and his associates in 1947 (Bing, 1954). The chemical composition of arterial blood entering the heart was compared with that of coronary sinus blood leaving the heart. Glucose, lactate and fatty acids were established as the heart's major sources of energy. According to the condition selected, each substrate could be the chief provider of energy.

A substrate is, strictly speaking, a molecule which

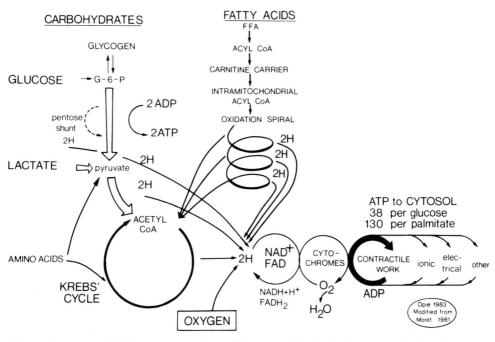

Fig. 9-1 The major myocardial fuels are carbohydrates (glucose and lactate) and non-esterified free fatty acids (FFA). Ultimately all fuels are broken down to acetyl CoA which produces hydrogen atoms (H) by various dehydrogenases to form NADH$_2$ (NADH + H$^+$) which interacts with the cytochrome chain to produce ATP. Fatty acids also produce FADH$_2$ from the oxidation spiral, which likewise enters the cytochrome chain.

an enzyme converts by its catalytic function to the products of the reaction. As each energy source— glucose, lactate, fatty acid—requires enzymatic conversion before further breakdown, the term "substrate" can be used to indicate a fuel of the heart (Fig. 9-1).

The uptake of various substrates by the heart is dependent on the arterial concentration of the fuel concerned, and increasing the contribution of any one substrate leads to a decrease contribution by the others. How did Bing's observations fit into general advances in the biological sciences?

Pasteur Effect and Anaerobic Glycolysis

In the nineteenth century Pasteur studied the oxygen metabolism of micro-organisms. When the oxygen supply was adequate there were low rates of glucose uptake, but when the oxygen supply was inadequate

"fermentation" was accelerated. Today we would regard fermentation as those processes which keep the cells alive in the absence of oxygen, i.e. anaerobic glycolysis.

When the oxygen supply to the heart is normal, the rate of glycolysis is inhibited by high levels of citrate and ATP formed by oxidative metabolism in the citrate cycle (Randle and Morgan, 1962). When there is anoxia, or severe hypoxia, then oxidative metabolism ceases, citrate and ATP levels fall and glycolysis is stimulated. This feedback mechanism is the Pasteur effect (Fig. 9-2). But when there is not only extreme hypoxia but also poor blood flow (ischemia) then products of glycolysis accumulate, the protons and lactate inhibit glycolysis (Fig. 9-2) and glucose utilization falls (Fig.9-3). Because glycolysis can provide energy even in the absence of oxygen (anaerobic energy), the inhibition of the Pasteur effect by severe ischemia limits the capacity of the tissue to survive the ischemic insult.

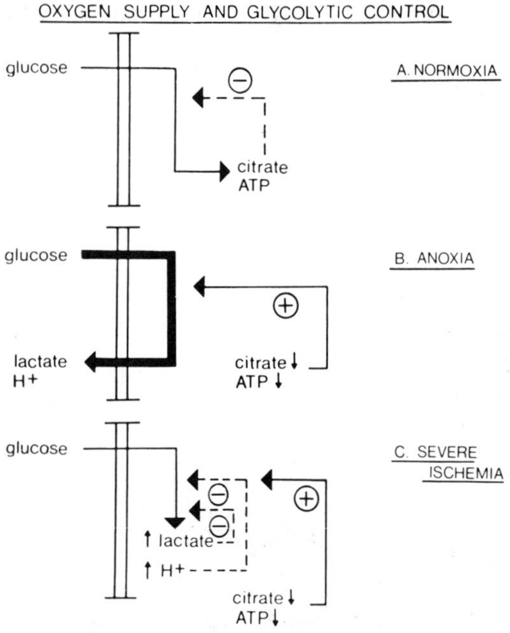

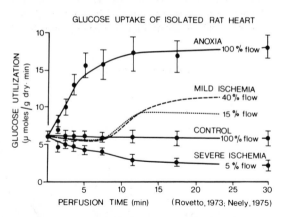

Fig. 9-3   Effect of coronary flow rate on glucose uptake of isolated perfused rat heart. Note the increased glucose uptake during anoxia with maintained coronary flow and washout of inhibitory metabolites (Panel B, Fig. 9-2). Coronary flow worsens and ischemia progresses; inhibitory products of anaerobic glycolysis accumulate so that the glucose uptake falls progressively. For data sources see Rovetto et al. (1973) and Neely et al. (1975). These approximate values for coronary flow, based on isolated rat heart data, cannot directly be extrapolated to man.

OXYGEN SUPPLY AND GLYCOLYTIC CONTROL

Fig. 9-2   A. In the normally oxygenated heart, tissue citrate and ATP are high and inhibit glycolysis. B. When oxygen is removed (hypoxia or anoxia) but the coronary flow rate allowed to increase, the Pasteur effect results. C. In severe ischemia (deprivation of both oxygen and coronary flow) the accumulation of lactate and protons inhibits glycolysis despite any tendency to acceleration by a low cardiac content of citrate and ATP.

Competition for Available Oxygen Supply

Fisher and Williamson (1961), working with Krebs, established an important general principle: in conditions when an adequate coronary flow ensures that the supplies of substrate and of oxygen to the heart were adequate, then the various substrates compete for oxygen. A specific example is that free fatty acids suppress the oxidation of glucose and are a major fuel of the human heart in the fasted state. High levels of tissue citrate, formed during fatty acid oxidation, inhibit the pathway of glycolysis (Fig. 9-2).

The principles of competition between fuels of the heart are ultimately based on the metabolic properties of red and white muscle (Opie, 1968).

Red versus white muscle
Muscles can be divided into two extreme types, red and white, the red muscles being used for continuous activity and the white for short bursts of intense activity. These have different metabolic, physiological and biochemical properties. The extreme example of white muscle is the chicken breast muscle, used rarely but then vigorously for a burst of flying. An extreme example of red muscle is the mammalian heart, called on to sustain high levels of muscular activity over a prolonged period. The activities of key enzymes of glycolysis are different in white and red muscles (Fig. 9-4). White muscle can function anaerobically and has the enzymes present for "reversed glycolysis" so that some of the products of a spurt of glycolysis can be removed by resynthesis of glycogen.

In white muscle, the activities of the enzymes of glycogen synthesis (fructose 1,6-bisphosphatase and phosphoenolpyruvate carboxykinase) are similar to those in liver and kidney cortex, which are the major gluconeogenic tissues of the body. In red muscle such as heart, the enzymes of glycolysis are lower in activity, glycolysis is a much less important source of energy and mitochondrial metabolism plays a correspondingly **more important role. There is no synthesis of glycogen from pyruvate because of the absence of the appropriate enzymes (Fig. 9-4). Substrates which only yield energy by mitochondrial metabolism, such as lactate and free fatty acids, are "preferred" as fuels to glucose which can yield additional energy by glycolysis.**

Substrate Oxidation

Oxygen extraction ratio

How did Bing know which substrates were most important for the oxidative metabolism of the heart? Taking the equations for full oxidation of the various substrates (Table 9-1), it is possible to calculate how much oxygen would be used up by the amount of each substrate extracted by the heart. The essential measurements required are the simultaneous arteriovenous differences (arterial vs coronary sinus blood) of glucose, lactate, pyruvate, free fatty acid and oxygen.

RED MUSCLE: ONE-WAY GLYCOLYSIS

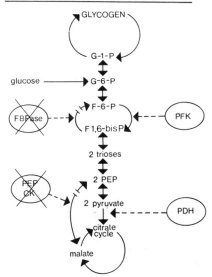

Fig. 9-4 In red muscle, of which the heart is an extreme example, there is "one-way" glycolysis. Note that enzymes for "two-way" glycolysis in white muscle are absent. G-1-P = glucose 1-phosphate; G-6-P = glucose 6-phosphate; F-6-P = fructose 6-phosphate; F1,6-bisP = fructose 1,6-bisphosphate; FBPase = fructose 1,6-bisphosphatase; PFK = phosphofructokinase; PEPCK = phosphoenolpyruvate carboxykinase; PDH = pyruvate dehydrogenase.

Table 9-1

Equations used in the calculation of oxygen extraction ratios

1. $C_6H_{12}O_6 + 6\,O_2 \longrightarrow 6\,CO_2 + 6\,H_2O$
2. $CH_3COCOOH + 2\tfrac{1}{2}\,O_2 \longrightarrow 2\,H_2O + 3\,CO_2$
3. $CH_3CHOHCOOH + 3\,O_2 \longrightarrow 3\,H_2O + 3\,CO_2$
4. $CH_3(CH_2)_{14}COOH + 23\,O_2 \longrightarrow 16\,CO_2 + 16\,H_2O$

1 = glucose, 2 = pyruvic acid, 3 = lactic acid, 4 = palmitic acid.

For convenience the un-ionized forms have been shown; in reality it is the ionized forms (e.g. lactate, pyruvate, palmitate) that are oxidized.

Respiratory quotient

A cruder estimate of the type of fuel used by the heart can be obtained by the respiratory quotient, which is calculated by comparing the rate of oxygen uptake with the rate of production of carbon dioxide. Thus a respiratory quotient of near to one implies oxidation of glucose and/or lactate (Table 9-2), whereas a low value implies fatty acid oxidation. Because the myocardial respiratory quotient was frequently low, early workers were alerted to the importance of oxidation of lipid even before blood fatty acid concentrations could be measured.

Table 9-2

Respiratory quotient (RQ) values for various substrates

Substrate	RQ
Glucose	1.0
Lactate	1.0
Pyruvate	0.83
Palmitate	0.70

Respiratory quotient = ratio of number of molecules of oxygen taken up to carbon dioxide produced; see Table 9-1.

Energy yield

Chemical equations can give yet another useful piece of information, namely the energy yield per molecule. Such data are calculated from a detailed analysis of the pathways of oxidation of each compound. Quite the highest yield of ATP per molecule is from a fatty acid such as palmitate (Table 9-3), which is easy to explain because many of the carbon atoms in carbohydrates are partially oxidized by virtue of the oxygen in the molecule (Table 9-1). The fatty acid

Table 9-3

Comparative energy yields of various fuels per molecule fully oxidized

Molecule	ATP yield per molecule	ATP yield per carbon atom	ATP yield per oxygen atom taken up
Glucose	38	6.3	3.17
Lactate	18	6.0	3.00
Pyruvate	15	5.0	3.00
Palmitate	129	8.0	2.80

SUBSTRATE METABOLISM: FASTING

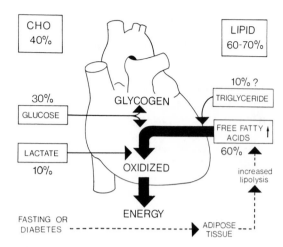

Fig. 9-5 Patterns of substrate metabolism when blood levels of free fatty acids are high as in the fasted state (or poorly controlled diabetes mellitus). High levels of blood free fatty acids are oxidized by the heart in preference to glucose and lactate. Utilization of lipid accounts for 60–70 percent of the oxygen uptake of the heart, whereas utilization of carbohydrate accounts for 40 percent. Potential errors in the indirect methods used mean that the sum of the oxidation extraction rations (Table 9-1) will not exactly equal 100 percent.

SUBSTRATE METABOLISM: GLUCOSE FEEDING

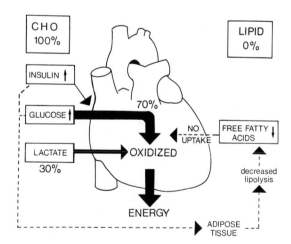

Fig. 9-6 After a high carbohydrate meal or glucose feeding, blood glucose and insulin are high and blood free fatty acids low. Glucose becomes the major fuel of the heart and carbohydrate can account for 100 percent of the oxygen uptake.

molecules contain little oxygen and therefore can yield more ATP for each carbon atom. The disadvantages of fatty acids as fuel is that for each molecule of ATP produced they need relatively more oxygen (Table 9-3). Experimentally, a heart using fatty acid alone would need about 17 percent more oxygen to produce the same amount of ATP than when using only glucose.

The molecular explanation for the relatively poor ATP yield of fatty acids per oxygen taken up, is that each turn of the fatty acid spiral yields equal amounts of $FADH_2$ and $NADH_2$. $FADH_2$ enters the respiratory chain further along than $NADH_2$ and yields less ATP (see Chapter 11). Such processes account for part of the "oxygen-wasting" capacity of fatty acids; in addition, when fatty acids are presented in excess to the heart or when fatty acids cannot be fully oxidized as in ischemia, then fatty acids can "waste" even more oxygen (Chapter 10).

Substrate Metabolism of Human Heart

In man, the major substrates are carbohydrates and lipids (Table 9-1). In the fasted state, blood free fatty acids are high. Rates of uptake of fatty acids are also high and inhibit the oxidation of glucose by the heart (Fig. 9-5), so that fatty acids become the major source of energy (Opie, 1968; Neely and Morgan, 1974). When fatty acids are oxidized the glucose taken is increasingly converted to glycogen—the "glucose-sparing" of fatty acid oxidation.

Little is known about the effect of feeding on the metabolism of the human heart; hence this situation must be inferred from animal data. In animals, an infusion of glucose raises the respiratory quotient to unity, which suggests total reliance on carbohydrate. When glucose and insulin are infused to represent the carbohydrate-fed state (Fig. 9-6), circulating fatty acid values are suppressed, the uptake of fatty acids by the heart falls, the inhibition of glycolysis by fatty acids is removed and glucose oxidation increases. In this way the heart can "see-saw" between carbohydrate in the carbohydrate-fed state and fatty acids in the fasted state as the major sources of energy.

In patients who have just taken a high-fat meal of cream and cheese, there is a marked rise in blood triglycerides during the post-prandial lipemia. Triglyceride is converted by the enzyme lipoprotein lipase to free fatty acids which then enter the pathways of fatty acid oxidation (Fig. 9-7). In these exceptional

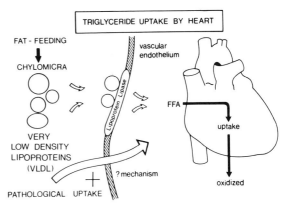

Fig. 9-7 After fat-feeding, there is a lipemia with increased circulating chylomicra and low-density lipoproteins, both converted by lipoprotein lipase to free fatty acids (FFA) which join the myocardial pathways for fatty acid metabolism. After infusions of ethanol and epinephrine there is increased uptake of triglyceride which must still be broken down to fatty acid to be metabolized.

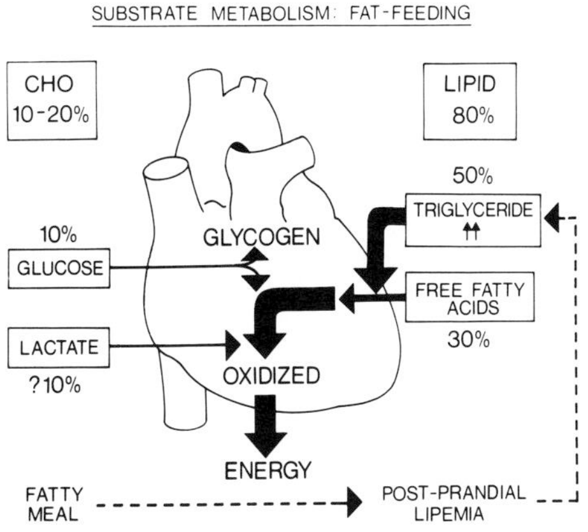

Fig. 9-8 After fat-feeding, or intravenous infusions of triglyceride, the myocardial metabolism shifts in favor of triglycerides which become the major fuel.

circumstances triglyceride becomes the major myocardial fuel (Fig. 9-8).

During exercise the blood lactate rises and lactate becomes the major fuel. Lactate inhibits the oxidation of glucose and the uptake of free fatty acids, each of which now contribute only 15–20 percent of the energy needs of the heart during exercise (Fig.9-9).

Ketone bodies are not a major substrate of the normal human heart. Even after an overnight fast, when the circulating ketone concentration is about 0.1–0.3 mM, the uptake of ketones can account for

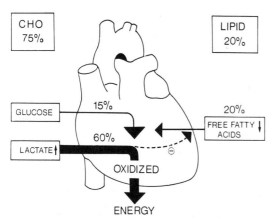

SUBSTRATE METABOLISM: EXERCISE

CHO 75%

LIPID 20%

GLUCOSE

LACTATE ↑

15%

60%

20%
FREE FATTY ACIDS ↓

OXIDIZED

ENERGY

Fig. 9-9 During acute exercise the blood lactate rises and lactate becomes the major fuel of the heart. Lactate inhibits the uptake of free fatty acids. Carbohydrate can account for 70 percent of the oxygen uptake. CHO = carbohydrate.

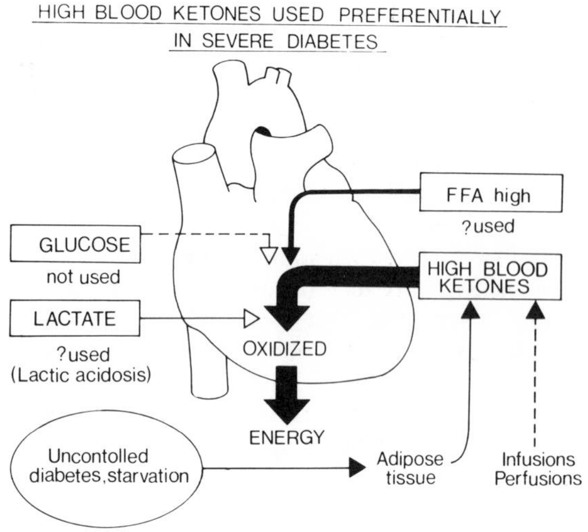

HIGH BLOOD KETONES USED PREFERENTIALLY IN SEVERE DIABETES

GLUCOSE
not used

LACTATE
?used
(Lactic acidosis)

FFA high
?used

HIGH BLOOD KETONES

OXIDIZED

ENERGY

Uncontolled diabetes, starvation

Adipose tissue   Infusions Perfusions

Fig. 9-10 Only when blood ketone body concentrations are very high, as in diabetic ketosis, are ketone bodies thought to be the major fuel of the human heart.

Table 9-4

Effect of nutritional state and exercise on fuel for oxidative metabolism of the human heart

Conditions	Glucose (OER %)	Pyruvate (OER %)	Lactate (OER %)	Total (CHO %)	FFA (OER %)	TG (OER %)	Ketones (OER %)	Amino acids (OER %)
Glucose + insulin; feeding	—	—	—	92	very low	—	—	—
Post-prandial	68	4	28	100	very low	—	—	—
Fasting few hours	31	2	28	61	34	—	—	—
Same, during exercise	16	0	61	77	21	—	—	—
Same, recovery from exercise	21	2	36	59	36	—	—	—
Resting, fasting overnight	17	1	11	38	59	14	very low	very low

For details, see Opie (1984).
— = absence of data; OER = oxygen extraction ratio; CHO = carbohydrate; FFA = free fatty acids = NEFA = non-esterified fatty acids; TG = triglyceride.

only 2–9 percent of the total myocardial oxygen uptake during rest and for even less during exercise. Probably ketones only contribute significantly to the energy metabolism of the heart in severe diabetic ketosis (Fig. 9-10).

It needs to be emphasized that such substrate "balance-sheets" depend on at least four measurements—an arterial and coronary sinus concentration of each substrate and of oxygen. Steady-state conditions are essential for correct analyses. Thus there are potential sources of error, especially during conditions such as exercise when arterial values may be changing rapidly. All the values shown in the Figures and in Table 9-4 are, therefore, only approximate and need not necessarily add up to 100 percent.

Summary

In certain well-defined situations, studies in steady-state conditions show that free fatty acids are the major fuel in the fasted state, glucose in the carbohydrate-fed state, triglyceride in the fast-fed state, lactate during acute exercise and ketones in ketotic diabetes.

The contribution of any given fuel to the oxidative metabolism of the heart varies throughout the day and probably even from minute to minute with changes of posture or exercise. In the case of glucose, the contribution to the energy needs of the heart might vary from 10 percent after a fat meal to 70 percent after a carbohydrate meal. To achieve such variations requires complex mechanisms to control the rate of glucose uptake and glycolysis, as will be considered in the next chapters.

References

Bing RJ (1954). The metabolism of the heart. Harvey Lecture Series 50: pp 27–70, Academic Press, Orlando, New York and London.

Fisher RB, Williamson JR (1961). The effects of insulin, adrenaline and nutrients on the oxygen uptake of the perfused rat heart. J Physiol 158: 102–112.

Neely JR, Morgan HE (1974). Relationship between carbohydrate and lipid metabolism and the energy balance of heart muscle. Ann Rev Physiol 36: 413–459.

Neely JR, Liedtke AJ, Whitmer JT, Rovetto MJ (1975). Relationship between coronary flow and adenosine triphosphate production from glycolysis and oxidative metabolism. In: Recent Advances in Studies on Cardiac Structure and Metabolism. Vol 8. The Sarcoplasm. Eds. PR Roy, P Harris, pp 301–321, University Park Press, Baltimore.

Opie LH (1968). Metabolism of the heart in health and disease. Am Heart J 76: 685–698.

Opie LH (1984). Substrate and energy metabolism of the heart. In: Function of the Heart in Normal and Pathological States. Ed. N. Sperelakis, pp 301–336, Martinus Nijhoff, New York.

Randle MJ, Morgan HE (1962). Regulation of glucose uptake by muscle. Vitamins Horm 20: 199–249.

Rovetto MJ, Whitmer JT, Neely JR (1973). Comparison of effects of anoxia and whole heart ischemia on carbohydrate utilization in isolated working rat hearts. Circ Res 22: 699–711.

New References

Opie LH (1984). Substrate and energy metabolism of the heart. In: Physiology and Pathophysiology of the Heart. Ed. N Sperelakis, pp 301–336, Nijhoff, Boston.

10 | Carbohydrates and Lipids

The heart is a scavenger, taking whatever fuel it can from the circulating blood according to what is delivered. There are complex intracellular control mechanisms which help to regulate the rates of the various pathways converting these fuels to acetyl CoA—the next step being further metabolism in the citrate cycle.

During the **uptake of glucose** by the heart from the bloodstream, its rate of transport across the sarcolemma is controlled by the **glucose carrier** which is stereospecific and "prefers" glucose to other circulating sugars. The carrier requires no energy for transport because the glucose concentration in the extracellular space is so much higher than in the cytosol. Rather, a small amount of energy seems to be required to keep glucose out of the cell (Randle and Smith, 1958). When glucose transport is increased by hypoxia, as in the Pasteur effect (see Fig. 9-2), or by increased heart work (Fig. 10-1), then it may be the breakdown of ATP that is the signal. In contrast, insulin increases the number of glucose carriers without involving ATP. Insulin binds to specific **insulin receptors** (Larner et al., 1981) thereby (it is thought) generating a "second messenger" peptide or acting on a membrane-bound protein kinase. As a result, the number of glucose carriers at the surface is increased at the expense of intracellular "masked" carriers.

The uptake of glucose increases whenever glucose transport into the cell rises as during hypoxia, increased heart work, or in the fed state. All these conditions also enhance glycolysis. Conversely, the uptake of glucose is reduced by all those factors inhibiting glycolysis—the fasted state, a low work load, severe ischemia and uncontrolled diabetes mellitus.

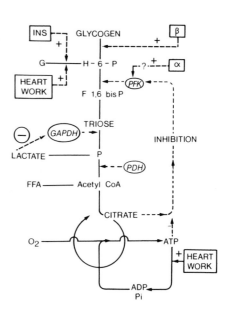

Fig. 10-1 In the well-oxygenated heart glucose uptake and glycolysis can be accelerated by heart work (substrate: glucose) and partially inhibited by fatty acid oxidation. G-6-P = glucose 6-phosphate; PFK = phosphofructokinase; PDH = pyruvate dehydrogenase; P = pyruvate; Ins = insulin; GAPDH = glyceraldehyde 3-biphosphate dehydrogenase; F 1,6 bisP = fructose 1,6-biphosphate; FFA = free fatty acids; G = glucose.

Pathways of Glycolysis

By glycolysis is generally meant that metabolic pathway common to glucose uptake and glycogen

Table 10-1

Reactions of glycolysis (the enzyme for each reaction is in brackets)

1. **Hexosephosphate pathways: utilization of ATP**
   1. Glucose + ATP → glucose 6-phosphate + ADP ....(hexokinase)
   2. Glucose 6-phosphate $\rightleftharpoons$ fructose 6-phosphate ....(hexosephosphate isomerase)
   3. Fructose 6-phosphate + ATP → fructose 1,6-bisphosphate + ADP.....................(phosphofructokinase)

2. **Triose pathways: production of O_2-independent ATP**
   1. Fructose 1,6-bisphosphate $\rightleftharpoons$ glyceraldehyde 3-P + dihydroxyacetone-P............................(aldolase)
   2. Glyceraldehye 3-P $\rightleftharpoons$ dihydroxyacetone-P..(triose phosphate isomerase)
   3. Two glyceraldehyde 3-phosphate + two NAD^+ + two P_i →
      two 1,3 diphosphoglycerate + two NADH + two H^+ ....(glyceraldehyde 3-phosphate dehydrogenase)
   4. Two 1,3-diphosphoglycerate + 2 ADP → 3-phosphoglycerate + 2 ATP..............(phosphoglycerate kinase)
   5. Two 3-phosphoglycerate $\rightleftharpoons$ two 2-phosphoglycerate................................(phosphoglyceromutase)
   6. Two 2-phosphoglycerate $\rightleftharpoons$ two phosphoenolpyruvate + H_2O ....(enolase)
   7. Two phosphoenolpyruvate + 2 ADP → two pyruvate + 2 ATP ....(pyruvate kinase)

3. **Anaerobic pathways: utilization of $NADH^+$ + H^+**
   1. Two pyruvate + 2 NADH + 2 H^+ → two lactate + 2 NAD^+ ....(lactate dehydrogenase)
   2. Two dihydroxyacetone-P + 2 NADH + 2 H^+ → two L-glycerol 3-phosphate + 2 NAD^+.....................
      ....|(glycerol phosphate dehydrogenase) (L-glycerol 3-phosphate = α-glycerol phosphate)

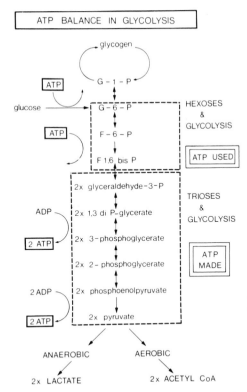

Fig. 10-2 Glycolysis produces 4 ATP per molecule of glucose 6-phosphate (G-6-P) converted to two molecules of pyruvate. Glycolysis uses up 2 molecules of ATP. Glycolysis from glycogen uses up one molecule of ATP.

breakdown which produces lactate in anaerobic conditions, or under conditions where the mitochondrial capacity to handle the glycogen flux is inadequate (Table 10-1). During normal oxidative metabolism, glycolysis yields pyruvate which is then broken down aerobically in the citrate cycle (adequate mitochondrial capacity); this process may be termed aerobic glycolysis. An important function of glycolysis is to produce ATP independently of oxygen.

The pathways of glycolysis can be divided into two stages (Fig. 10-2). Glycolysis first converts glucose 6-phosphate (rapidly formed from intracellular glucose by **hexokinase**) into a compound containing two phosphate groups, fructose 1,6-diphosphate(= fructose 1,6-bisphosphate). Thereafter, glycolysis converts each six carbon hexose-phosphate into two three-carbon triose-phosphates, eventually forming pyruvate. In the first stage, two molecules of ATP are used per glucose molecule converted to two triose-phosphate molecules. In the second stage, four molecules of ATP are made independently of oxygen for each glucose 6-phosphate ultimately converted to pyruvate.

Phosphofructokinase

The flow through glycolysis (glycolytic flux) can vary greatly by a factor of about 10-fold, comparing the potassium-arrested heart with that working maximally in the presence of insulin. Although many enzymes

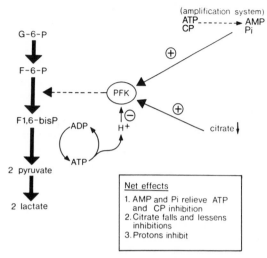

PHOSPHOFRUCTOKINASE (PFK) ACTIVITY:
LIMITED ACTIVATION IN SEVERE ISCHEMIA

Net effects
1. AMP and Pi relieve ATP and CP inhibition
2. Citrate falls and lessens inhibitions
3. Protons inhibit

Fig. 10-3 Phosphofructokinase (PFK) activity is stimulated by the fall of ATP and creatine phosphate (CP) in ischemia as well as by the rise of adenosine monophosphate (AMP) and of inorganic phosphate (P_i). The fall of citrate also stimulates, but accumulation of protons inhibits the enzyme.

participate in the reactions of the glycolytic pathway, only a few actually regulate the flux. Of great importance is the role of phosphofructokinase (PFK, Fig. 10-3); when its activity increases as in hypoxia, glucose 6-phosphate is converted at an increased rate via fructose 6-phosphate to fructose 1,6-bisphosphate:

$$glucose\ 6\text{-}phosphate \longrightarrow fructose\ 6\text{-}phosphate$$
$$fructose\ 6\text{-}phosphate + ATP \longrightarrow$$
$$fructose\ 1,6\ bisphosphate + ADP$$

The phosphofructokinase reaction, because it uses ATP, is not reversible, while the enzyme governing the reverse process, fructose 1,6-bisphosphate, is absent from the heart. Hence the activity of phosphofructokinase acts as a unidirectional valve to help regulate the rate of glycolysis. As increased activity of phosphofructokinase causes the cellular content of glucose 6-phosphate to fall, the normal inhibition of hexokinase by glucose 6-phosphate is lessened, more glucose is phosphorylated and more glucose is taken up. In contrast, the activity of phosphofructokinase can be inhibited when the oxidation of alternate fuels such as fatty acid or lactate produces excess **citrate** (Fig. 10-1), and the reverse series of events occurs.

Table 10-2

Major factors controlling glycolysis and sites of action

Conditions	Glucose uptake	Glyco-gen	Phos-pho-fructo-kinase	Pyru-vate dehydro-genase
Increased heart work	+	↓	+	+
Inotropic agents	+	↓	+	+
Fed state, insulin	+	↑	+	+
Starvation, fatty acids, ketones	–	↑	–	–
Hypoxia, mild ischemia	+	↓	+	–
Severe ischemia	–	↓	–	–

+ = stimulation; – = inhibition; ↓ = decreased content; ↑ = increased content.

There is thus co-ordinated intracellular control of glucose uptake, glucose phosphorylation and activity of phosphofructokinase which can all speed up or slow down simultaneously (Table 10-2).

The phosphofructokinase reaction is ideally suited for metabolic control of glycolysis because it is so sensitive to the energy status of the myocardial cells. Low molecular weight metabolites such as ATP, AMP, ADP and P_i interact with the enzyme at **allosteric sites** which are distant from the site of interaction between substrates and enzyme. During hypoxia and mild ischemia ATP levels fall, those of ADP and AMP rise, as does that of P_i (Fig. 10-3); these changes enhance the activity of the enzyme (increased anaerobic glycolysis). During severe ischemia, intracellular acidosis inhibits the enzyme thereby explaining the rapid inhibition of glycolysis (another factor being the inhibition of glyceraldehyde 3-phosphate dehydrogenase, see next section).

Glyceraldehyde 3-phosphate dehydrogenase

Initially the regulation of glycolysis was largely explained by altered regulation at the level of phosphofructokinase. Another important control step is that regulating the flow through glycolysis at the level of the enzyme glyceraldehyde 3-phosphate dehydrogenase (Mochizuki and Neely, 1979). Glyceraldehyde 3-phosphate is produced as fructose 1,6-bisphosphate is split by the enzyme **aldolase** into two triose-phosphate (three-carbon) units, the other triose being dihydroxyacetone phosphate. The rate of conversion of glyceraldehyde 3-phosphate to 1,3-diphosphoglycerate (= 3-phosphoglyceryl phosphate) is important because its activity in severely ischemic tissue is inhibited by the end products of anaerobic glycolysis such as lactate, protons and $NADH_2$ (Fig. 10-4).

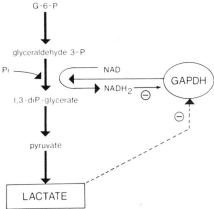

GLYCOLYSIS IN SEVERE ISCHEMIA LIMITED BY GLYCERALDEHYDE 3-P DEHYDROGENASE

Fig. 10-4 During severe ischemia, products of glycolysis (NADH, lactate) accumulate and inhibit glyceraldehyde 3-phosphate dehydrogenase (GAPDH).

Anaerobic Glycolysis and Disposal of NADH₂

One major difference between **anaerobic** (lacking oxygen) and oxidative metabolism is the method of disposal of $NADH_2$—the reduced form of the cofactor nicotinamide adenine dinucleotide (NAD) which can exist in either oxidized (NAD^+) or reduced ($NADH_2$) forms. The hydrogen atoms contained in fuels such as glucose must first convert NAD to $NADH_2$ before passing the electrons along the cytochrome chain to produce ATP (Fig. 10-5), and eventually to form water. Glycolysis produces two $NADH_2$ molecules (each of which ionizes at pH 7.0 into NAD^+ and H^+) for every molecule of glucose 6-phosphate ultimately converted to pyruvate. If $NADH_2$ accumulates, it will reduce pyruvate to lactate by means of the reaction catalyzed by lactate dehydrogenase and thereby prevent pyruvate oxidation. A much less important effect of $NADH_2$

accumulation is to convert dihydroxyacetone to alpha-glycerol phosphate which is a potential precursor for triglyceride formation (see Fig. 10-19). During normal aerobic respiration $NADH_2$ is transferred chiefly by the malate–aspartate shuttle to within the mitochondria so that NAD forms again by yielding 2H to the respiratory chain (Fig. 10-6).

NADH₂ during anaerobic glycolysis

In contrast, during anaerobic metabolism $NADH_2$ produced by glycolysis cannot be oxidized so that pyruvate is reduced to form lactate thus using up $NADH_2$ (Fig. 10-7):

Glycolysis + 2 NAD → 2 pyruvates + 2 $NADH_2$
2 Pyruvates + 2 $NADH_2$ → 2 lactates + 2 NAD

The natural tendency of the lactate–pyruvate reaction is to be at equilibrium. As lactate accumulates relative to pyruvate, so will $NADH_2$ rise relative to NAD to attempt to maintain equilibrium:

$$(L)/(P) = K (NADH)(H^+)/(NAD^+)$$

where K is the equilibrium constant. During anaerobiosis mitochondrial $NADH_2$ accumulates so that cytosolic $NADH_2$ mounts and cytosolic pyruvate is converted to lactate. Couples of compounds (like lactate and pyruvate) which react to the state of oxidation of the myocardium are called **redox couples**. Formation of lactate is therefore usually a sign of myocardial hypoxia. $NADH_2$ also convert dihydroxyacetone phosphate to alpha glycerol phosphate (Fig. 10-19).

Proton production by glycolysis

The above equations show that when lactate forms during anaerobic glycolysis, as much $NADH_2$ is used as is made. No hydrogen ions (protons) are produced. The change from NAD to $NADH_2$

$$2H + NAD \rightarrow NADH_2$$

is more correctly given as:

$$2H + NAD^+ \rightarrow NADH + H^+$$

Thus the reduction of NAD^+ requires the addition of two hydrogen atoms which are derived from glycolysis. The protons produced are handled together with NADH (hence the first equation is usually used in this book to avoid confusion). Why is anaerobic glycolysis usually held to be

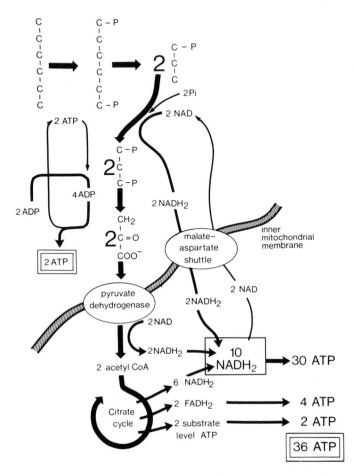

Fig. 10-5 Production of 38 ATP (36 in mitochondria, 2 in cytosol) during complete oxidative metabolism of glucose. Continued disposal of cytosolic NADH$_2$, formed by aerobic glycolysis, by transfer into mitochondria is required.

proton-producing and the potential cause of myocardial acidosis?

When all the charges are written into the individual glycolytic reactions and allowance is made for the probable degree of binding of ADP and ATP with magnesium and the intracellular pH, the following approximations are derived (Gevers, 1977):

$$\text{glucose} + 2 \text{ MgADP}^{1-} + 2 \text{ P}_1^{2-} \longrightarrow$$
$$2 \text{ lactate}^{1-} + 2 \text{ MgATP}^{2-}$$

In anaerobic conditions, all ATP produced will be broken down so that protons are produced from ATP:

$$2 \text{ MgATP}^{2-} \longrightarrow 2 \text{ MgADP}^{1-} + 2 \text{ P}_i^{2-} + 2 \text{ H}^+$$

Thus glycolytically made ATP (and not lactate) is the "source" of the protons produced during anaerobic glycolysis. Concomitant production of lactate and protons yields "lactic acid".

Function of Glycolysis in Normal Heart

In the normal well-oxygenated (aerobic) heart, free fatty acids or lactate can be the major source of energy

MALATE – ASPARTATE CYCLE

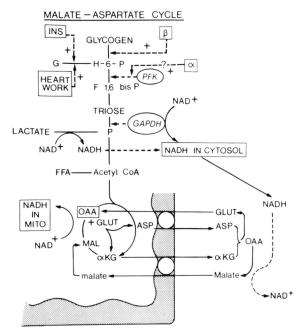

Fig. 10-6 Details of the malate–aspartate cycle. GLUT = glutamate; ASP = aspartate; OAA = oxaloacetate; αKG = alpha-ketoglutarate. For other abbreviations see Fig. 10-1. Taken from Opie (1984), with permission.

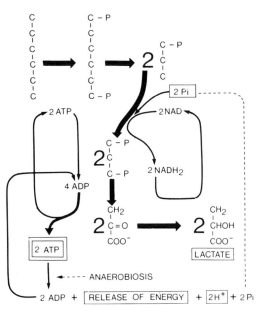

ENERGY BALANCE DURING ANAEROBIC METABOLISM OF GLUCOSE

Fig. 10-7 During anaerobic metabolism of glucose, 4 ATP molecules are made while 2 are used. $NADH_2$ is re-utilized in the conversion of pyruvate to lactate. Protons are produced by the breakdown of ATP.

and the function of such **aerobic glycolysis** may appear obscure. Yet even when glycolysis is inhibited by fatty acids or by lactate, glucose remains an important fuel for the heart, providing 30 percent of the energy needs of the heart in the fasted state and up to 70 percent after a carbohydrate meal. After a high fat meal glucose still accounts for about 10 percent of the oxygen uptake. It is not known if the low remaining rates of glycolytic flux have a function. This residual flux may merely keep the pathway open so as to accelerate more easily during the onset of a sudden increase of heart work.

A second possible function of glycolysis is to provide a rapid source of extra energy during sudden bursts of heart work. When heart work is increased by exercise, the rapid acceleration of glycolysis, calculated to start within 5 sec (Achs et al., 1982), leads to a correspondingly rapid rate of increase in the oxidation metabolism of glucose to yield 36 extra ATP units per molecule.

A more controversial function of glycolysis is to sustain maximal heart work. In a highly artificial situation when isolated hearts are perfused with glucose alone and then subjected to sustained and high

work loads, rates of glycolysis do not provide adequately for the energy needs of the heart (Kobayashi and Neely, 1979). The factor restricting glycolysis is that $NADH_2$ forms more rapidly than it can be transported to the mitochondria. When perfusion conditions are altered to give maximal work performance and maximal oxygen uptake, then the rate of mitochondrial metabolism is high enough to allow peak rates of glycolysis (in the presence of insulin) to provide enough energy for the heart (Noakes, 1981). In addition, glycolysis appears to promote the rate of relaxation (Anderson and Morris, 1978). Such studies with single substrates are chiefly of theoretical interest. In reality, during increased heart work as part of the physiological response to exercise, the coronary flow of normal man will always provide a variety of fuels including lactate and free fatty acids, besides glucose, together with sufficient oxygen for oxidative metabolism. An apparent exception is at the very start of severe heart work, when temporary ischemic changes develop in the electrocardiogram of some normal subjects undertaking exercise (Chapter 14).

It is then that the acute acceleration of glycolysis might be of most importance.

Energy production by glycolysis

When glucose is the source of glycolysis, the whole glycolytic path uses 2 ATP and produces 4 ATP, i.e. the net production is 2 (Fig. 10-2). When glycogen is the source, ATP production is 3 per six-carbon molecule passing through glycolysis. An important point is that glycolytic ATP will be made whenever glucose 6-phosphate is converted to pyruvate even during oxidative metabolism. For anaerobic glycolysis to produce as much ATP as during aerobic metabolism of glucose would require an acceleration of glycolysis by nearly 20 times — in contrast to the more modest acceleration that even total anoxia produces when coronary flow is maintained artificially. Thus the anaerobic heart develops a severe deficit of energy, unless arrested by potassium (Fig. 10-8) or hypothermia (see Fig. 25-1).

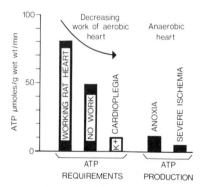

ANAEROBIC ATP CANNOT MEET
ENERGY NEEDS OF HEART
UNLESS CARDIOPLEGIC

Fig. 10-8 Anaerobic ATP cannot meet the energy needs of the heart, unless it is cardioplegic, even when produced at maximal rates (anoxia with sustained coronary flow, see Fig. 9-3). During total ischemia the rate of anaerobic glycolysis falls so that the best way of preserving the ischemic myocardium is by reducing the ATP demand (cardioplegia + hypothermia; see Fig. 25-1). For details of calculations, see Opie LH (1971). Cardiology 56: 2.

Pentose Shunt

The normal glycolytic pathway can in part be bypassed by the pentose shunt, which converts glucose 6-phosphate to riboses. The five-carbon pentose-phosphates can re-enter glycolysis, which explains the name pentose shunt. Alternatively, the ribose molecules can be used to form ribonucleic acids (RNA) required in the synthesis of proteins and lipids, or nucleotides such as ATP (see Fig. 11-13). In the normal adult myocardium, where the rate of protein synthesis is relatively low, the activity of the pentose shunt is also low. When much more protein synthesis is needed, as in the fetal and neonatal heart, or in the reparative phase of myocardial infarction, or during experiments with catecholamine stimulation (Zimmer, 1981), then the rate of activity of the shunt rises. Changes in the rate of the shunt are achieved by regulating the activity of the enzyme glucose 6-phosphate dehydrogenase.

Pyruvate

During normal aerobic metabolism, lactate is taken up by the heart and intracellular pyruvate is formed both from such uptake and from glycolysis. Sometimes pyruvate can also be formed by transamination from the amino acid alanine. In the anaerobic heart the end-state of glycolysis is the formation of lactate; a lesser fate is alanine (Fig. 10-9). In the aerobic heart the major fate of pyruvate is oxidative decarboxylation and entry into the citrate cycle which requires the activity of pyruvate dehydrogenase.

Before pyruvate can be oxidized fully in the Krebs citrate cycle, it must undergo oxidative decarboxylation through the action of the enzyme complex, **pyruvate dehydrogenase**, which is found in the inner mitochondrial membrane. The products of the multi-stage reaction (see Walsh et al., 1976) include acetyl CoA, which is ready to enter the citrate cycle, and $NADH_2$ which will form ATP by oxidative phosphorylation. Pyruvate dehydrogenase can exist in either active or inactive forms (Fig. 10-10). Normally only about 20 percent of the enzyme is active, but when glycolytic flux increases as during increased heart work, then 60–90 percent of the enzyme can be active. During stimulation by catecholamines and other inotropic agents, conversion to the active form is thought to be caused by an increased mitochondrial calcium concentration (McCormack et al., 1982). Whether the enzyme is in the active or inactive form depends on whether or not it is phosphorylated (which inactivates) or dephosphorylated (which activates). Such a phosphorylation–dephosphorylation cycle is quite a common mechanism for regulating enzyme

THREE PATHWAYS FOR PYRUVATE

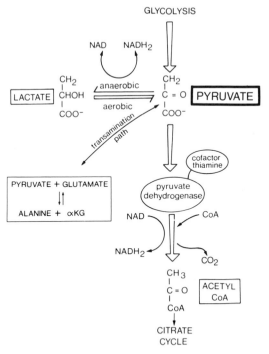

Fig. 10-9 The major fates of pyruvate. In the normal aerobic heart, lactate is taken up and converted to pyruvate, the major part of which enters the citrate cycle. Transamination is a pathway of minor significance. In the anaerobic heart, lactate is produced from pyruvate derived from glycolysis.

activity. The kinase (pyruvate dehydrogenase kinase) phosphorylating and inactivating the enzyme is itself "turned on" by various metabolic signals such as $NADH_2$, so that pyruvate dehydrogenase becomes inactive during ischemia and pyruvate now forms lactate.

A further metabolic pathway of uncertain significance is the addition of CO_2 or **pyruvate carboxylation** to form oxaloacetate, thereby potentially regenerating citrate cycle intermediates in certain experimental conditions (Peunkurinen and Hassinen, 1982).

Lactate

The uptake of lactate by the heart depends on a specific transport system because the sarcolemma is not freely permeable to lactate. Once taken up, intracellular lactate is converted into pyruvate by **lactate dehydrogenase** and thus joins the "pool" of pyruvate in the cytosol.

The reaction catalyzed by lactate dehydrogenase is freely reversible:

$$\text{Lactate} + NAD^+ \longrightarrow \text{pyruvate} + NADH + H^+$$

The myocardial activity of lactate dehydrogenase (LDH) is high enough to make it unlikely that it could be a controlling step for lactate metabolism by the heart. There are five **LDH isoenzymes** named in order

PYRUVATE DEHYDROGENASE: ACTIVATION

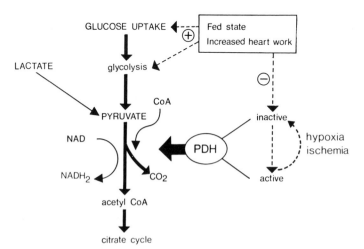

Fig. 10-10 Factors enhancing glycolysis also activate pyruvate dehydrogenase (PDH) to increase entry of pyruvate into the citrate cycle. Exceptions are hypoxia and ischemia which inactivate the enzyme.

of rapidity of their electrophoretic migrations; each isoenzyme is a tetrameric unit composed of four subunits of the H or M type. The H type, predominating in the heart muscle, is also known as LDH_1 or as alpha-hydroxybutyrate dehydrogenase because alpha-hydroxybutyrate can replace pyruvate as substrate. In acute myocardial infarction, an estimate of infarct size may be found by measuring the rate of appearance and disappearance of the LDH cardiac isoenzyme (LDH_1), which occurs later than that of creatine kinase so that peak values are reached 35–43 hours after the onset of symptoms (Hermens and Witteveen, 1977).

The contribution of lactate to the myocardial energy needs increases of up to 60 percent when the circulating lactate level is high, for example during and soon after exercise. Lactate is a much less important fuel when its circulating level is low, or when the circulating free fatty acid level is high. When the plasma lactate concentration is artificially elevated to above 4.5 mM (a level found in exercise in man), lactate is oxidized in preference to both glucose and free fatty acid (Drake et al., 1980). The mechanisms concerned probably include: (i) inhibition of glycolysis by citrate resulting from lactate oxidation; (ii) inhibition of glyceraldehyde 3-phosphate dehydrogenase by lactate and by $NADH_2$; and (iii) inhibition of the fatty acid activating enzyme, thiokinase. In resting man at normal blood levels of below 1 mM, lactate cannot be expected to be a major fuel. Anaerobic glycolysis changes the normal uptake of lactate to discharge (Fig. 10-11) so that the level in the coronary sinus may exceed that in arterial blood during angina pectoris.

Glycogen

Glycogen is a polysaccharide (i.e. a combination of many molecules of glucose) which forms large storage granules in the cytoplasm of the heart. Chemically, it resembles glycogen found in other organs such as the liver. Although frequently thought of as a "storage" carbohydrate, the large and restless glycogen molecules are in a constant state of turnover as a result of variable rates of synthesis and degradation. In contrast to the very detailed understanding of the complex chemical signals controlling glycogen synthesis and breakdown, the actual physiological function of cardiac glycogen is poorly understood. The pathways of glycogen synthesis function separately from those of glycogen breakdown because two different enzyme systems are involved. Glycogen synthesis (Fig. 10-12) thus proceeds at a high rate in the fed state under the influence of insulin, and also at a lower rate in the fasted state

LACTATE PRODUCTION BY HEART

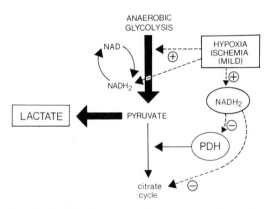

FACTORS PROMOTING GLYCOGEN
SYNTHESIS

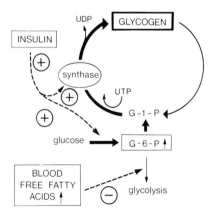

Fig. 10-11 Mechanisms of lactate production during anaerobic glycolysis, as occurs in anoxia with maintained coronary flow or mild ischemia (see Fig. 9-3). In contrast, accumulated products of anaerobic glycolysis (lactate, protons, $NADH_2$; see Figs 10-3 and 10-4) all inhibit glycolysis during severe ischemia. For definition of mild ischemia see Fig. 9-3.

Fig. 10-12 In the fed state, insulin is the stimulus to glycogen synthesis. In the fasted state, cardiac glucose 6-phosphate (G-6-P) rises as a result of the inhibition of glycolysis by fatty acids. In the process energy is used as uridine triphosphate (UTP) is converted to UDP. UTP in turn is made from ATP (Chapter 11).

despite the lack of insulin, because of high myocardial levels of glucose 6-phosphate. The energy required is derived from a special high-energy phosphate, UTP (uridine triphosphate, which is in turn formed from ATP).

The two major mechanisms for stimulating glycogen breakdown are activated either by cyclic AMP or, in anoxia, by a fall in high-energy phosphate levels (Fig.10-13). A rise in cyclic AMP promotes the cascade of events which eventually converts inactive glycogen **phosphorylase** *b* molecules to the highly active **phosphorylase** *a* by the well-known "cascade":

catecholamine stimulus $\longrightarrow$ beta-receptor $\longrightarrow$ adenylate cyclase $\longrightarrow$ cyclic AMP activation of protein kinase — activation of phosphorylase *b* kinase $\longrightarrow$ change of phosphorylase *b* to *a* $\longrightarrow$ breakdown of glycogen.

Calmodulin, the intracellular calcium-binding receptor protein, is one of the subunits of phosphorylase *b* kinase; hence calcium ions are required for the formation of phosphorylase *a* (Werth et al., 1982). Phosphorylase is the enzyme controlling the initial burst of glycogenolysis during hypoxia or ischemia, and thereafter the activity of the **debranching enzyme** becomes significant.

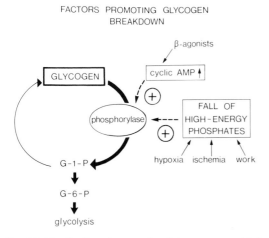

FACTORS PROMOTING GLYCOGEN BREAKDOWN

Fig. 10-13 Cardiac glycogen breakdown occurs chiefly as a result of stimulation by beta-adrenergic catecholamines. Increased intracellular formation of the second messenger, cyclic AMP, initiates the breakdown "cascade" (see text) which eventually converts phosphorylase *b* to the much more active form, *a*. In addition, phosphorylase *b* can have its activity increased by factors decreasing tissue high energy phosphate levels.

Function of cardiac glycogen

Cardiac glycogen is a potential source of myocardial energy, yet the cardiac glycogen content would have to be extremely high and glycogenolysis extremely rapid for glycogen to be the major fuel of the heart over a long period. Many workers have suspected but not proved that a measure of glycogen breakdown occurs with each cardiac cycle. There is little advance beyond the view of Evans (1934) that glycogen is reserved for anoxemic emergencies, such as the "fight or flight" reaction, which include the abrupt onset of much increased heart work (Achs et al., 1982). Apart from these specific situations, the sequential cascades for glycogen breakdown (controlled chiefly by adrenergic stimulation) and glycogen synthesis (controlled chiefly by insulin) are far more complex than the limited physiological use of glycogen appears to warrant. Possibly such complex mechanisms merely reflect the evolutionary inheritance of red heart muscle from the more primitive white skeletal muscle. It is equally possible that these complex mechanisms might have a function as yet undiscovered.

Glycogen storage disease of the heart

In the lysosomes of the heart the breakdown of some of the glycogen is mediated by a different pathway dependent on alpha-1,4 glucosidase (acid maltase).

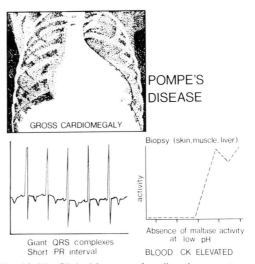

Fig. 10-14 Clinical features of cardiac glycogen storage disease of Pompe.

The congenital absence of this enzyme has drastic consequences because the heart cells become "stuffed" with glycogen, so that the fatal condition of cardiomegalic glycogenolysis or Pompe's disease results (Fig. 10-14). Cytoplasmic glycogenolysis, dependent on phosphorylase and the debrancher enzyme, proceeds normally in these cases. Because of distension of the lysosomes by glycogen, the lysosomal membranes rupture, presumably with destruction of heart muscle by the lysosomal enzymes.

Free Fatty Acids

The uptake of circulating free fatty acids (nonesterified fatty acids) by the myocardium increases as the circulating level rises, provided that all the steps leading to ultimate oxidation are proceeding freely. Eventually feedback systems will limit the uptake (Fig. 10-15). In man, the chief fatty acid taken up is oleic acid (Table 10-3). The first step in fatty acid oxidation is the activation of fatty acids so that CoA is gained

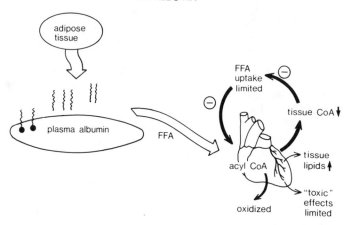

CIRCULATING FFA EXCEEDS TIGHT BINDING SITES ON ALBUMIN

Fig. 10-15 Uptake of free fatty acids (FFA) at high circulating levels, exceeding the tight binding sites on plasma albumin (● ●), is uncontrolled and may give rise to "toxic" effects. For details of tissue CoA and acyl CoA see Fig. 10-16.

Table 10-3

Myocardial uptake of plasma free fatty acids in fasting man

Fatty acid	Structure	Site of unsaturated bonds	Percentage of total plasma FFA[1,2]	Percentage of uptake of FFA by human heart
Palmitic	C16 : 0	—	About 25	16
Palmitoleic	C16 : 1	9	2	2
Stearic	C18 : 0	—	14	7
Oleic	C18 : 1	9	30–45	53
Linoleic	C18 : 2	9,12	10–14	7
Linolenic	C18 : 3	6,12,15	8 in guinea pig	No data
Arachidonic	C20 : 4	5,8,11,14	5	No data in man, no uptake in dog heart[3]
Erucic	C22 : 1	13	Normally low	No data but may increase with rape-seed ingestion

[1]Spector A (1971). Prog Biochem Pharm 6: 130.
[2]Calculated from data of Rothlin ME, Bing RJ (1961). J Clin Invest 40: 1380.
[3]Van der Vusse GJ et al. (1982). Circ Res 50: 538.

to form fatty acyl CoA derivatives; acyl CoA molecules are then transferred from the cytosol to within the mitochondria by a transfer system that requires carnitine; thereafter the long chain acyl CoA molecules are progressively broken into 2-carbon units of acetyl CoA by beta-oxidation; and finally acetyl CoA is oxidized in the citrate cycle. Any activated intracellular fatty acid not oxidized can be stored as triglycerides, or be transformed to structural lipids by lengthening and alterations in the degree of saturation to myocardial membrane lipids. Complex intracellular controls exist to prevent any undue accumulation of lipid intermediates which may have the "toxic" effects.

Activation of intracellular fatty acids

Being lipid-soluble, fatty acids can freely cross the sarcolemma to form intracellular fatty acids which must be activated prior to further metabolism by the enzyme thiokinase (Fig. 10-16). Using palmitate as an example:

$$\text{palmitate} + \text{CoA} + \text{ATP} \longrightarrow$$
$$\text{palmityl CoA} + \text{AMP} + \text{PPi}$$

Thereby the long-chain fatty acid is converted to a long-chain acyl CoA. Because the pathways of fatty acid oxidation need control to avoid the accumulation

ESSENTIAL ROLE OF CARNITINE CARRIER IN FATTY ACYL
TRANSPORT INTO MITOCHONDRIA

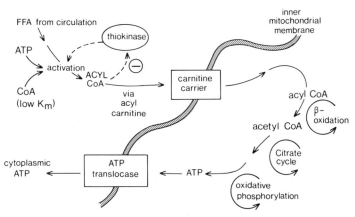

Fig. 10-16 The carnitine carrier functions to transfer activated fatty acid (acyl CoA) into the mitochondrial space for oxidation in the fatty acid oxidation space. Acyl CoA = long chain acyl CoA compounds; acyl carnitine = long chain acyl carnitine compounds.

UPTAKE OF "EXCESS FFA" LIMITED BY RATE OF ACTIVATION

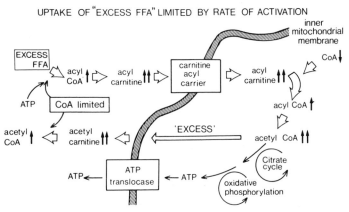

Fig. 10-17 Limitation of CoA in the cytosol will tend to inhibit the rates of fatty acid uptake and act as a brake to the accumulation of acyl CoA and acyl carnitine. Thus when circulating FFA are high (see Fig. 10-15), intracellular mechanisms exist to limit uptake and potential "toxicity" of accumulated lipid intermediates.

of detergent intermediates, it makes sense that the rate of activation is subject to careful regulation (Oram et al., 1975). When circulating fatty acids are high in concentration and are taken up at high rates, the rate of activation will also rise, but as more acyl CoA forms the cytosolic CoA falls to slow down the thiokinase reaction (Fig. 10-17). Conversely, during increased heart work the rate of mitochondrial oxidation rises, acyl CoA falls and fatty acid activation speeds up.

Acyl CoA and carnitine

Once formed, activated fatty acids in the form of acyl CoA have two possible fates: (i) transfer into the mitochondrial space or (ii) formation of triglyceride and other glycerides. The former mechanism depends on carnitine which is a relatively simple compound of widespread distribution with some properties resembling those of a vitamin. Its structure is:

$$(CH_3)_3N^+ . CH_2CH (OH) . CH_2 . COO^-$$

and the naturally occurring form is L(−).

The overall steps can be summarized as follows:

(a) extramitochondrial acyl CoA forms from fatty acid (Fig. 10-16);

(b) extramitochondrial acyl carnitine forms from extramitochondrial acyl CoA;

(c) carnitine–acyl carnitine translocase transfers extramitochondrial acyl carnitine to within the mitochondrial space;

(d) mitochondrial carnitine acyl transferase allows intramitochondrial acyl carnitine to react with CoA so as to liberate intramitochondrial acyl CoA and carnitine;

(e) intramitochondrial acyl CoA enters the fatty acid oxidation spiral;

(f) the carnitine–acyl carnitine translocase system transfers intramitochondrial carnitine formed in the fourth reaction to outside the mitochondria. Thus extracellular fatty acids are activated and transferred to become acyl CoA molecules within the mitochondria.

Beta-oxidation

Next beta-oxidation converts intramitochondrial long-chain acyl CoA to the two carbon fragment acetyl CoA. The fatty acid oxidation spiral continuously removes acetyl CoA from the carboxyl (−COOH) end of the chain (Fig. 10-18). The enzymes of

FATTY ACID OXIDATION SPIRAL

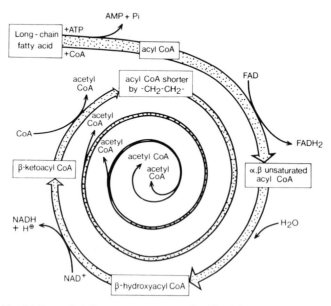

Fig. 10-18 The fatty acid oxidation spiral. Seven turns are required for full oxidation of palmitate, which produces 129 molecules of ATP.

beta-oxidation are loosely organized into a multi-enzyme complex in which the intermediates never leave the complex except for entering and departing. The products of each reaction are simply displaced by the arrival of fresh substrates for that reaction, to move on in the spiral (Hochachka et al., 1977).

During **increased heart work**, the mitochondria become more oxidized. Intramitochondrial levels of $NADH_2$ and presumably $FADH_2$ fall, and there is an increased turnover of the whole fatty acid oxidation spiral. Mitochondrial acetyl CoA also falls, as the citrate cycle accelerates. A series of events opposite to those shown in Fig. 10-17 help to "tell" the cytosol that the mitochondria need a higher rate of fatty acid activation during increased heart work (Idell-Wenger et al., 1982). Cytosolic acetyl CoA can enter the mitochondria after transformation to acetyl carnitine. Thereby free cytosolic CoA forms and the rate of fatty acid activation is enhanced. These events are more fully described elsewhere (Opie, 1984).

Conversely, **during anaerobiosis**, intramitochondrial $NADH_2$ rises as does $FADH_2$. The basic effect is probably impaired beta-oxidation due to decreased electron transport (Moore et al., 1982). Intermediates of fatty acid metabolism accumulate, including the hydrogen-containing beta-hydroxy-fatty acid compounds and acyl CoA itself.

Triglycerides

Triglycerides (triacylglycerols) can also be formed from acyl CoA molecules and alpha-glycerol phosphate, the latter being derived from glycolysis by the process of **esterification** (Fig. 10-19). True lipogenesis (for example, the formation of long-chain fatty acids from acetyl CoA) may also occur in the heart as the enzymes have been identified in this tissue. Nonetheless, it seems that esterification of exogenously derived fatty acids is the normal route for the synthesis of cardiac lipids. Thus fatty acids taken up from the circulation are the ultimate source of tissue lipids, sometimes after restructuring by chain elongation or altering the degree of saturation.

When the heart is deprived of external fuels there is breakdown of endogenous triglycerides (**lipolysis**) to provide energy. However, not all the triglyceride is available for such energetic purposes because about one-fifth is structural and remains even when the heart

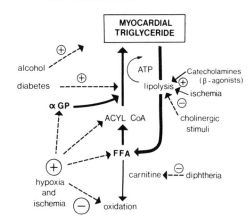

Fig. 10-19 Factors helping to form and break down triglyceride in the myocardium. FFA = tissue free fatty acids; αGP = alpha-glycerol phosphate derived from glycolysis in anaerobic conditions (page 121); in aerobic conditions, it can form from glycerol, liberated by triglyceride hydrolysis (enzyme glycerol kinase).

is exhausted by substrate depletion. For the normal heart, there is no evidence that endogenous lipid is an energy source with the possible exceptions of very intense exercise or prolonged fasting. Triglycerides are broken down by several enzymes (lipases) by a system which catecholamines stimulate and cholinergic stimulation inhibits. In general, fatty acids produced from lipolysis have the same effects as those taken up from the circulation.

Triglyceride accumulation in pathological states

Triglycerides accumulate in the heart cell in alcoholic heart disease, diabetes mellitus, ischemia, or diphtheria. The process is thought to be harmful to the heart because it is usually associated with increased formation of fibrous tissue (Shipp et al., 1973), yet it is difficult to separate causation from association. Theoretically, the continued synthesis of triglyceride and its breakdown could "waste" ATP, thereby setting the stage for focal deficits of ATP and a situation resembling a micro-infarct with a focus of fibrosis. It is equally possible that an energy deficit caused by ischemia or other metabolic excess prevents fatty acid oxidation with the accumulation of triglyceride as a by-product. In one extreme situation, that of erucic acid toxicity, triglycerides accumulate in great excess and physically impair normal myo-cardial structure.

Erucic acid is found in rape-seed oil, widely used for margarine. The cellular basis of erucic acid toxicity is the low rate of oxidation of this unphysiological long-chain polyunsaturated fatty acid, which under-goes esterification to form so much excess triglyceride that the mitochondria are damaged. Such animal experiments do not directly prove that dietary intake of erucic acid can cause heart disease in man, yet the theoretical dangers have prohibited the use of rape-seed oil for margarine in many countries.

Structural Lipids of the Heart

Phospholipids, the major structural lipids of the heart, form an important part of the various cell membranes, especially the mitochondrial membrane. In prolonged ischemia, all membranes are damaged and products of phospholipid breakdown are formed. One view is that ischemic injury become irreversible when the molecular structure of the cell membranes is damaged beyond repair. In phospholipid molecules both the free base group (choline or ethanolamine) and the phos-phate are charged, providing a "polar head" in contrast to the "non-polar tail" (Fig. 10-20). It is this polarity of the molecular which allows the formation of the **lipid-bilayer** of the cell membranes; the polar heads point outward, the non-polar tails inward. Into the lipid bilayer are inserted various complex proteins, including enzyme systems which may require specific phospholipids for optimal activity. Such **lipid–enzyme** complexes include adenylate cyclase and the sarcolemmal sodium–potassium pump.

Fatty Acids and Lipid Metabolites in Ischemic Injury

Oliver and co-workers (1968) made the important observation that patients with acute myocardial infarction with serious complications were more likely to have high blood fatty acid levels; the mortality appeared to be related to the fatty acid level. In early experimental infarction there is continued, albeit reduced, uptake of fatty acids (Opie et al., 1973) which may "drive" the oxygen consumption of those mitochondria still receiving oxygen (Pearce et al., 1979). Many other factors operate to contribute to the harmful effects of accumulated tissue fatty acids in ischemia (Liedtke, 1981).

Fatty Acyl CoA

Activated long-chain fatty acid (**acyl CoA**) may accumulate both within and without the mitochondria as the rate of mitochondrial oxidation falls (Fig. 10-21). In isolated sub-mitochondrial particles, long-chain fatty acyl CoA can inhibit the adenine nucleotide translocase from either outside or inside. The idea that accumulated acyl CoA impairs mitochondrial function during ischemia is widely accepted, yet a careful study

ORIGIN OF LYSOPHOSPHOLIPIDS

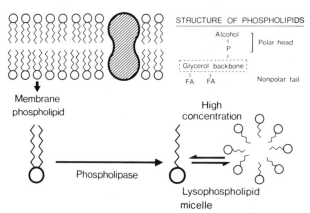

Fig. 10-20 Phospholipids of bilipid membranes may be broken down by phospholipases to yield lysophospholipids. High concentrations of the latter may form micelles (see also Fig. 10-22).

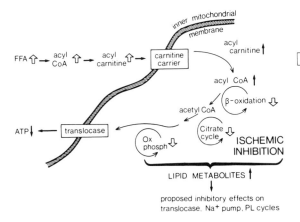

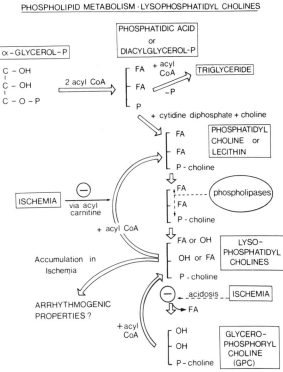

PHOSPHOLIPID METABOLISM · LYSOPHOSPHATIDYL CHOLINES

Fig. 10-21 The major effect of ischemia on pathways for FFA oxidation is on inhibition of oxidative metabolism so that acyl CoA, acyl carnitine, and FFA all accumulate in the ischemic tissue. Proposed effects are inhibition of the ATP/ADP translocase by acyl CoA, inhibition of the sodium pump by acyl carnitine and inhibition of phospholipid (PL) cycles with re-acylation of lysophosphatidyl choline.

has shown that acyl CoA is no higher in the ischemic than in normal tissue (Feuvray and Plouet, 1981).

It is now suspected that it is partly the accumulation of other lipid metabolites such as acyl carnitine which contribute to the detrimental effects. In the normal heart the cytosolic concentration of **acyl carnitine** is very low, being estimated at 25 μmol/L (Idell-Wenger et al., 1978) with none in the mitochondria. During ischemia the concentrations in both cytosol and mitochondria rise to about 2000 μmol/L. Such increases are very much more than those undergone by acyl CoA. Acyl carnitines have properties which are potentially arrhythmogenic (Corr et al., 1981). Acyl carnitines also inhibit the activity of the sodium–potassium pump at concentrations likely to be present in the ischemic tissue (Wood et al., 1977); the ensuing loss of potassium is also arrhythmogenic. Because accumulation of acyl carnitine cannot explain the inhibition of the critical adenine nucleotide translocase reaction (Pande and Blanchaer, 1971), many workers still believe that an accumulation of acyl CoA is a critical event despite the reservations outlined.

Lysophosphoglycerides are membrane-active fatty acids that are released from the phospholipids of the sarcolemma and other membranes during ischemia (Fig. 10-22). It is proposed that accumulated lysophosphatidyl choline (LPC) has arrhythmogenic properties (Corr et al., 1982).

Fig. 10-22 Pathways involved in the formation of lysophospholipids such as lysophosphatidyl cholines which hypothetically promote arrhythmias in experimental ischemia (see Corr et al., 1982).

"Oxygen-wastage"

When the heart is exposed to high circulating levels of circulating catecholamines and/or free fatty acids, the oxygen uptake may rise much more than expected from the change in respiratory quotient in switching from carbohydrate to fatty acids as fuel. This phenomenon, also found in man (Simonsen and Kjekshus, 1978), may in part be mediated by increased turnover of intracellular futile cycles, thereby "wasting" ATP. Alternatively, pathways of respiration producing not ATP but free oxygen radicals, may be enhanced (see page 144) with the potential for myocardial damage. Similar mechanisms may underlie the development of **lipid peroxides** (see page 356), which together with formation of phospholipids, free radicals and lipid intermediates, may all theoretically contribute to ischemic reperfusion damage (Meerson et al., 1982).

Summary

Glucose is not normally the major myocardial fuel, but can become so after a high carbohydrate meal. Glucose is converted to pyruvate by glycolysis which is the pathway common for the breakdown of glucose 6-phosphate formed either from the uptake of glucose or the breakdown of glycogen. Glycogen is not an important energy source except in emergency situations such as a sudden acceleration of heart work. Each glucose molecule converted to pyruvate gives a net yield of 2 ATP. Pyruvate can either be converted anaerobically to lactate (re-using $NADH_2$), or pyruvate can be converted aerobically to acetyl CoA by the enzyme pyruvate dehydrogenase which is located on the mitochondrial membrane. During oxidative metabolism, the $NADH_2$ produced by glycolysis enters the mitochondrial space by the malate–aspartate cycle, to join the $NADH_2$ produced by pyruvate dehydrogenase and citrate cycle activity. The additional energy yield is about 36 ATP molecules per glucose molecule, with a total yield of 38 ATP. In the severely ischemic heart, when both oxygen and coronary flow are decreased, protons, $NADH_2$ and lactate all accumulate and glycolysis is inhibited at the levels of glyceraldehyde 3-phosphate dehydrogenase and phosphofructokinase. An increased glycolytic flow in mildly ischemic or non-ischemic cells may be a mechanism to decrease cellular damage in regional ischemia.

Long-chain free fatty acids, usually the major myocardial fuel, are fat-soluble so that they easily pass through the sarcolemmal membrane before irreversible activation to acyl CoA, which cannot penetrate the mitochondrial barrier without a carnitine carrier system. Acyl CoA becomes acyl carnitine which is carried to within the mitochondria. There acyl CoA reforms to enter the pathways of beta-oxidation which chop off two carbon fractions one at a time to form acetyl CoA; the latter then enters the citrate cycle. The oxidation system is sufficiently active to keep very low the intracellular concentrations of free fatty acids, acyl CoA, and acyl carnitine, each of which is water-soluble only in very low concentrations. That part of the free fatty acid uptake which is not oxidized can form triglyceride and myocardial structural lipids, the latter by changes in the degree of saturation and chain length. In ischemia the rate of uptake of fatty acids exceeds the rate of disposal and intermediates of lipid metabolism such as intracellular free fatty acid, acyl CoA and acyl carnitine accumulate with potentially harmful effects.

References

Achs MJ, Garfinkel D, Opie LH (1982). Computer simulation of metabolism of glucose perfused rat heart in a work-jump. Am J Physiol 243: R389–R399.

Anderson GL, Morris RG (1978). Role of glycolysis in the relaxation process in mammalian cardiac muscle: comparison of the influence of glucose and 2-deoxyglucose on maintenance of resting tension. Life Sci 23: 23–32.

Corr PB, Snyder DW, Cain ME, Crafford WA Jr, Gross RW, Sobel BE (1981). Electrophysiological effects of amphiphiles on canine Purkinje fibers; implications for dysrhythmia secondary to ischemia. Circ Res 49: 354–363.

Corr PB, Gross RW, Sobel BE (1982). Arrhythmogenic amphiphilic lipids and the myocardial cell membrane. Editorial. J Molec Cell Cardiol 14: 619–626.

Drake AJ, Haines JR, Noble MIM (1980). Preferential uptake of lactate by the normal myocardium in dogs. Cardiovasc Res 14: 65–72.

Evans G (1934). The glycogen content of the rat heart. J Physiol 82: 468–480.

Feuvray D, Plouet J (1981). Relationship between structure and fatty acid metabolism in mitochondria isolated from ischemic rat heart. Circ Res 48: 740–747.

Gevers W (1977). Generation of protons by metabolic processes in heart cells. J Molec Cell Cardiol 11: 867–874.

Hermens WT, Witteveen SAGJ (1977). Problems in estimation of enzymatic infarct size. J Molec Med 2: 233–239.

Hochachka DW, Neely JR, Driedzic WR (1977). Integration of lipid utilization with Krebs cycle activity in muscle. Fed Proc 36: 2009–2014.

Idell-Wenger JA, Grotyohann LW, Neely JR (1978). Coenzyme A and carnitine distribution in normal and ischemic hearts. J Biol Chem 253: 4310–4318.

Idell-Wenger JA, Grotyohann LW, Neely JR (1982). Regulation of fatty acid utilization in heart. Role of carnitine-acetyl-CoA transferase and carnitine-acetyl carnitine translocase system. J Molec Cell Cardiol 14: 413–417.

Kobayashi K, Neely JR (1979). Control of maximum rates of glycolysis in rat cardiac muscle. Circ Res 44: 166–175.

Larner J, Cheng K, Huang L, Galaski G (1981). Insulin mediators and their control of covalent phosphorylation. Cold Spring Harbor Conferences 8: 727–733.

Liedtke AJ (1981). Alterations of carbohydrate and lipid metabolism in the acutely ischemic heart. Prog Cardiovasc Res 23: 321–336.

McCormack JG, Edge NJ, Denton RM (1982). Regulation of rat heart pyruvate dehydrogenase activity. Biochem J 202: 419–427.

Meerson FZ, Kagan VE, Kozlov YuP, Belkina LM, Arkhipenko YuV (1982). The role of lipid peroxidation in pathogenesis of ischemic damage and the antioxidant protection of the heart. Basic Res Cardiol 77: 465–485.

Mochizuki S, Neely JR (1979). Control of glyceraldehyde-3-phosphate dehydrogenase in cardiac muscle. J Molec Cell Cardiol 11: 221–236.

Moore KH, Radloff JE, Koen AE, Hull FE (1982). Incomplete fatty acid oxidation by heart mitochondria: beta-hydroxy fatty acid production. J Molec Cell Cardiol 14: 451–459.

Noakes TD (1981). Exercise and the heart. M.D. Thesis, University of Cape Town.

Oliver MF, Kurien VA, Greenwood TW (1968). Relation between serum free fatty acids and arrhythmias and death after myocardial infarction. Lancet i: 710–715.

Opie LH (1984). Substrate and energy metabolism of the heart. In: Function of the Heart in Normal and Pathological States, Ed. N Sperelakis, pp 301–336, Martinus Nijhoff Publishers, New York.

Opie LH, Owen P, Riemersma RA (1973). Relative rates of oxidation of glucose and free fatty acids by ischemic and non-ischemic myocardium after coronary artery ligation in the dog. Europ J Clin Invest 3: 419–435.

Oram JF, Wenger JI, Neely JR (1975). Regulation of long chain fatty acid activation in heart muscle. J Biol Chem 256: 73–78.

Pande SV, Blanchaer MC (1971). Reversible inhibition of mitochondrial adenosine diphosphate phosphorylation by long chain acyl CoA esters. J Biol Chem 246: 402–411.

Pearce FJ, Forster J, DeLeeuw G, Williamson JR, Tutwiler GF (1979). Inhibition of fatty acid oxidation in normal and hypoxic rat hearts by 2-tetradecylglycidic acid. J Molec Cell Cardiol 11: 893–915.

Peunkurinen KJ, Hassinen IE (1982). Pyruvate carboxylation as an anaplerotic mechanism in the isolated perfused rat heart. Biochem J 202: 67–76.

Randle PJ, Smith GH (1958). Regulation of glucose uptake by muscle. II. The effects of insulin, anaerobiosis and cell poison on the penetration of isolated rat diaphragm by sugars. Biochem J 70: 501–508.

Shipp JC, Menahan LA, Crass MF III, Chaudhuri SA (1973). Heart triglyceride in health and disease. In: Recent Advances in Studies on Cardiac Structure and Metabolism, Vol. 3, Myocardial Metabolism. Ed. NS Dhalla, G Rona, pp 179–204, University Park Press, Baltimore.

Simonsen S, Kjekshus JK (1978). The effect of free fatty acids on myocardial oxygen consumption during atrial pacing and catecholamine infusion in man. Circulation 58: 484–491.

Walsh DA, Cooper RH, Denton RM, Bridges BJ, Randle PJ (1976). The elementary reactions of the pig heart pyruvate dehydrogenase complex. A study of the inhibition by phosphorylation. Biochem J 157: 41–67.

Werth DK, Hathaway DR, Watanabe AM (1982). Regulation of phosphorylase kinase in rat ventricular myocardium. Role of calmodulin. Circ Res 51: 448–456.

Wood JM, Rush B, Pitts BJR, Schwartz A (1977). Inhibition of bovine heart Na$^+$, K$^+$-ATPase by palmitylcarnitine and palmityl CoA. Biochem Biophys Res Comm 74: 677–683.

Zimmer HG (1981). Rapid stimulation of the hexose monophosphate shunt in the isolated perfused rat heart: possible involvement of oxidized glutathione. J Molec Cell Cardiol 13: 531–535.

New References

Corr PB, Gross RW, Sobel BE (1984). Amphipathic metabolites and membrane dysfunction in ischemic myocardium. Circ Res 55:135–154.

Ferrari R, Katz AM, Shug A, Visioli O (1984). Myocardial ischemia and lipid metabolism. Plenum Press, New York.

Hütter JF, Piper HM, Spieckermann PG (1984). Kinetic analysis of myocardial fatty acid oxidation suggesting an albumin receptor mediated uptake process. J Molec Cell Cardiol 16: 219–226.

Kang ES, Mirvis DM (1984). Reversible, highly localized alterations in fatty acid metabolism in the chronically ischemic canine myocardium. Am J Cardiol 54: 411–414.

Lammerant J, Huynh-Thu T, Kolanowski J (1985). Inhibitory effects of the D(−) isomer of 3-hydroxybutyrate on cardiac non-esterified fatty acid uptake and oxygen demand induced by norepinephrine in the intact dog. J Molec Cell Cardiol 17: 421–433.

Neely JR, Grotyohann LW (1984). Role of glycolytic products in damage to ischemic myocardium. Dissociation of adenosine triphosphate levels and recovery of function of reperfused ischemic hearts. Circ Res 55: 816–824.

Schwaiger M, Schelbert HR, Ellison E, Hansen H, Yeatman L, Vinten-Johansen J, Selin C, Barrio J, Phelps ME (1985). Sustained regional abnormalities in cardiac metabolism after transient ischemia in the chronic dog model. J Am Coll Cardiol 6: 336–347.

Wisneski JA, Gertz EW, Neese RA, Gruenke LD, Cymerman Craig J (1985). Dual carbon-labeled isotope experiments using D-[6-^{14}C] glucose and L-[1,2,3-^{13}C$_3$] lactate: A new approach for investigating human myocardial metabolism during ischemia. J Am Coll Cardiol 5: 1138–1146.

11 | ATP Synthesis and Breakdown

The breakdown of ATP is the immediate source of energy for contraction, the maintenance of ion gradients and other vital functions. Metabolic pathways transform glucose, free fatty acids and lactate to acetyl CoA which enters the citrate cycle to produce $NADH_2$, which in turn yields the hydrogen atoms which flow along the cytochrome chain, where ADP is converted to ATP by oxidative phosphorylation (Fig. 11-1). Once produced in the mitochondria, ATP is transported outwards to the cytosol by the ATP/ADP transport system for utilization, chiefly in contraction, with formation of ADP. As cytosolic ATP is used it is replenished by synthesis from ADP in the mitochondria. The rates of synthesis and breakdown of ATP are therefore closely linked.

Citrate Cycle of Krebs

The rate at which the citrate cycle of Krebs (Fig. 11-2) operates is a major factor controlling the rate of

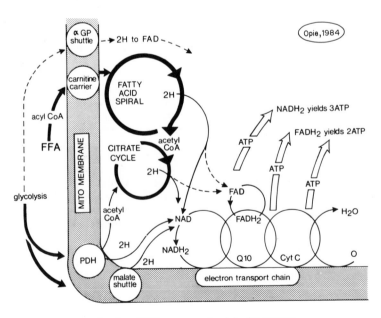

Fig. 11-1 Mitochondrial energy production. PDH = pyruvate dehydrogenase.

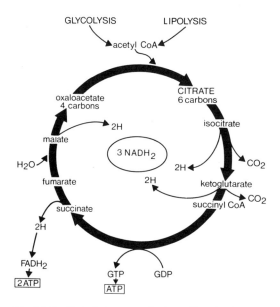

GLYCOLYSIS   LIPOLYSIS

acetyl CoA

CITRATE
6 carbons

oxaloacetate
4 carbons

isocitrate

2H

malate

$3 NADH_2$

H_2O

2H CO_2

fumarate

2H

ketoglutarate

succinate

succinyl CoA CO_2

2H

$FADH_2$

2ATP

GTP   GDP

ATP

Fig. 11-2 Krebs' citrate cycle. In reality, the following reactions are readily reversible: citrate → isocitrate; succinate → oxaloacetate via intervening reactions. The most important potential sites of control are citrate synthase, isocitrate dehydrogenase, alpha-ketoglutarate dehydrogenase, and malate dehydrogenase (by regulating the supply of oxaloacetate). These dehydrogenases respond to a decreased mitochondrial $NADH_2$ during increased heart work by increased activity.

production of ATP by the heart, because this cycle regulates the formation of $NADH_2$. An increased rate of the Krebs cycle occurs with increased heart work; conversely, decreased rates of operation of the cycle occur during states of oxygen deprivation such as anoxia, hypoxia and ischemia or during cardioplegic arrest.

Sir Hans Krebs was still actively leading his research team in Oxford at the age of 81 in 1981, when he died. He described the citrate cycle in 1938 in a famous paper which was rejected by *Nature* and published in *Experientia*. This work was done after Krebs had left Nazi Germany to work in England.

Each turn of the cycle produces twelve molecules of ATP (Table 11-1). How can the activity of the citrate cycle be matched to the energy requirements of the heart? The citrate cycle must receive acetyl CoA units from glycolysis or fatty acid breakdown at a rate sufficient to replenish the eventual breakdown of acetyl CoA to CO_2 and $NADH_2$. This input must be matched to the ouput of $NADH_2$, because it is the latter compound which is required to provide the electrons for transport along the electron transmitter chain during oxidative phosphorylation. Much regulation appears to occur through the ratio of NAD to $NADH_2$. As the heart works harder, more ATP is broken down to ADP to drive oxidative phosphorylation, which in turn uses H from $NADH_2$, so that the ratio $NAD/NADH_2$ within the mitochondria rises thereby stimulating the activity of certain key enzymes of the citrate cycle (isocitrate dehydrogenase, alpha-ketoglutarate dehydrogenase, malate dehydrogenase). The change in the mitochondrial $NAD/NADH_2$ ratio towards NAD also helps the formation of oxaloacetate from malate; oxaloacetate is one of the substrates for citrate synthase. The other substrate is acetyl CoA, the formation of which is also stimulated during increased heart work by increases in the rates of glycolysis and the fatty acid oxidation spiral. Conversely, during hypoxia, $NADH_2$ accumulates in the mitochondria to inhibit the citrate cycle.

Besides these mechanisms by which the citrate cycle

Table 11-1

Sites of production of H, CO_2 and high-energy phosphate in citrate cycle

Product	Sites of production	Fate
$4 \times 2H$ in total	1. Isocitrate dehydrogenase	Formation of NADH plus H^+ ($NADH_2$) and electron transport to produce 3 ATP
	2. α-Ketoglutarate dehydrogenase	3 ATP as above
	3. Succinate dehydrogenase	$FADH_2$ formation and electron transport via CoQ to produce 2 ATP
	4. Malate dehydrogenase	3 ATP as above
GTP	1. Succinate dehydrogenase by substrate level phosphorylation	Ultimate formation of 1 ATP
One turn of citrate cycle →	Various dehydrogenase reaction as above →	12 ATP

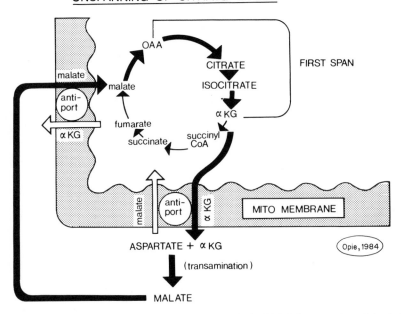

UNSPANNING OF CITRATE CYCLE

Fig. 11-3 The citrate cycle may operate in two spans, the second of which is bypassed as alpha-ketoglutarate (αKG) passes to the cytosol to be returned as malate. The proposal is that the cycle could be unspanned, so as to "bypass" the more slowly functioning second span (alpha-ketoglutarate to malate) at the start of a sudden increase in citrate cycle activity (see Neely et al., 1972).

responds to the mitochondrial $NAD/NADH_2$ ratio, it may be that the rate of part of the citrate cycle is just too slow for certain extreme situations, as during a sudden increase of heart work, when the cycle must spin very rapidly. The slow part of the cycle can then be "bypassed" (Fig. 11-3).

Transamination to replenish the citrate cycle

Every time the citrate cycle "spins" once, two molecules of CO_2 are formed; the loss of carbons is made good by provision of acetyl CoA derived from glycolysis or lipolysis. What happens if the citrate cycle suddenly speeds up due to a work jump, but glycolysis or lipolysis fail to deliver the required amount of acetyl CoA? Here the cardiac stores of amino acids can be used to form citrate cycle intermediates by transamination. Such reactions, "filling up" the citrate cycle, are called **anaplerotic** reactions.

Of the nine enzymes of the citrate cycle at least two help to adjust the rate of the cycle to the oxygen uptake. Both isocitrate dehydrogenase and alpha-ketoglutarate dehydrogenase convert NAD into

$NADH_2$; the latter compound exerts feedback control on both enzymes. When $NADH_2$ accumulates, as in hypoxia or ischemia, the activities of these dehydrogenases fall. Again when $NADH_2$ falls as a result of increased respiration and oxidative phosphorylation during increased heart work, the activities of the dehydrogenases rise and the citrate cycle spins faster. Another enzyme (citrate synthase) responds indirectly to a fall of $NADH_2$ which stimulates formation of oxaloacetate from malate (by altering the equilibrium of the malate dehydrogenase reaction). It is not so much the absolute amount of $NADH_2$ that regulates the citrate cycle enzymes, but the mitochondrial $NAD/NADH_2$ ratio (Fig. 11-4), which increases approximately four-fold when the heart work is suddenly increased (Opie and Owen, 1975).

Regulation of the citrate cycle by calcium

The above outline describes how the citrate cycle responds when the oxygen uptake of the heart is increased by a volume or a pressure load. When the

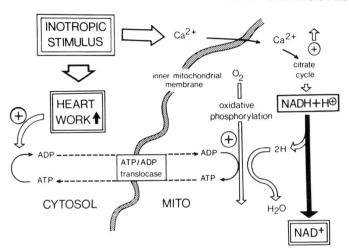

Fig. 11-4 During increased heart work, ADP is produced from ATP in the cytosol. ADP is transported inwards to the matrix space where it stimulates oxidative phosphorylation to convert NADH2 (NADH plus H+) to NAD (ionized form: NAD+). Note the proposed role of intramitochondrial calcium ions, rising in response to an inotropic stimulus, in increasing citrate cycle activity.

primary stimulus to increased heart work is increased contractility, associated with an increased cytosolic concentration of calcium ions, a new proposal is that the intramitochondrial calcium concentration also rises in response to the cytosolic increase. The end result is an increase in the rate of the citrate cycle (Fig. 11-4). There are two dehydrogenases of the citrate cycle, isocitrate dehydrogenase and alpha-ketoglutarate dehydrogenase, which are both sensitive to calcium ions in the range thought to be found in the cytosol. So also is pyruvate dehydrogenase sensitive to calcium which causes the conversion of the inactive to the active form. Calculations suggest that changes in the cytosolic Ca^{2+} of the order of $0 \cdot 1$–1 μM (in the range occurring in the cardiac cycle) could result in changes in intramitochondrial Ca^{2+} sufficient in magnitude to activate the dehydrogenase (Denton and McCormack, 1980; Coll et al., 1982).

Calcium Uptake and Release by Mitochondria

Calcium uptake by the mitochondria occurs by a "uniporter" system which is not linked to transport any other ion (Fig. 11-5). This uniporter transfers a double positive charge inwards with each calcium ion taken up so that the mitochondrial membrane tends to become depolarized. The mitochondrial matrix is normally negative (-180 mV) with respect to the cytosol (-90 mV) as a result of the outward pumping

of protons due to active mitochondrial respiration. Thus the uptake of calcium ions by the mitochondrial matrix effectively requires energy to pump the protons out to balance the charges brought in with calcium ions.

Calcium release occurs by an "antiporter" system, whereby sodium ions are taken up as calcium ions are released. This carrier system is electrically neutral so that two sodium ions are taken up for each calcium ion released. There are separate pathways and separate control mechanisms for calcium uptake and release; the operation of both at once leads to a constant cycling of calcium ions across the inner mitochondrial membrane. The flux of calcium ions can be varied in either direction so that the mitochondrial pool of calcium can act as a calcium buffer for the cytosol.

In conditions of **calcium overload** the uptake of excess calcium will ultimately impair the protein gradient across the mitochondrial membranes, thereby reducing the ability of mitochondria to synthesize ATP. The ultimate result is that there is less ATP production in comparison to the uptake of oxygen, so that the phosphorylation/oxidation (P/O) ratio falls (Fig. 11-6). Accumulation of Ca^{2+} by itself does not lead to permanent loss of mitochondrial function; simultaneous accumulation of inorganic phosphate is required for irreversible depolarization (Lotscher et al., 1980).

Calcium-mediated processes are the probable basis of reperfusion damage, when the mitochondria

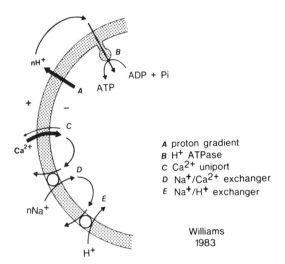

A proton gradient
B H⁺ ATPase
C Ca²⁺ uniport
D Na⁺/Ca²⁺ exchanger
E Na⁺/H⁺ exchanger

Williams
1983

Fig. 11-5 Calcium ions are transported into the mitochondrial matrix space in response to the proton gradient generated by respiration via a uniport system (C). Dissipation of the proton gradient may lead to an efflux of calcium by a reversal of the uniport. In contrast, calcium transport outwards is by a sodium–calcium exchange system (D), electrically neutral, which requires no energy. Sodium ions are then recycled out of the matrix by a sodium proton exchanger (E). Modified from Williams (1983), with permission.

become loaded with both calcium and phosphate, with about two calcium ions and one phosphate ion accumulating for each pair of electrons passing through each energy-conserving site of the respiratory chain. Calcium accumulates as insoluble calcium phosphate in the mitochondrial matrix to form **granular densities**.

Coupled Oxidative Phosphorylation

The exact mechanisms linking the oxidation of $NADH_2$ (formed from the activity of the citrate cycle or pathways of substrate breakdown) to the formation of ATP are still ill-understood, despite the obvious importance of this critical process. The basic **oxidative** reaction in coupled oxidative phosphorylation is the oxidation of $NADH_2$ (which equals NADH and H^+):

$$NADH + H^+ + O \rightarrow NAD^+ + H_2O$$

This is coupled to the **phosphorylation** of ADP

$$3\ ADP + 3\ P_i \rightarrow 3\ ATP$$

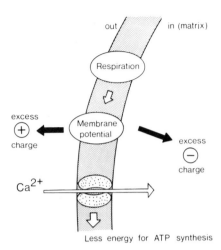

Less energy for ATP synthesis

Fig. 11-6 When calcium accumulates in the cytosol, respiration-driven uptake of calcium through the "uniporter" to the mitochondrial matrix is increased. Transport is electrophoretic, in that the positively charged calcium ions move to the side of the membrane with a relative excess of negative charges. This process consumes energy which would otherwise have been used for ATP synthesis by means of oxidative phosphorylation. Figure by courtesy of Prof. W Gevers.

in such a way that close to 3 molecules of ATP are formed for each atom or half-molecule of oxygen taken up (**P/O ratio** of 3). Depending on the substrate oxidized, the exact P/O ratio will vary from 2.83 to 3.17 (see Table 9-3). That means that the oxygen uptake can be changed by the nature of the substrate by a factor of just over 10 percent. The "physiological" variations in the P/O ratio simply reflect the number of O atoms in the substrate used. Thus, glucose, already containing some oxygen atoms in its structure, needs less oxygen added to produce H_2O than does fatty acid.

By **oxidation** is meant a process during which there is a transfer of electrons from an electron donor to an electron acceptor. Thus during oxidation, two processes occur:

(a) an electron donor donates e^-

(b) an electron acceptor accepts e^-

where e^- is the electron. Transfer of hydrogen is regarded as an equivalent process and the hydrogen atoms (H^+ plus e^-) are **reducing equivalents**. In the oxidation of $NADH_2$ the transfer of hydrogen atoms act as an overall reducing process by transferring electrons to oxygen to form water. Reduction of one molecule of oxygen (O_2) to water requires four electrons and, therefore, the components of the electron transport chain probably function in pairs.

Respiratory chain

Reducing equivalents, derived from $NADH_2$ (NADH + H^+), flow along the respiratory transport (or electron transmitter) chain as follows:

$$NADH + H^+ + flavoprotein \rightarrow$$
$$reduced\ flavoprotein + NAD^+$$

$$reduced\ flavoprotein + coenzyme\ Q \rightarrow$$
$$reduced\ coenzyme\ Q^* + flavoprotein$$

$$reduced\ coenzyme\ Q + cytochromes \rightarrow$$
$$reduced\ cytochromes + coenzyme\ Q$$

$$reduced\ cytochromes + oxygen \rightarrow$$
$$cytochromes + H_2O$$

(*coenzyme Q = ubiquinone = coenzyme Q_{10}).

Electrons are transferred through the cytochromes which are electron-transferring proteins containing iron porphyrin (heme) groups; the iron atoms undergo reversible changes in valency from the ferrous to the ferric form and vice versa. Heart mitochondria, with their high rate of respiration and extensive surface area of inner membranes, each contain 60 000–70 000 molecules of cytochrome in all, compared with 17 000 in each liver mitochondrion (Lehninger, 1975).

The respiratory chain may be divided into three spans, each associated with the production of ATP. **Site 1** is the span between NADH and coenzyme Q; **site 2** the span between cytochrome b and cytochrome c; and **site 3** is the span between cytochrome a and oxygen. Each of these sites yields one ATP and mitochondrial oxidation of NADH produced by the citrate cycle therefore yields three molecules of ATP per atom of oxygen reduced (a phosphorylation to oxygen uptake ratio or P/O ratio of 3). Other reactions (e.g. pyruvate dehydrogenase) forming $NADH_2$ will also have a P/O ratio of 3. But reactions feeding into the chain at the level of coenzyme Q will have a P/O ratio of 2 (succinate dehydrogenase produces $FADH_2$ which reacts with coenzyme Q).

Proton pumping

We have thus far concentrated on the transport of electrons; what of the accompanying **protons**? Thus:

$$Hydrogen\ atom = proton + electron$$
$$H = H^+ + e^-$$

There is thus an accompanying movement of protons together with electrons. According to Mitchell's theory of oxidative phosphorylation, protons are pumped outwards across the inner mitochondrial membrane, to yield a gradient of H^+ across them or within them (Fig. 11-7). This H^+ gradient is the driving force for phosphorylation of ADP, because protons re-enter the mitochondrial matrix through a complex of membrane proteins called the ATP synthetase, which is a protein ionophore. Formation of ATP is thus driven by proton

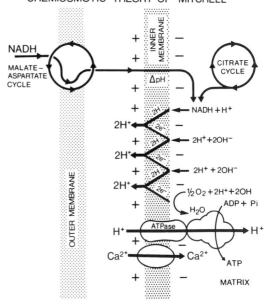

Fig. 11-7 Mitchell's chemiosmotic hypothesis, according to which the electron transfer components of the respiratory chain are arranged spatially and in sequence so that alternate electron and hydrogen atom (i.e. electron plus proton) transfers occur. The consequence of such an arrangement is that protons are transferred from the mitochondrial matrix space out across the inner membrane. The result is the establishment of an electrochemical proton gradient across the mitochondrial inner membrane (the proton motive force) made up of a proton concentration gradient and a charge separation or membrane potential. Coupling of the proton motive force to the synthesis of ATP from ADP and inorganic phosphate (P_i) occurs via a protein complex located in and on the inner mitochondrial membrane as protons re-enter the mitochondrial matrix. For further details, see Williams (1983). Figure by courtesy of Dr R Ferrari.

movements caused by the transmembrane proton gradient. The limitations of the Mitchell hypothesis and other hypotheses for oxidative phosphorylation have been discussed by Slater (1977) and Williamson (1979).

The Mitochondrial ADP–ATP Translocase

For oxidative phosphorylation to proceed requires a continuous supply of: (i) oxygen, delivered by the coronary circulation; (ii) protons and electrons, delivered by the citrate cycle; and (iii) ADP. Both ADP and ATP are large, highly charged molecules which must rapidly and continuously be transported across the impermeable inner mitochondrial membrane (Fig. 11-4). Such counter-exchange of ADP inwards and ATP outwards across the inner membrane occurs by the activity of a very active transport system, the ADP–ATP carrier or "antiporter", also called the **translocase**. Klingenberg (1979) calculates that the carrier constitutes 12 percent of the total protein in heart mitochondria, making it the most abundant protein of cardiac mitochondria. Metabolic considerations demand that this shuttle, together with the transport of inorganic phosphate, should be the most active system for moving metabolites across the mitochondrial membranes. The carrier system is highly selective, transporting only ADP and ATP; AMP and other nucleotides are not affected. The direction in which ADP and ATP are transported is determined by the properties of the translocase. The entry process of the translocase greatly prefers ADP to ATP, possibly by over 50 times. Hence as the cytosolic ATP is converted to ADP during increased heart work, ADP transport to within the mitochondrial matrix is encouraged. Thus in isolated heart mitochondria there is an inverse relation between the external ATP/ADP ratio and the oxygen uptake.

Inhibitors of ADP–ATP translocase

The activity of this translocase is vital to life of the heart, and hence compounds inhibiting the carrier can literally kill the heart. One such inhibitor is bongkrekate, a deadly poison produced by bacteria growing on coconut food products in Indonesia. Another inhibitor of pharmacological interest is **atractyloside** which is similar in structure to the physiological inhibitor acyl CoA. When infused into the coronary circulation, atractyloside can induce deficits of tissue high-energy phosphate compounds and an elevation of the ST-segment of the epicardial electrocardiogram, while bongkrekate causes cardiac failure.

ATP and Energy Status

A fall of ATP stimulates both the "primitive" energy supply systems of glycogenolysis and glycolysis, and also the oxidative systems (Fig. 11-8). Stimulation of the latter is assisted by an increased coronary blood flow via adenosine formation and means increased oxidative phosphorylation in the mitochondria. The detailed mechanisms whereby the decline in high-energy phosphate acts on the different pathways vary (Table 11-2), yet the principle is constant. It is not the level of ATP itself which regulates the "compensatory pathways", rather it is the formation of ATP breakdown products (adenosine monophosphate, inorganic phosphate, adenosine) which acts as the regulator. Breakdown of only a small amount of ATP can potentially markedly increase the cellular levels of the real regulators, such as AMP and adenosine.

Atkinson (1968) examined the general biological significance of the relation between adenine nucleotides and energy production. As less and less of the adenylate pool (ATP + ADP + AMP) exists in the form of ATP and more and more in the form of the breakdown products (ADP and AMP), so are many enzymes involved in energy production activated. He has proposed a complex (but frequently used) formation to represent the energy status of the cell:

$$E = \frac{1}{2} \frac{2\,ATP + ADP}{AMP + ADP + ATP}$$

where E = **energy charge**. Whether there is any real advantage to this complex formula still remains to be tested. In at least one situation—ischemic arrest during cardiopulmonary bypass (Foker et al., 1980)—marked loss of ATP is accompanied by an unchanged energy charge because ADP and AMP are utilized at the same rate as ATP. Hence the concept of "energy charge" may leave much to be desired when applied to the heart. The alternative term **"energy status"** refers to the balance between the high-energy phosphate compounds (ATP and CP) and their breakdown products.

The **phosphorylation potential** is another less complex formula, which has been evolved to relate change in high-energy phosphates to mitochondrial metabolism:

INFLUENCE OF O_2 SUPPLY ON
EXTENT OF ATP BREAKDOWN

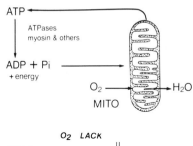

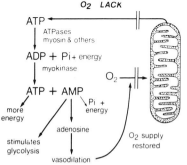

Fig. 11-8 The influence of oxygen supply on the extent of ATP breakdown. In normoxia ATP is broken down by heart work (myosin ATPase) to ADP and inorganic phosphate (P_i) which are resynthesized to ATP in the mitochondria. In hypoxia further breakdown yields more energy and stimulates glycolysis to provide anaerobic energy and causes a compensatory vasodilation (probably via adenosine).

$$\text{phosphorylation potential} = \frac{(ATP)}{(ADP)\,(P_i)}$$

AMP is omitted because it does not play a direct role in the regulation of mitochondrial respiration. The value of this ratio is that it is reciprocally related to the rate of mitochondrial oxidative metabolism (Sobell and Bunger, 1981). An even simpler approach is to think in terms of the cytosolic ADP concentration which is the major factor driving mitochondrial respiration. There is good correlation between the "phosphorylation potential" and the oxygen uptake of the isolated rat heart (Giesen and Kammermeier, 1980), provided that the problems of calculating the cytosolic ADP concentration (which is bound to proteins) are overcome. As ATP is broken down by increased heart work, oxidative phosphorylation is proportionately stimulated by the formation of the first stages of its breakdown products, ADP and inorganic phosphate.

Non-phosphorylation Respiration

Not all of the oxygen taken up by the heart is used in the production of ATP. Up to 10–20 percent of the oxygen uptake can be metabolized by pathways not producing ATP and sensitive to inhibition of oxidative phosphorylation such as cyanide or oligomycin. When the heart is "overloaded" with excess circulating fatty acids, or in hypermetabolic states such as catecholamine or thyroid stimulation, the percentage of such respiration rises (Challoner, 1966). The presumed mechanism of such oligomycin-insensitive respiration is by the newly described pathways whereby molecular oxygen is reduced by an unpaired electron to

Table 11-2

"Compensatory" metabolic pathways sensitive to falls of ATP and creatine phosphate (CP) and rises of ADP, AMP and inorganic phosphate (P_i)

Pathway	Site of regulation	Mode of regulation
Glycogenolysis	Phosphorylase	CP inhibits; AMP and P_i stimulate phosphorylase b
Glycolysis	Phosphofructokinase	ATP and CP inhibit; rise of AMP and P_i stimulates
Adenosine formation	5' nucleotidase	Fall in "energy status" activates
ATP synthesis	Oxidative phosphorylation	ADP and P_i stimulate mitochondrial oxidative phosphorylation

produce **free oxygen radicals** such as the superoxide anion:

$$\text{reduced flavin-enzyme} + O_2 \rightarrow$$
$$\text{flavin-enzyme} + O_2{}^-$$

Free radicals may also be produced by the xanthine oxidase reaction which is, however, not very active in the heart. Such free radicals are normally removed by various enzyme systems such as superoxide dismutase, which converts the superoxide anion into hydrogen peroxide; the latter is then acted on by catalase and peroxidase to yield water and molecular oxygen. **Glutathione reductase** also helps to remove spare electrons by aiding the formation of reduced glutathione. Because it is suspected that the increased formation of free radicals may contribute to ischemic and reperfusion damage, **scavenger** compounds have been used experimentally—such scavengers may include mannitol, glucose, coenzyme Q10 and α-tocopherol (Hess and Manson, 1984).

ATP Utilization

When the contractile activity of the heart is stopped by cardiac arrest or ventricular fibrillation, about 60–70 percent of the oxygen uptake ceases, showing that most of the high-energy phosphate production by oxidative phosphorylation is directed towards contractile activity (Fig. 11-9). Not all of such ATP is used directly for hydrolysis by the myosin heads, but some is used for uptake of calcium by the sarcoplasmic reticulum and for pumping sodium potassium and calcium ions across the sarcolemma. ATP may also be used in transporting ions into and out of the mitochondria. Smaller amounts of ATP may be required to maintain normal mitochondrial volume and structure. Further requirements of ATP are for (i) synthetic purposes (glycogen, triglyceride and protein synthesis) and (ii) to run "futile cycles".

"**Futile cycles**" use up ATP while cycling in two directions apparently without change in direction (Newsholme et al, 1984). An example is the constant turnover of glycogen. Another proposed cycle is the synthesis and breakdown of triglyceride in the triglyceride–fatty acid cycle. A third example of an apparently "futile cycle" is the constant uptake and release of Ca^{2+} by mitochondria, where the uptake is energy-dependent. Such "futile cycles" use ATP to maintain a low rate of turnover, but the cycles can suddenly be converted to one-way activity.

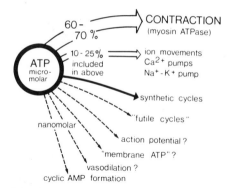

FUNCTIONS OF ATP

Fig. 11-9 Functions of ATP.

Except in the fetal heart, the rate of synthetic reactions is usually low. Nevertheless, as myocardial protein turns over at a relatively high rate, there must be a constant requirement for ATP for protein synthesis (Chapter 3).

Division of ATP utilization

Very rough estimates of the myocardial energy expenditure can be made. About 60–70 percent of myocardial oxygen uptake and ATP utilization is used for contractile purposes, including all the associated essential phenomena such as calcium uptake by the sarcoplasmic reticulum. About 10–15 percent of ATP may be used for active transport by the sodium–potassium pump (see Table 4-5). Very little (less than 5 percent) is used for the actual generation of the action potential or the conduction of the cardiac impulse. Some small amounts of ATP are needed to phosphorylate the proteins in response to the formation of cyclic AMP (Chapter 6). An ill-defined small percentage is used for the "futile cycles" of glycogen and triglyceride turnover and of mitochondrial calcium uptake and release, while a further small percentage is used for protein synthesis. In pathological states, ATP may be wasted if futile cycles speed up and if non-phosphorylating pathways of oxygen uptake are stimulated by excess free fatty acids ("oxygen-wastage").

In all these calculations it must be appreciated that the actual **energy** liberated by ATP hydrolysis is largely converted to heat. Thus only about 20–25 percent of the ATP used is actually converted into mechanical work. When allowance is made for the inevitable loss of heat, the heart is in fact very efficient in its ability to convert free energy into mechanical work plus heat.

Creatine Phosphate

At first sight it would appear that creatine phosphate (= phosphocreatine) rather than ATP is the immediate source of energy for contraction. In several types of heart failure, loss of creatine phosphate exceeds that of ATP. Yet the overall evidence is that it is ATP and not creatine phosphate that is used directly in muscular contraction, because it is ATP that causes isolated actomyosin threads to shorten. It is logical (and in agreement with the classical concepts of skeletal muscle physiology) that the ATP concentration in the myocardial cell should be maintained at the expense of creatine phosphate, with the pool of creatine phosphate suffering from more marked depletion than the pool of ATP. Very careful measurements show what is expected. Thus a small early fall of ATP precedes the large fall in creatine phosphate (Hearse, 1979) when all the coronary flow is abruptly stopped (global ischemia).

Energy transfer between ATP and CP

The transfer of energy from creatine phosphate to ATP occurs under the influence of creatine kinase (= CK = creatine phosphokinase = CPK), which catalyzes the following reaction:

$$CP + ADP \longrightarrow ATP + creatine$$

and the equilibrium favors formation of ATP by about 50 times. The function of creatine phosphate as a reserve of energy can be seen during an acute work jump in the isolated heart when creatine phosphate falls and ATP is kept constant. Why does the content of ADP rise rather than fall as would be expected from the above equation? This is partly because the initial event is ATP hydrolysis. Thus

$$ATP \xrightarrow{\text{myosin ATPase}} ADP + P_i + \text{free energy}$$

But ATP is reformed from creatine phosphate and ADP (see first equation above). Therefore, combining the above two equations, ATP should not fall at all:

$$CP \longrightarrow creatine + P_i + \text{free energy}$$

In reality ATP falls and ADP rises showing that the rate of ATP hydrolysis by the work jump exceeds

the rate at which ATP is formed from creatine phosphate.

Creatine kinase (or creatine phosphokinase)

The heart has a high content of creatine kinase and the loss of this enzyme in large amounts into the circulation is taken as proof of cell necrosis in acute myocardial infarction. The larger proportion of the cardiac creatine kinase exists in the cytosol as the **MB isoenzyme** (having one subunit of M muscle type and one of B brain type). The MM isoenzyme is present in small amounts in the myofibrils and possibly the microsomes. Different localization of isoenzymes within the extramitochondrial space could be one way in which "local" aliquots of energy are transferred from creatine phosphate to ATP, so that ATP can be used at various localized sites in the cytoplasm.

A mitochondrial CK isoenzyme is situated on the outside of the inner mitochondrial membrane where it is thought to be in close juxtaposition to the adenine nucleotide translocase (Fig. 11-10). The kinetic

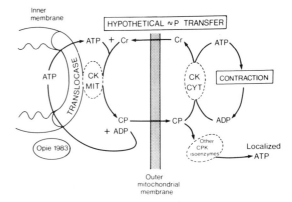

Fig. 11-10 Possible role of creatine phosphokinase (CPK), or creatine kinase isoenzymes in functional compartmentalization of ATP. According to the concepts of Saks et al. (1982), the mitochondrial CPK isoenzyme (CPK MIT) is situated between the inner and outer mitochondrial membranes to form creatine phosphate (CP) from creatine (CR). The outer mitochondrial membrane is freely permeable to creatine phosphate which can then reform ATP from ADP generated by cellular activity as, for example, contraction. This is the function of the cytoplasmic CPK isoenzyme (CPK CYT). Other CPK isoenzymes are also thought to produce "localized" ATP. For criticisms of this hypothesis see Altschuld and Brierley (1977).

properties of the enzyme support the role of enzyme in dealing with ATP newly synthesized and newly exported from mitochondria. ATP produced in the mitochondria by oxidative phosphorylation is thought to be transferred by the mitochondrial CK isoenzyme to cytoplasmic creatine phosphate. The latter compound then transfers high-energy phosphate bonds back to ATP at the site of ATP utilization, under the influence of a cytosolic isoenzyme of creatine kinase.

This doctrine of "privileged" access of mitochondrial ATP to mitochondrial creatine kinase is espoused by Saks and colleagues (Saks et al., 1982) but challenged by Altschuld and Brierley (1977). The latter authors propose that the cytoplasmic creatine kinases are so active that they promote rapid equilibrium of the substrate throughout the cytosol.

Whichever view is adopted, creatine kinase plays a vital role in the maintenance of cytosolic ATP at the expense of cytosolic creatine phosphate. By transferring energy-rich bonds from ATP emerging from the mitochondria to cytosolic creatine phosphate, and then back again to ATP, creatine kinase also controls the transport of energy in the cytosol.

Creatine phosphate as a source of inorganic phosphate

Besides its well-accepted function as a store of energy, creatine phosphate has other functions, such as being able to transfer energy from one ATP pool to another (Fig. 11-11). Creatine phosphate also functions as a "store" of inorganic phosphate (P_i) which is liberated in the formation of ATP without an increase in the total concentration of adenine nucleotides. Concomitant liberation of creatine will help to regulate the rate of energy production because ADP, formed from ATP and creatine, will stimulate oxidative phosphorylation. The rapid increase of inorganic phosphate is a striking feature of increased heart work or anoxia. Such increased inorganic phosphate can specifically stimulate phosphofructokinase and act as a substrate for phosphorylase *b* to stimulate glycogenolysis. When inorganic phosphate forms in the cytosol during a work jump, mitochondrial oxidative phosphorylation is stimulated.

Two mechanisms for the effect of P_i on mitochondrial respiration may operate. First, the extramitochondrial phosphorylation potential (ATP)/(ADP)(P_i) is altered so as to favor increased mitochondrial respiration; the reasons for this effect

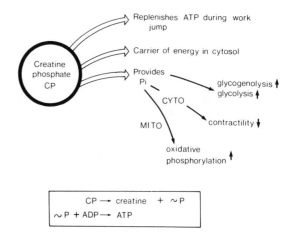

FUNCTIONS OF CREATINE PHOSPHATE

- Replenishes ATP during work jump
- Carrier of energy in cytosol
- Provides P_i
  - glycogenolysis ↑
  - glycolysis ↑
  - contractility ↓
  - oxidative phosphorylation ↑

$$CP \longrightarrow creatine + \sim P$$
$$\sim P + ADP \longrightarrow ATP$$

Fig. 11-11 Functions of creatine phosphate.

are very complex (Giesen and Kammermeier, 1980). Secondly, there probably is increased uptake of P_i by mitochondria which helps in the formation of ATP within the mitochondrial matrix (Altschuld and Brierley, 1977).

Formation of inorganic phosphate during heavy work can stimulate formation of energy. Also excess accumulation of inorganic phosphate during ischemia can paradoxically inhibit contractility and thereby diminish the oxygen demand (Kübler and Katz, 1977).

ATP Compartments

Mitochondrial versus cytoplasmic ATP

Compartmentation means that certain compounds are not uniformly distributed throughout the cell; rather, different concentrations are found in different compartments within the cell. Compartmentation of ATP between its site of production in mitochondria and its site of utilization in the cytoplasm is well-accepted. At least 90 percent of the ATP is found in the cytosol. During acute heart work it is the ATP in the cytosol which is broken down so that the very small amount of cytosolic ADP doubles. Cytosolic ADP will therefore rise with increased work to drive mitochondrial respiration, according to the classic concept that the rate of mitochondrial respiration is set by ADP.

Cytoplasmic subcompartments

The possibility of subcompartments of ATP within the cytoplasm provokes abundant controversy. Evidence **favoring** cytoplasmic subcompartmentation is as follows. First, unequal distribution of creatine kinase isoenzymes throughout the cytoplasm could form more ATP from creatine phosphate in specific cytosolic sites. Secondly, the existence of a small subcompartment of "rapid-turnover" ATP would explain those situations in which small changes in total ATP occur, but appear to have large effects — for example, the abrupt loss of contractile activity in ischemic hearts while the ATP is still relatively high (Gudbjarnason et al., 1970). Such low rates of fall of ATP in regional ischemia, compared with the much faster falls of creatine phosphate, have been shown by numerous workers. Hearse (1979) proposes that in the early seconds of ischemia, both ATP and creatine phosphate are lost. Depletion of only a small pool of ATP could cause contractile failure but it is equally possible that other factors such as a rise of tissue pCO_2 could cause the failure. Thirdly, ATP produced by glycolysis appears to have a special function in protecting the cell membrane (Bricknell and Opie, 1978) and in promoting relaxation of the heart. When ischemic contracture develops in under-perfused hearts, it is the source of ATP and not the total ATP which is important in preventing contracture. Thus ATP made by glycolysis is effective, while ATP from residual mitochondrial metabolism is not (Bricknell et al., 1981). Fourthly, ATP injected directly into altered cells helps to prolong the action potential duration (Taniguchi et al., 1983), suggesting a role of cytoplasmic ATP in electrogenesis.

Besides the possible role of glycolytically generated ATP on the sarcolemma threatened by anoxia, it also seems that ATP can interact directly with the cell membrane (Shukla et al., 1978). In ingenious experiments, red cell ghosts were lysed and resealed in media of varying ATP concentrations. The susceptibility of these ghosts to attack by phospholipases was studied. $MgATP^{2-}$ partially protected the ghosts — and only if it had access to the cytoplasmic surface of the membrane. A non-metabolizable analog of ATP gave as much protection as did ATP. One proposal is that the presence of ATP in the cytoplasm protected red cells against lysis by binding to a membrane glycoprotein on the cytoplasmic surface, thereby modulating the "local lipid environment".

Evidence arguing **against ATP compartments** chiefly relates to correlations found between the fall in the total ATP and the onset of irreversible ischemic injury (Kübler and Spieckermann, 1970; Hearse, 1979). An additional biochemical argument is that the cytosol can be viewed as in uniform space, throughout which creatine phosphate and ATP are in equilibrium (Altschuld and Brierley, 1977).

Localized formation of ATP in relation to myosin ATPase activity could be explained as the combined effects of ATP utilization and localized proton production, both events favoring the formation of ATP from creatine phosphate by the cytoplasmic creatine kinase system.

Breakdown of ATP

Adenosine diphosphate (ADP)

The best known products of ATP breakdown (Fig. 11-8) are ADP and inorganic phosphate, which normally form during the cardiac contraction cycle. Usually forgotten are the proton and the chelation of ATP to magnesium.

Thus the standard equation

$$ATP \longrightarrow ADP + P_i + \text{free energy}$$

becomes

$$MgATP^{2-} \longrightarrow MgADP^{1-} + Pi^{2-} + H^+ + \text{free energy}$$

The exact charges depend on the intracellular pH; ADP can (i) reform ATP via the creatine kinase reaction; or (ii) be further split to form ATP and AMP by the adenylate kinase reaction (see next section); or (iii) enter the mitochondria under the influence of the adenine nucleotide translocase to stimulate respiration.

The normal content of ADP in the heart is about 0.5–1 μmol/g wet wt. However, the real concentration dissolved in cell water (as opposed to the overall level) is difficult to assess because most ADP is bound to actin (Kohn et al., 1971), some to myosin and only a smaller portion is freely dissolved in the cytosol. In special experimental circumstances, ADP rises with each systole as ATP falls (Wikman-Coffelt et al., 1983). The breakdown of even small amounts of cytosolic ATP to ADP can markedly increase the concentration of "free" ADP in the cytosol (estimated at only 0.02 μmol/g wet wt), thereby stimulating mitochondrial metabolism.

Adenosine monophosphate (AMP)

Adenylate kinase (= AMP kinase = myokinase) allows the breakdown of ADP to proceed to AMP, thereby increasing the cardiac content of AMP:

$$2\ ADP \xrightarrow{\text{myokinase}} ATP + AMP$$

This reaction is reversible and will only proceed towards formation of AMP when ADP is elevated. Thus under the influence of myosin ATPase

$$2\ ATP \longrightarrow 2\ ADP + 2\ P_i + 2(\text{free energy})$$

and under the influence of myokinase

$$2\ ADP \longrightarrow ATP + AMP$$

and myosin ATPase again catalyzes

$$ATP \longrightarrow ADP + P_i + \text{free energy}$$

so that the overall reaction is

$$2\ ATP \longrightarrow ADP + AMP + 3\ P_i + 3(\text{free energy})$$

This overall equation liberates 1.5 times as much high-energy phosphate as does simple ATP hydrolysis (compare above equations).

Adenosine, inosine and hypoxanthine

Formation of AMP provides the substrate for the AMP deaminase reaction whereby AMP is broken down to IMP (inosine monophosphate; see Fig. 11-12). Another pathway of metabolism of AMP is also stimulated, since the decline in the "energy status" of the anaerobic cell activates 5′ nucleotidase (Fig. 11-12), the enzyme converting AMP to adenosine.

The extra energy provided by the added breakdown of ATP beyond ADP to AMP is bought only at the cost of further metabolism of AMP to IMP and adenosine (de Jong, 1979). Ultimately the adenine grouping will have to be resynthesized which will use ATP. Although some AMP forms within the heart cell at the start of severe stress, such as a sudden increase in heart work, such formation is only a temporary means of gaining added energy. A more important function is that of coronary vasodilation by adenosine. Once coronary flow is increased to meet the requirements of the new higher rate of oxygen uptake, tissue AMP returns virtually to normal. Thus it might be supposed that the processes breaking down ATP and related compounds normally stop at AMP. In reality deaminase enzymes must also be active because there

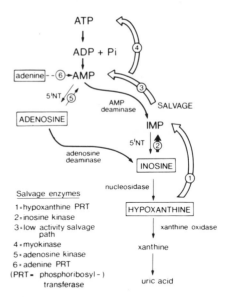

ADENINE NUCLEOTIDE SALVAGE PATHWAYS

Fig. 11-12 Pathways of adenine nucleotide salvage.

is production of small amounts of **ammonia** (NH_3) by the normal heart. Increased amounts of NH_3 are produced when ATP breakdown is pathologically accelerated as during ischemia. The rate of NH_3 formation probably becomes a good index of the activity of adenosine or AMP deaminase, because oxidative deamination (the alternative source of NH_3) is likely to be severely limited by $NADH_2$ accumulation in exhausted muscle.

Adenosine

Besides the critical role of adenosine in the regulation of coronary vasodilation to the Berne hypothesis (Chapter 12), adenosine has further interesting properties. It slows the sinus node and conduction through the AV node (Belardinelli et al., 1980) and hence is now being tested in the therapy of paroxysmal supraventricular tachycardias (DiMarco et al., 1983). **Adenosine also inhibits adenylate cyclase (Schrader et al., 1977), thereby providing potential protection** against excess beta-adrenergic stimulation. Adenosine may also protect against catecholamine-mediated damage by inhibition of entry of calcium ions by the slow channel. In ischemic cardiac arrest there is loss of total adenine nucleotides; successful efforts have been made to stimulate the rate of resynthesis of ATP during the recovery period by the therapeutic provision of adenosine, which acts provided that its breakdown is inhibited (Foker et al., 1980). In all these cases the adenosine concentrations achieved are probably far higher than the very low amount of adenosine found in the normal heart. Regulation of coronary flow therefore remains the major physiological role of adenosine.

Adenine Nucleotide Synthesis

There are two major pathways for synthesis of adenine nucleotides (for nomenclature see Table 11-3). First, the **salvage pathway** recovers the deaminated breakdown products such as inosine monophosphate or inosine, or even hypoxanthine (Fig. 11-11). Secondly, adenine nucleotides can be "freshly" made by **de novo synthesis**. Because of the loss of inosine and hypoxanthine from the ischemic myocardium (see next section), salvage pathways cannot fully restore adenine nucleotide levels. De novo synthesis (Fig. 11-13) probably operates in the post-ischemic recovery period. Not only is such de novo synthesis slow (taking hours or even days), but it is costly, requiring six high-energy phosphate bonds to manufacture one molecule of IMP from ribose phosphate (Murray, 1971). Hence delayed resynthesis of adenine nucleotides probably accounts, in part, for delayed recovery after reperfusion of the ischemic myocardium.

ATP Breakdown and Ischemia

When ATP is broken down acutely, as in hypoxia or ischemia, release of breakdown products from the heart can be expected. Thus during regional ischemia the concentration of inorganic phosphate in the coronary sinus rises; this phosphate is derived only in

PATHWAYS OF DE NOVO SYNTHESIS OF ADENINE NUCLEOTIDE

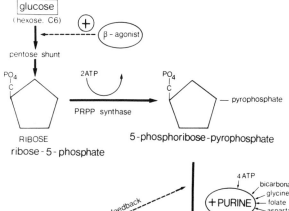

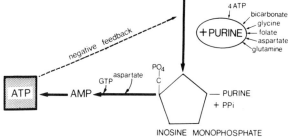

Fig. 11-13 Pathways of de novo ATP synthesis.

part from ATP, with a larger component coming from the breakdown of creatine phosphate. Adenosine, inosine and hypoxanthine can all cross the cell membrane and it is therefore not surprising that the ischemic myocardium releases these compounds (Fig. 11-14). All these changes are **indices of ischemia** indirectly indicating breakdown of high-energy phosphate compounds (as does release of inorganic phosphate). Generally, such breakdown will be accompanied by anaerobic glycolysis and lactate production. It is doubtful if the complex assays required for adenosine, inosine and hypoxanthine would warrant the added information gained, except

Table 11-3

Nomenclature of purines, nucleosides and nucleotides

Term	Definition	Example
Purine	Parent compound; heterocyclic; combination of 5- and 6-membered rings	—
Adenine	Purine + amino group = heterocyclic base	Adenine
Nucleoside	Heterocyclic compound + sugar	Adenosine, inosine
Nucleotide	Heterocyclic compound + sugar + phosphate = nucleoside phosphate. If sugar is ribose, then above = ribonucleoside phosphate	Adenine nucleotides (ATP, ADP, AMP); guanosine nucleotides; inosine nucleotides.

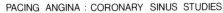

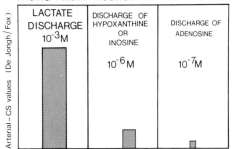

Fig. 11-14 Release of hypoxanthine, inosine and adenosine into coronary sinus blood during pacing-induced angina as a result of the breakdown of ATP. Note the much lower molar concentrations than of lactate, produced by anaerobic glycolysis. Based on data of de Jong (1979) and Fox et al. (1974).

as a research procedure. The chief value of measuring inosine and hypoxanthine is to confirm the changes in lactate.

Is there a critical level of ATP?

A simplistic view of cell death in ischemia would be that ATP falls to a critical level, vital functions cease and all is over. Considering the pains to which the cell goes to maintain and replenish its ATP, it would not be surprising if there was a critical level of ATP required to keep the cell alive.

In **surgical ischemic arrest**, Kübler and Spieckermann (1970) found that as ATP levels fell, there was a theoretical limit below which adequate cardiac function on reperfusion could not be regained. That limit was 3.5 μmol/g wet wt, below which glycolysis ceased. Hearse et al. (1977) have claimed a similar limit for recovery from **global ischemia** induced by aortic clamping, but set the value of ATP at about 12 μmol/g wet wt or about 2.4 μmol/g fresh wt. They did not find a link between the fall of ATP and the cessation of glycolysis. In **regional ischemia**, Jennings et al. (1978) have linked irreversible ultra-structural changes about 40 min after coronary artery occlusion to ATP levels of 2–3 μmol/g dry wt (= 0.4–0.6 μmol/g fresh wt). Similarly, the onset of rigor mortis could be linked to endocardial ATP values of 0.6 μmol/g fresh wt (Lowe et al., 1979). In **underperfused** heart, with acetate as a substrate (Bricknell et al., 1981), the development of ischemic contracture could be dissociated from the initial

pre-contracture ATP value. In the **non-ischemic zone** after coronary occlusion, there was an unexpected fall in the ATP content in some experiments. When it occurred, the fall in ATP and creatine phosphate reflected the severity of ischemic heart failure. Gudbjarnason et al. (1970) found that non-ischemic muscle contracted normally and survived at ATP values as low as 1.5–2.0 μmol/g wet wt. In **reperfusion** after ischemic arrest, Schaper et al. (1979) showed that ATP might fall as low as 1 μmol/g wet wt and the hearts could still survive.

The above evidence shows that it is very unlikely that there is a single "critical" level of ATP, especially because of the possibility of compartmentation of ATP. Furthermore, as cells die a great number of events besides loss of ATP takes place and the true cause of lethality could be the combination of depletion of ATP with the accumulation of potentially "toxic" metabolites, such as fatty acid derivatives, lactate, protons and CO_2. In any given experimental condition it seems easy to link a given ATP value with irreversibility. ATP depletion is harmful for ischemic cells but low ATP levels in well-oxygenated or reperfused cells can be withstood. Measurements of ATP are no substitute for direct measurements of irreversible ischemic injury such as ultrastructural changes or ischemic contracture.

ATP — an index of ischemic blood flow?

Another concept that needs consideration is whether or not the degree of depletion of ATP is an index of the severity of ischemia. If so, there should be a relationship between the fall of ATP and the deprivation of myocardial blood flow (Kloner and Braunwald, 1980). Several reasons have been advanced by Hearse (1984) against this simple empirical and apparently valid relationship. First, the depletion of ATP is not linear with time as could be expected because of complexities such as the reserve role of creatine phosphate, compartmentalization of ATP, and variable replenishment of ATP by glycolysis. Secondly, flow can be reduced up to about 50 percent without a detectable fall of ATP with flow falls to less than 20 percent. ATP decreases to about 30 percent of control within 45 min and then declines more slowly — such tissue is irreversibly damaged according to Hearse. It is in the intermediate flow value — to between 50 and 20 percent of normal — that the ischemia is "critical" and here there is a good relation between flow fall and ATP loss. Because many flow decreases in the dog heart with coronary occlusion are in this neighborhood, the relationship described by Kloner and Braunwald has empirical validity for that model.

ATP and arrhythmias

Given intravenously, ATP is effective against supraventricular re-entrant tachycardias (Belhassen et al., 1983). The probable mechanism is by conversion of ATP to adenosine, which in turn inhibits the AV node.

Non-ATP Nucleotides

From the point of view of nucleic acid biosynthesis, ATP occupies no more important a position than do its "sister" ribonucleoside triphosphates (guanosine triphosphate, uridine triphosphate, and cytidine triphosphate) or the deoxyribonucleotide triphosphates (dATP, dGTP, dCTP). Yet all these other substances are present at much lower concentrations in the cytoplasm of cardiac cells and are, in a sense, "slaves" to the prevailing status of the ATP pool. The ratio of ATP to ADP is reflected in each case in the prevailing ratio, at an actual concentration level 10 or 100 times lower, of the triphosphate and diphosphate forms of the other species.

Guanosine triphosphate (GTP) is necessary for initiation, elongation and termination steps in protein biosynthesis (Chapter 3). It is also an essential cofactor of the adenylate cyclase system (see Fig. 6-2) where it binds to the "regulator" protein which assists in transducing the effects of hormone–receptor interaction (e.g. in the case of beta-adrenergic receptors) into cyclic AMP formation. **Uridine triphosphate** (UTP) is a general co-factor for polysaccharide biosynthesis, and is required for the formation of UDPG (from glucose 1-phosphate), to act as the substrate for glycogen synthesis (see Fig. 10-12). In the case of phospholipid biosynthetic pathways, **cytidine triphosphate** (CTP) activates free bases such as choline or ethanolamine, or converts phosphatidate into an activated form for the formation of some membrane phospholipids (see Fig. 10-22).

Summary

The citrate cycle functions within the mitochondrial matrix to produce both CO_2 and hydrogen atoms and ultimately ATP by oxidative phosphorylation. The latter process takes place as hydrogen atoms are transferred along a chain of redox carriers (respiratory chain). The reducing equivalents pass through the respiratory chain while high-energy phosphate compounds are produced, normally three ATP molecules to every O atom taken up (P/O ratio of 3). Regulation of the citrate cycle is complex because its activity takes place in at least two spans and because part of the cycle can be bypassed by transamination reactions. An important mechanism regulating the activity of the citrate cycle is the mitochondrial ratio of $NAD/NADH_2$ (the redox state) which falls during increased heart work, when more cytosolic ATP is also broken down to ADP per unit time. The increased supply of cytosolic ADP is transferred to within the mitochondria by the ADP–ATP translocase, and this stimulates mitochondrial oxidative phosphorylation, using up both reducing equivalents and oxygen to form ATP and H_2O.

During inotropic stimulation, an increased cytosolic calcium ion concentration may also directly stimulate some dehydrogenases by increasing the intramitochondrial calcium. Simultaneous vasodilation (as a result of the formation of adenosine) brings the required extra supply of oxygen and substrates to the heart cells. When oxidative metabolism is impaired by ischemia the use of ATP falls dramatically. The ATP content also falls, but less rapidly, because ischemic arrest of contractility decreases utilization of ATP, and because of replenishment from creatine phosphate. As ATP falls, the level of breakdown products rises and the "energy charge" of the cell falls to stimulate restorative processes. During anaerobic states, there is formation of adenosine to cause a compensatory coronary vasodilation. Other eventual breakdown products are inosine and hypoxanthine. In the phase of recovery from ischemic arrest (as after cardiac surgery), ATP can be reformed either by salvage pathways or by de novo synthesis. The maximal rates of activity of the pathways are limited, so that post-ischemic recovery of ATP is aided by the addition of precursors for ATP recovery. It seems unlikely that there is a fixed critical ATP level below which the cell dies, although ATP is always low in dying cells.

References

Altschuld RA, Brierley GP (1977). Interaction between the creatine kinase of heart mitochondria and oxidative phosphorylation. J Molec Cell Cardiol 9: 875–896.

Atkinson DE (1968). Energy charge of the adenylate pool as a regulatory parameter: interaction with feedback modifiers. Biochemistry 7: 4030–4034.

Belardinelli L, Belloni FL, Rubio R, Berne RM (1980). Atrioventricular conduction disturbances during hypoxia: possible role of adenosine in rabbit and pig heart. Circ Res 47: 684–691.

Belhassen B, Pelleg A, Shoshani D, Geva B, Laniado S (1983). Electrophysiological effects of adenosine-5′-triphosphate on atrioventricular reentrant tachycardia. Circulation 68: 827–833.

Bricknell OL, Opie LH (1978). Effects of substrates on tissue metabolic changes in the isolated rat heart during underperfusion and on release of lactate dehydrogenase and arrhythmias during reperfusion. Circ Res 43: 102–115.

Bricknell OL, Daries PS, Opie LH (1981). A relationship between adenosine triphosphate, glycolysis and ischaemic contracture in the isolated rat heart. J Molec Cell Cardiol 13: 941–945.

Coll KE, Joseph SK, Corkey BE, Williamson JR (1982). Determination of the matrix free Ca^{2+} concentration and kinetics of Ca^{2+} efflux in liver and heart mitochondria. J Biol Chem 257: 8696–8704.

de Jong JW (1979). Biochemistry of acutely ischemic myocardium. In: The Pathophysiology of Myocardial Perfusion. Ed. W Schaper, pp 719–750, Elsevier/North Holland.

Denton RM, McCormack JG (1980). The role of calcium in the regulation of mitochondrial metabolism. Biochem Soc Transac 8: 266–268.

DiMarco JP, Sellers TD, Berne RM, West GA, Belardinelli L (1983). Adenosine: electrophysiologic effects and therapeutic use for terminating supraventricular tachycardia. Circulation 68: 1254–1263.

Foker JE, Einzig S, Wang T (1980). Adenosine metabolism and myocardial preservation. J Thor Cardiovasc Surg 80: 506–516.

Fox AC, Reed GE, Glassman E, Kaltman AJ, Silk BB (1974). Release of adenosine from human hearts during angina produced by rapid atrial pacing. J Clin Invest 53: 1447–1457.

Giesen J, Kammermeier H (1980). Relationship of phosphorylation potential and oxygen consumption in isolated perfused rat hearts. J Molec Cell Cardiol 12: 891–907.

Gudbjarnason S, Mathes P, Ravens KG (1970). Functional compartmentation of ATP and creatine phosphate in heart muscle. J Molec Cell Cardiol 1: 325–339.

Hearse DJ (1979). Oxygen deprivation and early myocardial contractile failure: A reassessment of the possible role of adenosine triphosphate. Am J Cardiol 44: 1115–1121.

Hearse DJ (1984). Critical distinctions in the modification of myocardial cell injury. In: Calcium-Antagonists and Cardiovascular Diseases. Ed LH Opie, pp 129–145, Raven Press, New York.

Hearse DJ, Garlick PB, Humphrey SM (1977). Ischemic contracture of the myocardium: mechanisms and prevention. Am J Cardiol 39: 986–993.

Hess ML, Manson NH (1984). Molecular oxygen: friend and foe. J Molec Cell Cardiol 16: 969–985.

Jennings RB, Hawkins HK, Lowe JE, Hill ML, Klotman S, Reimer KA (1978). Relation between high energy phosphate and lethal injury in myocardial ischemia in the dog. Am J Pathol 92: 187–207.

Klingenberg M (1979). The ADP, ATP shuttle of the mitochondrion. Trends Biochem Sci 4: 249–252.

Kloner RA, Braunwald E (1980). Observations on experimental myocardial ischemia. Cardiovasc Res 14: 371–395.

Kohn MC, Achs MJ, Garfinkel D (1977). Distribution of adenine nucleotides in the perfused rat heart. Am J Physiol 232: 158–163.

Kübler W, Spieckermann PG (1970). Regulation of glycolysis in the ischemic and the anoxic myocardium. J Molec Cell Cardiol 1: 351–377.

Kübler W, Katz AM (1977). Mechanism of early "pump" failure of the ischemic heart: possible role of adenosine triphosphate depletion and inorganic phosphate accumulation. Am J Cardiol 40: 467–471.

Lehninger AL (1975). Biochemistry, 2nd Edition, p 513, Worth Publishers, New York.

Lotscher HR, Winterhalter KH, Carafoli E, Richter C (1980). The energy-state of mitochondria during the transport of Ca^{2+}. Europ J Biochem 110: 211–216.

Lowe JE, Jennings RB, Reimer KA (1979). Cardiac rigor mortis in dogs. J Molec Cell Cardiol 11: 1017–1031.

Murray AW (1971). The biological significance of purine salvage. Ann Rev Biochem 40: 773–826.

Neely JR, Denton RM, England PJ, Randle PJ (1972). The effects of increased heart work on the tricarboxylate cycle and its interactions with glycolysis in the perfused rat heart. Biochem J 128: 147–159.

Opie LH, Owen P (1975). Assessment of mitochondrial free $NAD^+/NADH$ ratios and oxaloacetate concentrations during increased mechanical work in isolated perfused rat heart during production or uptake of ketone bodies. Biochem J 148: 403–415.

Saks VA, Kupriyanov VV, Preobrazhenskii AN, Jacobus WE (1982). Creatine kinase and protein kinase reactions of cardiac cell membranes. J Molec Cell Cardiol 14: Suppl 3: 1–12.

Schaper J, Mulch J, Winkler B, Schaper W (1979). Ultrastructural, functional, and biochemical criteria for estimation of reversibility of ischemic injury: a study on the effects of global ischemia on the isolated dog heart. J Molec Cell Cardiol 11: 521–541.

Schrader J, Baumann G, Gerlach E (1977). Adenosine as inhibitor of myocardial effects of catecholamines. Pflügers Arch 372: 29–35.

Shukla SD, Billah MM, Coleman R, Finean JB, Michell RH (1978). Modulation of the organization of erythrocyte membrane phospholipids by cytoplasmic ATP. The susceptibility of isotonic human erythrocyte ghosts to attack by detergents and phospholipase C. Biochim Biophys Acta 509: 48–57.

Slater EC (1977). Mechanism of oxidative phosphorylation. Ann Rev Biochem 46: 1015–1026.

Sobell S, Bunger R (1981). Compartmentation of adenine nucleotides in the isolated working guinea pig heart stimulated by noradrenaline. Hoppe-Seyler's Z Physiol Chem 362: 125–132.

Taniguchi J, Noma A, Irisawa H (1983). Modification of the cardiac action potential by intracellular injection of adenosine triphosphate and related substances in guinea pig single ventricular cells. Circ Res 53: 131–139.

Wikman-Coffelt J, Sievers R, Coffelt RJ, Parmley WW (1983). The cardiac cycle: regulation and energy oscillations. Am J Physiol 245: H354–H362.

Williams A (1983). Mitochondria. In: Cardiac Metabolism. Ed AJ Drake-Holland, MIM Noble, pp 151–171, John Wiley, New York.

Williamson JR (1979). Mitochondrial function in the heart. Ann Rev Physiol 41: 485–506.

New References

Newsholme EA, Challiss RAJ, Crabtree B (1984). Substrate cycles: their role in improving sensitivity in metabolic control. Trends Biochem Sci 9: 277–280.

Piper HM, Sezer O, Schleyer M, Schwartz P, Hütter JF, Spieckermann PG (1985). Development of ischemia-induced damage in defined mitochondrial subpopulations. J Molec Cell Cardiol 17: 885–896.

Zimmer HG, Ibel H (1984). Ribose accelerates the repletion of the ATP pool during recovery from reversible ischemia of the rat myocardium. J Molec Cell Cardiol 16: 863–866.

12 | Oxygen Supply: Coronary Flow

Because the work and the energy production of the heart vary so much from rest to exercise, there must be some system of variable oxygen delivery to the myocardium. It is a variable coronary flow rate which controls the delivery of oxygen. Blood leaving the heart in the coronary sinus is markedly deoxygenated and black in color; hence, in response to myocardial hypoxia, little further extraction of oxygen is possible. When the heart needs more oxygen (as during exercise), it is the coronary flow that must increase.

Berne (1964) has proposed that the myocardium communicates its oxygen requirements to the coronary arteries by the rate of production of adenosine. According to this hypothesis, when the heart cell lacks

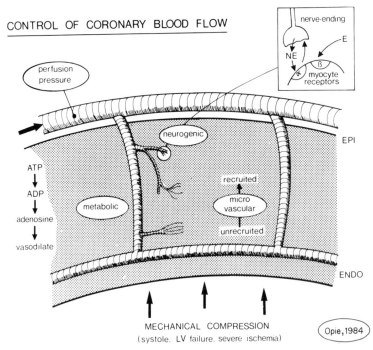

Fig. 12-1 Metabolic versus neurogenic control of the coronary circulation. Metabolic control is the basic mechanism, whereas neurogenic control is ancillary. EPI = epicardial; ENDO = endocardial

oxygen (as during vigorous work) the breakdown of only a small quantity of high-energy phosphate compounds produces enough adenosine for powerful coronary vasodilation. The link between the myocardium and the coronary circulation most probably lies in the factors regulating the production of adenosine (Feigl, 1983), although other theories emphasize the possible role of prostaglandins or other vasoactive compounds such as potassium and lactate. More recently the neurogenic theory for control of the coronary circulation has stressed that activity of the autonomic nervous system plays an important ancillary role (Fig. 12-1).

Coronary Circulation

The two major coronary arteries run from the base of the aorta to the left and right ventricles respectively, before giving off branches which track down the heart towards the apex. It is the left coronary artery which usually supplies the left ventricular wall; its major branch is the left anterior descending coronary artery (= anterior interventricular artery) which supplies part of the septum. This pattern is variable from species to species, as well as from individual to individual. In man, the coronary arteries have attracted popular attention because when partially or completely occluded by coronary atherosclerosis (= coronary artery disease), the myocardial oxygen supply becomes inadequate. The result is **myocardial ischemia**— an imbalance between the oxygen supply and demand, whereby demand exceeds the supply and the myocardium starts to suffer from the effects of lack of oxygen. The control of the myocardial oxygen supply resides in the small, narrow terminal branches of the coronary arteries, the coronary arterioles, which keep on branching (Fig. 12-2) until the very small, thin-walled capillaries are formed. The microcirculation is that part of the coronary circulation concerned with the regulation of the terminal arterioles and capillaries, directly responsible for the transfer of oxygen from the oxygenated arterial blood to the myocardial tissues.

Capillary anatomy

In the normal heart, there are over 2000 capillaries per cubic millimeter, of which only between 3/5 and 4/5 function normally (Winbury et al., 1969). The number of functioning capillaries increases by recruitment if

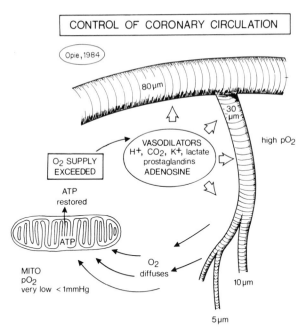

Fig. 12-2 The role of adenosine in local metabolic control of the coronary circulation. mito = mitochondria.

Table 12-1

Micro-anatomy of oxygen supply of myocardial cell

Capillaries per mm² left ventricle	about 2500
Muscle fibers (myocytes) per mm²	about 2500
Muscle fiber diameter, μm	17–18
Fiber–capillary ratio	1.0
Mean capillary diameter, μm	17
Intercapillary distance, μm	17
Diffusion distance, μm (half of intercapillary)	8.5

Data sources:
Bourdeau-Martini J et al. (1974). Am J Physiol 226: 800–810.
Honig CR and Bordeau-Martini J (1974). Circ Res Suppl 2: 34, 35: 97–103.
Kreuzer F and Turek Z (1979). In: Oxygen Supply of Heart and Brain, Eds Tenhoor et al., pp 48–62, Dutch Heart Foundation, The Hague.
Tomanek RJ et al. (1982). Circ Res 51: 295–304.
Wittenburg JB (1970). Physiol Rev 50: 559–636.

the arterial oxygen tension falls (Tables 12-1 and 12-2). The myocardium accommodates this "astonishing abundance of open capillaries" because each capillary is extremely narrow (Bourdeau-Martini et al., 1974). With a mean capillary diameter of about 3–7 μm, less than 5 percent of tissue volume is occupied. The

Table 12-2

Recruitment of capillaries

	Intercapillary distance (μm)	Diffusion distance (μm)
Normal	17	8.5
Exercise, estimated	14	7.0
Hypoxia	14.5	7.3
Prolonged anoxia	11	5.5
Maximal recruitment	6.5	3.3

For data sources, see footnote to Table 12-1.

normal intercapillary distance is about 17 μm (Table 12-1). During arterial hypoxia, the precapillary sphincters relax and more capillaries are recruited; now the intercapillary distance shrinks to 14.5 μm (Table 12-2). Prolonged anoxia reduces the distance further to 11 μm. These findings support Krogh's early idea (Krogh, 1919) of the regulation of capillary density by the metabolic demands of the tissue. In exercise, the coronary blood flow might double, but unless there is recruitment of capillaries with a reduction of intercapillary distance the oxygen demands of the tissue cannot be met. Even reducing the intercapillary distance from 17 to 14 μm allows the oxygen to diffuse to an additional 1.5 μm, which is an important adjustment to avoid tissue anoxia. Bing's group has used a new technique of transillumination to study the capillary pattern of the cat atrial muscle (Chang et al., 1982); different values for capillary size were found, but the principles of capillary control stay the same. Only after such microvascular changes have occurred, and oxygen-deprivation is still severe, are the reserves of oxygen dissolved in the tissue and in myoglobin used up.

Myoglobin

Myoglobin is an oxygen-binding hemoglobin-like compound found only in low concentrations in the heart, being about 0.25 mM or 0.4 g/100 g. Even the small amounts of oxygen associated with myoglobin may be important in intracellular oxygen transport (Wittenberg, 1970) because the partial presence of oxygen required for half maximal saturation of myoglobin is very low (2.4 mmHg). In the normal heart, oxygen bound to myoglobin or dissolved in the tissues can maintain the heart for about 8 sec or

8 contractions in the absence of any coronary blood flow (Kübler and Spieckermann, 1970). Whether myoglobin is not only a reservoir for small amounts of oxygen but also facilitates the transport of oxygen, as suggested by Wittenberg, still awaits direct proof.

Oxygen diffusion

In 1919 Krogh predicted that the oxygen tension of the tissue would fall as the distance from the capillary lumen increased. Thus oxygen could diffuse along its gradient of partial pressure from the site of supply, the capillary, to the site of utilization in the mitochondria. An implicit assumption was that oxygen could diffuse freely through the capillary by its lipid solubility or through pores (Pappenheimer et al., 1951).

It still remains possible that the capillary wall is not freely permeable to oxygen, thereby explaining why the oxygen tension in coronary venous blood is higher than in the tissue (Whalen, 1971), and why the tissue pO_2 appears to fall more than the coronary venous pO_2 after coronary occlusion. Another explanation of this phenomenon is that there are substantial arteriovenous anastamoses bypassing foci of low tissue pO_2. Counter-current exchange of oxygen between arterial and venous vessels, which would give the same effect as an arteriovenous shunt, is unusual in the heart where the dominant pattern (at least in atrial muscle) is an asymmetrical distribution (Chang et al., 1982).

Tissue oxygen tension

The cytochrome oxidase system where oxygen acts in the mitochondria (Chapter 11) requires a remarkably low oxygen tension of below 0.05 mmHg (O_2 concentration 10^{-7} M); this is the minimal effective tissue oxygen tension for oxidative phosphorylation (Chance, 1976). The oxygen tension required for mitochondrial function is about 2000 times less than that in arterial blood (say 100 mmHg). The average myocardial tissue pO_2 (oxygen tension) should lie between these values. To measure tissue oxygen tension with a needle microelectrode requires intracellular penetration and trauma, which can be circumvented by measuring pO_2 on the surface of the beating heart or calculated from the hemoglobin oxygen saturation measured in frozen myocardium. The same message emerges irrespective of the technique: there is a marked variation both in the oxygen content of the capillary hemoglobin and in the oxygen tension of myocardial tissue, with some values apparently approaching zero. Because of the wide variety of tissue pO_2 values, any given state of oxygenation is best described as a histogram. As the pO_2 falls, so does the histogram change until the majority of tissue oxygen tensions are less than 5 mmHg.

None of these techniques can measure the existence of possible oxygen gradients within the myocardial cell. Chance and his colleagues (Tamura et al., 1978) analyzed the state of oxygenation of various intracellular respiratory pigments to show the probable existence of an intracellular gradient of oxygen tension from the cytosol to the mitochondria.

The phasic patency of precapillary sphincters suggest that at any given overall level of capillary recruitment, capillaries are opening and closing all the time. The concept of temporarily dormant mitochondria waiting for recruitment of capillaries or for relaxation of precapillary sphincters to provide enough oxygen is not impossible; it is not known how many of the mitochondria of any given heart cell need to be functioning at any given time.

Metabolic Vasodilation

Adenosine

Adenosine plays a critical but probably not solitary role in the local metabolic regulation of the coronary circulation. As a result of hypoxia, ischemia or increased heart work, high-energy phosphate compounds are broken down; as the ATP falls there are rises in ADP (adenosine diphosphate), AMP (adenosine monophosphate) and inorganic phosphate (Chapter 11). This change in the energy status of the myocardial cell is thought to lead to activation of the enzyme 5'-nucleotidase with production of adenosine (Fig. 12-3) from AMP (Berne and Rubio, 1980).

The enzyme 5'-nucleotidase converts AMP to adenosine at the sarcolemma; any adenosine which returns to the cell interior is rephosphorylated to AMP while adenosine leaving the cell reaches the extracellular space where it is able to accumulate and act on the arteriolar vessel wall. Adenosine does not have to penetrate the vascular cell to vasodilate; it dilates even when firmly attached to molecules that cannot penetrate into the coronary artery cell.

Once adenosine has penetrated through the vessel

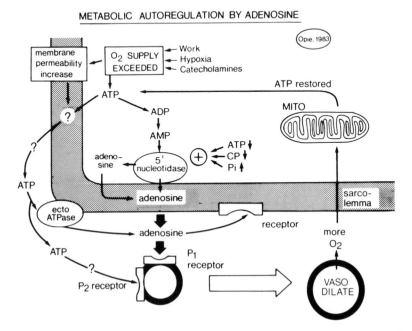

METABOLIC AUTOREGULATION BY ADENOSINE

Fig. 12-3 Adenosine, formed from ATP in conditions of increased myocardial work or hypoxia, is thought to interact with a vascular receptor (P_1, Table 6-1) to cause vasodilation. CP = creatine phosphate; P_i = inorganic phosphate.

into the intravascular space, it is broken down by adenosine deaminase present both in red cells and in the vessel wall. Agents such as dipyridamole (Persantine) and lidoflazine inhibit adenosine deaminase, allow adenosine to accumulate and increase coronary vasodilation. On the other hand, theophylline competes with adenosine for the vascular sites, so that it inhibits the vasodilation caused by exogenous adenosine.

Other vasodilatory metabolites

Many other metabolites besides adenosine may also control the coronary circulation, but for none is the case as strong as for adenosine.

Protons produced by anaerobic metabolism have a direct effect in causing coronary vasodilation and also sensitize the coronary arteries to the effects of added adenosine. The vasodilating effect of lactic acid could, in part, be explained by the effect of protons.

Certain concentrations of **potassium** are vasodilators and very high values vasoconstrict. Potassium modulates alpha- and beta-adrenergic effects and helps to regulate the rate of release of neurotransmitters from the coronary nerves in isolated coronary arteries.

Normally ATP is found within the cell and does not cross the sarcolemma. An unexpected and controversial proposal is that **ATP** is released in minute amounts by hypoxic or working heart muscle into the circulation, to have a vasodilating effect (Clemens and Forrester, 1980). In other tissues, purinergic nerve terminals are thought to release intracellular ATP by exocytosis. If this system were found in the heart it would provide a theoretical basis for ATP as a vasodilator.

Prostaglandins

During pacing angina, prostaglandins are released into coronary venous blood, so it is not surprising that prostaglandins have been regarded as physiological vasodilators. These early observations have been supported by the recent isolation of prostacyclin (PGI_2) which powerfully relaxes coronary arteries as well as inhibiting platelet aggregation. Drug interactions with prostaglandins are also being described; nitrates increase and indomethacin inhibits the formation of vasodilating prostaglandins. Yet the real role, if any, for prostaglandins in control of the coronary circulation is still unknown.

Autonomic Control

Sympathetic stimulation activates vasoconstricting alpha-adrenergic receptors in the coronary arteries (Fig. 12-4), while increasing the myocardial oxygen uptake by the positively inotropic effect. The alpha-mediated tendency to vasoconstriction prevents the full response to metabolic demands by about one-third (Mohrman and Feigl, 1978). During exercise, such alpha-mediated vasoconstrictor tone is withdrawn. A useful proposal is that alpha-mediated vaso-

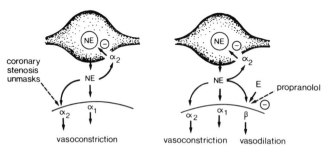

Fig. 12-4 The role of sympathetically mediated vasoconstriction, as may be important in genesis of coronary artery spasm. Norepinephrine (NE) released from the varicosities of the terminal nerve-endings (see Fig. 16-4), is thought to cause vasoconstriction by two types of post-synaptic alpha-adrenergic receptors, alpha-1 and alpha-2. The current proposal is that increasing coronary stenosis unmasks alpha-2-mediated vasoconstriction, whereas beta-adrenergic blockade by propranolol inhibits vasodilation mediated by norepinephrine and circulating epinephrine (E) to allow unopposed vasoconstriction which is alpha-2-mediated (Heusch and Deussen, 1983). For the further concept that calcium antagonists act to inhibit alpha-2-vasoconstriction, see Fig. 17-3.

constriction helps to keep metabolic vasodilation to the minimum required by the metabolic demands of the myocardium (Bassenge et al., 1978) so as to avoid "overloading" the myocardium with blood and thereby increasing the systolic work of the heart.

An abnormal increase in alpha-adrenergic tone may be a cause of coronary spasm during exposure to cold or emotional stress (Fig. 12-4).

Other autonomic effects

By analogy with arteries elsewhere, the coronary arteries should respond to beta-adrenergic stimulation by vasodilation. Although the beta-receptor effect is weak in coronary arteries, the expected vasodilatory effect can be unmasked by alpha-adrenergic blockade (Vlahakes et al., 1982). Hence the clinical concept that beta-adrenergic blockade could indirectly promote coronary vasoconstriction (by unopposed alpha-mediated activity) receives experimental support. The role of the parasympathetic system in the physiological control of the coronary circulation is not very significant.

Reactive Hyperemia

Reactive hyperemia is a phenomenon not well explained by either the metabolic or the neurogenic theories of coronary control. When the coronary arteries are transiently occluded and then reperfused, there is a period of apparent overperfusion as the blood flow rises substantially for a short period. Such reactive hyperemia is not inhibited by theophylline, as it would be if adenosine were involved. It is possible that during reactive hyperemia, protons are washed out from the heart cell and such protons increase the ability of adenosine to vasodilate to such an extent that the theophylline effect is no longer noted. Alternatively, a vasodilator other than adenosine (such as ATP) could be responsible for reactive hyperemia.

Reactive hyperemia can be found in patients in whom the coronary artery is briefly occluded during percutaneous transluminal angioplasty, a procedure used increasingly in selected patients with coronary artery disease. The effects of transient occlusion in patients seem to be less severe than in animals, possibly owing to a more abundant collateral formation in humans (Rothman et al., 1982).

Coronary Vascular Reserve

The mechanisms whereby the coronary blood flow can increase several-fold to meet the metabolic needs of exercise have been outlined. Such potential for vasodilation is called the coronary vascular reserve. Methods of achieving maximal flow include intracoronary administration of dipyridamole which inhibits the breakdown of adenosine and the maximal hyperemia flow found in response to the transient ischemia caused by injection of the radio-opaque contrast material used for coronary angiography. Coronary vascular reserve is reduced in ischemic heart disease, by chronic smoking (Klein et al., 1983) and in the hypertrophied heart of hypertension (Chapter 20).

Phasic Coronary Flow

Thus far we have not considered the implications of the pressure alterations during the cardiac cycle. An important current hypothesis is that systolic blood flow in the subendocardium falls as left ventricular pressure rises because the arteriolar flow is compressed. Conversely, subendocardial blood flow increases in diastole. In endocardial tissue, blood flow in systole stops as the pressure within the left ventricle rises. Of the total coronary flow, 85 percent occurs in diastole; the remaining 15 percent occurs in systole but only in the epicardial zone (Winbury and Howe, 1979).

The "Garden-hose" and "Erectile" Effects

The accepted view is that the coronary arteries dilate in response to an increased myocardial oxygen demand. Although the evidence for this supposition is good, there is also some evidence for an opposite sequence of events showing that an increased delivery of oxygen from the circulation can increase the myocardial oxygen uptake.

Gregg (1963) has commented on the possibility that in man the rate of coronary flow could regulate myocardial oxygen uptake rather than vice versa. Evidence has gradually hardened against the above point of view, which has even been called "Gregg's folly", but we should not lightly discard Gregg's ideas that excess coronary flow could cause an inotropic effect.

In 1965, Opie showed that increasing the perfusion

pressure of the coronary arteries of the isolated "non-working" heart led to an increased coronary flow and oxygen uptake. A simple explanation later provided by the Morgan–Neely group, was that the aortic perfused heart was not entirely empty but contained some fluid which probably reached the left ventricular cavity by the Thebesian vessels. This fluid could be ejected from the left ventricle against the pressure in the aorta, i.e. the perfusion pressure. Therefore, as the perfusion pressure increased, so would the heart rate rise as would the oxygen uptake. However, another factor was involved; in a classic paper by Arnold et al. (1968), it was shown that even at a constant coronary flow, an increase in perfusion pressure caused by a high viscosity perfusate could increase the oxygen uptake. They called this phenomenon the "garden-hose" effect (increased intraluminal pressure→stiffer hose→more rigid myocardial walls→more heart work). The blood within the arterial wall is thought to distend the artery with an "erectile" effect which in turn increases diastolic stiffness and heart work (Vogel et al., 1982). Conversely when an artery is empty of blood, a decreased erectile effect may contribute to decreased contractility.

Besides the "garden-hose" effect, the increased blood supply accompanying increased oxygen delivery could act by recruitment of vessels otherwise not patent. Yet another possible mechanism is that the local oxygen tension (increased by high coronary flow rates) could directly influence the oxygen uptake and mechanical performance (Whalen and Fangman, 1963; Frezza and Bing, 1976).

A possible example of Gregg's mechanism in man could be the effect of intracoronary nitrates on myocardial contractile activity. In one study, nitrates increased the maximal rate of pressure development (max dP/dt) at the same time as causing coronary vasodilation (Hood et al., 1980). This phenomenon, which could not be explained by the authors, could be an example of the "erectile effect".

Transmural Oxygen Gradients

A traditional point of view has been that the subendocardial zone of the heart has a lower oxygen tension and a more anaerobic type of metabolism. The lower oxygen tension could cause a lower oxygen uptake. When the coronary flow is reduced, the endocardial zone suffers from even lower values of

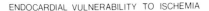

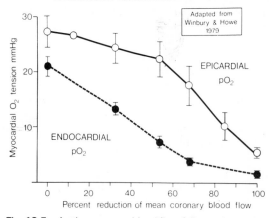

Fig. 12-5 As the coronary blood flow falls, so the oxygen tension in the endocardial zone falls more than in the epicardium. Data adapted from Winbury and Howe (1979).

Table 12-3

Comparative metabolism of subendocardial and subepicardial zones in normal hearts and in sustained ischemia.

	Subendocardial zone	Subepicardial zone
Normal[a]		
Blood flow, ml/100 g/min	71	57
O$_2$ uptake, ml/100 g/min	10.1	6.4
Developing infarction (2 hours)[b,c]		
Blood flow, ml/100 g/min	19	43
O$_2$ uptake, ml/100 g/min	1.3	2.5

[a]Holtz I et al. (1977). Pflügers Arch 370: 253–258.
[b]Weiss MR (1980); ligation of left ventricular descending coronary artery in dog.
[c]Ratio of flow in subendocardial to subepicardial zones is 0.44 vs 1.24 in non-ischemic zone.

oxygen tension (Fig. 12-5) and there is greater depletion of creatine phosphate and more accumulation of lactate.

More recent data show that the inner myocardial layers actually have higher, not lower, rates of oxidative metabolism (Table 12-3). Subendocardial layers, being subject to greater mechanical stress, require an increased oxygen uptake which accounts for the lower tissue oxygen tension. A higher rather than lower capillary density in the endocardial zones (Myers and Honig, 1964) also supports the idea of a higher rate of oxidative metabolism in the subendocardium.

Coronary Stenosis

Increasing coronary stenosis has two ultimate effects. First, the direct effect decreases the perfusion pressure. Secondly, the indirect effect of tissue ischemia causes contractile failure, thereby increasing the left ventricular end-diastolic pressure which in turn compresses subendocardial tissue and reduces coronary perfusion.

To reduce coronary flow by stenosis requires a very large reduction in arterial lumen (Gregg and Bedynek, 1978). The most important factor is the severity of the stenosis and the consequent increase in resistance to blood flow across the stenosis (Klocke, 1983). The resistance increases by a power of four as the radius decreases (Poiseuille's law, Chapter 21) so that reducing the internal diameter from 80 to 90 percent dramatically elevates the resistance (Fig. 12-6). Resting flow is not affected until the stenosis is very severe, so that one estimate is that a 70 percent reduction of internal diameter with a 90–95 percent fall in luminal area is required for basal coronary flow to fall (Gregg and Bedynek, 1978). In response to stimuli causing maximal vasodilation, flow starts to fail to achieve maximal values when the internal diameter is reduced beyond 30 percent and the internal luminal area by over 50 percent (Klocke, 1983).

For a given severity of stenosis, the longer the stenotic segment, the more marked the effects of any given degree of occlusion (Fig. 12-7). For any given degree of **fixed coronary stenosis**, there are complex additional factors such as the degree of turbulence across the stenosis and added vascular spasm which may decrease the flow as the demand rises during exercise (**dynamic stenosis**). In severe stenosis, the post-stenotic pressure can fall below a certain critical value of about 50 mmHg required for normal vasodilation and autoregulation (Klocke, 1983). The failure of compensatory vasodilation further robs the already ischemic myocardium of blood flow. Severe subendocardial or even transmural ischemia causes left ventricular failure by increasing the intracavity pressure, and further decreases the actual perfusion (driving) pressure across the stenosis.

Such experimental data show why the relationship

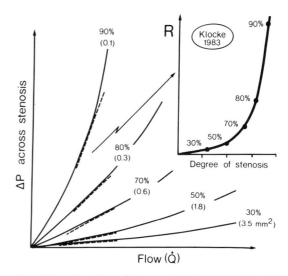

Fig. 12-6 The effect of the severity of coronary stenosis (internal diameter) on vascular resistance (R). From Klocke (1983), with permission.

EFFECT OF CORONARY FLOW ON 'CRITICAL' STENOSIS

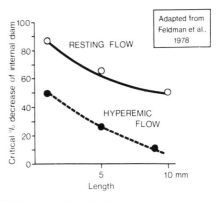

Fig. 12-7 As the length of stenosis of the coronary artery increases, so does a smaller internal diameter have a greater effect in reducing blood flow. As the flow rises in reactive hyperemia, a milder degree of stenosis becomes more serious. Data adapted from Feldman et al. (1978).

between the severity of coronary stenosis and the degree of ischemia produced in patients is not easy to predict — especially when irregular atherosclerotic plaques, various degrees of collateral circulation and pre-existing myocardial dilation might well alter the effects of any given degree of stenosis. The anatomical site of the occluded artery also determines the effect, with greater effects when a main left coronary artery is restricted than a branch—probably because collateral flow is better maintained with smaller ischemic lesions. Once subendocardial ischemia has occurred, left ventricular failure compresses the coronary arteries further so that an advancing "wave-front" phenomenon occurs and the epicardial zones are eventually involved (Fig. 12-8).

With branch arterial occlusions, subendocardial flow falls first at about 25 percent occlusion, with metabolic changes developing at about 60 percent and contractility and ECG changes at 75 percent (Gregg and Bedynek, 1978). With major artery occlusions, such events occur at about 25–40 percent flow reduction.

ADVANCING SUBENDOCARDIAL ISCHEMIA

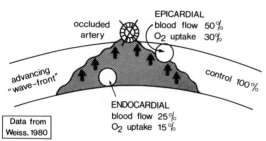

Fig. 12-8 With complete coronary occlusion, subendocardial tissue is damaged first; a "wave-front" phenomenon then involves the epicardial zones according to the model of Reimer et al. (1977). The mechanism is probably by a progressive increase in subendocardial pressure as the left ventricle fails. Blood flow data from Weiss (1980).

Coronary Artery Spasm

An alternative mechanism of coronary artery narrowing is by focal spasm, usually in the large epicardial arteries and frequently superimposed on anatomical stenosis. The added component of stenosis caused by the spasm is called **dynamic stenosis** because it can be relieved by coronary vasodilators. Clinically, coronary spasm is thought to have a wide range of expression, varying from asymptomatic ST-deviations on the electrocardiogram (page 341), to transmural ischemia with severe chest pain at rest and the typical ST-segment elevation of Prinzmetal's angina (see Fig. 24-6). There are two explanations for the association of spasm and organic stenosis. First, platelet thrombi

may form at the stenotic site to liberate vasoconstrictive agents such as serotonin and thromboxane A_2; also white cells may liberate leukotrienes (Chapter 17). Secondly, coronary atheroma damages the vascular endothelium, which is required for the action of some vasodilators (page 236). Thus endothelial damage may remove some physiological vasodilatory influences to allow an excess of vasoconstrictive stimuli. By such mechanisms the arteries are thought to become sensitized to vasoconstrictive alpha-adrenergic stimuli and to potential circulating vasoconstrictors such as histamine, serotonin and thromboxane A_2.

Coronary artery spasm frequently occurs at night, in part because decreased body metabolism leads to an increase of blood pH and an increased ionized calcium concentration in the blood; the latter change promotes spasm (Yasue, 1984). Parasympathetic vasoconstrictor stimuli, which normally are not very strong, may also play a role at night when parasympathetic tone is highest. The alpha-adrenergic receptors involved in spasm are probably alpha-2 in nature, which explains why calcium antagonists rather than alpha-1-blockers such as prazosin are effective in the therapy of coronary artery spasm (page 347).

Coronary Flow in Humans

Among the techniques used for measuring coronary flow in humans (Table 12-4), xenon washout is of special interest because modern imaging techniques allow non-invasive observation on **regional myocardial blood flow**. For example, reduced flow in a post-stenotic zone can be enhanced by coronary vasodilators such as nitrates and calcium-antagonists (Lichtlen et al., 1984). The technique is complex and subject to some inherent limitations, especially those of tracer recirculation and the problem of interpreting the multiple anatomical and physiological compartments that the tracer reaches and from which the washout occurs.

The technique most commonly used is **coronary angiography** which gives only an approximate idea of the degree of coronary narrowing, but is very valuable in localizing the site of obstruction and in planning for operative intervention. Today, multiple projections and special enlargements allow for a quantitative determination of the percent of the artery stenosed and of the effects of nitrates thereon (Lichtlen et al., 1984).

Table 12-4

Coronary blood flow in man in various conditions (as mean values ± SD, or range)

Species	Condition	Method	Left ventricular blood flow (ml/100 g/min)
Man	Rest	Xenon[1]	64–79
		Nitrous oxide[2]	83 ± 28
		Tritiated water[3]	97 ± 37
		Antipyrine[4]	106
	Heavy exercise	Nitrous oxide[5]	300?
		Xenon	240?
		Tritiated water[5]	260
	Coronary vasodilation	Xenon[1]	about 190
Man	**Disease**		
	Cardiomyopathy	Xenon[1]	43
	Severe aortic stenosis	Xenon[1]	49
	Single vessel disease	Xenon[1]	59
	Double-triple vessel disease	Xenon[1]	45–53
Man	**Regional flow** (in patients with normal arteriograms)		
	LV flow	Xenon[1]	**64 ± 14 (LV)**
	RV flow	Xenon[1]	**47 ± 11 (RV)**
	Rt atrial flow	Xenon[1]	**34 ± 10 (RA)**
Dog	Anesthetized	Xenon[6]	110 ± 46
		Microspheres[6]	114 ± 50
		Microspheres[7]	119 ± 26
	Regional ischemia, 60 min		
	Inner layer	Microspheres[7]	9 ± 4
	Outer layer	Microspheres[7]	32 ± 10

LV = left ventricular; RV = right ventricular.

In man, xenon values are consistently lower than most other methods due to tracer recirculation and retention in epicardial fat. See L'Abbate A et al. (1981). Circ Res 49: 41.

[1]Cannon PJ et al. (1977). Prog Cardiovasc Dis 20: 95.
[2]Rowe G (1972). In: Myocardial Blood Flow in Man. Ed. A Maseri, p 297, Minerva Medicine, Turin.
[3]L'Abbate A et al. (1979). Circulation 60: 776.
[4]Maseri A et al. (1974). Circ Res 35: 826.
[5]Jorgensen CR. In Cannon et al. (1977). p 251.
[6]Sciacca RR (1979). Cardiovasc Res 13: 330.
[7]Becker LC et al. (1975). Cardiovasc Res 9: 178.

Summary

The myocardium has a very rich supply of capillaries with about one capillary for each myofiber. Normally, not all the capillaries are open. Recruitment, or opening up of capillaries, occurs when the myocardial oxygen demand rises during exercise. Recruitment also occurs as the capillaries dilate in response to hypoxia, so that the available oxygen has a shorter distance to diffuse to the mitochondria where it is required. The mechanism for such vasodilation is chiefly metabolic. A small fraction of the ATP broken down by exercise or hypoxia is ultimately converted to the vasodilator adenosine; other vasodilators may include the prostaglandins. Catecholamines cause a secondary vasodilation due to release of adenosine or other metabolites from the myocardial cells as a consequence of the simultaneous positive inotropic effect. The major direct effect of catecholamine stimulation on the coronary arteries is vasoconstriction, mediated by alpha-adrenergic receptors, which opposes the metabolic vasodilation. The latter is normally powerful enough to overcome the alpha-mediated effects. Hemodynamic factors determine the greater oxygen demand of the subendocardial zones, which are the first to suffer when the blood supply is diminished as in coronary artery stenosis. The smaller the cross-sectional area of the lumen, the more severe is the resultant ischemia.

References

Arnold G, Kosche F, Miessner E, Neitzert A, Lochner W (1968). The importance of the perfusion pressure in the coronary arteries for the contractility and the oxygen consumption of the heart. Pflügers Arch 299: 339–356.

Bassenge E, Holtz, J, Restorff W (1978). What is the physiological significance of sympathetic coronary innervation? In: Primary and Secondary Angina Pectoris. Eds A Maseri, GA Klassen, M Lesch, pp 201–210, Grune and Stratton, Orlando, New York and London.

Berne RM (1964). Regulation of coronary blood flow. Physiol Rev 44: 1–29.

Berne RM, Rubio R (1980). Coronary circulation. In: Handbook of Physiology. The Cardiovascular System. I. The Heart. Ed. RM Berne, pp 873–952, American Physiological Society, Bethesda, Maryland, 1979.

Bourdeau-Martini J, Odoroff CL, Honig CR (1974). Dual effect of oxygen on magnitude and uniformity of coronary intercapillary distance. Am J Physiol 226: 800–810.

Chance B (1976). Pyridine nucleotide as an indicator of the oxygen requirements for energy-linked functions of mitochondria. Circ Res 38 Suppl 1: 131–138.

Chang B-L, Yamakawa T, Nuccio J, Pace R, Bing RJ (1982). Micro-circulation of left atrial muscle, cerebral cortex and mesentery of the cat. Circ Res 50: 240–249.

Clemens MG, Forrester T (1980). Appearance of adenosine triphosphate in the coronary sinus effluent from isolated working rat heart in response to hypoxia. J Physiol 312: 143–158.

Feigl E (1983). Coronary physiology. Physiol Rev 1–203.

Feldman RL, Nichols WW, Peipine CJ, Conti CR (1978). Hemodynamic significance of length of a coronary arterial narrowing. Am J Cardiol 41: 865–871.

Frezza WA, Bing OHL (1976). PO$_2$-modulated performance of cardiac muscle. Am J Physiol 231: 1620–1624.

Gregg DE (1963). Effect of coronary perfusion pressure or coronary flow on oxygen usage of the myocardium. Circ Res 13: 497–500.

Gregg DE, Bedynek JL (1978). Compensatory changes in the heart during progressive coronary artery stenosis. In: Primary and Secondary Angina Pectoris. Eds A Maseri, GA Klassen, M Lesch, pp 3–11, Grune and Stratton, Orlando, New York and London.

Heusch G, Deussen A (1983). The effects of cardiac sympathetic nerve stimulation on perfusion of stenotic coronary arteries in dog. Circ Res 53: 8–15.

Hood WP Jr, Amende I, Simon R, Lichtlen P (1980). The effects of intracoronary nitroglycerin on left ventricular systolic and diastolic function in man. Circulation 61: 1098–1104.

Klein LW, Pichard AD, Holt J, Smith H, Gorlin R, Teichholz LE (1983). Effects of chronic tobacco smoking on the coronary circulation. J Am Coll Cardiol 1: 421–426.

Klocke FJ (1983). Measurements of coronary blood flow and degree of stenosis: current clinical implications and continuing uncertainties. J Am Coll Cardiol 1: 31–41.

Krogh A (1919). The supply of oxygen to the tissues and the regulation of the capillary circulation. J Physiol (London) 52: 457–474.

Kübler W, Spieckermann PG (1970). Regulation of glycolysis in the ischemic and anoxic myocardium. J Molec Cell Cardiol 1: 351–357.

Lichtlen R, Engel H-J, Rafflenbul, W (1984). Calcium entry blockers, especially nifedipine in angina of effort. Possible mechanisms and clinical implications. In: Calcium-Antagonists and Cardiovascular Diseases. Ed. LH Opie, pp 221–236, Raven Press, New York.

Mohrman DE, Feigl EO (1978). Competition between sympathetic vasoconstriction and metabolic vasodilation in the canine coronary circulation. Circ Res 42: 79–86.

Myers WW, Honig CR (1964). Number and distribution of capillaries as determinants of myocardial oxygen tension. Am J Physiol 207: 653–660.

Opie LH (1965). Coronary flow rate and perfusion pressure as determinants of mechanical function and oxydative metabolism of isolated perfused rat heart. J Physiol 180: 529–541.

Pappenheimer JR, Renkin EM, Borrero LM (1951). Filtration, diffusion and molecular sieving through peripheral capillary membranes. Am J Physiol 167: 13–46.

Reimer KA, Lower JE, Rasmussen MM, Jennings RB (1977). The wavefront phenomenon of ischemic cell death. I. Myocardial infarct size vs duration of coronary occlusion in dogs. Circulation 56: 786–794.

Rothman MT, Bairn DS, Simpson JB, Harrison DC (1982). Coronary hemodynamics during percutaneous transluminal coronary angioplasty. Am J Cardiol 49: 1615–1631.

Skolasinska K, Harbig K, Lübbers DW, Wodick R (1978). PO$_2$ and microflow histograms of the beating heart in response to changes in arterial PO$_2$. Bas Res Cardiol 73: 307–319.

Tamura M, Oshino N, Chance B, Silver IA (1978). Optical measurements of intracellular oxygen concentration of rat heart in vitro. Arch Biochem Biophys 191: 8–22.

Vlahakes GJ, Baer RW, Uhlig PN, Verrier ED, Bristow JD, Hoffman JIE (1982). Adrenergic influence in the coronary circulation of conscious dogs during maximal vasodilation in adenosine. Circ Res 51: 371–384.

Vogel WM, Apstein CS, Briggs LL, Gaasch WH, Ahn J (1982). Acute alterations in left ventricular chamber stiffness. Role of the "erectile" effect of coronary arterial pressure and flow in normal and damaged hearts. Circ Res 51: 465–478.

Weiss HR (1980). Effect of coronary artery occlusion on regional arterial and venous O_2 saturation, O_2 extraction, blood flow, and O_2 consumption in the dog heart. Circ Res 47: 400–407.

Whalen WJ (1971). Intracellular PO_2 in heart and skeletal muscle. Physiologist 14: 69–82.

Whalen WJ, Fangman J (1963). Respiration of heart muscle as affected by oxygen tensions. Science 141: 274–275.

Winbury MM, Howe BB (1979). Stenosis: regional myocardial ischemia and reserve. In: Ischemic Myocardium and Antianginal Drugs. Eds MM Winbury, Y Abiko, pp 55–76, Raven Press, New York.

Winbury MM, Howe BB, Hefner MM (1969). Effect of nitrates and other coronary dilators on large and small coronary vessels: an hypothesis for the mechanism of action of nitrates. J Pharmacol Exp Ther 168: 70–95.

Wittenberg JB (1970). Myoglobin-facilitated oxygen diffusion: role of myoglobin in oxygen entry into muscle. Physiol Rev 50: 559–636.

Yasue H (1984). Coronary artery spasm and calcium ions. In: Calcium-Antagonists and Cardiovascular Disease. Ed. LH Opie, pp 117–128, Raven Press, New York.

New References

Houston DS, Shepherd JT, Vanhoutte PM (1985). Adenine nucleotides, serotonin, and endothelium-dependent relaxations to platelets. Am J Physiol 248: H389–H395.

Lamping KG, Marcus ML, Dole WP (1985). Removal of the endothelium potentiates canine large coronary artery constrictor responses to 5-hydroxytryptamine in vivo. Circ Res 57: 46–54.

Nuutinen EM, Wilson DF, Erecinska M (1985). The effect of cholinergic agonists on coronary flow rate and oxygen consumption in isolated perfused rat heart. J Molec Cell Cardiol 17: 31–42.

Sparks HV Jr, Wangler RD, DeWitt DF (1984). Control of the coronary circulation. In: Physiology and Pathophysiology of the Heart. Ed. N Sperelakis, pp 797–817, Nijhoff, Boston.

Uhlig PN, Baer RW, Vlahakes GJ, Hanley FL, Messina LM, Hoffman JIE (1984). Arterial and venous coronary pressure-flow relations in anesthetized dogs. Circ Res 55: 238–248.

13 | Oxygen Demand: Ventricular Function

The contractile mechanisms already described serve as the molecular basis of the pumping activity of the heart. From the point of view of the rest of the body, it matters not how the myosin heads interact with the thin actin filaments so long as the tissue requirement for oxygen is met. In order to adjust the cardiac output to the needs of the body the pumping function must be appropriately regulated. It is, in turn, the energy required for this process that largely determines the oxygen uptake of the heart.

The Cardiac Cycle

Wiggers' diagram is one of the most reproduced and modified figures in cardiology. Its message is so important that Wiggers' cycle must be committed to memory by every student of cardiology. Although the cycle seems to be composed of several arbitrary phases which can be difficult to remember, the basis is simple: (i) the left ventricle (LV) contracts; (ii) the LV relaxes; and (iii) during the later part of relaxation, the LV fills (Table 13-1). These events generate the pressure to propel blood received from the lungs to the body via the aorta (Fig. 13-1). Similarly right ventricular contraction propels blood to the lungs and thence to the left heart. For simplicity, we shall focus on events in the left side of the heart where the pressure changes are greatest and the ventricle correspondingly thicker. This increased wall thickness is a natural adaptation to the higher pressures in aorta and left

Table 13-1

The cardiac cycle

LV contraction
— isovolumic contraction (c)
— maximal ejection (d)
— reduced ejection (e)
LV relaxation
— isovolumic relaxation (f)
— rapid LV filling and (?) suction (g)
— slow LV filling (diastasis) (a)
— atrial booster (b)

The letters a–g refer to the phases of the cardiac cycle shown in Wiggers' diagram (Fig. 13-1).

ventricle than in pulmonary artery and right ventricle; a thicker wall decreases the wall stress (see later).

The ventricle contracts

Left ventricular pressure starts to build up with the arrival of calcium as the contractile elements "turn on" the cross-bridge interaction. Because the heart has been resting, the communication between the receiving chamber (left atrium) and pumping chamber (left ventricle) is open—the mitral leaflets are far apart. As the cross-bridges start to interact, the ventricular pressure rises to exceed that in the left atrium. The left atrial pressure is similar to that in the capillaries

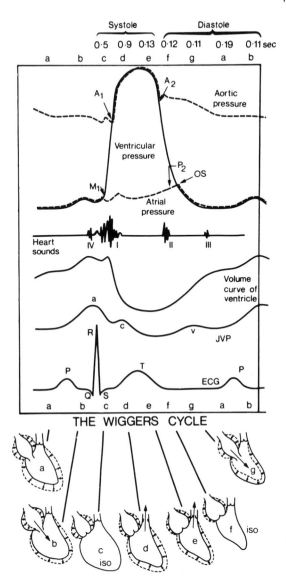

Fig. 13-1 Wiggers' diagram which explains the mechanical events in the cardiac cycle. It has been modified and reproduced more than any other diagram in cardiology. This modification shows the components of the heart sounds. The visual phases of the ventricular cycle are taken with permission from Shepherd and Vanhoutte, The Human Cardiovascular System, Raven Press, New York, 1979, p 68. For explanation of phases a to g see Table 13-1.

of the lungs, and normally not more than 10–15 mmHg. The left ventricular pressure must rise to much higher values to exceed that in the arterial tree,

which is normally about 120 mmHg as blood is being ejected into it, and 80 mmHg during the resting diastolic phase (i.e. the blood pressure is about 120/80 mmHg). As the left ventricular pressure exceeds that in the left atrium, the mitral valve abruptly closes to create the audible mitral component of the first sound (M_1).

Now the volume of the contracting ventricle is fixed (**isovolumic contraction**) because both aortic and mitral valves are shut. Pressure builds up until that in the left ventricle exceeds that in the aorta, whereupon the aortic valve opens (aortic component of first sound, A_1, possibly caused by sudden distension of aortic root structures). Blood flows rapidly from left ventricle to aorta during this phase of **rapid ejection**; both ventricular and aortic pressures rise to peaks which will be the same.

In the meantime the sarcoplasmic reticulum has been actively sucking up calcium ions (because of the rise in calcium concentration during systole) and the myocardium enters the **relaxation phase**, so that left ventricular and aortic pressures start falling from peak values. The rate of ejection of blood falls (phase of **reduced ejection**) until the pressure in the aorta exceeds the falling left ventricular pressure and the aortic valve closes (creating the first component of the second sound, A_2). The second audible component of the second sound comes when the pulmonary valve closes abruptly (pulmonary component of second sound, P_2) as the right ventricular pressure drops to below that in the pulmonary artery.

The ventricle continues to relax while both aortic and mitral valves are closed in the phase of **isovolumic relaxation** until the ventricular pressure falls further to be below that in the left atrium so that the mitral valve opens. This opening is normally silent, probably because the bicuspid mitral valve gradually drifts open; in contrast, there is a snap-like opening sound in mitral stenosis.

The ventricle fills

First ventricular filling is purely passive as the left atrial pressure exceeds that in the left ventricle. The left ventricle distends quite rapidly (phase of rapid filling which accounts for 80 percent of ventricular filling) and soon pressures in the atrium and ventricle equalize so that filling stops (the name diastasis for this phase is little used in practice). To fill further requires that the pressure gradient from atrium to ventricle must increase further. There are only two ways of doing this—the left atrium must contract or the left ventricle must relax. Therefore either the atrial pressure must increase and/or the left ventricle must help by "sucking". Probably both mechanisms are at work. A **left ventricular suction** effect has been found by carefully comparing left ventricular and left atrial pressures, and it occurs especially in the phase of rapid filling (at the end of ventricular relaxation). The sucking effect is probably of most importance in mitral stenosis (Sabbah et al., 1980). During catecholamine stimulation, the rate of relaxation may increase to enhance the sucking effect and to prolong the period of filling.

Until recently, the role of the **left atrial booster** (= "kick") contraction was in dispute. Some believed that' the inco-ordinate atrial contractions found in atrial fibrillation made no difference, so long as the time for diastolic filling was adequate. Now it is known that the left atrial booster effect, which accounts for 20 percent of ventricular filling, is important especially when a high cardiac output is demanded as during exercise. The timing of this booster contraction is shown by the P wave of an electrocardiogram. The wave of excitation then travels through the atria to reach the atrioventricular node and very shortly thereafter very rapid conduction by the Purkinje fibers spreads over the ventricles to cause the QRS wave, which is followed immediately by ventricular contraction. Now the cardiac cycle restarts.

Systole and diastole

Systole is when the heart contracts, and diastole when it relaxes. Contraction and relaxation of the contractile protein must be distinguished from systole and diastole as understood by the cardiologist, whose diastole stretches from when the aortic valve closes (A_2) to when the mitral valve shuts (M_1, Fig. 13-1). In contrast, the phase when the cytosolic calcium ion concentration is rising and cross-bridge interaction increasing, lasts only till the peak of the ventricular pressure wave. Thereafter cytosolic calcium falls until relaxation is complete. The term **protodiastolic** (= early diastole) for the physiologist is the early part of the relaxation phase from when aortic flow begins to fall until when the aortic valve shuts. For the cardiologist, protodiastole includes the period of rapid filling and is the early phase of cardiological diastole, which extends from the second sound to the next first sound. Hence a **protodiastolic gallop** indicates an audible S_3 at the time of rapid ventricular filling. For obvious reasons, the term protodiastolic is best avoided.

Heart Sounds

The relations between ventricular pressure and the opening and closing of valves have long ceased to be of purely academic interest. In mitral stenosis, besides the rumbling murmur made by turbulence across the mitral valve as the left ventricle fills, the increased atrial pressure means that the ventricular pressure must rise more than usual to close the valve which then shuts with a bang (loud M_1). Any factor increasing the inotropic state—catecholamines, digitalis, thyrotoxicosis—will also increase the mitral component of the first sound (M_1) because the left ventricle accelerates as it contracts. Conversely, a soft M_1 results from decreased contractility as in congestive heart failure, cardiomyopathy and acute myocardial infarction. M_1 is also influenced by the position of the mitral valve (a nearly closed mitral valve lessens M_1 when the PR interval is prolonged). Before using the loudness of M_1 as a rough index of the inotropic state of the left ventricle, mitral stenosis or abnormal PR intervals must be excluded.

A_2 will be loud if the pressure in the aorta is abnormally high or in systemic hypertension, or loud and ringing if the aorta is dilated (hypertension, aneurysm, syphilis). The second sound reverberates through the "cavern" of the dilated aorta.

P_2 will be abnormally loud if the pulmonary artery pressure is too high (pulmonary hypertension). Conversely, P_2 will be soft when the pulmonary valve is stenosed. To distinguish P_2 from a mitral opening snap, the A_2–P_2 interval can be prolonged by inspiration.

Besides the mitral opening snap, opening of valves may produce clicks (Table 13-2). In systole, between the first and second sounds, there may be a variety of **systolic clicks** produced by abnormal aortic or mitral valves, as in aortic stenosis or when the mitral valve balloons as part of the click–murmur syndrome (Chapter 21). The aortic ejection click will only be produced if the valve itself is stenosed and not if the stenosis is above (supravalvular) or below (subaortic) the valve. If thick and calcified as in aortic stenosis of the elderly, there also will be no aortic ejection click.

Table 13-2

Added heart sounds

1. Opening events
   — opening snap of mitral stenosis
   — early systolic ejection click of aortic stenosis
   — mid-systolic click of billowing mitral valve

2. Filling events
   — 4th heart sound — increased atrial booster
   — 3rd heart sound — abnormal ventricular filling

Besides the first and second heart sounds, there may be added third and fourth sounds (S_3 and S_4). When either is present, the added sound causes a **triple rhythm**, usually a sign of a diseased heart. The cadence of the three successive sounds is like that of a galloping horse, making a **gallop rhythm**. Depending on the cause of the extra sound, it may be determined as an S_3 gallop or S_4 gallop. S_3 is also called a proto-diastolic gallop. When both S_3 and S_4 are heard, there is a **quadruple rhythm**.

When the phase of filling of the ventricle is abnormal, then S_3 may be produced by a mechanism still unknown. A practical approach is to ascribe S_3 to abnormalities of the ventricle which either fails to expand during rapid filling (as in constrictive pericarditis), or to a high left atrial filling pressure so that rapid filling is enhanced. Sometimes an S_3 results from torrential blood flow into the ventricle, as in mitral regurgitation or some types of congenital heart disease. In young people an S_3 may be physiological, possibly because of more rapid blood flow. So also may enhanced sympathetic tone, as in anxiety or thyrotoxicosis, cause an S_3.

The cause of the S_4 gallop sound (= atrial gallop = presystolic gallop) is also poorly understood. Generally the left ventricle has become stiff (loss of compliance) as in hypertrophic cardiomyopathy, hypertension or aortic stenosis, or diffusely altered as in ischemic heart disease (especially in acute infarction). The atrium contracts more vigorously to produce S_4. The extra force of atrial contraction may cause a stronger ventricular contraction by Starling's law, so that the patient with an S_4 may be relatively symptom-free; the patient with an S_3 will be more likely to be symptomatic (high left atrial pressure).

Ventricular Work

As the ventricles pump they perform work and use up oxygen. **Work** is performed as the ventricles eject a volume of blood against a pressure. Only part of the oxygen uptake and ATP production of the contracting heart is translated into mechanical work. A great deal is spent on heat production which contributes to the heat required to keep the temperature of the body above environmental values. Thus the efficiency of work of the heart is only about 12–20 percent (Gibbs, 1974) where

$$\text{Efficiency} = \frac{\text{work performed}}{\text{maximum work possible}}$$

The work performed (or power production) is the sum of the kinetic work and the pressure work, where the **pressure work** is the larger component and is the product of the cardiac output and the peak systolic pressure. The **kinetic work** is that component required to move the blood against the pressure of the arterial system; kinetic work depends on the cardiac output, the density of the blood, the cross-sectional area of the major resistance site (e.g. the aortic valve) and the ejection time. Normally kinetic work is only a fraction of the total work (Kannengiesser et al., 1979). In aortic stenosis, kinetic work increases sharply as the cross-sectional area narrows while pressure work increases as the gradient across the aortic valve rises.

The formulae for work production are as follows (Kannengieser et al., 1979)

$$\text{Pressure power} = K_1 \times Ps \times CO$$

$$\text{Kinetic power} = K_2 \times \frac{(CO)^3}{A^2} \times \frac{(T)^2}{Te}$$

where Ps = peak systolic pressure in mmHg; CO = cardiac output in mL/min; A = area of aortic valve in cm^2; T = total cycle time; Te = ejection time (sum of rapid and reduced periods); and the units for power are milliWatts, i.e. mJoules/sec. Instead of the peak systolic pressure, another formula uses the mean systolic pressure. Even these formulae are simplifications, because in reality the pressure power is the product of the integrated sum of the instantaneous arterial pressure which changes all the time, and the instantaneous aortic flow (also changing). In clinical practice, a frequent approximation is

work = systolic (or mean) aortic pressure × CO

where CO is the cardiac output in liters/min.

Heat production

Another way of looking at the fate of the myocardial oxygen uptake is by measuring heat production. To measure heat production precisely would require careful calorimetric measurements across the heart; such measurements are not easily obtained. In isolated muscle, however, the heat of contraction and of relaxation can be measured more readily. The sum of heat and work is the **enthalpy**. There is a high correlation between enthalpy and the load placed on the muscle (more load, more enthalpy).

Further analyses of heat production are of most use when trying to marry the analyses of skeletal muscle mechanics by A. V. Hill and his followers, to the much more complex mechanics of cardiac muscle. From the metabolic view, however, all "heat" production is nothing other than the utilization of ATP, partially for contraction and relaxation, but also for ionic movements, with the production of heat as the major product of ATP hydrolysis.

Ventricular Function and Myocardial Oxygen Uptake

Heart work and oxygen uptake

There are two reasons why heart work is not a direct index of the myocardial oxygen uptake. First, cardiac output can increase without any increase in oxygen demand when the afterload (see page 174) is reduced, as when vasodilator therapy is used for congestive heart failure. Secondly, as already considered, much more of the myocardial oxygen uptake is used for heat production than for mechanical work. Usually the more the mechanical work, the more the heat production; however, the ratio between these two can vary. The higher the efficiency, the greater the mechanical work for any given oxygen uptake. Experimentally, efficiency falls with high external fatty acids as the sole fuel, or after coronary artery ligation; clinically, variations in the efficiency of work have not yet been recognized as being of practical importance.

Determinants of myocardial oxygen uptake

Instead of trying to relate heart work to oxygen uptake, a more sound approach is to study those factors which are the prime determinants of the

myocardial oxygen uptake. Such an indirect approach is much more useful for the clinician than having to measure the oxygen uptake, which requires measurements of the oxygen content of the arterial blood, of coronary sinus blood, and of the coronary flow rate. All of these are difficult to obtain. In current terms, therefore, the major determinants of the oxygen uptake are: (i) heart rate; (ii) wall stress; and (iii) contractility (Fig. 13-2). In certain pathological circumstances there may also be metabolic "oxygen-wastage". Thus the mechanical work of the heart is not in itself a determinant of the oxygen uptake; rather it expresses itself by alterations of heart rate, wall stress and contractility, each of which is now examined.

MAJOR DETERMINANTS OF O_2 DEMAND OF HEART

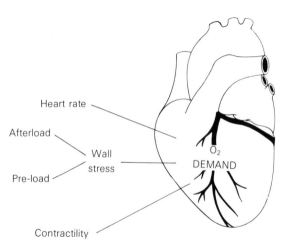

Fig. 13-2 Major determinants of the oxygen demand of the normal heart are heart rate, wall stress and contractility.

Heart Rate and Oxygen Uptake

Each cycle of contraction and relaxation performs a certain amount of work and takes up a certain amount of oxygen. The faster the heart rate, the higher the cardiac output and the higher the oxygen uptake. Exceptions occur (i) when the heart rate is extremely fast, as may occur during a paroxysmal tachycardia, because an inadequate time for diastolic filling decreases the cardiac output; and (ii) when a less severe tachycardia occurs in the presence of coronary artery disease. Another way by which the heart rate can increase the oxygen uptake is as follows.

Force–interval relation

An increased heart rate progressively increases the force of ventricular contraction, even in an isolated papillary muscle preparation (**Bowditch staircase phenomenon**). Alternative names are the **treppe** (German for steps) phenomenon or **positive inotropic effect of activation** or **force–frequency** relation. Conversely, a decreased heart rate has a negative staircase effect (Fig. 13-3). During rapid stimulation, more sodium and calcium enter the myocardial cell than can be handled by the sodium pump and the mechanisms for calcium exit. The increased intracellular sodium concentration exchanges outwards to admit more calcium, which in turn is the probable cause of the staircase—according to one proposal the time taken for these adjustments explains the delayed onset of the peak inotropic effect (**sodium pump "lag" effect**, Langer, 1983). This "lag" may explain why contractility has a "memory" and is a function of the intervals between past contractions (Johnson, 1979).

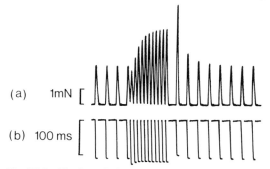

(a)   1mN

(b)   100 ms

Fig. 13-3 The Bowditch or treppe phenomenon. The top panel shows tension developed by rapid papillary muscle and the bottom panel the action potential duration shown on an analog analyzer. mN = milliNewtons. Reproduced with permission from Noble (1983).

An alternative explanation rests on the possible inhibition of calcium ion entry by the amount of calcium in what is held to be a "release compartment" (Noble, 1983). The first contraction after the shortened interval is less than normal, because the cardiac calcium cycles do not have enough time for full uptake of calcium via the release compartment (probably the sarcoplasmic reticulum). The incomplete cycle exerts less inhibitory feedback on calcium ion entry, which is therefore enhanced to increase contractile force. Once again the shortened interval fails to inhibit calcium entry and the contractile force increases until a plateau is reached. After the frequency is slowed

down, the greater filling of the release compartment means that more calcium is released when the next stimulus arrives. To explain the decreased contractile force in the subsequent contractions, it is held that calcium ion entry is decreased by the feedback mechanism (for effects of internal calcium on I_{si}, see page 95).

Post-extrasystolic potentiation and the inotropic effect of **paired pacing** can be explained by the same model, again assuming an enhanced contractile state after the prolonged interval between beats (for an alternative theory, see page 103).

Opposing the force–frequency relation is the positive inotropic effect of prolonged filling, where the longer the interval, the better the ventricular filling and the stronger the subsequent contraction. This phenomenon can be shown in patients with mitral stenosis and a variable filling interval as a result of atrial fibrillation (Schneider et al., 1983).

Overdrive suppression is a different relation between heart rate and contraction referring to the slowness of the heart to resume pacemaker activity after a tachycardia (see page 64). It must be recalled that overdrive suppression relates to the pacemaking activity of the heart and not to the contractile state.

Wall Stress or Tension

At a fixed heart rate, the myocardial wall tension is the major determinant of the oxygen uptake. When the myofilaments slide over each other during cardiac contraction they are ultimately squeezing blood out of the ventricles into the circulation. An analogy is the human effort required to squeeze a ball in the palm of the hand (Fig. 13-4). A small rubber ball can easily be compressed; a larger rubber ball (tennis ball in size) is compressed less readily; two large rubber balls—or one really large ball—could be compressed only with the greatest difficulty. As the size of the object in the hand increases, so does the force required to compress it. At this point it is appropriate to deviate briefly into a description of force, tension and wall stress.

"**Force**" is a term frequently used in studies of muscle mechanics. Strictly

$$force = mass \times acceleration$$

Thus when a load is suspended from one end of a muscle as the muscle contracts it is exerting force against that load. A relationship between force and

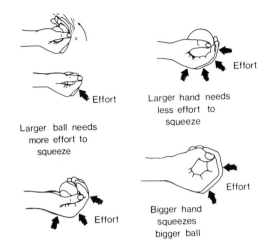

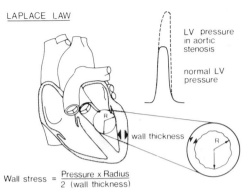

Wall stress = $\dfrac{\text{Pressure} \times \text{Radius}}{2 \,(\text{wall thickness})}$

Fig. 13-5 Wall stress increases as the afterload increases. Thus there is more stress in acute aortic stenosis until the wall hypertrophies to decrease the bottom component of the equation.

Fig. 13-4 The effort required to squeeze a ball in the hand has some analogies to the development of wall tension in the heart. When the volume of blood in the ventricle is increased, then the wall stress increases (analogy: left hand side of figure). When the heart hypertrophies the wall tension decreases and a larger volume of blood in the ventricle can more easily be ejected (analogy: right hand side).

velocity is also one between load and velocity. In many cases it is not possible to define force with such exactitude but, in general, force has the following properties (Cromer, 1977). First, force is always applied by one object (such as muscle) on another object (such as a load). Secondly, force is characterized both by the direction in which it acts, and its magnitude; hence it is a vector. Thus the effect of a combination of forces can be established by the principle of vectors. Thirdly, each object exerts a force on the other, so that force and counter-force are equal and opposite (Newton's third law of motion).

Tension exists when the two forces are applied to an object so that the forces tend to pull the object apart (Cromer, 1977). Thus when a spring is pulled by a force, tension is exerted; when more force is applied, the spring stretches and the tension increases.

Stress develops when tension is applied to a cross-sectional area, and the units are force per unit area. In **Laplace's law** it is wall stress and not tension which regulates the myocardial oxygen uptake (Fig. 13-5):

$$\text{Wall stress} = \frac{\text{pressure} \times \text{radius}}{2 \times \text{wall thickness}}$$

This equation, although useful, is an over-simplification.

For either a spherical or ellipsoidal model, the stress acting parallel to the long axis of the heart, known as the meridional stress, is expressed by the more complex formula (Grossman et al., 1975):

$$\text{Wall stress} = \frac{P \times R_\mathrm{i}}{2\,h\,(1 + h/2\,R_\mathrm{i})}$$

where P = pressure; R_i = internal radius; h = wall thickness. Hefner's (1962) equation, simpler to remember, also gives the meridional stress:

Wall stress = P × cross-sectional area of cavity

In ellipsoidal models, to which the left ventricle corresponds more closely, more complex formulations are required (Walker et al., 1971).

In **cardiac hypertrophy**, Laplace's law explains the changes in wall thickness. Whereas an acute pressure load increases the myocardial oxygen uptake more than an acute volume load, in chronic pressure overload (as in aortic stenosis, see Fig. 21-2), the wall thickness in diastole increases so that the myocardial oxygen demand remains normal despite the greatly increased systolic pressure. The increased wall thickness due to hypertrophy balances the increased pressure so that the wall stress remains unchanged during the phase of compensatory hypertrophy (see Fig. 15-4). In congestive heart failure, the heart dilates to increase the radius factor, thereby elevating wall stress.

The "**time–tension**" index of Sarnoff considers the time for which pressure is maintained on the myocardial wall (Fig. 13-6, Table 13-3). The use of the term "tension" is strictly incorrect; it is the

Table 13-3

Indices of myocardial oxygen uptake

Index	Advantage	Comment
Double product		
Pressure-rate, systolic pressure × heart rate	Non-invasive, easy	No allowance for contractile state
Triple product		
Above × systolic ejection time	Non-invasive, more difficult	Some allowance for contractility
Time–tension index	Invasive	Should be called "time–pressure" index

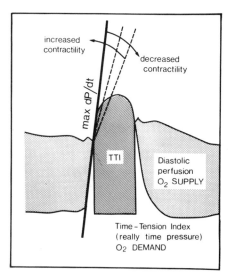

Fig. 13-6 Two indices derived from Wiggers' diagram. The maximal rate of pressure development (max d P/dt) is an index of contractility, whereas the "time–tension" index is closely related to the myocardial oxygen uptake. The latter should really be a "time–pressure" index. Note the effects of modifications of the index of contractility, d P/dt, so that catecholamine beta-stimulation enhances the contractile state and congestive heart failure decreases the contractile state.

pressure that is measured. Pressure can be translated into tension only if wall thickness and radius (or cross-sectional area) are known.

Clinical measurement of wall stress

To calculate wall stress throughout the cardiac cycle needs concurrent measurements of left ventricular pressure, dimensions and wall thickness, which can be achieved by a combination of left ventricular pressure measurements and echocardiography (see

later). Because invasive measurements on patients are avoided whenever possible, a more practical clinical approach is to measure two important determinants of the wall stress, namely the preload and the afterload.

Preload and wall stress

The preload is the load "before" the heart, or the pressure which fills the heart—the **left ventricular filling pressure**, which is only slightly below the left atrial pressure (Fig. 13-1). Thus the left atrial pressure is a good approximation of the left ventricular filling pressure. The left atrial pressure can be measured indirectly by the pulmonary capillary wedge pressure, using a **Swan–Ganz catheter** (see Fig. 1-10). Here a catheter with a balloon cuff is put in through the great veins in the neck (a bedside procedure for experienced cardiologists), advanced into the terminal pulmonary arteries, and the balloon inflated. The pressure at the tip of the catheter is the **pulmonary capillary wedge pressure** (or simply "wedge pressure") and is a good reflection of the left atrial pressure. As the wedge pressure rises, so does the preload on the myocardial fibers. An increased diastolic volume should increase the heart work and stroke volume (SV) by the Starling law (see page 7). At a fixed heart rate, the cardiac output (SV × HR) will rise. The Swan–Ganz catheter measures the **cardiac output** by a temperature-sensitive device at the tip of the catheter (see page 192). With such techniques it is possible to relate the cardiac output (or stroke volume) to the venous filling pressure.

Swan, co-inventor of the catheter, and Head of Cardiology at Cedar's Sinai Medical Center at UCLA, tells of how he watched yachts at sail in the Los Angeles Bay on a rare smog-free day. He saw the spinnakers loom outwards to carry the yachts forward.

Why not allow a catheter to float from the great veins in the neck into the pulmonary artery? Hence the balloon was placed on the end of the catheter. When it has floated to the pulmonary artery through the right side of the heart, it is expanded and the catheter tip senses only the pressure in the capillary bed, i.e. the pulmonary capillary wedge pressure. This is a good index of the left ventricular filling pressure (see Fig. 1-10).

It must not be supposed that it is easy to distinguish the exact hemodynamic status of the patient. While an elevated **pulmonary capillary wedge pressure** (above an arbitrary value of 12–18 mmHg) indicates left ventricular or "backward" failure, and a low cardiac output indicates "forward failure", it is not easy from one single determination to be sure whether or not the inotropic state of the heart has changed. Furthermore, it is sometimes difficult to know whether an agent is improving the cardiac output by reduction of the afterload or by improving the inotropic state of the heart or having both actions. Thus two drugs acting in two entirely different ways, for example a vasodilator such as nitroprusside or an inotropic agent such as digitalis, may have similar effects in moving the stroke volume upwards while the left ventricular filling pressure decreases. Thus much of what is known about the effects of drugs on the failing heart is extrapolated from their basic pharmacological properties (which make it quite obvious how nitroprusside and digitalis differ).

Afterload and wall stress

The afterload is the load "after" the heart, and includes all the factors against which the heart must work. Most prominent is the **systemic** or **peripheral vascular resistance**—the resistance to outflow of blood from the heart caused by the small arterioles (see Fig. 17-1). At a fixed cardiac output, an increase of peripheral resistance produced by alpha-adrenergic stimulation will increase the blood pressure. Hence it is the arterial blood pressure which is largely equated with the afterload by many clinical cardiologists. However, if the aortic valve is stenosed, then it becomes the major source of the afterload. Either hypertension or aortic stenosis will require the myocardium to contract more vigorously in systole and thereby primarily increase systolic wall tension. When the myocardium fails it cannot produce enough systolic force to overcome the afterload, and the

amount of blood ejected (ejection fraction, see page 178) falls. As blood accumulates in the ventricle the end-diastolic pressure rises, as does the preload. In this way afterload and preload are indirectly linked. The primary reason for the decreased myocardial performance in heart failure is the depressed contractile state (Chapter 22). A secondary development is the increased peripheral vascular resistance, related chiefly to an increased sympathetic drive; now the poorly functioning myocardium cannot cope with the afterload which for it is excessive (see Fig. 22-2), and the failure becomes even more severe.

Contractility or the Inotropic State

The problems of definition and measurement of contractility have already been put in historical perspective in Chapter 1. For practical purposes, increased contractility explains a greater velocity of contraction which reaches a greater peak tension or pressure, when other factors influencing myocardial oxygen uptake such as the wall stress and heart rate are kept constant. Contractility (or the inotropic state as it is also called) is therefore an important regulator of the myocardial oxygen uptake; yet its effects can be explained entirely by an increase in wall stress which is therefore the fundamental factor. Factors which increase contractility are: adrenergic stimulation, digitalis and other inotropic agents. Contractility also rises as the heart rate increases (especially in isolated heart preparations) and during "post-systolic potentiation". A useful hypothesis is that the factor common to all these situations is an increased cytosolic calcium ion concentration. Contractility is decreased when energy is depleted by anoxia or ischemia, or by antiarrhythmic agents (a poorly understood mechanism), or when the myocardium is damaged by ischemic fibrosis or by chronic congestive heart failure.

Contractility is independent of load

Implicit in the concept of contractility is that it is possible to separate the effects of fiber length on contraction (which operates by the Starling mechanism) from true changes in the contractile state which can be found at a fixed length. Both preload and afterload influence the internal radius and the wall stress (see above). Such a change in myocardial oxygen uptake is load-dependent. In contrast, the concept of contractility implies a load-independent quality. On this basis it has been traditional to separate the Starling law (load-dependent performance) from the contractile state. Yet it now appears that much of the decrease in tension at shorter sarcomere lengths results from incomplete activation of the muscle (Jewell, 1977) (activation includes all the chemical processes required for muscular contraction). As the initial length of isolated papillary muscle increases, so does the tension develop; yet the cytosolic calcium rises to the same extent (Ter Keurs, 1983) (Fig. 13-7). Hence there must be some mechanism whereby an increasing muscle length sensitizes the contractile mechanism to the same amount of calcium (Allen and Kurihara, 1982). Thus muscle length can influence contractility and the traditional separation of length and inotropic state into two independent regulators of cardiac muscle performance is no longer entirely true if the end result is considered. Nevertheless, it still remains useful to separate the effects of a primary increase of muscle length (length–tension relation) from a primary change in contractility (force–velocity relation).

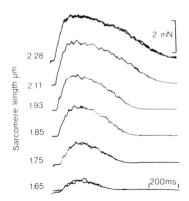

Fig. 13-7   The time course of force development versus sarcomere length (SL). The sarcomere length was kept constant at the value shown by a complex self-regulating mechanism. Note that with increasing sarcomere length there is increasing peak force development and increasing rate of force development. Reproduced with permission from Van Heuningen et al. (1982).

Length–tension relation in skeletal muscle: a useful model

Either tension or force can be related to the initial muscle length. It is useful first to analyze the length–tension relation of skeletal muscle. Maximum tension

is reached when the muscle is stimulated to contract during isometric conditions at approximately the same muscle length as found in the body. The muscle is length-dependent because shorter or longer muscle lengths lead to a decline in the tension developed. **L Max** is the resting length of the muscle at which subsequent development of tension is maximal. An analogy exists with the work of a spring. As the spring is stimulated by an increasing load, more work is done until excessive loads overstretch the spring and the work performance falls. Because of such major effects of variations in the load on the tension achieved and work performed, skeletal muscle functions as an **afterload-dependent** muscle.

Papillary muscle length–tension relation

Data have been published showing the apparent fall off of tension as sarcomere length of papillary muscle increases beyond an "optimal" value of 2.2 μm. Now it is known that many of the preparations used contained a zone of dead or only partially active tissue at the clamped ends. To measure the sarcomere length in the viable central zones requires sophisticated techniques such as laser light diffraction (Gordon and Pollack, 1980; Van Heuningen et al., 1982). Force can be measured at the ends of the preparation provided that the changes are not too rapid. Using such techniques (Ter Keurs, 1983) force continuously increases over the sarcomere length at which the muscle operates (1.55–2.35 μm) with a peak at 2.4 μm. At greater lengths, the passive or resting tension rises steeply to alter the basic relation (Fig. 13-8). Neither a plateau nor a descending limb is found when relating sarcomere length to active tension and ignoring passive tension.

Increasing the external calcium concentration (range 0.5–2.5 mM) increases the tension at any given length, which suggests that the cytosolic calcium concentration enhances the degree of cross-bridge interaction for any given muscle length.

Force–velocity curve and V_{max}

The force–velocity curve aims to define two extreme conditions—the maximal rate of shortening in unloaded muscle (i.e. when the load on the muscle is rapidly removed), and the force developed when muscle is isometric and undergoing no shortening at all (Fig. 13-9).

The V_{max} of muscle contraction is an idealized concept, defined as the **maximal velocity** of **contraction** when there is no load on the isolated

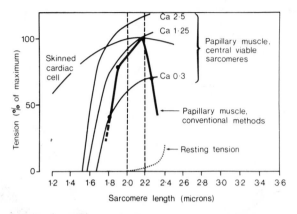

Fig. 13-8 The relation between sarcomere lengths and tension for cardiac muscle. Note (i) the effect of increasing calcium ion concentration, (ii) the absence of any decrease of tension at maximal sarcomere lengths, so that there is no basis for the descending limb of the Starling curve. Taken from data of Ter Keurs (1983) and Gordon and Pollack (1980). The sophisticated laser-diffraction techniques used by these workers invalidate previous curves based on apparent sarcomere length–tension relationships.

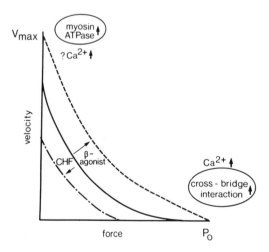

Fig. 13-9 Two fundamental properties of isolated muscle preparations, P_0 and V_{max} can provisionally be explained in cellular terms. P_0 is also termed F_0, and the other name for V_{max} is V_0 (Murphy, 1983). Note the contrasting effects of catecholamines and congestive heart failure (CHF).

muscle, or no afterload to prevent maximal rates of cardiac ejection. V_{max} cannot be directly measured but is an extrapolated value of the peak mechanical function obtained from the intercept on the velocity axis; it is also called V_0 (the maximum velocity at zero load). This type of V_{max} differs from the V_{max} of an enzymatic reaction which is measured during the initially maximal rate of that reaction. An important link exists between the mechanical V_{max} of muscle and the enzymatic V_{max} of the myosin ATPase activity (Chapter 8), which both increase in the same direction. In another extreme condition there is no muscle shortening at all (zero shortening) and all the energy goes into development of pressure (P_0) or force (F_0). Some analogy can be drawn with the weight-lifter (Fig. 13-10). When the weight is very light he can pick it up very fast, thereby approaching V_{max} when all his energy can be put into the speed of lifting. When the weight is excessively heavy the distressed weight-lifter cannot move the weight and his muscles cannot shorten (P_0), although much energy is used in the attempt. The heavier the weight, the greater the initial pressure development (P_0 rises).

The force–velocity relationship has been subject to much debate chiefly because of the technical difficulty in defining V_{max}. By careful measurement of the velocity of shortening of central sarcomeres in maximally unloaded muscle, Ter Keurs (1983) found that V_{max} is the same at sarcomere lengths between 1.85 and 2.35 μm, although decreasing at shorter lengths to become zero at 1.6 μm. Thus it seems as if V_{max} is indeed length-independent at the more physiological sarcomere lengths. The paradox is that in the loaded state fiber length does influence force

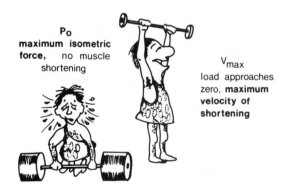

Fig. 13-10 Current concepts of cardiac contractility have evolved from those of skeletal muscle mechanics, as shown in this cartoon of a weight-lifter.

(or tension) development (Fig. 13-7), and increases the velocity of shortening at any given load so that length influences contractility; in contrast, in unloaded conditions the intrinsic contractility as assessed by V_{max} does not change with initial fiber length. With these observations in mind it is now useful to distinguish between **true contractility** which is independent of length but very difficult to measure, and the **apparent contractility** or **contractile state** of loaded muscle which is length-dependent. The true contractility is influenced by the external calcium concentration which can increase both V_{max} and P_0. The mechanism of such calcium-dependence of velocity could be either control of the myosin ATPase (Chapter 8) or alteration of the internal viscosity of the sarcomere (Ter Keurs, 1983). Adrenergic stimulation markedly increases V_{max} and P_0, presumably acting by an increased cytosolic calcium concentration. At any given load, increasing either external calcium or catecholamine beta-stimulation increases the velocity of shortening (Fig. 13-9).

The force–velocity curve should really be a straight line; the reasons for deviations are given by Katz (1977). The major defect of the V_{max} concept is the near-impossibility of its application to the heart as a whole.

Force–velocity–length relation

To combine the length–force and force–velocity relations requires a complex three-dimensional plot. Although theoretically useful (Braunwald and Ross, 1979), this triple plot has not yet come into general use. The additional dimension given is length–velocity. An inotropic stimulus increases the velocity of shortening for any given muscle length. A corresponding three-dimensional plot in patients is wall tension–velocity–circumference, obtained from a catheter tip velocity meter in the aorta. From the practical point of view, it seems simpler and as accurate to continue to think in terms of separate length–force and force–velocity plots.

Clinical Assessment of Inotropic State

Whereas it is relatively easy for the clinician to define the preload or the afterload of the heart by measuring the left ventricular filling pressure and the peripheral resistance, and also to measure the stroke volume (see

Fig. 1-10), it is very difficult to assess the inotropic state (or the contractile state) of the myocardium. For clinical purposes, the contractile state of the myocardium may be described as **the quality that determines the force and velocity of myocardial contraction, in conditions of constant preload, afterload and heart rate**. In relation to Wiggers' cycle, it is easiest to consider left ventricular function during the period of isovolumic contraction. During this period, the preload and afterload are constant and therefore the rate of pressure generation should be an index of the inotropic state (Table 13-4)

$$\text{Inotropic index} = \max \, dP/dt$$

This index has stood the test of years and gives some absolute values. Bearing in mind that left ventricular pressure is changing during the period of isovolumic contraction, some workers prefer to make a correction for the change in pressure by dividing the above expression by a fixed developed pressure, e.g. $dP/dt(DP_{40})$, or by the pressure at the instant of the maximal rate of pressure development, $(dP/dt)/P$. Such corrections add little (Braunwald and Ross, 1979; Noble, 1979).

The measurements required for dP/dt can only be obtained by left ventricular catheterization; ideally direct left ventricular puncture or a special catheter is required to eliminate the unwanted "noise" and "dampening" effect of an ordinary catheter introduced from the femoral artery through the aorta into the left ventricle. Therefore, this index is not ideal in clinical practice.

Exact force–velocity relations are even more difficult to measure, and require a combination of cineangiography and very accurate measurements of intraventricular pressure. V_{max} is therefore very seldom estimated in clinical work.

Contractile element velocity (V_{CE})

The skeletal muscle model of A. V. Hill is used to estimate contractile element velocity. The two components are the **contractile element** and the **series elastic element**. During isovolumic contraction, V_{CE} is explained by changes in the contractile element alone, whereas during shortening (ejection phase), V_{CE} is the sum of the rate of shortening and an expression which is inversely proportional to the

Table 13-4

Some indices of myocardial contractility (inotropic state)

Index	Advantage	Comment
max($+$)dP/dt	Easy provided invasive monitoring accepted	Classical invasive index
max($+$)dP/dt corrected for ventricular pressure	As above	Supposedly allows for changes in ventricular pressure during isovolumic contraction
max($-$)dP/dt	As above	Index of maximal rate of relaxation; influenced by aortic impedance
Systolic time intervals	Non-invasive	Influenced by many anatomic factors
Velocity of circumferential fiber shortening (V_{cf})	Non-invasive echocardiographic technique	Calculated from end-systolic and end-diastolic diameters and ejection time
Percent fractional shortening	Simple non-invasive echocardiographic technique	(EDD − ESD)/(EDD) as defined in Fig. 13-12
Ejection fraction	Non-invasive radionuclide MUGA scan	Volume ejected during systole compared with initial ventricular volume; widely used to assess left ventricular function
Pressure–volume loop	Invasive for full loop; non-invasive for part	Increased slope indicates increased contractility; also measures ventricular compliance

stiffness of the series elastic component. For example, V_{CE} can be calculated as (dP/dt)/kP where k is the stiffness constant of the series elastic element. V_{CE} can be plotted against the instantaneous wall stress (measured by angiography) during the isovolumic phase; if V_{CE} is extrapolated to zero stress that is thought to be V_{max}. This complex approach is not widely used.

The rate of change of power, the **isovolumic power production**, as the isovolumic ventricle compresses blood within it, may give another viable index of contractility (Stein and Sabbah, 1975). Undoubtedly the numerous indices of contractility in clinical use reflect the impossibility of directly measuring this idealized concept. In practice, ejection phase indices are widely used.

Ejection phase indices of contractile state

During the ejection phase, the left ventricle contracts against the afterload. Hence all indices of function in this period are afterload-dependent, although not directly influenced by the preload. As congestive heart failure develops and myocardial contractility decreases, there is increasing sensitivity to the afterload. This change is used to monitor indirectly the myocardial contractile state by indices related to the ejection phase. Such indices can be obtained non-invasively and are widely used by clinicians, whereas the direct indices of the inotropic state, such as dP/dt_{max}, are used less and less.

The **ejection fraction** of the left ventricle, measured by radionuclide techniques, is one of the most frequently used indices of left ventricular pump function. The ejection fraction relates stroke volume to end-diastolic volume and is, therefore, an index of the extent of left ventricular fiber shortening. It is particularly useful in evaluating the course of chronic heart disease when the preload and the afterload are approximately unchanged. The theory is relatively simple—the end-systolic volume when compared with the end-diastolic volume by a multiple gated blood pool technique (MUGA; Fig. 13-11) gives an indirect index of the inotropic state. The higher the ejection fraction for a given end-diastolic volume, the higher the inotropic state. The end-systolic volume occurs at the peak of the left ventricular pressure curve (see Wiggers' diagram) after the opening of the aortic valve, and so the characteristics of the afterload will influence the degree of emptying. The ejection fraction is, therefore, an index of the contractile behavior of

Echocardiographic indices of contractile state

The echocardiogram is used increasingly to provide an indirect index of the inotropic state of the myocardium. Ultrasound waves are passed through the chest wall to reach the myocardium and the valves and then reflected and recorded visually (Fig. 13-12). The ultrasound may be passed through the heart at a specific site, so that each part of the heart caught in the beam creates an echo; thus an enlarged ventricular wall will create a wider than normal distance between the echoes from the inner and outer layers. This technique is known as M-mode (M for motion) echocardiography. In **two-dimensional echocardiography** the ultrasonic beam is moved very rapidly so that a cross-sectional view of cardiac shape and motion is obtained. To obtain an idea of blood flow within the heart **Doppler echocardiography** makes use of the shift in the frequency of the ultrasonic wave as it is reflected from the moving blood, the ultrasonic energy being reflected by the moving red cells. This emerging technique may be able to help detect abnormalities of blood flow in valvular heart disease.

Conventional echocardiography is especially useful in diagnosing the extent and site of ventricular wall thickening in hypertrophy (in hypertrophic subaortic stenosis there is a specific thickening of the ventricular septum and here the finding on the echocardiogram is virtually diagnostic). Abnormal valve movements can also be detected as well as abnormal thickening. A very accurate idea of the pumping function of the heart can be obtained with the echocardiogram. In particular, the velocity at which the circumference of the heart in its minor axis changes during systole, is a useful index of myocardial contractility. The mean **velocity of circumferential fiber shortening** (mean V_{cf}) can be determined from echocardiographic measurements of the end-diastolic and end-systolic sizes. The difference between the calculated circumferences is divided by the duration of shortening which is the ejection time. The mean V_{cf} compares favorably with more sophisticated invasive measurements of the contractile state. In these determinations the minor axis of the heart is measured as the distance from the left side of the septum to the posterior endocardial wall.

If left ventricular pressure measurements are also made, then the wall tension can be calculated either at the end of diastole (preload), or at the end of isovolumic systole (afterload), from the left ventricular

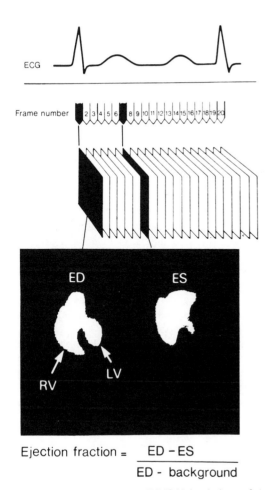

Ejection fraction = $\dfrac{ED - ES}{ED - background}$

Fig. 13-11 Multiple gated (MUGA) technique for measurement of ejection fraction using technetium-99m labeled erythrocytes. The patient's electrocardiogram is used to "gate" the counts so that repetitive cardiac cycles are analyzed to give end-diastolic (ED) and end-systolic (ES) dimension. If the stroke volume is also known, then LV end-diastolic volume can be calculated: EDV = SV/EF. Modified from Willerson J (1984). J Molec Cell Cardiol 16: 697, with permission.

the heart throughout systole, rather than a "pure" index of contractility. Because it relates the systolic emptying to the diastolic volume without measuring that volume, the left ventricle would theoretically be markedly enlarged and yet have reasonable systolic function. Thus the correlation between the degree of clinical heart failure and the ejection fraction is often only imperfect.

dimensions and measurements of the wall thickness using echocardiography.

The ejection fraction can also be measured by echocardiography, which gives the diameter of the heart (Fig. 13-12). Now the problem is to determine the ejection fraction and here only an index can be used—the percentage change of the minor axis in systole.

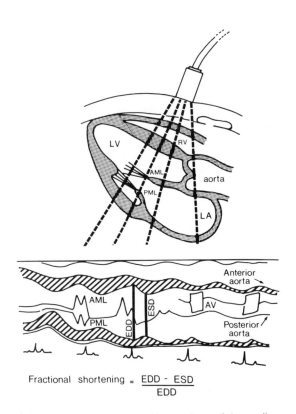

Fractional shortening $= \dfrac{EDD - ESD}{EDD}$

Fig. 13-12 Echocardiographic correlates of the cardiac structures. The transducer (T) is directed from the apex to the base of the heart. AML = anterior mitral leaflet; Ao = aorta; Ao(a) = aorta, anterior wall; Ao(p) = aorta, posterior wall; ARV = anterior right ventricular wall; AV = aortic valve; Ch = chordae tendinae; CW = chest wall; ECG = electrocardiogram; EDD = end-diastolic diameter; EFS = echo-free space; En = endocardium; Ep = epicardium; ESD = end-systolic diameter; IVS = interventricular septum; LA = left atrium; LV = left ventricle; P = pericardium; PML = posterior mitral leaflet; PW = posterior wall; RV = right ventricle; S = sternum. From Krasnow N and Stein PD (1978). Cardiovasc Med 3: 797, with permission.

Other non-invasive procedures of contractile state

The **apex cardiogram** (ACG) is a graphic record of the precordial chest wall movements during the cardiac cycle. It can be recorded simultaneously with the heart sounds (phonocardiogram), the electrocardiogram, and the carotid pulse. With present sophisticated instrumentation the ACG is being used more and more to gain an idea of left ventricular function in relation to the rest of the cardiac cycle. The ACG may show abnormalities of the upstroke, which is when the heart is contracting and the apex displaced outwards, or of the downstroke, which corresponds to the period of ventricular emptying or ejection. For example, in ischemic heart disease the upstroke may be prolonged and there may be a poor downstroke or even an abnormal upward movement during the ejection period. This late systolic bulge is thought to be caused by asynergy of contraction and very frequently occurs in acute myocardial infarction.

Systolic time intervals are useful for objective non-invasive measurements of the above bedside principles. The left ventricular ejection time starts with systole and ends with the closure of the aortic valve; it is measured on the carotid pulse. The **pre-ejection period** is the time from the start of electrical activation of the ventricles (start of QRS on the electrocardiogram) till the opening of the aortic valve on the phonocardiogram; the period of isovolumic contraction is included. The total time of systole, from the start of QRS to A_2, may be measured from the ECG and the carotid pulse and the ejection time subtracted to give the pre-ejection period. In heart failure, the pre-ejection period (index of dP/dt) is lengthened and ejection time shortened so that the total contraction time is unchanged. Conversely, beta-adrenergic stimulation, digitalis and thyrotoxicosis all shorten the pre-ejection time. When allowing for the influence of other factors which also influence these times, a useful non-invasive index of contractility is achieved.

Pressure–volume loops and contractile state

Measurements of pressure–volume loops are a new approach to the assessment of contractility in the human heart (Fig. 13-13), and can be estimated in part from the arterial systolic pressure and the end-systolic echocardiographic dimension (Borow et al., 1982).

Invasive measurements of the left ventricular pressure are required for the full loop, which is an indirect measure of the relationship between the force (as measured by the pressure) and the muscle length (measured indirectly by the volume). As contractile force develops in the left ventricular wall in systole, **so does the pressure build up in the cavity (a → b in Fig. 13-13) until the moment when the aortic valve** opens to eject the blood, and the isovolumic phase of left ventricular contraction is over. The intraventricular pressure is highest just before the aortic valve opens (point b); when the aortic valves open, the flow of blood commences, the ventricular pressure **decreases, and the volume falls (b → c). In early diastole, the heart relaxes, the pressure drops nearly to zero (c → d), while the ventricle is nearly empty.** Then, as the mitral valve opens and the left ventricle fills, the volume rises as the pressure stays low (d + a). When systole starts, the cycle is repeated. It is proposed that conditions associated with a higher contractile activity (increased inotropic state) will have higher end-systolic pressures for a given end-systolic volume, and have correspondingly higher oxygen uptakes.

When the preload and afterload of the heart are both reduced by nitroglycerin, then the pressure-volume loop shifts downwards and to the left, while theoretically there is no change in the inotropic state. The reduction in preload is particularly striking, so

that the initial heart volume and ventricular pressure are both much less (Magorien et al., 1983). Interventions which alter ventricular volume can be separated by such pressure-volume loops from those which alter the inotropic state.

Left ventricular angiography

All non-invasive techniques are generally compared with left ventricular angiography which remains the "gold standard". Although "angio" means blood vessel, the term is used to describe the cinematic technique which outlines left ventricular activity in the various phases of the cardiac cycle. Ventricular volumes can be estimated and the difference between end-systolic and end-diastolic volumes used to calculate the angiographic ejection fraction (which should correspond to that measured by radionuclide techniques). Left ventricular function is usually first studied non-invasively by radionuclide ventriculography and two-dimensional echocardiography. Although the left ventricular angiogram is an invasive procedure it has had three advantages: visualization of regional or segmental ventricular dysfunction which is common in ischemic heart disease, concurrent **coronary angiography** to delineate coronary artery disease, and sensitive detection of valvular regurgitation (for example, a small aortic leak causes a reflux of dye from the aorta to the left ventricle in diastole). Two-dimensional echocardiography and radionuclide angiography, which are completely non-invasive techniques, are now taking the place of invasive angiography when the aim is to visualize the depressed function of regions of the myocardium which are ischemic (left ventricular **segmental dysfunction**).

Where Does Starling Fit In?

Starling related the venous filling pressure of the heart (preload) or the volume of the heart (fiber length) to the output of the heart (see page 7). The links between the length of the muscle fiber and the tension developed have suggested to many that the sarcomere length and degree of "overlap" of thin and thick filaments can explain the **ascending limb** of the Starling relationship (more venous filling leading to a higher cardiac output). The conventional concept has been that of "optimal" overlap between thick and thin filaments, occurring at sarcomere lengths of about

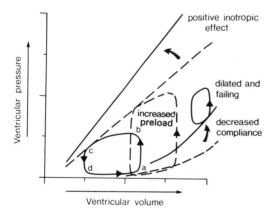

Fig. 13-13 The modern pressure–volume loop. A positively inotropic intervention increases the peak pressure reached at the same initial volume. An increased afterload increases the volume and pressure but leaves the inotropic slope unchanged. A decreased compliance increases the pressure at any given volume. In a dilated and failing myocardium the volume change is much less (small ejection fraction) and the compliance is decreased.

2.2 μm. Shorter lengths give inadequate cross-bridge contact so that the force generation decreases, especially below 1.6 μm (Fig. 13-8), where "double overlap" is the proposed explanation. Excessive sarcomere lengths reduce the overlap to give the descending limb of the Starling curve. Now it is known that the sarcomere length–force relation when correctly measured by laser diffraction does not go into a downward decline. An alternative explanation for the ascending limb of the Starling curve is that at larger fiber lengths the cross-bridges become more sensitive to the prevailing cytosolic calcium ion concentration. Where the ascending limb of the Starling curve could be explained by more optimal cross-bridge overlap is in the very short sarcomere range which is of little physiological importance.

As the venous filling pressure continues to increase the cardiac output reaches a **plateau**. This part of the Starling curve does not appear to be explained by the properties of the individual sarcomeres (Fig. 13-8), even though a plateau of tension development is found in intact papillary muscle preparations. The following explanations may be offered. First, the sarcomeres are incapable of stretching beyond 2.35 or 2.4 μm, when they exert maximum tension (Crozathier et al., 1977). Increasing the papillary muscle length further increases resting tension while the active tension (total tension – resting tension) does not rise. In the intact heart, as the left ventricular end-diastolic pressure rises further, the sarcomere length reaches a limit as does left ventricular end-diastolic diameter or volume (Fig. 13-14). Increasing left ventricular filling pressure or volume further will only increase the resting tension while leaving the stroke volume unchanged, thus giving the plateau of the curve. If the filling pressure is high enough subendocardial ischemia will tend to decrease the stroke volume (next paragraph).

Whether there really is a **descending limb** of the Starling curve is highly controversial. Such a decline is a clinical reality because as venous pressure keeps on rising, cardiac output actually starts to fall (see Fig. 22-2). Yet numerous careful animal experiments have failed to confirm that the descending limb is part of the inherent properties of cardiac muscle. In the failing human heart the descending limb appears to apply (see Fig. 1-10) largely because of (i) the development of subendocardial ischemia and mitral incompetence at large heart volumes and high wall tensions; (ii) "fiber-slippage"; and (iii) increased afterload caused by peripheral vasoconstriction. In developing myocardial infarction, a true stretch of the

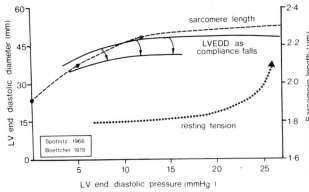

Fig. 13-14 As the left ventricular end-diastolic pressure increases, the left ventricular end-diastolic volume (here measured as left ventricular end-diastolic diameter or LVEDD) increases over low pressures but rapidly reaches a maximum. Similarly sarcomere length also reaches a maximum. If the left ventricular end-diastolic pressure is increased beyond the physiological limit of about 12 mmHg, resting tension starts to rise and will impair subendocardial myocardial perfusion. If the compliance of the ventricle is decreased, as after myocardial infarction, then dV/d P falls so that there is a lesser volume rise for a given pressure rise. These relations can explain some aspects of the Starling curve. Original data based on Spotnitz (1966) and Boettcher (1978).

sarcomeres up to 3.6 μm may occur, probably as result of fragmentation of the thin filaments (Crozathier et al., 1977). Such an alteration of myocardial fiber properties probably leads to a decreased inotropic state. In clinical terms, a large dilated heart contracts poorly and if the filling pressure rises more then myocardial function is more likely to be impaired. When the subendocardial tension is relieved by reduction of the preload by nitrates, the stroke volume stays the same or improves as the venous filling pressure falls. When the afterload is reduced by vasodilator therapy then myocardial performance also improves.

In contrast to the obvious relevance of the Starling relation to congestive heart failure, its significance to the healthy conscious animal is questioned. When the left ventricular end-diastolic diameter is already near maximal (Boettcher et al., 1978) an increased venous return simply elevates the left ventricular end-diastolic pressure without increasing the heart volume. Thus in exercising dogs (Chapter 14) the increased venous return is largely dealt with by an increased heart rate and an increased inotropic state rather than by the Starling law. In recumbent man, the Starling relation plays a more important role, as shown by a considerable increase in heart volume during vigorous exercise (Chapter 14). The difference may lie not in the species but in the posture, because the Starling law is less important in the upright position (see page 190). Presumably the venous return in the upright position is more governed by the pressure generated by the heart which ultimately has to drive the blood "uphill" from the exercising limbs to the right heart.

Ventricular function curves

Clinically, the symptoms of an increased filling pressure and "**backward failure**" (shortness of breath, signs of pulmonary congestion) can be related to poor left ventricular output ("**forward failure**"); despite an increased left ventricular filling pressure, the cardiac output is not enough because the inotropic state is decreased and there is myocardial failure (see Fig. 22-2). Under therapy with positively inotropic agents such as digitalis (inhibition of the sodium pump, Chapter 4), the signs of congestion and of forward failure should lessen. This improvement is not caused by a change in the filling pressure, the Starling law is therefore not in operation and the inotropic state has improved. For each inotropic state there is one characteristic relationship between the filling pressure and the output, producing a **family of Starling curves**, each reflecting its own inotropic state (see Fig. 1-10).

Non-invasive assessment of the preload

Soon non-invasive assessment of ventricular function curves may be possible. Doppler measurements of the cardiac output (Chapter 14) could then be linked to echocardiographic determination of the left ventricular filling pressure. The theory for the latter is simple. In mitral stenosis the interval between the second sound and the opening snap lengthens, whereas the interval between the onset of the QRS and the first sound (M_1) lengthens as the size of the mitral valve orifice decreases and the left atrial pressure rises. A similar relation holds even in the absence of mitral stenosis, so the pulmonary wedge pressure can be determined from intervals measured by the echocardiogram (Fig. 13-15). The critical points are the time between aortic valve closure and the maximum opening of the mitral valve (first sound interval), and from the start of QRS to mitral valve closure (Askenazi et al., 1981). By this

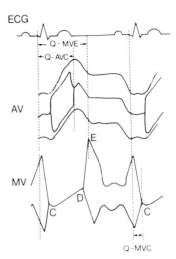

Fig. 13-15 Schematic drawing showing the measurements of the interval from the Q wave on the electrocardiogram to the echo of the mitral valve (MV) leaflets' coaptation point (C) in early systole (MVC), from Q to the point of early maximum diastolic opening of the anterior mitral valve leaflet (MVE) and from Q to the echo of the aortic valve closure point (AVC). The ratio Q-MVC/ACV-E is an indirect index of the left ventricular filling pressure. From Askenazi et al. (1981), with permission.

technique, left ventricular filling pressure may be measured indirectly in various types of non-valvular heart disease as well as in mitral stenosis.

Circumferential fiber length–stress relation

Another sophisticated approach to the Starling law in man is to relate the volume of the contracting heart to the force or stress generated. Because circumferentially orientated fibers predominate in the left ventricular myocardium, a representative fiber length, the **mid-wall circumferential fiber length** can be calculated and compared with the "net wall force" or stress (Weber et al., 1982). When the left ventricle is contracting isovolumically (no change in chamber volume, see phase C of Wiggers' cycle, Fig. 13-1), the developed force does not reach a plateau over the whole physiologic range of filling volumes at filling pressures of 0–25 mmHg. Only when supraphysiologic pressures of about 50 mmHg are reached is there a plateau in isovolumic conditions; therefore the intact healthy ventricle works only in the ascending limb of the Starling curve, in keeping with the recent model of the length–tension relationship in isolated cardiac muscle. The **slope** of the idealized length–stress (length–force) relation is an index of the contractile state of the myocardium. Adrenergic stimulation shifts the slope upward and to the left, whereas propranolol, ischemia or myocardial failure shift the relation downwards and to the right. These changes correspond to those shown for the ascending limb of the Starling curve.

The way ahead

Now that echocardiography can accurately determine dimensions of the ventricle, and the volume of the heart can be found using multiple gated ventriculography, it is only a question of time before the Starling relation will be more easily assessed by non-invasive techniques. The hold-up will be the accurate non-invasive measurement of cardiac output (Chapter 14).

Length-dependent vs inotropic changes

To summarize: both an increasing initial fiber length and a positive inotropic intervention can increase the force **and** the velocity of contraction. Although these two effects can still be separated by very exactly measuring the maximal velocity of contraction (V_{max}) of rapidly unloaded muscle (Fig. 13-9), in practice there is a close similarity between the ultimate results of increasing fiber length and increasing the contractile state. Currently the effect of length is explained as an increased sensitivity of the cross-bridges to the prevailing calcium ion concentration; the exact mechanism involved is still unclear and some rôle for optimal cross-bridge overlap cannot be excluded. A reasonable hypothesis relates to the contractile state of the healthy myocardium to the peak cytosolic calcium ion concentration. Therefore, theoretically, a length-dependent increase in the contractile state could be additive to a length-independent increase caused by a positive inotropic agent. The former would increase contractile sensitivity to the prevailing calcium ion concentration; the latter would primarily increase the cytosolic calcium. In the failing heart, the cause of the decreased contractility is very complex and not yet well understood (Chapter 22).

Ventricular Relaxation

Thus far the relation between systolic force generation and the contractile state has been emphasized, yet impaired contractility can also depress the rate of

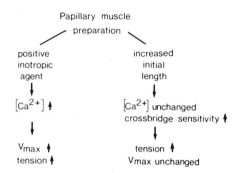

Fig. 13-16 Both increased inotropic stimulation and increased fiber length act to enhance the degree of tension developed at any given muscle length. The inotropic stimulus increases the prevailing cytosolic calcium ion concentration, whereas an increased length sensitizes the cross-bridges to a given calcium ion concentration.

relaxation. The recent realization that impaired relaxation is an early event in angina pectoris has revived interest in this phase of the contractile cycle. In angina, a proposed metabolic explanation is that there is impaired generation of energy, which diminishes the supply of ATP required for the early diastolic uptake of calcium by the sarcoplasmic reticulum. The result is that the cytosolic calcium, at a peak in systole, delays its return to normal in the early diastolic period. Theoretically the rate of relaxation during the phase of isovolumic relaxation (phase F) of Wiggers' cycle (Fig. 13-1) is independent of muscle length. In reality, longer sarcomere lengths "order" and delay the rate of relaxation (Krueger and Farber, 1980). The factor concerned is an intrinsic property of the elements of the contractile lattice. Clinically, too, the end-systolic volume may influence the peak rate of relaxation (Cohn et al., 1972), just as the end-diastolic heart volume can alter the inotropic index, maximum positive dP/dt. The rate of ventricular relaxation can be obtained non-invasively by computer analysis of the relaxation phase as visualized by echocardiography or radionuclide MUGA scanning. In left ventricular hypertrophy, such non-invasive indices as the **diastolic time index** are determined by so many factors that invasive measurements (Fig. 13-17) are preferable.

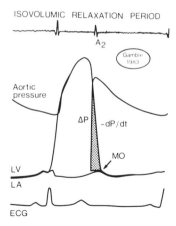

Fig. 13-17 The isovolumic relaxation phase of the cardiac cycle is shaded in. It extends from the aortic second sound (A₂) to the cross-over point between the left ventricular and left atrial pressures (MO = mitral valve opening; see also point OS in Fig. 13-1). The rate of relaxation is given by $-dP/dt$ (contrast with Fig. 13-6). A_2 = aortic second sound, which in normal hearts occurs at the onset of isovolumic relaxation. From Gamble et al. (1983) Circulation 68: 76, with permission from the author and the American Heart Association.

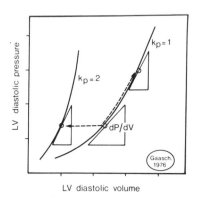

Fig. 13-18 The compliance reflects the relation between the increase in heart volume for a given increase in pressure (dP/dV). On the right, the heart has become stiffer because it operates at a higher end-diastolic pressure (Fig. 13-14). On the left, the compliance is decreased, because the modulus of chamber stiffness (k_p) is increased; such a true increase of stiffness can occur in acute myocardial infarction. From Gaasch et al. (1976) Am J Cardiol 38: 645, with permission.

Compliance

The diastolic volume of the heart is influenced not only by the loading conditions but also by the elastic properties of the myocardium. **Elasticity** means that the myocardium recovers its normal shape after removal of the systolic stress. Compliance is strictly defined as the relation between the change in stress and the resultant **strain** (percentage change in dimension or size); in clinical practice it is taken as the ratio of dP/dV, that is, the rate of pressure change divided by the rate of volume change. The relation is curvilinear so the initial slope of the change is gentle; then as the pressure increases more, the volume increases less and less so that there is a considerable increase of pressure for only a small increase of volume (Fig. 13-18). This relation is in some ways similar to that between sarcomere length and tension and the plateau of the Starling curve.

Whereas resting skeletal muscle relation is truly in a state of relaxation (so that the resting tension is close to zero), the heart has a very high resting tension. Resting **stiffness** may in part be attributed to the unique myocardial collagen network, thought to counter the high systolic pressure normally developed in the ventricles (Borg and Caulfield, 1979). Pathological loss of compliance is usually due to abnormalities of the myocardium. In **myocardial hypertrophy** there is an apparent loss of muscular compliance, so that the pressure rises more for any given volume increase (the thicker the wall the more intraluminal pressure is needed to make it stretch). But when corrected for the increased mass the muscular compliance in myocardial hypertrophy is close to normal. Another approach is to plot left ventricular stress against volume, so that there is an in-built compensation for the increased wall thickness.

A true loss of muscular compliance occurs from a variety of causes — acute ischemia as in angina, fibrosis as develops after myocardial infarction, and infiltrations causing a restrictive cardiomyopathy. In angina the increased stiffness is probably a combination of a rise of intracellular calcium and of altered myocardial properties (Lewis et al., 1980). In myocardial infarction the connective tissue undergoes changes after 40 min of occlusion (Sato et al., 1983); eventually healing and fibrosis increases stiffness permanently. All such causes of muscle stiffness will also increase **chamber stiffness**. When functioning of the chambers is indirectly impaired by constrictive pericarditis, a hemodynamic situation similar to restrictive cardiomyopathy may arise, but the basic cause is extracardiac so that the fall of compliance is more apparent than real.

The compliance of the heart will influence both the Starling curve and the pressure–volume loop. A stiffer heart will be on a lower Starling curve, and the baseline of the pressure–volume loop will rise upwards more steeply. For these reasons, compliance is a fundamental mechanical property of the heart.

Summary

The activity of the contractile proteins of the sarcomeres explains the pumping action of the heart. The chief factors determining the mechanical function and the oxygen uptake of the heart are the heart rate, the stress on the myocardial wall and the contractility (or inotropic state). The wall stress is in turn determined by the afterload (largely the arterial blood pressure) and the preload (the left atrial filling pressure). When the preload increases (Starling's law) the ventricular filling improves, end-diastolic volume rises, and so does stroke volume. The mechanism involved was held to be a more optimal positioning of cross-bridges; now length-dependent activation is invoked. Although Starling's law applies to many animal preparations and in the failing human heart, its application to the normal non-failing heart is limited because the left ventricle end-diastolic volume cannot acutely increase beyond a certain amount. At a fixed muscle length (diastolic heart volume unchanged), an increased inotropic stimulus such as adrenergic stimulation will increase stroke volume. In clinical practice it is not easy to measure the inotropic state. Various indices, both invasive and non-invasive are therefore used. Increasingly popular are the non-invasive ejection phase indices such as the ejection fraction. These are afterload-dependent, so that they are of most use in congestive heart failure when the increasing afterload limits left ventricular performance. Left ventricular function curves can be obtained by Swan–Ganz catheterization. When the preload and afterload are fixed, an increase of stroke volume reflects an increased inotropic state. Positively inotropic drugs, such as digitalis or catecholamines, should improve the inotropic state of the failing myocardium by moving the myocardium to a more favorable left ventricular function curve.

References

Allen DG, Kurihara S (1982). The effects of muscle length on intracellular calcium transients in mammalian cardiac muscle. J Physiol 327: 79–94.

Askenazi J, Koenigsberg DI, Ziegler JH, Lesch M (1981). Echocardiographic estimates of pulmonary artery wedge pressure. N Eng J Med 26: 1566–1568.

Boettcher DH, Vatner SF, Heyndrickx GR, Braunwald E (1978). Extent of utilization of the Frank-Starling mechanism in conscious dogs. Am J Physiol 234: H338–H345.

Borg TK, Caulfield JB (1979). The collagen network of the heart. Lab Invest 40: 364–372.

Borow KM, Neumann A, Wynne J (1982). Sensitivity of pressure–dimension and pressure–volume relations to the inotropic state in humans. Circulation 65: 988–997.

Braunwald E, Ross J Jr (1979). Control of cardiac performance. In: Handbook of Physiology, Section 2: The Cardiovascular System, Volume 1. The Heart. Eds R Berne, N Sperelakis, SR Geiser, pp 533–580, Am Physiol Soc.

Cohn PF, Liedtke AJ, Serur J, Sonnenblick EH, Urschel CW (1972). Maximal rate of pressure fall (peak negative dP/dt) during ventricular relaxation. Cardiovasc Res 6: 263–267.

Cromer AH (1977). Physics for the Life Sciences, pp 17–38, McGraw-Hill, New York.

Crozathier B, Ashraf M, Franklin D, Ross J Jr (1977). Sarcomere length in experimental myocardial infarction: evidence for sarcomere overstretch in dyskinetic ventricular regions. J Molec Cell Cardiol 9: 785–797.

Gibbs CL (1974). Cardiac energetics. In: The Mammalian Myocardium. Eds GA Langer, AJ Brady, pp 105–133, Wiley, New York.

Gordon AM, Pollack GH (1980). Effects of calcium on the sarcomere length–tension relation in rat cardiac muscle: implications for the Frank Starling mechanism. Circ Res 47: 610–619.

Grossman W, Jones D, McLaurin L (1975). Wall stress and patterns of hypertrophy in the human left ventricle. J Clin Invest 56: 56–64.

Hefner LL, Sheffield LT, Cobbs GC, Klip W (1962). Relation between mural force and pressure in the left ventricle of the dog. Circ Res 11: 654–663.

Jewell BR (1977). A re-examination of the influence of muscle length on myocardial performance. Circ Res 40: 221–230.

Johnson E (1979). Force-interval relationship of cardiac muscle. In: Handbook of Physiology. The Cardiovascular System 1. Ed RM Berne, pp 475–494, Am Physiol Soc.

Kannengiesser GJ, Opie LH, Van der Werff TJ (1979). Impaired cardiac work and oxygen uptake after reperfusion of regionally ischaemic myocardium. J Molec Cell Cardiol 11: 197–207.

Katz AM (1977). Physiology of the Heart. Raven Press, New York.

Krueger JW, Farber S (1980). Sarcomere length "orders" relaxation in cardiac muscle. Europ Heart J 1: Suppl A: 37–47.

Langer GA (1983). The "sodium pump lag" revisited. J Molec Cell Cardiol 15: 647–651.

Lewis MJ, Housmans P, Claes VA, Brutsaert DL, Henderson AH (1980). Myocardial stiffness during hypoxic and reoxygenation contracture. Cardiovasc Res 14: 339–344.

Magorien DJ, Shaffer P, Bush CA, Magorien RD, Kolibash AJ, Leier CV, Bashore TM (1983). Assessment of left ventricular pressure–volume relations using gated radio-nuclide angiography, echocardiogrpahy, and micromano-meter pressure recordings. Circulation 67: 844–853.

Murphy R (1983). Contraction of muscle cells. In: Physiology. Eds RM Berne, MN Levy, pp 359–386, CV Mosby, St Louis.

Noble MIM (1979). The Cardiac Cycle. Blackwell Scientific Publications, Oxford.

Noble MIM (1983). Excitation–contraction coupling. In: Cardiac Metabolism. Eds AJ Drake-Holland, MIM Noble, pp 49–71, John Wiley, Chichester.

Sabbah HN, Anbe DT, Stein PD (1980). Negative intraventricular diastolic pressure in patients with mitral stenosis: evidence of left ventricular diastolic suction. Am J Cardiol 45: 562–566.

Sarnoff SJ, Braunwald E, Welch GH Jr, Case RB, Stainsby WM, Macraz R (1958). Hemodynamic determinants of oxygen consumption of the heart with special reference to the tension–time index. Am J Physiol 192: 148–156.

Sato S, Ashraf M, Millard RW, Fujiwara H, Schwartz A (1983). Connective tissue changes in early ischemia of porcine myocardium: an ultrastructural study. J Molec Cell Cardiol 15: 261–275.

Schneider J, Berger HJ, Sands MJ, Lachman AB, Zaret BL (1983). Beat-to-beat ventricular performance in atrial fibrillation: radionuclide assessment with the computerized nuclear probe. Am J Cardiol 51: 1189–1195.

Spotnitz HM, Sonnenblick EH, Spiro D (1966). Relation of ultrastructure to function in the intact heart. Circ Res 18: 49–66.

Stein PD, Sabbah HH (1975). Ventricular performance in

patients based upon rate of change of power during isovolumic contraction. Am J Cardiol 35: 258–263.

Ter Keurs HEDJ (1983). Calcium and contractility. In: Cardiac Metabolism. Eds AJ Drake-Holland, MIM Noble, pp 73–99, John Wiley, Chichester.

Van Heuningen R, Rijnsburger WH, Ter Keurs HEDJ (1982). Sarcomere length control in striated muscle. Amer J Physiol 242: H411–H420.

Walker ML Jr, Hawthorne EW, Sandler H (1971). Methods for assessing performance for the intact hypertrophied heart. In: Cardiac Hypertrophy, Ed. NR Alpert, pp 387–405, Academic Press, Orlando, New York and London.

Weber KT, Janicki JS, Hunter WC, Shroff S, Pearlman ES, Fishman AP (1982). The contractile behavior of the heart and its functional coupling to the circulation. Prog Cardiovasc Dis 5: 375–399.

Wiggers CJ (1949). Physiology in Health and Disease. 5th edition. Lea & Febiger, Philadelphia.

New References

Allen DG, Kentish JC (1985). The cellular basis of the length-tension relation in cardiac muscle. J Molec Cell Cardiol 17: 821–840.

Goldman ME (1985). Emerging importance of the right ventricle. J Am Coll Cardiol 5: 925–927.

Lecarpentier Y, Martin J-L, Claes V, Chambaret J-P, Migus A, Antonetti A, Hatt P-Y (1985). Real-time kinetics of sarcomere relaxation by laser diffraction. Circ Res 56: 331–339.

Poliner LR, Farber SH, Glaeser DH, Nylaan L, Verani MS, Roberts R (1984). Alteration of diastolic filling rate during exercise radionuclide angiography: a highly sensitive technique for detection of coronary artery disease. Circulation 70: 942–950.

Suga H, Goto Y, Yamada O, Igarashi Y (1984). Independence of myocardial oxygen consumption from pressure-volume trajectory during diastole in canine left ventricle. Circ Res 55: 734–739.

14   Cardiac Output and Exercise

Only a sustained increase of the work load on the heart gives rise to hypertrophy. Acute work loads can be handled successfully by other adaptations, which augment the cardiac output by increasing heart rate and stroke volume. During the complex integrated response to acute bodily exercise, the venous return increases and the cardiac output rises. When exercise is frequent or sustained, then it may result in physiological hypertrophy.

Autoregulation

The effect of venous return on the stroke volume can readily be established in an isolated working heart model—if the left atrial pressure is abruptly increased, then the stroke volume rises within seconds. The heart rate also increases, possibly because of catecholamine discharge or because of an effect of stretch on the pacemaker tissue (Blinks, 1956). The cardiac output (stroke volume × heart rate) increases because both stroke volume and heart rate rise. As the peripheral **vascular resistance (PVR) is fixed in an isolated heart model, an increased cardiac output (CO) must result in an increased aortic pressure:**

$$\text{aortic pressure} = CO \times PVR$$

This in turn abruptly increases the aortic pressure, evoking the Anrep effect and other autoregulation mechanisms.

Anrep effect

When the aortic pressure is elevated abruptly a positive inotropic effect follows within one or two minutes. This used to be called **homeometric autoregulation** (homeo = the same; metric = length), because it was apparently independent of muscle length and by definition a true inotropic effect. Two possible explanations are: (i) transient subendocardial ischemia results from the abrupt increase in left ventricular wall tension (Vatner et al., 1974); (ii) the "erectile" properties of the coronary arteries are involved; when the coronary arteries are distended by an increased aortic perfusion pressure, left ventricular work increases even in empty isolated hearts (Vogel et al., 1982).

Bainbridge reflex

When the heart is normally connected to the central nervous system, additional reflexes come into play. The Bainbridge reflex increases the heart rate. It is thought that distension of the right atrium and great veins stimulates receptors which transmit impulses to the vasomotor center by different vagal fibers. This mechanism is in addition to the increase of heart rate, found in the isolated heart ("Blinks' effect"), and the increased circulating catecholamines found during exercise. The increased heart rate may call forth a further inotropic response—the Bowditch effect (Chapter 13).

The combination of Anrep, Bainbridge and

Bowditch effects is such that an increase in venous return can invoke a positive inotropic effect quite apart from and in addition to the Starling mechanism. However, changes in the inotropic state are probably not as important as changes in the venous return in increasing the output of the healthy heart.

Venous Return

The venous return to the right atrium must be the result of the difference between the **central venous pressure** (CVP) and the higher peripheral venous pressure. Generally the peripheral venous pressure is about 5–10 cmH$_2$O higher than the central value. The CVP can readily be measured by a catheter; it is an index of the intrathoracic pressure and is normally very low (only a few mmHg), and with deep inspiration falls to below zero. The gradient for venous return to the central veins rises during inspiration. For this blood to enter the right ventricle from the right atrium, where the pressure might be very low, is best explained by a combination of right atrial contraction and right ventricular "suction". The central venous pulse is influenced by systemic vasoconstriction, muscular activity and the blood volume, and right ventricular intrathoracic pressure.

Systemic venous capacity

When the veins are vasoconstricted, as during catecholamine stimulation, the blood is squeezed out of the venous reservoirs and the venous return increases. Conversely, with vasodilator therapy the **venous capacitance** increases, decreasing the venous return and relieving the preload. About half of the circulating blood volume (4–5 L, slightly lower than the cardiac output) is normally present in the capacitance veins; vasodilators would increase this by about 1 liter or more whereas vasoconstrictors could decrease this by about 1 liter.

During systemic exercise the muscles contract on the peripheral veins to help increase the venous return despite the tendency to vasodilate (exercise produces vasodilatory metabolites).

When the **blood volume** is abruptly increased by an infusion, the cardiac output can temporarily double for a short time. However, the increased volume rapidly disappears as a result of: (i) hydrostatic pressure into the tissues; (ii) increased venous distension; and after a while (iii) a diuresis, to restore the blood volume.

When the blood volume abruptly falls, as in **hemorrhagic shock**, then the cardiac output falls as the venous return is less; the blood pressure is sustained by an increase of peripheral arterial resistance (arterial vasoconstriction) until a continued loss of blood leads to hypotension. In the hypovolumic patient, large amounts of fluid can be given without a rise of central venous pressure (which would otherwise rise).

Right ventricular function

Normally the right ventricle can cope easily with the venous return and need not generate as much pressure as the left because of the low resistance in the pulmonary arteries. In left sided failure, back-pressure causes pulmonary venous hypertension and the right ventricle gradually fails. The result is that the right atrial, central venous and jugular venous pressures all rise. Thus an increased filling pressure is required for the same stroke volume—the right ventricle is on an unfavorable Starling curve. As the filling pressure (preload) continues to rise, tricuspid regurgitation will cause the central venous pressure to rise much more. Over-distension of the ventricle requires removal of the preload by diuresis or vasodilator therapy.

Right ventricular impairment is not necessarily caused only by venous back-pressure. The **Bernheim effect** is the result of left ventricular dilation pressing on the right side in such a way that venous filling is impaired (so the jugular venous pressure rises) while there is no interference with right ventricular outflow.

Intrathoracic pressure

The intrathoracic pressure varies with the site of measurement—either the central veins, the pleural cavity (negative) or esophagus. It is highly dependent on respiration. In emphysema the jugular venous pressure rises on expiration in contrast to the normal fall. Thus the blood pressure will tend to fall on inspiration. When the thoracic pressure is sustained by the **Valsalva maneuver** (forced expiration against a closed glottis), the venous return must fall as must the blood pressure despite a reflex tachycardia. On release, there is a sudden fall of intrathoracic and blood pressure, with a subsequent overshoot of blood pressure which causes a bradycardia mediated by the baroreceptors. The phase of bradycardia is mediated by the vagus, and an enhanced vagal tone is one method of terminating an attack of supraventricular tachycardia. In congestive heart failure or in diabetic autonomic neuropathy, the reflex changes in the heart rate do not occur.

Right ventricular function in disease

Right heart mechanics can be monitored by inspection of the neck veins. The **jugular venous pressure** normally is only apparent in the recumbent position (low venous pressure) and rises in right sided failure. Right atrial contraction produces the **A wave**, thereafter right ventricular contraction produces the **C wave** by closing and bulging the tricuspid valve and by a carotid artefact (C = carotid). As ventricular systole occurs, the ring to which the tricuspid valve is attached is pulled down (like a fist contracting) and the right atrial volume falls to produce the **X descent**. Much later, during systole, the right atrial pressure builds up to cause the **V wave** (V for ventricular systolic contraction). As the tricuspid valve opens the V wave falls (**Y descent**) and the fall is so rapid that right ventricular suction is probably helping the ventricle to fill. If the tricuspid valve is incompetent (**tricuspid regurgitation**) the combined enhanced C waves are now caused by systolic ejection of blood into the atrium to overcome the X descent; C and V waves fuse so that the venous pulse is "ventricularized".

Right Ventricular Response

The venous return to the left heart governs the left atrial filling pressure and is clinically monitored by the pulmonary wedge pressure. The venous return from the lungs must be the same as output of the right ventricle, which is determined by the same factors as the left ventricle (heart rate, preload, afterload and contractility). The pulmonary artery does not undergo the same major increase in its resistance that occur in the peripheral vascular resistance, for obvious reasons — blood flow to the lungs must continue at all times, and in response to cold or heat there is no need for physiological vasoconstriction or dilation of the pulmonary arterioles to regulate the body temperature. Physiologically, the most important adaptation is pulmonary artery vasodilation—the pulmonary

arterial system is very compliant so that blood flow can increase several-fold without any increase in pressure. This change, together with the tachycardia, occurs in exercise, and results in an increase in ventricular stroke volume as the venous return increases to the right atrium. Pathologically, the pulmonary vascular resistance can increase in response to hypoxia, a cause of reflex **pulmonary hypertension**. If the pulmonary artery flow rises substantially over a long period, as in congenital heart disease with a left-to-right shunt, the pulmonary artery pressure (normal 15–25/5–10 mmHg) also rises to cause pulmonary hypertension (other causes: chronic left-sided heart failure and tight mitral stenosis). Sustained pulmonary artery pressures (e.g. above 40 mmHg systolic) will first cause hypertrophy and then failure of the right ventricle.

Exercise: Heart Rate vs Starling's Law

The above analysis emphasizes the effects of venous return in regulating right and therefore left ventricular function in normal man. However, the major adaptation to exercise is probably achieved by an increased heart rate. The expected increase in fiber length may in part be annulled by increased contractility. Animal experiments have suggested that the Starling relationship only comes into play with very low filling pressures (hemorrhagic shock, dehydration) or as a beat-to-beat regulatory mechanism in response to respiratory variation in the intrathoracic pressure. Tachycardia therefore should contribute more than does an altered venous filling pressure to the normal response to exercise. These patterns are also held to be correct for human subjects exercising in the recumbent position (Fig. 14-1). In the upright position, there is a greater contribution of the Starling mechanism, as shown by an increased end-diastolic volume (Fig. 14-2).

An increased adrenergic drive at the start of vigorous exercise can explain why the heart rate may double during exercise. Even in the presence of beta-adrenergic blockade, the heart rate can still double during maximal exercise—although the absolute heart rates reached are much reduced. Unexpectedly, in dogs with cardiac denervation (Donald and Shepherd, 1963), the heart rate can still rise although it does so more slowly and less than in controls. Here increased circulating catecholamines are the major stimulus (Fig. 14-3).

RELATIVE INFLUENCE OF
FACTORS AFFECTING MV̇O₂ IN THE
NORMAL HEART

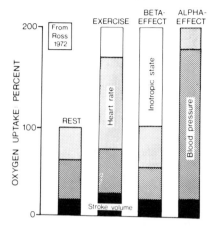

Fig. 14-1 During mild exercise in the upright position, the major factor increasing the myocardial oxygen uptake is the tachycardia (Kitamura et al., 1972). During infusion of a beta-adrenergic stimulant a positive inotropic effect becomes more important. During infusion of an alpha-adrenergic agonist the increase in blood pressure becomes more important. Note that the component marked "stroke volume" represents the oxygen required for shortening against a load (**Fenn effect**) which stays relatively constant throughout. Redrawn from Ross (1972), with permission.

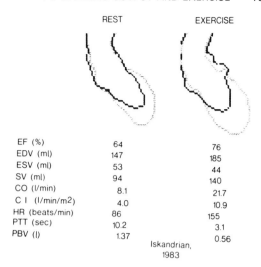

	REST	EXERCISE
EF (%)	64	76
EDV (ml)	147	185
ESV (ml)	53	44
SV (ml)	94	140
CO (l/min)	8.1	21.7
CI (l/min/m2)	4.0	10.9
HR (beats/min)	86	155
PTT (sec)	10.2	3.1
PBV (l)	1.37	0.56

Iskandrian, 1983

Fig. 14-2 First-pass radionuclide ventriculograms obtained at rest and during exercise in a normal subject in the upright position. The images show superimposed end-diastolic (light) and end-systolic (dark) perimeters. EF = ejection fraction; EDV = end-diastolic volume; ESV = end-systolic volume; SV = stroke volume; CO = cardiac output; CI = cardiac index; HR = heart rate; PTT = mean pulmonary transit time; PBV = pulmonary blood volume. Note that the large increase of 267 percent in cardiac output is obtained predominantly by an increased heart rate (180 percent). There is also a smaller rise in end-diastolic volume (126 percent) showing the operation of the Starling law. From Iskandrian et al. (1983), with permission from the Journal of the American College of Cardiology.

The circulatory and cardiac changes in response to exercise can now be traced out, taking the example of a runner and making some simplifying assumptions. When bodily exercise starts the leg muscles contract to increase the venous return which increases the right ventricular filling pressure and the volume of the ventricle. The major stimulus to the tachycardia of exercise comes from increased activity of the autonomic nervous system, probably in response to central arousal mechanisms which are activated by the runner's "readiness to go". The release of norepinephrine into the synaptic clefts within the heart stimulates the beta-1-adrenoceptors around the sinus node, the pacemaker currents respond and a tachycardia results. Release of epinephrine from the adrenal gland contributes to the cardiac beta-1-response. Sustained exercise leads to more release of catecholamines. Heart rate increases as does the myocardial oxygen uptake (Fig. 14-1).

That there is adrenergic stimulation during exercise is proved by the doubling of the plasma value of norepinephrine (Chidsey et al., 1962) and by the discharge of norepinephrine from the heart into the coronary sinus (Cousineau et al., 1977). Not surprisingly, when beta-adrenergic blocking agents are given the degree of exercise activity that can be reached is impaired so that when normal subjects are exercised to their limit, the cardiac output falls by about 25 percent after beta-blockade (Epstein et al., 1965). As in exercising denervated greyhounds (Fig. 14-3), the contribution of the Starling mechanism increases as the contribution of an increased heart rate diminishes.

As myocardial beta-1-receptors are occupied, so a series of events increases contractility (Chapter 6). First, adenylate cyclase is stimulated (withdrawal of vagal tone enhances the response at this point). Cyclic AMP "opens" calcium channels, perhaps by phosphorylation of a sarcolemmal protein; the enhanced calcium influx triggers the release of more intracellular calcium which increases the contractility. Cyclic AMP also phosphorylates two other proteins which enhance the rate of relaxation (troponin I and

RACING CAPACITY OF DENERVATED GREYHOUNDS

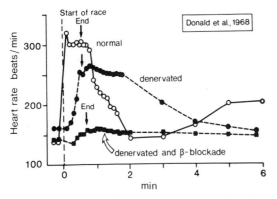

Fig. 14-3 After cardiac denervation in dogs there is a markedly reduced tachycardia in response to exercise. The residual response is the result of increased circulating catecholamines, and is almost completely abolished by beta-adrenergic blockade. As the heart rate falls, increased stroke volume maintains the cardiac output by the Starling mechanism. Redrawn from Donald et al. (1968), with permission.

phospholamban). The phosphorylation of troponin I in response to cyclic AMP decreases the interaction between actin and myosin which is apparently in opposition with the other effects of calcium. A conciliatory hypothesis proposes that an increased rate of relaxation and the increased max $-\,\mathrm{d}P/\mathrm{d}t$ result from the overall effects of catecholamine beta-adrenergic stimulation. Hence both contraction and relaxation are enhanced. Thus contractility increases while still allowing adequate time for the filling of the left ventricle during diastole despite the tachycardia.

That increased contractility occurs during exercise is shown in both man and animals (Fig. 14-1). In man the volume of the heart first increases as the venous return rises, and then during prolonged exercise (Holmgren and Ovenfors, 1960), despite the higher cardiac output, the decreased heart volume indicates that contractility increases. During very severe exercise in dogs the end-diastolic heart size increases slightly but the major increase is in contractility and in heart rate (Vatner et al., 1972).

The cardiac output increases to meet the oxygen demands of the exercising leg muscles as both heart rate and stroke volume increase, because

cardiac output = stroke volume × heart rate

The stroke volume (volume of blood ejected from

the left ventricle during each beat) increases due to the enhanced contractility with a small contribution from the Starling mechanism.

Measurement of Cardiac Output

The classic method has been the **Fick** principle. The arteriovenous difference of oxygen is obtained by arterial puncture and a mixed central venous sample; the oxygen uptake is determined by spirometry; the cardiac output is the volume of blood needed to account for the oxygen uptake.

The **indicator-dilution** method uses a dye such as indocyanine green which is injected centrally into the superior vena cava; turbulence mixes the dye with blood within the ventricles, and the rate of appearance and disappearance of the dye in the aorta depends on the cardiac output. During exercise the peak concentration of dye in the arterial circulation is less, and the dye appears and disappears more rapidly.

Thermodilution is now widely used with Swan–Ganz catheterization. A known amount of ice-cold saline is injected into the central venous circulation; the temperature fall at the tip of the catheter is converted to cardiac output values.

Doppler determinations of cardiac output have the great advantage of being non-invasive, although only at an early stage of perfection. An ultrasound beam is directed onto the stream of blood passing through the mitral valve. The signal returning to the sound-receiving crystal is shifted in frequency in response to the velocity of flow. The area of the mitral valve orifice is determined by two-dimensional echocardiography. The cardiac output is calculated from the mean velocity of blood flow and the diastolic mitral valve area (Fisher et al., 1983).

Using such techniques, the cardiac output during exercise can rise from the normal resting value of 6–7 L/min to 14 L/min in mild exercise, and 25 L/min during severe exercise (Fig. 14-2). In congestive heart failure the cardiac output is slow with inadequate tissue perfusion during exercise; in cardiogenic shock the cardiac output is so low that the tissues are inadequately perfused even at rest and life is threatened.

Isometric vs Isotonic Exercise

In experimental systems "volume work" is better tolerated than "pressure work". The counterpart of this situation in man is the contrast between isotonic and isometric exercise. Isotonic (= aerobic) exercise includes running, walking and related sports, where regular muscular activity occurs but against a light load. Isometric exercise includes activities like carrying a suitcase or weight-lifting, where muscle tension develops but there is little or no displacement of the object worked against. During isotonic exercise the total peripheral resistance decreases dramatically as a result of exercise-induced dilation of arterioles in skeletal muscle; the blood pressure increases simultaneously. During isometric exercise both heart rate and blood pressure (systolic and diastolic) rise within seconds; through reflex mechanisms, peripheral vascular resistance tends to rise rather than fall, especially when large muscle masses are involved (Mitchell et al., 1980). Reflexes are probably involved—sensory receptors in the muscles stimulate the vasomotor center to cause some reflex vasoconstriction of the arterioles (**somatic pressor reflex**) which opposes the effect of metabolic vasodilation. Thus isometric exercise is a different form of stress on the heart to isotonic. The fall in peripheral resistance during isotonic exercise tends to "unload" the heart as the venous filling pressure rises, so that the rise in blood pressure is less. In isometric exercise both heart rate and blood pressure rise, each of which increases the afterload and the wall stress.

Transient "ischemia" in normal subjects

In the isolated heart exposed to a work-jump, biochemical features of transient ischemia appear, such as a breakdown of high-energy phosphate compounds. In contrast to true ischemia, the mitochondrial state of oxygenation improves as $NADH_2$ is abruptly oxidized as the rate of oxidative phosphorylation increases. There can be transient subendocardial "ischemia", coupled with ST-depression on the electrocardiogram (Monroe et al., 1972). In man, too, transient "ischemia" can occur in some subjects, as judged by electrocardiographic signs (Barnard et al., 1973).

One possible explanation for this phenomenon is that coronary vasodilation lags some seconds behind the increased heart work which causes an immediate increased demand for oxygen, so that a sudden rise in oxygen uptake gives subendocardial ischemia. With warm-up the peak arterial pressures developed are lower and the time–tension index less. Such transient "ischemia", elicited by sudden extreme exercise in some normal subjects, must be distinguished from true clinical ischemia which is invoked by near maximal treadmill exercise in patients with ischemic heart disease (Chapter 24).

Energy Metabolism

Patterns of substrate metabolism of the human heart during exercise can be defined by the use of coronary sinus catheterization. There is a marked increase of the contribution of lactate to the oxidative metabolism of the heart during a short burst of exercise (Fig. 14-4). Thus the heart takes up and oxidizes the lactate which is being produced anaerobically by the peripheral muscles.

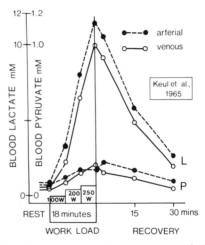

Fig. 14-4 During vigorous exercise over several minutes, the arterial lactate concentration rises. There is an increase in the arteriovenous difference across the heart and lactate becomes the major myocardial fuel. Redrawn from Keul et al. (1965), with permission. For oxygen extraction ratios during acute exercise, see Fig. 9-9.

Metabolic response

The oxygen uptake of the myocardium must rise as each of the determinants—heart rate, contractility and wall stress—rises. The latter rises in response to the increased afterload as the blood pressure rises. Cellular metabolic signals are set off by increased work to ensure that an adequate flow of substrates is ultimately metabolized by the citrate cycle to produce enough ATP. As cytosolic ATP is rapidly converted by

INCREASED WORK STIMULATES CITRATE CYCLE

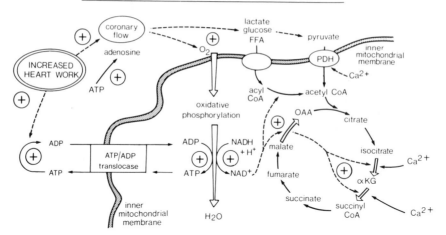

Fig. 14-5 The proposed effects of increased heart work in providing an increased supply of circulating substrates and in stimulating oxidative phosphorylation and citrate cycle activity. FFA = free fatty acids; PDH = pyruvate dehydrogenase; αkg = alpha ketoglutarate. See also Figs 10-10 and 11-4.

contraction to ADP, mitochondrial oxygen uptake and ATP formation are stimulated; $NADH_2$ is converted to NAD, the citrate cycle is stimulated and the uptake of glucose, lactate and free fatty acids is enhanced (Fig. 14-5). These fuels are converted to acetyl CoA to enter the citrate cycle. Thus enough ATP will always be made when heart work is increased during exercise — if the coronary arteries are normal and the supply of oxygen is adequate. The signal to coronary vasodilation is generally regarded as an increased formation of adenosine from the breakdown of ATP. At the very start of increased heart work, when coronary vasodilation is delayed for a few seconds, energy may be provided by the breakdown of glycogen.

Prolonged exercise

As exercise is prolonged beyond about 30 min, the blood lactate falls and arterial free fatty acids rise (Keul, 1971) so that after 120 min of exercise, free fatty acids are once again the major source of myocardial energy production (Table 14-1). Therefore, oxidative metabolism of lactate in acute exercise is replaced by that of free fatty acids during prolonged exercise.

Isolated heart vs human exercise

In the isolated heart perfused with glucose as the only exogenous substrate, a striking finding is the much

Table 14-1

Effect of sustained exercise on myocardial substrate metabolism

	Rest	Sustained exercise
Arterial concentrations		
Glucose, mmol/L	4.1	3.4
Lactate, mmol/L	0.65	1.35
Free fatty acids, mmol/L	0.62	1.28
Triglyceride fatty acid, mmol/L	1.02	0.96
Oxygen extraction ratios (percent)		
Glucose	25	13
Lactate	8	16
Pyruvate	0	1
Free fatty acid	49	49
Triglycerides	15	9
Endogenous fuel[a]	0	"12"
Total	97	100

[a]During sustained exercise there is release of glycerol, blocked by nicotinic acid, and presumably indicating enhanced endogenous lipolysis: oxygen extraction ratio deduced by subtraction of values for all other substrates from 100 percent; glycogenolysis cannot be excluded.
Data from Kaijser et al. (1972). J Appl Physiol 32: 847.

increased glucose uptake with increased heart work. Heart work accelerates glucose transport into the cell and stimulates glycolysis at multiple sites (Chapter 10).

Hence the absolute uptake of glucose rises so much that glucose oxidation can account for all the oxygen uptake of the heart. Not so in the human heart; both in acute and in sustained exercise, glucose only accounts for a part of the oxygen uptake. Because coronary flow is increased, glucose uptake in exercising man is increased in absolute terms. However, when compared with other fuels, the relative contribution of glucose to the energy metabolism falls (Table 14-1) because of the increased blood levels and uptake of lactate during acute exercise and fatty acids during sustained exercise.

The exercising heart, like the normal heart, consumes what it is given. The exception may be at the very onset of severe exercise, when the heart is not given enough external substrate and glycogen is transiently broken down.

Exercise Training

Conditioning of the heart

How does the heart adapt to exercise training? Adaptation of the coronary arteries seemed likely when the coronary arteries of Mr Marathon, a Boston runner who had completed numerous marathons, were found to be very large. The techniques then used to assess the size of coronary arteries would not be accepted today. Despite numerous studies of the coronary arterial tree, the effect of exercise training on the blood supply is an open question. Some studies favor the view that exercise training tends to improve the collateral circulation in patients with ischemic heart disease. To assess the direct effect of exercise training on the myocardium requires the use of a model such as the swimming or running rat. Such animals subjected to prolonged training are said to be conditioned; they then have higher myosin ATPase activities (Scheuer and Tipton, 1977).

Exercise training improves the Ca^{2+}-dependent ATPase activity of actomyosin, myosin and heavy meromyosin of rats conditioned by swimming training. There are molecular changes in the structure of the contractile proteins, especially in the sulfydryl group located near the active site of the ATPase. An additional finding is increased phosphorylation of myosin light chains (Resink et al., 1981). Changes in the composition of the sarcolemma may increase Ca^{2+} availability to the contractile elements. The greater myosin ATPase activity of the hearts of conditioned rats should allow higher contractile activity (for example, increased values of LV max dP/dt).

Exercise training and the heart rate

With training, the heart rate falls as a result of an alteration of the balance between the sympathetic and parasympathetic neural stimulation to the heart. Reduction of the resting heart rate and of the heart rate during submaximal exercise are two of the basic signs of exercise training. After training, beta-adrenergic blockade has less effect in reducing the heart rate both at rest and during exercise (Ekblom et al., 1973). Thus exercise has some effects similar to beta-adrenergic blockade (Brundin et al., 1976).

The athlete's heart

The increased vagal tone (either absolute or relative) of the athlete can give rise to bradycardia with prolonged conduction between atria and ventricles (prolonged PR interval) and abnormalities of repolarization. In some rare cases the sinus node function is suppressed so that some heart beats fail to develop and even hypotensive episodes result. Sometimes conduction through the AV node is so delayed that the **Wenkebach** phenomenon (see Fig. 5-9) develops. Such diseases of over-training can be cured by less exercise. Bradycardia is one explanation for the apparent increased size of the heart found in highly conditioned athletes, the mechanism being an increased diastolic filling time. True "physiologic" **hypertrophy occurs (Ikäheimo et al., 1979) and must be distinguished from the rare condition of hyper**trophic cardiomyopathy (Chapter 21) which can cause sudden death in young athletes. It is not known whether the stimulus to hypertrophy in endurance athletes is prolonged work load or prolonged stimulation by catecholamines.

Exercise rehabilitation

Does the widespread practice of exercise rehabilitation after myocardial infarction have any scientific basis? The patient may feel much better as a result of the rehabilitation program and will be physically fitter, while the profile of risk factors may be modified.

Reductions in the heart rate and blood pressure after training account for the increased exercise tolerance in patients with angina pectoris (Ferguson et al., 1980). As yet there is no good evidence that exercise training fundamentally improves the prognosis of patients after myocardial infarction.

Exercise as prophylaxis

Explanations for the apparent beneficial effect of exercise in preventing ischemic heart disease are as follows. First, exercise training could act in a non-specific way to modify the risk factors such as by increasing the ratio of circulating high density to low density lipoproteins (Heath et al., 1983). Secondly, exercise training need have no direct effect on the development of coronary artery disease but rather on the response of the myocardium to a given extent of coronary disease; for example, the arrhythmogenic effect of coronary artery occlusion could be decreased (Noakes et al., 1983). The decreased release of catecholamines from the heart after exercise training (Cousineau et al., 1977) is the sort of change that could be operating. Thirdly, exercise may open up coronary collateral vessels. In dogs it is only the epicardial collaterals which develop and their functional significance is open to question (Neill and Oxendine, 1979).

Summary

Three basic events account for the increased cardiac output during exercise. First, the heart rate increases. Secondly, the venous return from the exercising skeletal muscle increases. Thirdly, an increased contractile activity (inotropic state) occurs due to beta-adrenergic stimulation. The Starling mechanism only plays a minor role except in recumbent exercise. When the heart has been conditioned by prolonged exercise training, certain intrinsic metabolic qualities change so that a higher inotropic state develops during exercise. It is unlikely that such changes in the contractile properties directly protect against ischemic heart disease; rather, the lifestyle of an athlete appears to confer protective qualities.

References

Barnard RJ, MacAlpin R, Kattus AA, Buckberg GD (1973). Ischemic response to sudden strenuous exercise in healthy men. Circulation 48: 936–942.

Blinks JR (1956). Positive chronotropic effect of increasing right atrial pressure in the isolated mammalian heart. Am J Physiol 186: 209–303.

Brundin T, Edhag O, Lundman T (1976). Effects remaining after withdrawal of long-term beta-receptor blockade. Brit Heart J 38: 1065–1072.

Chidsey CA, Harrison DC, Braunwald E (1962). Augmentation of the plasma norepinephrine response to exercise in patients with congestive failure. N Eng J Med 267: 650–654.

Cousineau D, Ferguson RJ, de Champlian J, Cauthier P, Côté P, Bourassa M (1977). Catecholamines in coronary sinus during exercise in man before and after training. J Appl Physiol 43: 801–806.

Donald DE, Shepherd JT (1963). Response to exercise in dogs with cardiac denervation. Am J Physiol 205: 393–400.

Donald DE, Ferguson DA, Milburn SE (1968). Effect of beta-adrenergic receptor blockade on racing performance of greyhounds with normal and with denervated hearts. Circ Res 22: 127–134.

Ekblom B, Kilblom A, Soltysiak J (1973). Physical training bradycardia and autonomic nervous system. Scand J Clin Lab Invest 32: 251–256.

Epstein SE, Robinson BF, Kahler RL, Braunwald E (1965). Effects of beta-adrenergic blockade on the cardiac response to maximal and submaximal exercise in man. J. Clin Invest 44: 1745–1753.

Ferguson RJ, Cote P, Gauthier P, Bourassa MG (1980). Changes in exercise coronary sinus blood flow with training in patients with angina pectoris. Circulation 58: 41–47.

Fisher DC, Sahn DJ, Friedman MJ, Larson D, Valdes-Cruz LM, Horowitz S, Goldberg SJ, Allen HD (1983). The mitral valve orifice method for noninvasive two-dimensional echo Doppler determinations of cardiac output. Circulation 67: 872–877.

Heath GW, Ehsani AA, Hagberg JM, Hinderliter JM, Goldberg AP (1983). Exercise training improves lipoprotein lipid profiles in patients with coronary artery disease. Am Heart J 105: 889–895.

Holmgren A, Ovenfors CO (1960). Heart volume at rest and during muscular work in the supine and in the sitting position. Acta Med Scand 167: 267–277.

Iskandrian AS, Hakki A-H, DePace NL, Manno B, Segal BL (1983). Evaluation of left ventricular function by radionuclide angiography during exercise in normal subjects and in patients with chronic coronary heart disease. J Am Coll Cardiol 1: 1518–1529.

Keul J (1971). Myocardial metabolism in athletes. In: Muscle Metabolism During Exercise. Eds B Pernow, B Saltin, pp 447–455, Plenum Press, New York and London.

Keul J, Doll E, Steim H, Homburger H, Kern H, Reindell H (1965). Uber den Stoffwechsel des menschlichen Herzens. I. Die Substratversorgung des gesunden menschlichen Herzens in Ruhe, wahrend und nach korperlicher Arbeit. Pflügers Arch 282: 1–27.

Kitamura K, Jorgensen CR, Gobel FL, Taylor HL, Wang Y (1972). Hemodynamic correlates of myocardial oxygen consumption during upright exercise. J Appl Physiol 32: 516–522.

Mitchell JH, Payne FC, Saltin B, Schibye B (1980). The role of muscle mass in the cardiovascular response to static conditions. J Physiol 309: 45–54.

Monroe RG, Gamble WJ, La Farge CC, Kumar AE, Stark J, Sanders GL, Phornphutkul C, Davies M (1972). The Anrep effect reconsidered. J Clin Invest 51: 2573–2584.

Neill WA, Oxendine JM (1979). Exercise can improve coronary collateral development without improving perfusion of ischemic myocardium. Circulation 60: 1513–1519.

Noakes TD, Higginson L, Opie LH (1983). Physical training increases ventricular fibrillation thresholds of isolated rat hearts during normoxia, hypoxia and regional ischemia. Circulation 67: 24–30.

Resink TJ, Gevers W, Noakes TD, Opie LH (1981). Increased cardiac myosin ATPase activity as a biochemical adaptation to running training: enhanced response to catecholamines and a role for myosin phosphorylation. J Molec Cell Cardiol 13: 679–694.

Ross J Jr (1972). Factors regulating the oxygen consumption of the heart. In: Changing Concepts in Cardiovascular Disease. Eds HI Russel, BL Zohman, pp 20–31, Williams and Wilkins, Baltimore.

Scheuer J, Tipton CM (1977). Cardiovascular adaptations to physical training. Ann Rev Physiol 39: 221–251.

Ikäheimo MJ, Palatsi IJ, Takkunen JT (1979). Noninvasive evaluation of the athletic heart: sprinters versus endurance runners. Am J Cardiol 44: 24–30.

Vatner SF, Franklin D, Higgins DB, Patrick T, Braunwald E (1972). Left ventricular response to severe exertion in untethered dogs. J Clin Invest 51: 3052–3060.

Vatner SF, Monroe RG, McRitchie RJ (1974). Effects of anesthesia, tachycardia, and autonomic blockade on the Anrep effect in intact dogs. Am J Physiol 226: 1450–1456.

Vogel WM, Apstein CS, Briggs LL, Gaasch WH, Ahn J (1982). Acute alterations in left ventricular diastolic chamber stiffness: role of 'erectile' effect of coronary arterial pressure and flow in normal and damaged hearts. Circ Res 51: 465–478.

New References

Brooks GA, Fahey TD (1984). Exercise Physiology: Human bioenergetics and its applications, p 726. John Wiley & Sons, New York.

Mitchell JH (1985). Cardiovascular control during exercise: central and reflex neural mechanisms. Am J Cardiol 55: 34D–41D.

Cardiac Hypertrophy and Atrophy

R. Zak

Normal Development of the Heart

Growth of the heart is closely related to its hemodynamic workload. This relation can be found throughout the life of an individual and when species of different life styles are compared. Examples are the dramatic increase in the growth of the left ventricle following birth, or the cardiac enlargement accompanying valvular lesions. In different animal species, the biggest hearts (relative to body size) are found in those animals whose survival requires endurance exertion rather than short bursts of activity. Breeding for speed results in genetically larger hearts (greyhound vs domestic dog); domestication is accompanied by decreased size of the myocardium.

To a biologist, cardiac development and growth represent a system controlled by two sets of factors. First, intrinsic factors are not related to functional demands; an example is the cardiac morphogenesis prior to the development of the circulatory system. Secondly, extrinsic factors can be related to contractile activity. The main challenge is to delineate the differences between physiological and pathological limits of hemodynamic function, and to understand their respective effects on cardiac growth. The enlargement of the heart induced by hemodynamic overload is an adaptive response which allows the individual to survive. Nevertheless, when the overload is prolonged or exceeds an as yet undetermined limit, cardiac growth changes the organization and properties of myocardial cells with decreased contractile function and eventual heart failure.

In this chapter, the normal growth of the myocardium will be presented first, followed by examples of hemodynamic loads which deviate from physiological limits. Finally, we shall analyze the properties of the hypertrophied myocardium.

Cytodifferentiation of cardiac myocytes

The first stage of development (Fig. 15-1) consists in the proliferation of overtly undifferentiated cells (**presumptive myoblasts** or **premyoblasts**) which eventually acquire cross-striation and start to contract (now they are referred to as **myocytes**). The presumptive myoblasts are derived from splanchnic (precardiac) mesoderm. At first they appear as rounded, mononucleated cells with pronounced mitotic activity. The structure of such early cells is by no means typical of a muscle, but rather resembles undifferentiated cells of any tissue.

The myofibrillar mass accumulates within the spindle-shaped developing myocytes which are gradually transformed into cylindrical, fully functioning adult myocytes. In the heart presumptive myoblasts at a certain stage of development initiate synthesis of contractile proteins but continue to divide by mitosis. This division of mature myocytes has been shown conclusively by electron micrographs. In sharp contrast, in skeletal muscle only presumptive

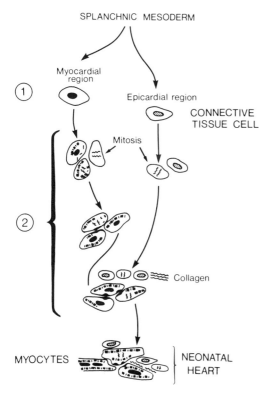

Fig. 15-1 Scheme of myocardial development. (1) Presumptive myoblasts (cells which do not exhibit the cardiac muscle cells phenotype); (2) developing myocytes (overtly differentiated muscle cells which contain various amounts of muscle-specific proteins). From Zak et al. (1979).

myoblasts proliferate. The various stages of myogenesis are governed by intrinsic, time-dependent factors because the circulatory system has not yet developed, and consequently hemodynamic forces are absent.

Cardiac morphogenesis

Heart formation in the chick (a convenient experimental model) begins with the inward movement of two folds of precardiac mesoderm. These two folds eventually come together, fuse and form the tubular heart rudiment. Next the tubular heart acquires morphological asymmetry through its bending and rotation to the right—a transformation referred to as **looping**. The process of looping coincides with first contractions (which in the chick occur at about 30 hours of

incubation). When contractions and the heart beat are blocked by placing the explanted embryos into a medium of a high concentration of potassium, the looping still progresses normally. On the other hand, looping depends on a critical mass of myofilament and can be prevented by inhibition of protein synthesis or of sarcomere assembly (Manasek et al., 1978).

During looping the heart consists of a pure population of developing myocytes. In the stages that follow a variety of non-muscle cells invade the myocardium which gradually becomes a heterogeneous cell population. (The non-muscle cells proliferate rapidly so that in the adult heart they outnumber muscle cells three to one.) With advancing cardiac development, the fraction of cell volume occupied by the mass of myofilaments increases up to a point where the cells lose their plasticity and cannot change their shape as they could during looping. The accumulating products of synthetic activities of non-muscle cells (such as collagen) further increase stiffness of the heart. As a consequence, the growth and morphological transformation are carried out mainly by increases in cell number (**hyperplasia**) or size (**hypertrophy**). At first, the increase in the number of cells by means of division is the principal feature of cardiac growth. As the development progresses, particularly during the late gestation period, the number of dividing cells rapidly decreases and the hypertrophy of existing myocytes becomes the mode of cardiac enlargement (Fig. 15-2). The accompanying changes in shape are a consequence of uneven growth rates in various regions of the heart. In addition, death of myocardial cells may also contribute to the morphological transformations.

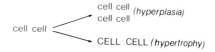

Fig. 15-2 Scheme of the cellular basis of growth. An organ can enlarge either by multiplication of cells without change in their volume (hyperplasia) or by increase in the volume of existing cells (hypertrophy).

Postnatal cardiac development

Myocytes in the myocardium continue to show substantial mitotic activity at birth. The trend of a decreasing rate of cellular division established in the embryonic period persists, so that only about 2 percent of rat myocytes are still dividing at birth. A similar trend is seen in cardiac non-muscle cells as well as in cells of any organ whose size approaches a limit in the adult organism, such as liver or kidney. Besides the decreasing rate of mitoses, the nature of mitotic events also appears to change after birth. Whereas in the embryonic period every nuclear division leads to two daughter cells, in the period following birth not every nuclear division is accompanied by cellular division. Thus, the population of cells containing more than one nucleus (see Fig. 15-3) increases during the neonatal period (Katzberg et al., 1977). Despite the low and declining proliferative activity, the number of cardiac myocytes in the heart doubles during the first 3–4 weeks of life. Thereafter, the normal growth of the heart is accomplished solely by the enlargement of existing cells. The diameter of myocytes increases from about 5 μm at birth to 12–17 μm in the adult heart (Table 15-1). Ventricular myocytes of various mammals appear to have the same diameter irrespective of animal size. The number of muscle cells thus varies directly with the size of the heart; a rat heart has 9×10^7 cells, while a blue whale has 2×10^{13} cells.

In contrast to the embryonic period, cell death is seen very rarely in the healthy heart and the myocytes therefore must have the same life span as the entire organism. The elements of connective tissue increase in mass by hyperplasia of their cells which remain mononucleated throughout their entire life.

Growth of the Heart under Altered Hemodynamic Load

The adjustment of cardiac mass to hemodynamic load is a fundamental characteristic of the heart. Any change in the hemodynamic function due either to physiological activity, or to pathological alterations in the cardiovascular system, eventually leads to changes in the heart : body weight ratio. The observed enlargement and reduction in heart size are commonly referred to as hypertrophy and atrophy respectively. In studies of congenital heart disease the term **hypoplasia** is used to indicate that the heart, or a part of the heart, is smaller than the control. These terms will be used not as they are by biologists to refer to the size and number of the heart's constituent cells, but to refer to the entire organ.

The common denominator of work-induced cardiac growth is the extent of energy utilization during actin–myosin interaction. The characteristics of the compensatory growth response vary widely depending on the experimental situation. Severity, duration and

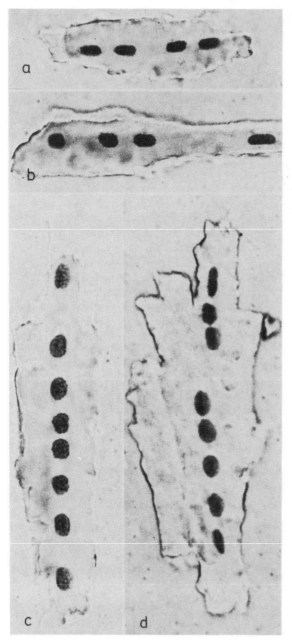

Fig. 15-3 Number of nuclei in isolated myocardial cells of pigs. Isolated cells stained with gallocyanine showing 4 (a,b) and 8 (c,d) diploid nuclei. From Grabner and Pfitzer (1974).

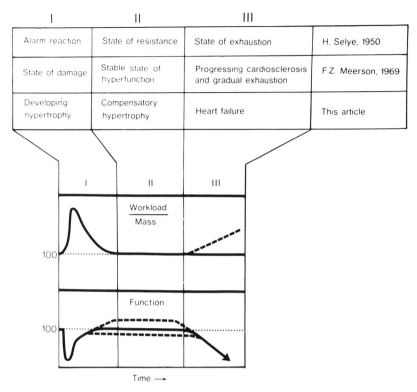

I	II	III	
Alarm reaction	State of resistance	State of exhaustion	H. Selye, 1950
State of damage	Stable state of hyperfunction	Progressing cardiosclerosis and gradual exhaustion	F.Z. Meerson, 1969
Developing hypertrophy	Compensatory hypertrophy	Heart failure	This article

Fig. 15-4 Phases of cardiac overload. In the bottom part of the diagram, 100 represents the normal control value. The dotted line gives the control reference value; the dashed line indicates that conflicting data have been reported in the literature (i.e. either no change, increase or decrease).

type of overload (pressure vs volume); the rate of overload application (acute aortic constriction vs slow onset of stenosis); the contractile state of the myocardium; the age and species of the animal, are all recognized as experimental variables. Meerson (1969) divided hypertrophy into three stages corresponding to Selye's phases of general stress syndrome: stage of damage (alarm reaction); stable state of hyperfunction (stage of resistance); and progressing cardiosclerosis and gradual exhaustion (stage of exhaustion). The major drawback of these generalized stages is the lack of unequivocal and measurable indices of growth response of the heart, such as the extent of damage, hyperfunction, resistance, or

Table 15-1

Contribution of muscle cell hypertrophy to cardiac enlargement

Species	Heart weight adult : newborn (approximate ratio)	Cell diameter (μm)		
		Newborn	Adult	Pathological hypertrophy
Man	16	6	14	20
Rat	35	5	12	23
Rabbit	35	7	17	23
Dog	40	7	15	—
Cattle	10	11 (calf)	15	—

From Zak (1974).

exhaustion. Therefore, we shall adhere to a terminology compatible with experimental description (Fig. 15-4).

Phase I: **Developing hypertrophy**, a period when the workload exceeds the normal work output of the mass of the heart.

Phase II: **Compensatory hypertrophy**, a period when the work-induced growth of the heart compensates for the increased workload : cardiac mass ratio set in Phase I. Depending on the experimental model, the contractile function per unit of cardiac mass might be unchanged, increased, or decreased.

Phase III: **Heart failure**, a period when the workload per unit cardiac mass increases again due to the progressively decreasing force-generation ability of the heart.

The duration of these three stages, as well as the progression from one to the next, depends on several variables, of which magnitude and type of overload are the most important. Generally, acute pressure-overload results in the earliest onset and the fastest rate of compensatory growth which is frequently accompanied by necrotic lesions within the cardiac tissue. Thus the comparison between various models of altered hemodynamic load should be attempted only after careful examination of experimental variables.

Cardiac Hypertrophy

A great variety of models have been used to study the effects of hemodynamic load on cardiac growth (Table 15-2). An investigator might choose from interventions which approximate valvular insufficiency, or from interventions which approximate stenosis. Each of these models can be further subdivided by the speed

of overload onset—whether acute or gradual. The degree of cardiac enlargement observed in animal models is generally smaller than that seen clinically. For example, a combination of both volume and pressure overload is required to double a rat's heart mass.

There are several complicating factors in experimental design. One is the change in body size which follows some experimental interventions, such as nutritional anemia, thyrotoxicosis, or carbon monoxide poisoning. Consequently, the absolute cardiac enlargement might not be detected, and one must rely on estimates of **heart : body-weight ratios**. The possible fallacy of this approach is demonstrated by development of cardiac "hypertrophy" during starvation when body weight decreases at a rate faster than that of the heart. A second complication is when rapid hemodynamic overload is accompanied by necrotic changes within the heart, with disintegration of myofibrils, proliferation of fibroblasts and accumulation of collagen. Those procedures which result in an acceptably minimal extent of necroses frequently also have such a slow rate of cardiac enlargement that it is difficult to observe a change in a given parameter. Thus the intervention has to be carefully chosen to best suit the question asked.

Cellular basis of cardiac enlargement

The evaluation of the mode of cardiac enlargement (hyperplasia vs hypertrophy) is a difficult task. Measurement of cell proliferation by DNA synthesis alone has several serious limitations, since the number of nuclei per cell might change and DNA replication or repair might occur without necessarily indicating

Table 15-2

Examples of experimental models of cardiac hypertrophy

Pressure overload	Volume overload	Overload due to multiple factors

Aortic stenosis
  Ascending or descending aorta,
  acute or gradual
Pulmonary stenosis
	Aortic insufficiency
	Arteriovenous fistula
	Sideropenic anemia
	Bradycardia
		Hyperthyroidism
		Hypoxia (simulated high altitude)
		
		Exercise
		Administration of isoproterenol
		Administration of norepinephrine

Hypertension
  Nephrectomy
  Implantation of DOCA pellet
  Spontaneous, congenital
		Cardiomyopathy

cell or nuclear division. Estimation of the total number of cells prior to and after cardiac enlargement is technically difficult.

Despite some uncertainty, it seems that compensatory cardiac enlargement depends largely on the ability of myocytes to synthesize DNA. In young rats where nuclear DNA synthesis still takes place (though at a very low rate), the heart enlargement produced both by volume (nutritional anemia) and by pressure overload (aortic constriction) is accompanied by activation of DNA synthesis. This activation is demonstrated by the incorporation of labeled precursors such as ^{3}H-thymidine into muscle nuclei and by the increase in the activity of DNA polymerase (Zak et al., 1979). The compensatory enlargement of hearts in young animals is a combination of hypertrophy and hyperplasia (Korecky and Rakusan, 1978). In contrast, similar stimuli applied to the adult animal (where DNA synthesis is already repressed), result in labeling of nuclei of connective cells only, and the growth of the heart is carried out by hypertrophy of myocytes (Zak, 1974). The capacity to synthesize DNA is not necessarily lost even in the adult. In some species, notably primates (including man), many myocytes may contain more than two sets of chromosomes (**polyploid nuclei**). Compensatory growth is accompanied by a marked shift to nuclei with a high degree of ploidy (Adler, 1976), which is

probably associated with amitotic cell division. The above data give support to Linzbach's (1952) original conclusion that cardiac enlargement above a certain critical size is supplemented by the addition of new cells which possibly originate from the splitting of polyploid nuclei. That stage is reached when the heart has about doubled its weight to reach 500 g and the left ventricular free wall height is about 250 g (Astorri et al., 1977). At about that weight, the cell diameter reaches a peak and then declines because of myocyte division. Cell length, on the other hand, keeps on increasing. Thus in extremely large hearts there is both hyperplasia and hypertrophy (Fig. 15-5).

Cellular organelles in the hypertrophic heart

Growth accompanied by co-ordinated accumulation of all cellular components might be expected to maintain cell organization and function similar to that of a normal state. The data available indicate that this is not so. Both quantitative electron microscopic description and biochemical analysis of enlarged hearts indicate a preferential increase of mitochondria during the earliest stages of developing hypertrophy. The volume of mitochondria relative to cell volume increases within the first day of pressure overload and progressively decreases later on. In contrast, the

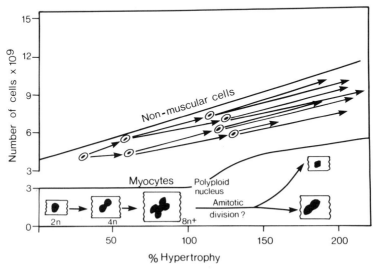

Fig. 15-5 Cell growth in cardiac overload in man. As hypertrophy occurs polypoid nuclei become more common and may undergo amitotic division. Evidence for an increasing number of myocytes in the human heart at a certain "critical" level is based on Astorri et al. (1977) and Linzbach (1952). Note that non-muscular cells undergo mitotic division over the whole range of growth. From Swynghedauw and Delcayre (1982) Pathobiol Ann 12: 137–183, with permission.

relationship between plasmalemma and cell volume, as well as between sarcotubular membrane area and myofibrillar volume, remain constant during left ventricular hypertrophy.

The preferential accumulation of mitochondrial components is only transient. During the subsequent phase of compensatory growth, myofibrils accumulate more rapidly. This sequence appears to be a characteristic response only to some forms of overload. When the heart enlarges due to volume overload or to gradually imposed pressure overload, the early relative increase in mitochondrial mass is not detected.

The early increase in mitochondrial volume in some models results from mitochondrial replication, since it is accompanied by synthesis of mitochondrial DNA (mtDNA; Rajamanickam et al., 1979). The relationship between the level of mtDNA and the rates of growth of the mitochondria is not a simple one. During the first 24 hours of aortic constriction, selected markers of inner mitochondrial membranes (cytochromes c, b and aa_3) all accumulate at the same rate but more slowly than mtDNA. During the later phases of developing hypertrophy the rate of mtDNA increment outstrips that of cytochromes. Thus the regulation of mitochondrial replication, transcription and translation is still poorly understood, just as in the whole cell.

Gene expression in the hemodynamically overloaded heart

An increase in the synthesis of RNA is perhaps the best documented and most striking change in the enlarging heart (Zak and Rabinowitz, 1979). The labeling of all classes of RNA increases several hours after imposition of a work overload. The rate of RNA transcription can be altered in two ways — by changing the activity of RNA polymerase, or by changing the amount of DNA template available for transcription. The early rise in transcription seems to be caused by activation of template while polymerase activity increases later (Cutilletta et al., 1978). However, rigorous demonstration of the preferential synthesis of mRNA in enlarging hearts has not yet been shown. Our present information only represents an initial description, necessary for future analysis of the relationship between hemodynamic events and translation of genetic information.

Cardiac Unloading

Unloading of the heart can occur in two situations: first, during chronically decreased hemodynamic activity, such as disease-associated bedrest; and secondly, following correction of hemodynamic overload, such as the closure of an arteriovenous fistula. The loss of cardiac mass which occurs in an otherwise healthy heart is usually referred to as atrophy, whereas the change which follows removal of hemodynamic overload is referred to as regression of cardiac hypertrophy. The division of the causes of cardiac unloading is useful because of the differences in their etiologies and clinical implications.

Atrophy

Atrophy can be viewed as the opposite of hypertrophy, as a decrease in the size of an organ and/or a loss of the number of constituent cells. Most of the descriptions of cardiac atrophy associated with decreased hemodynamic load concern clinical observations, such as cases of restrictive pericardial disease, chronic reduction in the mean arterial pressure, Addison's disease, or the decrease in the body mass due to starvation. In the case of ageing, cardiac atrophy is frequently suspected, although cardiomegaly in association with hypertension is more frequent. A common observation in the studies of cardiac atrophy is that the loss of mass is accompanied by a decrease in the diameter of muscle cells so that the number of muscle nuclei per cross-sectional area increases (Gottdiener et al., 1978).

In addition to mechanical unloading, other factors (such as hormone levels) also contribute to some of the situations mentioned above (starvation, Addison's disease).

Experimental studies in which the mechanical unloading can be induced without additional factors have been attempted only recently. In right ventricular papillary muscles, transection of their chordae tendineae was followed by a rapid decrease in cardiac mass, accompanied by a decrease in size of muscle cells, accumulation of collagen, partial disorientation of myofilaments and infiltration with fibroblasts and macrophages (Tomanek et al., 1981). The mechanical properties of these muscles also deteriorated, as demonstrated by the shifts in the force–velocity relationship and by decreased tension development. In contrast, oxygen consumption was unchanged.

Some aspects of cardiac atrophy appear to be not unlike a degenerative process.

Regression of cardiac hypertrophy

The return of the enlarged myocardium to the control heart weight : body weight ratio occurs in a variety of experimental models, such as removal of experimental aortic constriction, closure of arteriovenous shunt, re-establishment of normal blood pressure, or upon cessation of various pathological states (hyperthyroidism, excess catecholamines, high-altitude hypoxia). In contrast to unequivocal regression of experimental cardiac hypertrophy, results of corrective heart surgery are less conclusive. Repair of ventricular septal defects in children may achieve regression of left heart volume and mass (Jarmakani et al., 1971). Regression is not found in other studies (Behrendt and Austen, 1973), probably because of different characteristics of hypertrophic hearts prior to corrective surgery.

Contractile Activity as a Determinant of Cardiac Growth

The size of the heart is closely and effectively matched to changes in the hemodynamic requirements of an individual. Functional demands—ultimately reflected in the activity of myosin cross-bridges—must provide some kind of growth-regulating signal. Despite numerous hypotheses, however, the nature of the link between function and cardiac size remains as elusive as the factor(s) controlling the growth process. The following feed-back signals between the wall tension and growth of the heart have been proposed; none has been universally accepted.

ATP depletion theory

Increased rate of ATP utilization results in a temporary depletion of energy stores. This depletion is in turn thought to be sensed by a process which determines the mass of cellular components, including both synthetic as well as degradative pathways. Compensatory growth ensures energy, and the energy stores are eventually returned to normal values (Meerson and Pomoinitsky, 1972). The basic postulate of this theory of Meerson receives wide support from numerous investigators who have noted that many,

if not all, situations leading to cardiac enlargement are accompanied by increased oxygen consumption and ATP hydrolysis. Therefore, a finite drop in the energy potential of myocardial cells (i.e. the concentration ratio of ATP to ADP plus inorganic phosphate) must occur. The magnitude of this decrease and its temporal correlation to the growth activity, however, are disputed. It may rather be that a breakdown product of energy-utilization such as creatine provides the specific stimulus (Ingwall, 1976); creatine rises as creatine phosphate falls in acute heart work.

A specific problem with the energy depletion theory is that a "high" energy status is required for the activity of both the initiation and the elongation factors in protein synthesis (Chapter 3). In general, a "low" energy state would cause a fall in the ratio of guanosine triphosphate to diphosphate (GTP/GDP) which would decrease rates of protein synthesis. Besides numerous other inconsistent aspects, the energy depletion theory reveals nothing about the way the growth stimulus is affected.

Hypoxia as growth stimulus

There is a theory which postulates that increased ventricular wall stress results in myocardial hypoxia; a decreased partial oxygen tension in the tissue then derepresses biosynthetic activities. An increased oxygen tension can repress protein synthesis. For example, heart cells derived from chicken embryos incorporate progressively less radiolabeled precursors of protein and nucleic acid as the concentration of oxygen in the gas phase increases from 5 to 80 percent (Hollenberg, 1971). A second argument for the hypoxia theory is that the growth of the heart decreases after birth when the oxygen tension in arterial blood increases dramatically. Arguing against any simple effect of oxygen tension on biosynthesis is that the rate of tissue growth declines exponentially during both the late embryonic and postnatal period while the values of blood oxygen tension change in a stepwise fashion. Also, the growth rates of the two ventricles change disproportionately after birth.

Stretch theory

The enhanced preload and afterload of the overloaded myocardium results in the stretch of muscle cells; stretch induces compensatory growth. This theory has its origin in the classic observations of Feng et al. (1962) who demonstrated that stretching of skeletal muscle increased its oxygen consumption. Passive stretch may result in muscle growth. When the wing of a chicken is so fixed that the dorsal muscles are stretched, a substantial and rapid growth of those muscles results (Feng et al., 1962). Other examples of passive mechanical forces effecting growth include the stretching of skeletal muscle by the action of its antagonist, rhythmical stretching of a denervated hemidiaphragm by its functioning contralateral half and the extension of the uterus by the insertion of a rubber ball. Stretching skeletal muscle can influence the rates of protein degradation and synthesis (Etlinger et al., 1980). As far as the heart is concerned it must still be proved that chronic stretching of the ventricular wall mediates compensatory enlargement.

Humoral growth factors

There are several examples of humoral factors involved in the regulation of cardiac growth, the most dramatic being cardiac hypertrophy accompanying thyrotoxicosis. Although there is no doubt that large doses of thyroid hormone have profound effects on cardiac growth, it is also clear that the heart can undergo enlargement in the absence of any changes in the level of the hormone.

Cardiac enlargement can be induced by chronic infusion of norepinephrine in doses which do not lead to hypertension (Laks et al., 1976). Circulating levels of norepinephrine increase within 30 min after aortic constriction and the catecholamine content of the failing heart is dramatically reduced. Nonetheless, hypertrophy can occur even in pressure-loaded hearts in the presence of beta-adrenergic blockade (Zimmer and Gerlach, 1982).

Non-mechanical factors

Although unsupported by in-depth analysis, it has been frequently hinted that both hemodynamically overloaded as well as non-overloaded chambers of the heart undergo enlargement after experimental intervention. The adrenergic nervous system may be important, because in spontaneously hypertensive rats cardiac enlargement develops with time even when the hypertension has been adequately treated (Sen et al., 1976).

Growth control by cell degradation products

According to the theory that cell degradation products control growth, increased contractile activity of myocardial cells results in wear and tear of their components; the degradation products serve as activators of the growth process. This theory has so far received no direct support. The tissue damage that accompanies many forms of cardiac overload is related to the abrupt onset of hypertrophy, rather than to the growth process itself. When a more gradual onset of work overload is achieved cardiac enlargement takes place in the absence of any cellular damage.

Other signals to hypertrophy

Polyamines are derivatives of the amino acid, ornithine, which stimulate several enzymes involved in protein synthesis (Chapter 3). The content of polyamines in myocardial cells is elevated in many (practically all) models of hypertrophy. However, thyroxine treatment can cause hypertrophy even when an inhibitor of ornithine decarboxylase is present, so that tissue levels of polyamines stay normal (Pegg, 1981).

Cyclic nucleotides (cyclic AMP or cyclic GMP) rise in the heart tissue of some models; a causative role remains to be established.

Evaluation of hypotheses

Although the above hypotheses represent quite reasonable interpretations of an impressive volume of experimental data, none of them is fully compatible with all aspects of cardiac growth. This should not discourage future investigators interested in the fact that the heart is able to translate signals generated by hemodynamic activity—essentially a physical phenomenon—into language understood by its biochemical machinery.

Characteristics of the Hypertrophied Heart

The model chosen to show characteristics of the hypertrophied heart is important. When aortic constriction is induced in dogs an initial period of dilation of the left ventricle means that the wall stress (see Fig. 13-5) increases until a compensatory wall thickening develops to change the LaPlace relationship; eventually wall stress returns nearly to normal. The stage of compensatory hypertrophy (Meerson stage 2, Fig. 15-5) can be established in less than 3 weeks.

Hearts with stable hypertrophy have mechanical properties apparently similar to those of normal hearts. If so, it should be possible to detect a phase of cardiomegaly without heart failure in patients with chronic left ventricular overload. Such is the case in arterial hypertension, where mechanical function may actually be supranormal as judged by some indices such as the ejection fraction. There are superficial similarities to the "physiological hypertrophy" of the athlete's heart (Wikman-Coffelt et al., 1979). Theoretically these situations can be differentiated by studying the **myosin isoenzyme patterns** (see Chapter 8). In the pressure-overloaded rat heart abnormal patterns of myosin isoenzymes are associated with a decreased myosin ATPase activity and velocity of shortening, whereas in rats trained by swimming these parameters increase (Fig. 15-6). The decreased ATPase activity may be seen as a compensatory mechanism

because the decreased shortening velocity leads to less heat production and a more efficient contraction. In man, V_1 and V_3 myosin isoenzymes are also found, but shifts from V_1 to V_3 (Fig. 15-6) are not important in the adaptation to a pressure load (Mercadier et al., 1983).

While the hypertrophied left ventricle may have normal mechanical function, such a state might be achieved at the cost of "outgrowing" the blood supply. Estimations of the micro-anatomy of the hypertrophied cell show that the capillary surface area cell volume drops substantially during hypertrophy (Fig. 15-7). The distance between capillaries also increases until the slower growth of the capillary bed catches up (Tomanek et al., 1982); whether a completely normal situation is reached or not is a matter of dispute.

A useful hypothesis is that the hypertrophied heart has a normal myocardial blood flow, but not enough reserve in the coronary circulation to meet the added oxygen demands of tachycardia or an increased

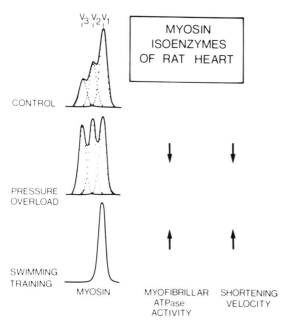

Fig. 15-6 Contrasting effects of pressure overload and swimming training on myosin isoenzyme patterns of rat heart. From Jacob et al. (1983). In: Advances in Myocardiology, Vol 4, Eds. E Chazov, V Saks, G Rona, p 70, Plenum, New York, with permission.

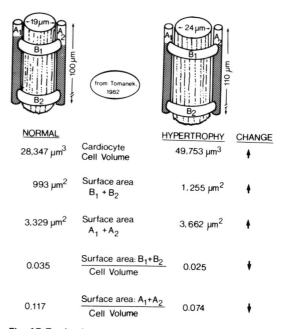

Fig. 15-7 As the myocyte enlarges by hypertrophy the capillary surface area falls in relation to the myocyte volume, unless there is an increase in capillary diameter and/or number of anastomoses. The result is threatened ischemia when the myocardial oxygen demand is much increased. For assumptions made in the calculation, see Tomanek et al. (1982). Reproduced with permission from the American Heart Association.

afterload (Bache et al., 1981). Such a situation may explain why patients with massively enlarged ventricles as a result of **hypertrophic cardiomyopathy** may develop angina pectoris and even myocardial infarction in the total absence of coronary artery disease.

Left ventricular stiffness

Whatever the stimulus to hypertrophy of myocardial cells, the same stimulus can stimulate the formation of collagen. Usually the rate of collagen formation "keeps up", yet sometimes it is too much and the myocardium becomes stiffer and less compliant, with impaired mechanical properties. The probable cause is increased **interstitial fibrosis**, which in turn reflects increased formation of collagen and related proteins. If linkage of the cross-bridges binding collagen and elastin fibers is prevented by a specific inhibitor (a lathyrogen) then hypertrophy develops without stiffness (Gaasch et al., 1982). At a cellular level, the increase of total cardiac DNA occurring during heart hypertrophy is almost entirely accounted for by proliferation of endothelial and interstitial cells, without true mitosis of cardiac myocytes. The increase of collagen can be monitored by an increase in hydroxyproline. When a pressure load is relieved left ventricular hydroxyproline and DNA levels remain unchanged (Cutiletta et al., 1975), presumably because the collagen is the result of true cellular hyperplasia and is situated in the interstitial fluid where it may be inaccessible to normal breakdown. This permanency of collagen can have severe consequences.

Summary

In the healthy heart the energy demands associated with acutely increased workload are adequately met by increased mitochondrial respiration. When the increased level of hemodynamic load is sustained either another slower response is activated or biosynthetic **pathways are de-repressed. The functional mass of muscle cells and their components increase. The** reserve capacity of the heart is maintained and the heart's ability to respond to acute overload is preserved.

Since the functional load of the heart is ultimately reflected in the rate of ATP hydrolysis during the cross-bridge cycle, it follows that the extent of energy consumption is coupled (in some yet unspecified way) to the genetic activities of the myocardial cell. Elucidation of this growth-regulating signal is an outstanding challenge.

In the compensated hypertrophied state the myocardium can have apparently normal mechanical function, as an increased wall thickness compensates for the increased wall stress caused by the increased afterload. Whether the capillary bed can grow sufficiently to keep a normal blood supply is an open question. One reasonable hypothesis is that the blood supply at rest is adequate, while subendocardial ischemia develops when a marked tachycardia or an increased afterload substantially increases the oxygen demand.

References

Adler CP (1976). DNA in growing hearts of children. Biochemical and cytophotometric investigations. Beitrage Pathol 158: 173–202.

Astorri E, Bolognesi B, Colla B, Chizzola, Visioli O (1977). Left ventricular hypertrophy: a cytometric study on 42 human hearts. J Molec Cell Cardiol 9: 763–775.

Bache RJ, Brobel TR, Arentzen CE, Ring WS (1981). Effect of maximal coronary vasodilation on transmural myocardial perfusion during tachycardia in dogs with left ventricular hypertrophy. Circ Res 49: 742–750.

Behrendt DM, Austen WG (1973). Current status of prosthetics for heart valve replacement. Prog Cardiovasc Dis 15: 369–401.

Cutilletta AF, Rudnik M, Zak R (1978). Muscle and non-muscle cell RNA polymerase activity during the development of myocardial hypertrophy. J Molec Cell Cardiol 10: 677–687.

Etlinger JD, Kameyama T, Toner K, van der Westhuyzen D, Matsumoto K (1980). Calcium and stretch-dependent regulation of protein turnover and myofibrillar diassembly in muscle. In: Plasticity of Muscle, Ed. D Pette, pp 541–557, Walter de Gruyter, Berlin.

Feng TP, Jung HW, Wu WY (1962). The contrasting trophic changes of the anterior and posterior latissimus dorsi of the chick following denervation. Acta Physiologica Sinica 25: 431–441.

Gaasch WH, Bing OHL, Mirsky I (1982). Chamber compliance and myocardial stiffness in left ventricular hypertrophy. Europ Heart J 3, Suppl A: 139–145.

Gottdiener JS, Gross HA, Henry WL, Borer JS, Ebert MH (1978). Effects of self-induced starvation on cardiac size and function in anorexia nervosa. Circulation 58: 425–433.

Grabner W, Pfitzer P (1974). Number of nuclei in isolated myocardial cells of pigs. Virch Arch (Abt. B) 25: 279–294.

Hollenberg M (1971). Effect of oxygen on growth of cultured myocardial cells. Circ Res 28: 148–157.

Ingwall, JS (1976). Creatine and control of muscle-specific protein synthesis in cardiac and skeletal muscle. Circ Res 38, Suppl 1:115–123.

Jarmakani JMM, Graham TP, Canent RV Jr, Capp MP (1971). The effect of corrective surgery on left heart volume and mass in children with ventricular septal defect. Am J Cardiol 27: 254–258.

Katzberg AA, Farmer BB, Harris RA (1977). The predominance of binucleation in isolated rat heart myocytes. Am J Anatomy 149: 489–499.

Korecky B, Rakusan K (1978). Normal and hypertrophic growth of the rat heart: changes in cell dimensions and number. Am J Physiol 234: H123–H128.

Laks NN, Morady F, Swan HJC (1976). Myocardial hypertrophy produced by chronic infusion of subhypertensive doses of norepinephrine in the dog. Chest 64: 75–78.

Linzbach AJ (1952). Die Anzahl der Herzmuskelkerne in normalen, überlasteten, atrophischen und mit Corhormon behandelten Herzkammern. Zeit Kreislaufforsch 41: 641–658.

Manasek FJ, Kulikowski R, Fitzpatrick L (1978). Cytodifferentiation: a causal antecedent of looping? Birth Defects 14: 161–178.

Meerson FZ (1969). The myocardium in hyperfunction, hypertrophy and heart failure. Circ Res 25, Suppl 2: 1–163.

Meerson FZ, Pomoinitsky VD (1972). The role of high-energy phosphate compounds in the development of cardiac hypertrophy. J Molec Cell Cardiol 4: 571–597.

Mercadier JJ, Bouveret P, Gorza L, Schiaffino S, Clark WA, Zak R, Swynghedauw B, Schwartz K (1983). Myosin isoenzymes in normal and hypertrophied human ventricular myocardium. Circ Res 53: 52–62.

Pegg AE (1981). Effect of alpha-difluoromethylornithine on cardiac polyamine content and hypertrophy. J Molec Cell Cardiol 13: 881–887.

Rajamanickam C, Merten S, Kwiatkowska-Patzer B, Chuang C, Zak R, Rabinowitz M (1979). Changes in mitochondrial DNA in cardiac hypertrophy in the rat. Circ Res 45: 505–515.

Sen S, Tartazi RC, Bumpus FM (1976). Biochemical changes associated with development and reversal of cardiac hypertrophy in spontaneously hypertensive rats. Cardiovasc Res 10: 254–261.

Tomanek RJ, Cooper G, Ehrhardt JC, Marcus MJ (1981). Chronic progressive pressure overload of the cat right ventricle. Circ Res 48: 488–497.

Tomanek RJ, Searls JC, Lachenbruch PA (1982). Quantitative changes in the capillary bed during developing, peak and stabilized cardiac hypertrophy in the spontaneously hypertensive rat. Circ Res 51: 295–304.

Wikman-Coffelt J, Parmley WW, Mason DT (1979). The cardiac hypertrophy process. Analyses of factors determining pathological vs physiological development. Circ Res 45: 697–707.

Zak R (1974). Development and proliferative capacity of cardiac muscle cells. Circ Res 35: 17–26.

Zak R, Rabinowitz M (1979). Molecular aspects of cardiac hypertrophy. Ann Rev Physiol 41: 539–552.

Zak R, Kizu A, Bugaisky L (1979). Cardiac hypertrophy: its characteristics as a growth process. Am J Cardiol 44: 941–946.

Zimmer HG, Gerlach E (1982). Some metabolic features of the development of experimentally-induced cardiac hypertrophy. Europ Heart J 3, Suppl A: 83–92.

New References

Anversa P, Beghi C, Levicky V, McDonald SL, Kikkawa Y, Olivetti G (1985). Effects of strenuous exercise on the quantitative morphology of left ventricular myocardium in the rat. J Molec Cell Cardiol 17: 587–595.

Kent RL, Uboh CE, Thompson EW, Gordon SS, Marino TA, Hoober JK, Cooper G (1985). Biochemical and structural correlates in unloaded and reloaded cat myocardium. J Molec Cell Cardiol 17: 153–165.

Simpson P (1985). Stimulation of hypertrophy of cultured neonatal rat heart cells through an alpha$_1$-adrenergic receptor and induction of beating through an alpha$_1$- and beta$_1$-adrenergic receptor interaction. Circ Res 56: 884–894.

Ten Eick RE, Bassett AL (1984). Cardiac hypertrophy and altered cellular electrical activity of the myocardium. In: Physiology and Pathophysiology of the Heart. Ed. N Sperelakis, pp 521–542, Nijhoff, Boston.

Wigle ED, Sasson Z, Henderson MA, Ruddy TD, Fulop J, Rakowski H, Williams WG (1985). Hypertrophic cardiomyopathy. The importance of the site and the extent of hypertrophy. A review. Prog Cardiovasc Dis 28: 1–83.

III | Pharmacology: Drug Action

Autonomic Nervous System. Beta- and Alpha-adrenoceptor Antagonism

The close links between the cardiac contraction cycle and the movements of calcium ions into and within the myocardial cell have already been emphasized. However, the heart does not function in isolation; rather, its activity must be closely co-ordinated with the demands of the body as a whole. That link is achieved by the activity of the autonomic nervous system (Fig. 16-1), so that the heart "knows" what the demands of the periphery are and can adapt accordingly. For example, the heart rate has to increase during exercise and decrease during rest. This chapter first outlines the neural control of the heart, which leads into a description of those pharmacological agents acting on the adrenergic receptors and neuro-transmitters to exert beneficial effects in specific types of heart disease such as angina pectoris, hypertension and arrhythmias.

Neurotransmitters

The overall effects of sympathetic stimulation closely resemble those of the adrenergic hormones. Of the many changes, tachycardia and an increased inotropic effect are among the best recognized. Hence the sympathetic system (Fig. 16-2) is frequently referred to as the **adrenergic system**. At a cellular level, many of the beta-effects can be explained by formation of cyclic AMP as second messenger whereas alpha-effects are

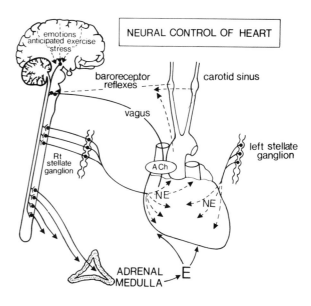

Fig. 16-1 Overall pattern of the neural control of the heart. Adrenergic stimulation is achieved by a combination of (i) neurotransmitter (NE = norepinephrine) release from the terminal nerve varicosities of postganglionic fibers running from left or right stellate ganglia; or (ii) epinephrine (E) release from the adrenal medulla. The parasympathetic system acts through the vagal nerve to release acetyl choline (ACh) which in general opposes the effects of sympathetic stimulation.

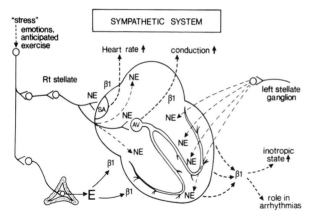

Fig. 16-2 Details of the effects of sympathetic stimulation, acting via (i) right stellate ganglion chiefly to increase release of norepinephrine (NE) to areas of sinus (SA) and atrioventricular (AV) nodes; (ii) left stellate ganglion to increase release of norepinephrine to left ventricle; and (iii) adrenal medulla to release epinephrine (E) to all parts of the heart.

still not well understood. In general, stimulation of the parasympathetic nervous system (Fig. 16-3) has effects resembling the effects of acetyl choline; hence the alternative name of **cholinergic system.**

Sympathetic–parasympathetic interaction

In view of the opposing adrenergic and cholinergic effects on heart rate and contractile state, the changes found during exercise could reflect either (i) increased sympathetic activity, (ii) decreased vagal activity, or both.

A **reflex bradycardia** can normally be expected during an acute elevation of arterial blood pressure (as occurs during exercise) as a result of stimulation of the baroreceptors and a parasympathetic efferent stimulus. This reflex bradycardia is almost totally abolished during exercise (Pickering et al., 1972). A blunting of the reflex bradycardia in response to a **blood pressure elevation** also occurs in heart failure; another situation where there is increased adrenergic activity. Hence ''considerable evidence exists that in states of heightened adrenergic tone, parasympathetic reflexes are attenuated'' (Higgins et al., 1973).

Cardiac Reflexes

It would be a serious over-simplification to regard the sympathetic–parasympathetic interaction as a simple ''push–pull'' system, with the idea that the opposing

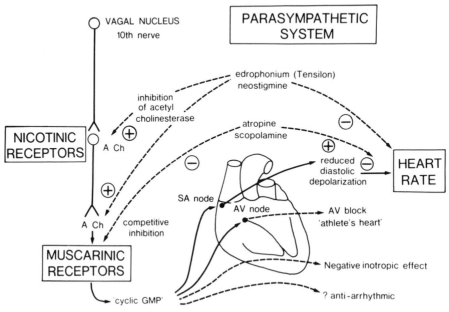

Fig. 16-3 The parasympathetic system, acting via nicotinic and muscarinic receptors may achieve its effects via prejunctional (= presynaptic) inhibition of release of norepinephrine and inhibition of formation of cyclic AMP. Activity of the parasympathetic system can be increased by agents inhibiting acetylcholinesterase, or decreased by agents competing with acetylcholine for the muscarinic receptor. Cyclic GMP is hypothetically the possible second messenger of acetylcholine.

effects always work together to achieve the aim of, for example, an increased heart rate. Rather, the efferent stimuli of the autonomic nervous system respond continuously to numerous afferent reflex stimuli. The best known of these reflexes arise in the baroreceptors of the aortic arch and the carotid sinuses. Every clinician is familiar with the bradycardiac effect of **carotid sinus massage**; the afferent stimuli travel to the vagal nucleus to stimulate the efferent limb so that there is increased vagal inhibition of sinus and atrioventricular nodes which can be induced to terminate a supraventricular tachycardia. It is also the baroreceptors which respond to peripheral vasodilation with a reflex tachycardia. Many other reflexes exist—Sleight (1975) lists 16 concerned with cardiovascular control. Our understanding of the cardiac reflexes is still in its infancy. The basic functions of these reflexes is to integrate the function of the heart with the physiological demands of the peripheral circulation and the rest of the body. Thus during exposure to cold, reflex vasoconstriction would unduly increase the blood pressure if not opposed by increased reflex vagal discharge. During sudden assumption of the erect posture, sympathetically mediated peripheral vasoconstriction is required to prevent postural hypotension; the effects of such sympathetic activation can be smoothed by vagal inhibition of the heart.

> It is not generally realized how effective is heart rate control in buffering sudden surges in blood pressure
> Sleight (1975)

At low levels of sympathetic activity, most of the control of the circulation is mediated by changes in the parasympathetic outflow; so sensitive is the mechanism that information gained in one beat can influence the next. At high levels of sympathetic activity most control is exerted by variations in the level of sympathetic discharge.

Sympathetic Response

During the sympathetic adrenergic response there are two main sources of catecholamines—first, release at the terminal varicosities of the adrenergic neurons, and secondly, the adrenal medulla. The adrenergic terminals release norepinephrine, synthesized in the varicosities via dopa and dopamine, and ultimately from tyrosine which is taken up from the circulation (Fig. 16-4). Norepinephrine is stored in the storage granules to be released upon stimulation by a nervous impulse. Thus, when central stimulation increases during excitement or exercise, then an increased number of impulses liberate an increased amount of norepinephrine from the terminals. Most of the released norepinephrine is taken up again by the nerve terminal varicosities to re-enter the storage vesicles or to be metabolized. At least some of the released norepinephrine interacts with specific receptors (beta or alpha) on the sarcolemmal membrane, and another fraction enters the circulation to account for the increased blood norepinephrine levels found during states of excitement or stress or exercise. Even in isolated hearts, norepinephrine can be made from tyrosine via dopa and dopamine using the following sequential enzymes:

tyrosine hydroxylase (which is rate-limiting) →
aromatic amino acid decarboxylase →
dopamine-beta-hydroxylase

Such synthesis takes place in the sympathetic nerve fibers, not the ordinary myocardial cells. Some norepinephrine is taken up from the circulation and may also be physiologically active.

Storage granules

Anatomically, the catecholamines are stored in granulated storage vesicles (= dense core vesicles = neurosecretory vesicles) of about 30–60 nm in size which are located in the varicosities of the preterminal peripheral adrenergic fibers. The varicosities are in close apposition to the receptor-containing effector sites in the sarcolemma. Norepinephrine is concentrated about 35 times in these vesicles as a stable complex with ATP. The chief factors controlling the activity of norepinephrine are the rates of release and re-uptake into the terminal varicosities and the rate of synthesis to keep pace with norepinephrine metabolized in the tissues. This picture is, however, oversimplified because it now seems that epinephrine can also be taken up into the terminal varicosities to be released with norepinephrine as a co-transmitter (Majewski et al., 1981).

Release of norepinephrine

Release of norepinephrine from the storage vesicles occurs with the arrival of the wave of depolarization

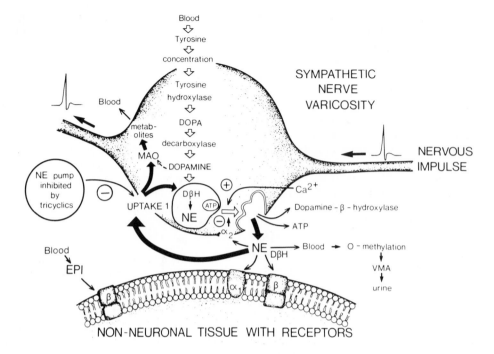

Fig. 16-4 Synthesis and release of norepinephrine from storage vesicles in the terminal sympathetic nerve varicosities (= terminal neurons). Norepinephrine is released by a calcium-mediated mechanism together with dopamine-beta-hydroxylase (DβH) and ATP. Most norepinephrine is taken back into the varicosity by uptake 1, which requires the activity of the norepinephrine pump. Some of the norepinephrine taken up by the pump is metabolized by monoamine oxidase (MAO); the rest re-enters the storage vesicle. Blood-borne epinephrine (EPI) is shown here stimulating a different population of beta-receptors from those stimulated by released neurotransmitter, according to the hypothesis of Baker and Potter (1980).

which liberates intracellular calcium, in turn to cause the vesicles to migrate to the neuronal plasma-lemma, there to liberate the enclosed norepinephrine. Pharmacologically, large scale release occurs after the administration of vasoactive amines such as tyramine and dopamine, by the stimulation of cardiac sympathetic nerves during markedly increased systolic pressures, and during chemical sympathectomy by reserpine. Anoxia followed by reoxygenation, or ischemia followed by reperfusion, are both procedures which release large amounts of norepinephrine. During sustained coronary occlusion there may be transient release of norepinephrine in the first 10 min. Because of the large amounts of catecholamines that potentially can be released from the heart it has even been proposed that the heart has the capacity to act as a neuroendocrine organ.

Re-uptake of norepinephrine

"Free" norepinephrine released from the vesicles into the junctional clefts has several possible fates (Fig. 16-4). First, the fate of most (perhaps 80 percent) of the released norepinephrine is "re-uptake" by **uptake 1** back into the sympathetic terminal neurons. This uptake 1 is energy-dependent and transports norepinephrine against a gradient which would explain the greater release of norepinephrine during anoxia. The process of uptake is inhibited competitively by the **tricyclic antidepressants.** Of that taken up, some goes back to the vesicles for re-storage but the remainder is inactivated by monoamine oxidase (intraneuronal inactivation). Small amounts of extraneuronal uptake (**uptake 2**) are physiological and include the interaction of norepinephrine with the alpha- and beta-adrenergic receptors of the effector cells. Thirdly, some norepinephrine is released into the blood stream and is eventually inactivated by *O*-methylation (COMT—catecholamine-*O*-methyl transferase activity) in various tissues including distal organs such as the liver. The combination of the activities of the catecholamine-*O*-methyl transferase and of monoamine oxidase activity in the liver converts the **circulating catecholamines to breakdown products such as metanephrines and vanillylmandelic acid.**

Neuromodulation

This relatively new concept provides for "smoothing" excess autonomic activity (Fig. 16-5). The site of action is at the level of the presynaptic receptors. For example, acetyl choline inhibits the release of norepinephrine from adrenergic terminal neurons. A second example is the facilitation of release of norepinephrine by epinephrine, acting on a presynaptic

beta-adrenergic receptor (Majewski et al., 1981). A third example is a negative feedback loop whereby released norepinephrine acts on a presynaptic site (alpha-2) to inhibit its own further release. Yet other presynaptic modulators are described which are especially important in controlling peripheral vascular resistance. Given a constant activity of the sympathetic neurons the amount of norepinephrine released can be either augmented or decreased by substances which bind on the neuronal membrane. The most important facilitatory modulator of adrenergic neurotransmission in vascular smooth muscle is the powerful vasoconstrictor, angiotensin II. Among the inhibitory modulators are acetyl choline, the products of cellular metabolism (such as adenosine, ATP, protons and potassium), histamine, 5-hydroxytryptamine and prostaglandins of the E series (Shepherd et al., 1978).

Thus the presynaptic terminal neuron is able to exert neuromodulation by multiple receptor sites which govern the rate of release of norepinephrine.

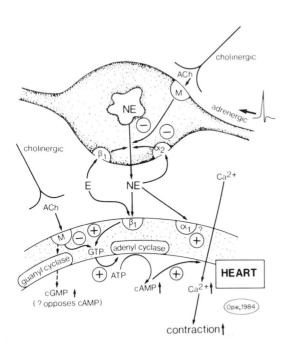

Fig. 16-5 Proposed role of neuromodulation in regulating release of norepinephrine (NE) from terminal varicosities in adrenergic neurons of the heart. Note the proposed effects of acetyl choline (ACh) in interacting with muscarinic (M) receptors to inhibit the cellular effects of norepinephrine (NE).

Drugs Acting on the Sympathetic Nervous System

Sympathomimetic drugs act on the cardiac beta-adrenergic receptors or the vascular alpha- or beta-adrenergic receptors (Table 16-1). The myocardial alpha-adrenergic receptors, being low in number, are not yet a specific site for drug action. The naturally occurring catecholamines have their expected beta-adrenergic agonist inotropic and chronotropic effect, with norepinephrine also vasoconstricting by stimulating vascular alpha-adrenergic receptors. Epinephrine dilates peripheral vessels by stimulating vascular beta-2-adrenergic receptors. If an intravenous positively inotropic agent is required to give acute support to the failing heart, the usual choice is one **of the new catecholamines, dopamine or dobutamine (Chapter 19).**

Sympatholytic agents (Table 16-1) decrease adrenergic activity and are especially used in the therapy of hypertension when specific reduction of the sympathetic outflow to the heart is required. The choice may fall on a beta-adrenergic antagonist (beta-blocker, see later in this chapter) which leaves the rest of the sympathetic system, including the alpha responses, unimpaired.

Table 16-1

Effects of agents acting on the sympathetic nervous system

Category	Examples	Comments
Increased sympathetic activity = sympathomimetic = adrenergic		
Combined α- and β-agonists	Norepinephrine (noradrenaline)	Peripheral α, cardiac β
	Epinephrine (adrenaline)	Dominant β ($\beta_1 > \beta_2$)
	Ephedrine	α and β
	NE-releasing agents	α and β
	Dopamine	α and β; dopaminergic
β-Agonists	Dobutamine, pirbuterol	$\beta_1 > \beta_2$
	Salbutamol, rimiterol	$\beta_2 > \beta_1$
	Metaproterenol (orciprenaline)	Dominant β_2
	Isoproterenol (isoprenaline)	Pure β ($\beta_1 + \beta_2$)
	Prenalterol	β_1
α-Agonists	Phenylephrine	α_1; slight high-dose β
	Methoxamine	α_1; slight high-dose β
Decreased sympathetic activity = sympatholytic = anti-adrenergic		
Central	Clonidine	**Central alpha$_2$-stimulation (see page 283)**
	Methyldopa	decreased peripheral α_1-tone; side-effect: drowsiness
Neuron-blocking agents	Guanethidine	Can cause some autonomic blockade with postural hypotension and impotence
Peripheral β-antagonist agents	Propranolol and others	Non-selective
	Atenolol, metoprolol and acebutolol	Selective ($\beta_1 > \beta_2$)
Peripheral α-antagonist agents	Prazosin	Inhibition of α_1 receptors
	Labetalol	Combined α- and β-antagonism
Catecholamine-depleting	Reserpine	Discharge of stored norepinephrine from terminal sympathetic nerve endings; marked central side-effects

α = alpha-adrenergic receptor; β = beta-adrenergic receptor; NE = norepinephrine.

Drugs Acting on the Parasympathetic Nervous System

The effect of the neurotransmitter acetyl choline can be enhanced by agents which either reduce the rate of its breakdown by inhibiting the cholinesterase, or by the parasympathomimetic **cholinergic** drugs which structurally resemble acetyl choline (Table 16-2). The end result is bradycardia and slowed atrioventricular conduction. Similar effects result when the vagal nucleus is reflexly stimulated by drugs causing acute hypertension or by digitalis. The **anti-cholinergic** agent atropine may be used in acute myocardial infarction to treat sinus bradycardia when it is severe enough to cause hypotension, or when there is significant atrioventricular conduction block of the Wenkebach type. Side-effects of the antiarrhythmic agents quinidine and disopyramide are to inhibit the interaction

of acetyl choline with the muscarinic receptors; such inhibition is much weaker than that caused by atropine (Table 16-3), yet frequently causes tachycardia or other side-effects.

An important proposal is that drugs stimulating the muscarinic receptor exert their effects chiefly by decreasing tissue cyclic AMP levels acting both at the level of neuromodulation and by an effect on adenylate cyclase (Fig. 16-5).

Drugs Acting on Neurotransmission

Reserpine

Altered rates of release or uptake of adrenergic neurotransmitters can explain the action of the antihypertensive drug reserpine, obtained from Rauwolfia root and originally used in India for its

Table 16-2

Effects of agents acting on the parasympathetic nervous system.

Category	Examples	Comments
Increased parasympathetic activity = cholinergic		
Cholinesterase inhibitors	Edrophonium	**Edrophonium short-acting, used in supraventricular tachycardias and myasthenia gravis**
	Prostigmine	
	Neostigmine	
Parasympathomimetic drugs (resembling acetyl choline)	Carbachol	**Previously used to provoke coronary spasm**
	Methacholine	
Indirect vagal stimulation	Digitalis	Added direct inotropic effect by inhibition of $Na^+-K^+-ATPase$
Reflex vagal stimulation	α-Agonists such as phenylephrine, methoxamine	Acute hypertension causes reflex bradycardia
	Carotid sinus pressure	Reflex bradycardia by direct stimulation of baroreceptors
Decreased parasympathetic activity = anticholinergic		
Inhibition of acetyl choline	Atropine	Competitive inhibition of acetyl choline; some low dose agonist effects. Used for sinus bradycardia or heart block
	Quinidine	Antiarrhythmics with anticholinergic side-effects
	Disopyramide	
	Methylscopolamine (= hyoscine methylbromine)	Similar to atropine but fewer agonist and fewer central effects
	Belladonna	The original "beautiful, big-eyed lady effect" due to atropine content

Table 16-3

Muscarinic receptor. Anticholinergic side-effects of group 1A antiarrhythmic compounds (see page 326)

	Inhibitor constant (K_i) for binding to muscarinic receptor
Atropine	1.2×10^{-9} M
Disopyramide	8.5×10^{-7} M
Quinidine	2.8×10^{-6} M
Procainamide	5.6×10^{-5} M

The K_i is derived from the ability to displace labeled quinuclidinyl benzilate from muscarinic binding sites. Data from Mirro et al. (1980). Circ Res 47: 855.

tranquillizing effects. Reserpine acts to prevent uptake of norepinephrine into the storage vesicle, so that progressive depletion of the stores occurs. Such reserpine-treated hearts lose about 85 percent of the myocardial stores of norepinephrine so that reserpine has vasodilatory properties. Depletion of norepinephrine stores can be found within one hour of intravenous administration and takes about 24 hours to develop fully; a prolonged period is required for recovery when the drug is stopped. The high clinical doses previously used caused excess depletion of cerebral catecholamines with severe depression sometimes leading to suicide. When given in appropriate low doses, reserpine has fewer central effects than does methyldopa (Gibb et al., 1970).

Indirect sympathomimetics

Stimulation of the release of norepinephrine results from drugs which displace the stored norepinephrine from the storage vesicles: tyramine, mephentermine, ephedrine and amphetamine. These agents are amines but lack the full catechol nucleus. Ephedrine has been used for bronchial asthma acting via the beta-effect of released adrenergic neurotransmitter. Amphetamine has as its chief site of action the central nervous system; it acts as an appetite suppressant which because of its stimulatory effects can be habit-forming. Sympathomimetic cardiac side-effects are frequent.

Psychotropic agents

Although psychotropic agents have their major effects on the central nervous system, prominent cardiovascular effects can be found. The **tricyclic antidepressants** block the re-uptake of norepinephrine through competitive binding, thereby raising the levels of circulating catecholamines and exerting their antidepressant effect. Anticholinergic side-effects also contribute to the tachycardia. **Phenothiazines** such as chlorpromazine also block the re-uptake mechanisms; in addition chlorpromazine has a marked peripheral alpha-blocking effect so large doses can cause severe hypotension. **Monoaminase oxidase inhibitors increase available neurotransmitter by inhibiting the** metabolism by the monoamine oxidase system both within the varicosities and in the liver. When such agents are being used, any catecholamine-like agents given, whether for cardiovascular or pulmonary therapy, may have excessive effects—the normal "dampening" uptake of circulating catecholamines into the terminal varicosities being hindered.

False transmitters

The pump which takes up released norepinephrine back into the terminal varicosity is not very selective in its effects. Thus drugs such as **guanethidine** and others (bethanidine, debrisoquine) are taken up into the storage vesicles. Once enough has accumulated, the storage vesicle no longer responds to stimulation by depolarization and hypotension results. Thus these agents have acted as false transmitters. The antihypertensive agent **methyldopa** is known to have its chief site of action in the central nervous system, acting like clonidine by stimulating central alpha-receptors which in turn inhibit outflow along the sympathetic nervous system. It also is incorporated into the terminal varicosities, and enters the synthetic pathways to form alpha-methyl norepinephrine which is then stored in the vesicles. Later, when released, this compound can act as a mildly effective competitor with norepinephrine for vascular alpha-receptors.

Drugs Acting on Cardiovascular Adrenergic Receptors

The two chief categories of agents are the beta-adrenergic receptor antagonist and alpha-adrenergic receptor antagonist. The chief physiological role of the beta-adrenergic receptors is on the heart, increasing heart rate, conduction and contractility; hence the antagonists have chiefly a cardiac effect. The chief physiological role of alpha-adrenergic receptors is in causing vascular contraction, hence the antagonists have mainly a vasodilator effect (Chapter 17). Although it is scientifically inexact to use the terms "beta-blockade" or "alpha-blockade" these abbreviations are now so imbedded in clinical terminology that they will sometimes be used here.

In differentiating the receptor subtypes the important differences are in the rank-orders of responses to a variety of agonist and antagonist agents which allow a descriptive differentiation of the two beta- and three alpha-adrenergic receptor subtypes (Table 16-4).

Beta-adrenergic Receptor Antagonists ("Beta-blockers")

Beta-adrenergic antagonists are defined as agents with the common property of competitive inhibition of the effects of isoproterenol on the heart (Fig. 16-6); isoproterenol is taken as that catecholamine with exclusively beta-adrenergic properties. Common properties to all beta-adrenergic antagonists are

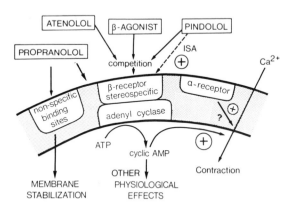

Fig. 16-6 Propranolol, the "gold-standard" beta-adrenergic blocker, competes with beta-agonists for the stereospecific beta-adrenergic receptor site. Propranolol also has non-specific binding sites which may be concerned with "membrane stabilization". Atenolol is an example of a cardioselective beta-adrenergic blocker, while the non-selective agent pindolol also partially stimulates the receptor besides its blocking effect (ISA = intrinsic sympathomimetic activity). Modified from Opie (1983). Am J Cardiol, 52: 2D–9D, with permission.

Table 16-4

Cardiovascular adrenoceptor subtypes; agonists, antagonists and putative messengers

Receptor	Site	Agonist	Antagonist	Putative messenger
β_1	Myocardial and nodal	Iso > E > NE	Atenolol, Metoprolol	Cyclic AMP (Ca^{2+})
β_2	Vascular	Iso > E > NE	Propranolol and other non-selective agents	Cyclic AMP (Ca^{2+})
α_1	**Vascular (Postsynaptic)**	NE > E > Iso[1] Methoxamine[2] Phenylephrine Midodrine[4]	Prazosin Nicergoline[3] Labetalol WB-4101[5]	Ca^{2+} (indirect effect)
α_2	Presynaptic	NE > E > Iso Clonidine Circazoline Xylazine[1]	Yohimbine Rauwolscine[1]	Unknown; possibly Ca^{2+}
α_2	**Vascular (Postsynaptic)**	NE > E > Iso B-HT 920[2,6] α_2-presynaptic agents	Ca^{2+}-antagonists[2,6] (non-specific effect) α_2-presynaptic agents	Ca^{2+}

α = alpha-adrenergic receptor; β = beta-adrenergic receptor; NE = norepinephrine = noradrenaline; E = epinephrine = adrenaline; Iso = isoproterenol = isoprenaline; WB-4101 = 2-(2′6′-dimethyl-phenoxyethalamino)-methylbenzodioxane; B-HT 920 = 2-amino-6-allyl-tetrahydro-thiazolo-azepin.

[1]McGrath JC (1981). In: Vasodilatation. Ed. Vanhoutte and Leusen, p 97, Raven Press, New York.
[2]Kobinger W and Pichler L (1980). Europ J Pharmacol 65: 393.
[3]Huchet A et al. (1981). J Cardiovasc Pharmacol 3: 677.
[4]Pittner H et al. (1976). Arzeim-Forsch 26: 2145.
[5]U'Prichard DC and Snyder SH (1979). Life Sci 24: 79.
[6]Van Meel JCA et al. (1981). Europ J Pharmacol 69: 205.

slowing of the heart rate and a negative inotropic effect. Their antihypertensive effect is another shared property. The properties distinguishing the various beta-blockers (Fig. 16-7) from each other include: (i) cardioselectivity; (ii) intrinsic sympathomimetic activity; (iii) membrane stabilizing activity; and (iv) pharmacokinetic properties including variable formation of active metabolites. In addition: (v) some beta-adrenergic antagonists have added vasodilator properties; (vi) claims have been made for different effects on renal blood flow; (vii) anti-renin effects could differ; and (viii) antiplatelet effects are found with propranolol.

Cardioselectivity

Non-selective beta-blockers, of which propranolol is the prototype, will antagonize both cardiac beta-1-receptors and the non-cardiac beta-2-receptors. In contrast, cardioselective agents bind about 100 times more avidly to beta-1- than to beta-2-receptors (Fig. 16-8). Cardioselectivity is lost at high concentrations. Thus

bronchospasm is more likely to develop with non-selective blockers (Fig. 16-9). Less well-established are differences on vascular tissue. Unopposed peripheral alpha-activity should be more marked with non-selective agents which may cause vasospasm, a fall in

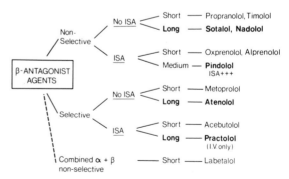

Fig. 16-7 Classification of some beta-adrenergic blocking agents (heavy type = long-acting agents; ISA = intrinsic sympathomimetic activity; IV = intravenous; α = alpha-adrenergic blocking activity). Reproduced with permission from Opie (1980). Drugs and the Heart, p 1, The Lancet, London.

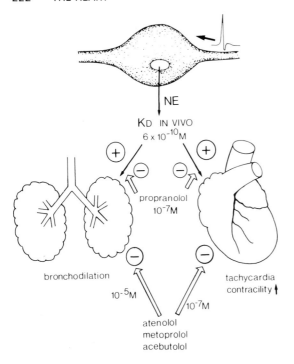

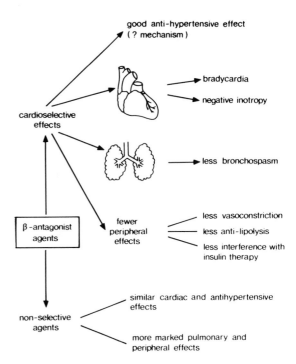

Fig. 16-8 Role of antagonism of beta-1- and beta-2-adrenergic receptors in explaining cardioselectivity. Note that cardioselective agents (atenolol, metoprolol and acebutolol) can have an action on the bronchial beta-2-receptors but at much higher concentrations. NE = norepinephrine released from the terminal varicosities (see Fig. 16-4); K_D = apparent dissociation constant (see Fig. 6-3).

Fig. 16-9 Beta-blockers may be either cardioselective or non-cardioselective. Reproduced with permission from Opie (1980). Drugs and the Heart, p 1, The Lancet, London.

skin blood flow and Raynaud's phenomenon (McSorley and Warren, 1978). Through this mechanism the non-selective agents may actually temporarily exaggerate hypertension when given intravenously, because of an increased alpha-mediated arterial spasm. This danger is especially marked in pheochromocytoma when there are already excess circulating catecholamines with both alpha- and beta-agonist properties. Theoretically, propranolol is more likely to precipitate coronary vasospasm and vasospastic angina than are the cardioselective agents.

There are **metabolic differences** between cardioselective and non-selective agents. The metabolic response to the hypoglycemia induced by insulin is dependent on beta-2-stimulation in response to an outpouring of circulating catecholamines, which in turn cause glycogen breakdown in the liver and reverse the hypoglycemia. This whole sequence of events is dampened by propranolol when compared with atenolol or metoprolol (Lager et al., 1979) and the hypoglycemia persists for longer (Deacon et al., 1977). Recently McLeod et al. (1983) have shown that receptors mediating lipolysis are beta-1 in nature. Therefore cardioselective agents will inhibit lipolysis, with possible benefit in ischemia (Chapter 12), while leaving hepatic carbohydrate metabolism unimpaired.

Whether **plasma lipids** are differentially altered by selective and non-selective agents is not clear. In patients with peripheral vascular disease, there was a greater rise in plasma triglyceride caused by propranolol than by atenolol (Day et al., 1979); such effects on plasma lipids are poorly understood and variable (Berchtold and Berger, 1980). In contrast, the alpha-adrenergic blocker prazosin is thought to have no such effects on plasma lipids.

Cardioselective vs non-selective agents

Not all cardioselective agents are equally selective. Thus using the degree of exercise-induced bronchospasm as a criterion, atenolol was slightly more cardio-selective than metoprolol and both were more selective than acebutolol (Decalmer et al., 1978). In the case of both angina of effort and hypertension, cardio-selective blockers are as effective therapeutic agents as are the non-selective agents (e.g. atenolol vs propranolol; metoprolol vs propranolol). Are there any arguments left for the use of non-selective blockers such as propranolol and others?

First, propranolol has generally been used for longer than any other agent and thus clinical experience is much wider. In certain conditions (for example, in hypertrophic obstructive cardiomyopathy) there is now very considerable clinical experience with propranolol but there has not been the same experience with other agents. Secondly, the vasoconstrictive effect on the

vascular system may be of specific benefit in the case of migraine where propranolol has documented benefit. Other non-cardiac conditions in which propranolol has been well-evaluated include anxiety states, thyrotoxicosis and tremor. Cardioselective agents in general also seem to work in these situations but their use is less well-documented. Thirdly, propranolol is better than the selective agents in suppressing renin levels (Harms et al., 1978) which could be important in the high-renin hypertension of renal disease. Finally, propranolol has been used for so long that all its side-effects are well-understood.

The modern trend is to use the cardioselective beta-antagonists more and more, especially for angina pectoris and hypertension; cardioselective agents are used preferentially in patients with bronchospasm or

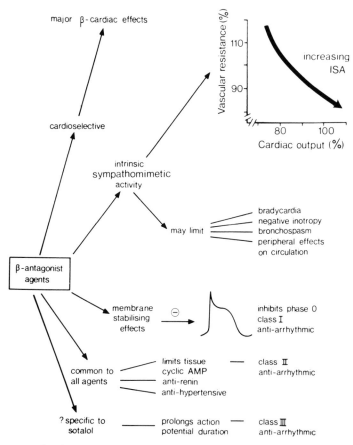

Fig. 16-10 In addition to cardioselectivity other properties of individual beta-blockers include intrinsic sympathomimetic activity (ISA) and membrane stabilization. While ISA may have useful properties it can also cause cramps as a side-effect. Membrane stabilization may not be a clinically relevant property. Reproduced from Opie et al. (1984). In: Drugs for the Heart, Ed. Opie, p 16. American Edition, Grune & Stratton, Orlando, New York and London.

diabetes mellitus requiring insulin. The case in peripheral vascular disease is less clear. Nevertheless, no beta-antagonist, not even a cardioselective one, may be given to patients with asthma or a history of asthma unless under careful hospital supervision.

Intrinsic sympathomimetic activity

Intrinsic sympathomimetic activity (= ISA = **partial agonist activity**) is that property whereby a positive inotropic or chronotropic effect can be found in catecholamine-depleted preparations (Nayler, 1972); the explanation is that the molecular structure of the beta-antagonist partially resembles that of the beta-agonist (there must be at least similarity of a small part of the molecule to allow the "fit" of the beta-antagonist into the beta-receptor). Possession of ISA (Fig. 16-10) may theoretically diminish the degree of cardiac depression caused by beta-blockade. By stimulation of beta-2-receptors, ISA may also reduce the degree of bronchospasm or peripheral vaso-constriction found in some patients as a side-effect of beta-blockade; however, the therapeutic response to added beta-2-stimulation by the bronchodilator salbutamol is correspondingly low. ISA may stimulate the sympathetic tone when it is low, as at night, while depressing the tone when it is increased, as during exercise, thereby minimizing the natural swings in sympathetic tone. In practice, the various beta-blocking agents are equally effective against angina of effort because the exercise rate is similarly reduced (Thadani et al., 1979).

Membrane-stabilizing activity (MSA)

This property is of importance in animal preparations when, in high concentrations, certain beta-blockers have a quinidine-like, membrane-stabilizing effect. The competition between beta-adrenergic drugs and beta-antagonist drugs for the binding sites on the cell membrane is typical of beta-responses and involves a stereospecific phenomenon. In the case of propranolol, binding to heart tissue involves not only stereospecific sites but also a large number of non-specific sites, the latter presumably reflecting "membrane-stabilizing activity". It is usually held that membrane-stabilizing activity is of no clinical significance even in the therapy of arrhythmias, yet the ischemic myocardium is considerably more

sensitive to membrane-stabilizing activity than is the non-ischemic myocardium (Vaughan Williams, 1978). Membrane-stabilizing activity may also explain why 3-methyl propranolol, with no beta-antagonist effects, is nearly as effective as propranolol itself in hindering the development of experimental acute myocardial infarction (Ku and Lucchesi, 1978; Gross et al., 1978).

Myocardial depression

Beta-blockers may be required in the therapy of ischemic conditions except when myocardial function is already depressed or when there is the risk of heart failure being precipitated by beta-blockade. Much effort has therefore been spent to determine the relative cardiodepressant effects of various beta-blockers. Basically, by inhibiting the formation of cyclic AMP, all beta-blockers must have a negative inotropic effect which is part of their therapeutic effect in angina of effort. The real question is whether the possession of ancillary qualities other than beta-receptor antagonism can modify the degree of cardiodepression that results.

First, the degree of intrinsic sympathomimetic activity should logically alter the degree of cardio-depression. In reality, the differences are not striking unless there is sufficient ISA to allow the agent to act as a positively inotropic agent (Chapter 19). Secondly, a popular theory is that beta-blockers with membrane-stabilizing activity (such as propranolol) are more likely to cause cardiodepression than other beta-blockers. At first sight, membrane-stabilization and depression of hemodynamic activity are expressions of completely different pharmacological properties. There is, however, a link in that high concentrations of propranolol (3×10^{-5} M) cause inhibition of the fast sodium channel (Tarr et al., 1973) which in turn could be cardiodepressant by a secondary failure to "open" the calcium gate normally. The concentrations of propranolol inhibiting the sodium channel are, however, considerably above those normally found. With top doses of propranolol of up to 1000 mg daily, as used in some resistant arrhythmias (Woosley et al., 1979), the plasma concentration is likely to be about 1000 ng/mL or nearly 10^{-5} M (Walle et al., 1978) which should depress fast channel activity. In doses used for angina pectoris propranolol is no more cardiodepressant than therapeutically equivalent doses of nadolol (Turner et al., 1978) or timolol. A third possibility is that some beta-blockers such as propranolol have a non-specific calcium-antagonist effect (Grun et al., 1972). As this quality is elicited only at very high concentrations of propranolol (above 10^{-5} M) and is not shared by oxprenolol or pindolol, a non-specific membrane effect may well be involved.

Stereospecificity

Beta-blocking effects are associated with a stereo-specific membrane receptor; membrane-stabilizing effects do not have stereospecificity. If membrane-stabilization is linked to cardiodepression at high doses then two ways to minimize the depression of myocardial function would be: (i) to develop agents without membrane-stabilization; and (ii) to develop agents with only ($-$) specificity. The latter approach has been used in the design of ($-$) penbutolol, an agent otherwise similar to propranolol. Whether or not these properties matter at clinically relevant concentrations of beta-blockers must still be proven.

Lipophilicity

Lipophilicity is determined from the comparative distribution in octanol and water with a high partition coefficient indicating lipophilicity and a low coefficient hydrophilicity (Cruickshank, 1980). Propranolol is the prototype of lipophilic beta-blockers; because of its high lipid-solubility it readily penetrates the brain, hence explaining the unpleasant dreams which may occur, and it is also metabolized by the liver. The prototype of hydrophilic beta-blockers is atenolol, which does not penetrate the central nervous system (neither into brain nor cerebrospinal fluid in any amounts), nor is it metabolized by the liver. Excretion of the unchanged compound is by the kidney. Nadolol and sotalol have similar hydrophilic properties.

Vasodilating properties of some beta-antagonists

The natural tendency of beta-blockers is to cause peripheral vasoconstriction, which is especially marked in the case of the non-selective agents such as propranolol, but is found even with selective agents. Vasoconstriction might theoretically oppose the hypotensive effects of beta-antagonists. To overcome this potential disadvantage beta-blockade can be combined with ISA, yet there is no evidence that the agent pindolol containing high amounts of ISA is more effective as an antihypertensive agent than other beta-blockers. Another approach is to combine beta-blockade with alpha-blockade as in labetolol; this agent gives a more acute hypotensive effect than does a conventional beta-blocker, but during chronic therapy high doses may be required to exert the alpha-blocking effect. Some new molecules like bucindolol have a hydralazine-like component built in.

Labetalol is a combined alpha- and beta-adrenergic receptor antagonist already available in most countries (also in the U.S.A.). Its alpha-antagonist effect is theoretically much less potent than its beta-effect (Greenslade et al., 1979). In reality the alpha-effect is sufficiently powerful that an intravenous injection causes the blood pressure to fall within minutes, in marked contrast to the effects of propranolol or atenolol (see Fig. 20-5).

Renal blood flow

Generally beta-blockers decrease renal blood flow because they decrease the cardiac output. Several agents may, it is claimed, "protect" renal function during therapy of hypertension. Atenolol, nadolol, pindolol and penbutolol might all have this apparent advantage, as might other as yet untested beta-blockers. There is no evidence that any of these agents actually improve renal impairment in the therapy of hypertension. Even in the case of propranolol there is a distinction between renal blood flow, which falls, and renal function measured by creatinine clearance, which does not fall (Bauer and Brooks, 1979).

Effects on renin

Renin, liberated especially from the ischemic kidney, promotes the formation of the vasoconstrictor angiotensin. The non-selective beta-blockers have a greater effect in depressing resting renin levels (Amery et al., 1977) and in antagonizing the isoproterenol-induced increases in plasma renin activity (Harms et al., 1978) than the non-selective agents. It is no longer held that the antihypertensive effect of beta-blockers bears a direct relation to the anti-renin effect.

Effects on platelets

Platelets are thought to contribute to myocardial ischemia in several ways. Platelet aggregates may (i) promote the formation of damage to arterial walls as in atherosclerosis; and (ii) help ischemia to extend. It might be thought that, by inhibiting formation of platelet cyclic AMP, propranolol should promote platelet aggregation. In reality, therapeutic doses inhibit platelet aggregation (Frishman et al., 1974) with an effect additive to that of aspirin (Keber et al., 1979). Presumably it acts by membrane-stabilization.

Therapeutic Spectrum of Beta-adrenergic Antagonists

Hypertension

Beta-antagonists have both direct cardiac effects (negative inotropic and chronotropic effects) and indirect cardiac effects, exerted by effects on the blood pressure and the peripheral circulation. If beta-antagonists tend to cause vasoconstriction, why do they decrease the arterial pressure when given chronically? The answer to this vexed question is still not clear. The antihypertensive effects of beta-antagonists were first discovered accidentally in patients treated for angina pectoris. Multiple mechanisms are thought to be involved: the cardiac output falls as a result of the negative inotropic and chronic effects; hence the blood pressure can fall despite the increased peripheral resistance. Decreased circulating renin activity plays an important role according to Laragh. The central effect, as emphasized by some workers, is difficult to accept because of the poor penetration of atenolol into the central nervous system despite its antihypertensive efficacy. A very new theory is that a presynaptic beta-receptor plays a role in the release of norepinephrine. Whereas only some beta-antagonists cause hypotension when given acutely and intravenously, all beta-antagonists are effective antihypertensive agents when given chronically.

Antiarrhythmic effect of beta-antagonists

Beta-antagonists should be especially effective in those arrhythmias in the genesis of which cyclic AMP is thought to play an important role, such as ventricular tachycardia and fibrillation in the very early phases of acute myocardial infarction. Intravenous beta-blockade is now being evaluated in such patients and an effect in preventing ventricular fibrillation has been found. Beta-antagonists are also effective in those arrhythmias caused by increased circulating catecholamines (pheochromocytoma, anxiety, exercise) or by thyrotoxicosis. The effect in mitral valve prolapse may be explained in part by the increased blood catecholamine concentrations in that condition. The inhibitory effects on the sinus node make beta-antagonists the ideal therapy for the sinus tachycardia of anxiety states. A similar inhibitory effect on the atrioventricular node leads to the use of beta-antagonists for paroxysmal supraventricular tachycardias. An interesting effect of sotalol is to increase the action potential duration (class 3 activity) thereby theoretically exerting an additional antiarrhythmic effect by prolonging the effective refractory period (Fig. 16-10).

Beta-blockade for angina pectoris

The effects of beta-antagonists in **angina of effort** are best viewed in relation to the factors influencing the oxygen balance of the ischemic myocardium. Beta-antagonists will beneficially influence most of the factors influencing the oxygen demand of the heart, and especially the double product (heart rate × blood pressure) during exercise, as well as decreasing the contractility. There may also be an improved oxygen supply by an improved diastolic coronary perfusion, as a result of the prolonged diastolic period. On the other hand, when beta-antagonists cause clinical heart failure the preload will increase and the oxygen demand will rise; heart failure will therefore need vigorous treatment for beta-antagonists to be effective.

Coronary spasm can either occur in the absence of coronary artery disease or be imposed on pre-existing atherosclerosis. When the condition is extreme and results in severe transmural ischemia, it is called Prinzmetal's variant angina. Lesser degrees of coronary spasm may also contribute to the ischemia in angina at rest. Beta-antagonism is either ineffective or possibly harmful in the therapy of conditions caused by coronary spasm, because the unopposed alpha-activity of catecholamines can now cause coronary vasoconstriction (see Fig. 18-3).

Exertional coronary artery spasm is a newly described entity in which the sympathetic response to exercise precipitates spasm. As expected, beta-antagonism is either ineffective or only partially effective; the calcium inhibitors are the agents of choice.

Potential use in acute myocardial infarction

The use of beta-blockers in this context is still controversial. When carefully given intravenously to patients with acute myocardial infarction, the benefits include reduced chest pain, decreased heart failure and less ventricular arrhythmias. Current evidence suggests that intravenous beta-blockers given within 4–6 hours of the onset of symptoms may reduce infarct size in patients. When given later they may still be antiarrhythmic but without reducing infarct size.

Rebound effects on the ischemic heart

Withdrawal rebound is the development of new symptoms of angina or even infarction following abrupt withdrawal of beta-blockade. Possibly the danger has been exaggerated, especially in hospitalized patients in whom abrupt discontinuation is safe (Shiroff et al., 1978). Clinical prudence still requires that patients given beta-blockade therapy should be warned against the risk of abrupt discontinuation. The mechanism of the effects of abrupt withdrawal is of interest. First, prolonged administration of propranolol increases the number of beta-adrenergic receptors (Glubiger and Lefkowitz, 1977), hence theoretically explaining hypersensitivity to normal circulating concentrations of catecholamines. Circulating catecholamine levels (elevated during propranolol therapy) stay raised for up to 9–10 days, during which time there is danger of rebound events (Nattel et al., 1979).

Post-infarct prophylaxis

If sympathetic stimulation harmfully effects myocardial ischemia then prolonged beta-blockade can be expected to have a beneficial effect when given after myocardial infarction. This expectation has now been realized in the case of propranolol, timolol, and metoprolol with suggestive evidence for atenolol. Practolol is no longer used. In the case of oxprenolol, data are conflicting. It may be that beta-blockers without ISA are best. The usual contra-indications must be observed when selecting patients (heart failure, conduction delay and especially asthma).

Hypercontractile states

In certain specific conditions the inhibitory effect of beta-antagonists on the heart rate is less important than that on contractility. Patients with hypertrophic cardiomyopathy (idiopathic hypertrophic subaortic stenosis = asymmetrical septal hypertrophy) have an increased contractile activity, typically with a high ejection fraction of the heart. Upon infusion of isoproterenol the contractility increases still further and the gradient across the hypertrophied and obstructive ventricular septum increases. Hence the therapeutic aim is to reduce contractility. Propranolol is now standard therapy for hypertrophic obstructive cardiomyopathy, although recently challenged by verapamil. Propranolol is usually effective against the cyanotic spells of Fallot's tetralogy, acting by inhibiting right ventricular contractility.

Non-cardiac indications for beta-blockade

Beta-blockers and especially propranolol are used for non-cardiac indications: tremor, migraine and anxiety states. The use of very high doses of propranolol for schizophrenia depends on a drug interaction in the liver whereby blood levels of other antipsychotic agents such as chlorpromazine are enhanced. Some relief of the chemical features of hyperparathyroidism can be obtained. In thyrotoxicosis beta-blockade is used to control the cardiovascular features such as tachycardia and palpitations, as well as tremor.

Side-effects

The major side-effects include lack of energy and fatigue; there is possibly a combination of central effects and decreased muscle blood flow involved. Bradycardia, myocardial failure and heart block are all readily explicable. Bronchospasm is especially likely to occur with non-selective agents. Rapid death from refractory bronchospasm has occurred rarely and when non-selective agents have been given to asthmatics.

Summary

The autonomic nervous system is the link between the central nervous system and the mechanical activity of the heart (heart rate and contractility). The sympathetic system both releases norepinephrine at the terminal nerve endings in myocardium and coronary vessels, and increases blood epinephrine concentrations by stimulation of the adrenal medulla. The parasympathetic system regulates the mechanical activity of the heart in the opposite direction to the sympathetic. Pharmacologically, the activity of the sympathetic system can be enhanced by sympathomimetic agents such as the beta-adrenergic agonists isoproterenol and dobutamine, or the alpha-adrenergic agonists phenylephrine and methoxamine. Sympatholytic drugs include the specific antagonists acting at the alpha- or beta-receptors, as well as centrally acting agents and neuron-blocking drugs. Cholinergic agents include edrophonium and digitalis. The chief anticholinergic agent is atropine; the quinidine group of antiarrhythmic agents exerts less inhibition on the muscarinic receptor. Thus potentially profound changes in myocardial function can be achieved by pharmacological measures.

Exercise-induced increases in heart rate and contractility can be lessened by inhibition of the cardiac beta-adrenergic receptors using beta-antagonist compounds such as propranolol, which has beneficial effects in angina of effort. Although there are marked pharmacological and pharmacokinetic differences between beta-antagonists, in practice these matter little. A property of practical consequence is cardioselectivity, whereby cardiac beta-1-receptors are inhibited in preference to smooth muscle beta-2-receptors. Added intrinsic sympathomimetic activity may prevent undue negative inotropic or chronotropic effects during therapy; more evidence on this theory is required. In the therapy of hypertension, selective and non-selective beta-adrenergic receptor antagonist are equally effective.

References

Amery A, Lijnen P, Fogard R, Reybrouck T (1977). Atenolol and plasma renin concentration in hypertensive patients. Postgrad Med J 53: Suppl 3, 116–119.

Baker S, Potter LJ (1980). Biochemical studies of cardiac beta-receptors and of their clinical significance. Circ Res 1: 38–42.

Bauer JH, Brooks CA (1979). The long-term effect of propranolol therapy on renal function. Am J Med 66: 405–410.

Berchtold P, Berger M (1980). Metabolic effects of beta-blockers: an overview. In: Advances in Beta-blocker Therapy, Eds. H Roskamm, KH Graefe, pp 32–45, Excerpta Medica, Amsterdam.

Cruickshank JM (1980). The clinical importance of cardioselectivity and lipophilicity in beta blockers. Am Heart J 100: 160–178.

Day JL, Simpson N, Metcalfe J, Page RL (1979). Metabolic consequences of atenolol and propranolol in treatment of essential hypertension. Brit Med J 1: 77–80.

Deacon SP, Karunanayke A, Barnett D (1977). Acebutolol, atenolol and propranolol and metabolic responses to acute hypoglycaemia in diabetics. Brit Med J 2: 1255–1257.

Decalmer PBS, Chatterjee SS, Cruickshank JM, Benson MK, Sterling GM (1978). Beta-blockers and asthma. Brit Heart J 40: 184–189.

Frishman WH, Weksler B, Christodoulou JP, Smithen C, Killip T (1974). Reversal of abnormal platelet aggregability and change in exercise tolerance in patients with angina pectoris following oral propranolol. Circulation 50: 887–896.

Gibb WE, Malpas JS, Turner P, White RJ (1970). Comparison of bethanidine, alpha-methyldopa, and reserpine in essential hypertension. Lancet ii: 275–277.

Glaubiger G, Lefkowitz RJ (1977). Elevated beta-adrenergic receptor number after chronic propranolol treatment. Biochem Biophys Res Comm 78: 720–725.

Greenslade FC, Tobia AJ, Madison SM, Krider KM, Newquist KL (1979). Labetalol binding to specific alpha- and beta-adrenergic sites in vivo and its antagonism of adrenergic responses in vivo. J Molec Cell Cardiol 11: 803–811.

Gross GJ, Warltier DC, Hardman HF (1978). Beneficial actions of N-dimethyl propranolol on myocardial oxygen balance and transmural perfusion gradients distal to a severe coronary artery stenosis in the canine heart. Circulation 58: 663–669.

Grun G, Byon KY, Kaufmann R, Fleckenstein A (1972). Discrimination between beta-adrenolytic and Ca^{2+}-antagonist effects of agents showing beta-receptor blocking activity in cardiac smooth muscle with special reference to Trasicor. Arzt Forsch 26: 369–378.

Harms HH, Gooren L, Spoelstra AJG, Hesse CJ, Verschoor L (1978). Blockade of isoprenaline-induced changed in plasma free fatty acids, immunoreactive insulin levels and plasma renin activity in healthy human subjects by propranolol, pindolol, practolol, atenolol, metoprolol and acebutolol. Brit J Clin Pharm 5: 19–26.

Higgins CB, Vatner SF, Braunwald E (1973). Parasympathetic control of the heart. Pharmacol Rev 25: 119–155.

Keber I, Jerse M, Keber D, Stegnar M (1979). The influence of combined treatment with propranolol and acetylsalicylic acid on platelet aggregation in coronary heart disease. Brit J Clin Pharm 7: 287–291.

Ku DD, Lucchesi BR (1978). Effects of dimethyl propranolol (UM-272; SC-27761) on myocardial ischemic injury in the canine heart after temporary coronary artery occlusion. Circulation 57: 541–548.

Lager I, Blohme G, Smith U (1979). Effect of cardioselective and non-selective beta-blockade on the hypoglycaemic response in insulin-dependent diabetics. Lancet i: 458–462.

McLeod AA, Brown JE, Kuhn C, Kilzhell BB, Sedor FA, Sanders Williams R, Shand DG (1983). Differentiation of hemodynamic, humoral and metabolic responses to beta$_1$- and beta$_2$-adrenergic stimulation in man using atenolol and propranolol. Circulation 67: 1076–1084.

McSorley PD, Warren DJ (1978). Effects of propranolol and metoprolol on the peripheral circulation. Brit Med J 2: 1598–1600.

Majewski H, Rand MJ, Tung LH (1981). Activation of prejunctional beta-adrenoceptors in rat atria by adrenaline applied exogenously or released as co-transmitter. Brit J Pharm 73: 669–679.

Nattel S, Rangno RE, Van Loon G (1979). Mechanism of propranolol withdrawal phenomena. Circulation 59: 1158–1164.

Nayler WG (1972). Comparative partial agonist activity of beta-adrenoceptor antagonists. Brit J Pharm 45: 382–384.

Pickering TG, Gribbin B, Strange Petersen E, Cunningham DJC, Sleight P (1972). Effects of autonomic blockade on the baroreflex in man at rest and during exercise. Circ Res 30: 177–185.

Shepherd JT, Lorenz RR, Tyce GM, Vanhoutte PM (1978). Acetyl choline-inhibition of transmitter release from adrenergic nerve terminals mediated by muscarinic receptors. Fed Proc 37: 191–194.

Shiroff RA, Mathis J, Zelis MD (1978). Propranolol rebound—a retrospective study. Am J Cardiol 41: 778–780.

Sleight P (1975). Neural control of the cardiovascular system. In: Modern Trends in Cardiology. Vol 3, Ed. MF Oliver, pp 1–43, Butterworths, London.

Tarr M, Luckstead EF, Jurewicz PA, Haas HG (1973). Effect of propranolol on the fast inward sodium current in frog atrial muscle. J Pharm Exp Therap 184: 599–610.

Thadani U, Davidson C, Singleton W, Taylor SH (1979). Comparison of the immediate effects of five beta-adreno-ceptor-blocking drugs with different ancillary properties in angina pectoris. N Eng J Med 300: 750–755.

Turner GG, Nelson RR, Nordstrom LA, Diefenthal HC, Gobel FL (1978). Comparative effects of nadolol and propranolol on exercise tolerance in patients with angina pectoris. Brit Heart J 40: 1361–1370.

Vaughan Williams EM (1978). Some factors that influence the activity of antiarrhythmic drugs. Brit Heart J 40: Suppl, 52–61.

Walle T, Conradi FC, Walle UK, Fagan TC, Gaffney TE (1978). The predictable relationship between plasma levels and dose during chronic propranolol therapy. Clin Pharm Therap 24: 668–677.

Woosley RL, Kornhauser D, Smith R, Reele S, Higgins SB, Nies AS, Shand DG, Oates JA (1979). Suppression of chronic ventricular arrhythmias with propranolol. Circulation 60: 819–827.

New References

Bristow MR, Kantrowitz NE, Ginsburg R, Fowler MB (1985). Beta-adrenergic function in heart muscle disease and heart failure. J Molec Cell Cardiol 17 (Suppl 2): 41–52.

Floras JS, Hassan O, Jones JV, Sleight P (1985). Cardioselective and nonselective beta-adrenoceptor blocking drugs in hypertension: A comparison of their effect on blood pressure during mental and physical activity. J Am Coll Cardiol 6: 186–195.

Gebhardt VA, Wisenberg G (1985). The role of beta blockade, with and without intrinsic sympathomimetic activity, in preserving compromised left ventricular function in patients with ischemic heart disease. Am Heart J 109: 1013–1020.

Levy MN, Martin PJ (1984). Neural control of the heart. In: Physiology and Pathophysiology of the Heart. Ed. N Sperelakis, pp 337–354, Nijhoff, Boston.

Vasodilators and Vascular Smooth Muscle

Peripheral Circulation

The arterial bed serves to carry blood from the aorta to the peripheral tissues, while the venous bed returns the blood to the heart and the capillaries function as the site of gas exchange. From the point of view of the heart, the critical site of regulation lies in the peripheral arteries, because they control the peripheral resistance which in turn regulates the work of the heart (Fig. 17-1). Of the three layers of the blood vessel, the intima, the muscular layer and the adventitia, it is the middle layer which is of fundamental importance in regulating the peripheral vascular resistance. It is here that the opposing vasoconstrictor and vasodilator influences work (Table 17-1).

Blood flow

Blood flow through the artery occurs because the pressure gradient at the arterial end is lower than at the capillary end. Apart from the pressure differences, a very important factor is the radius (r) of the blood vessel—the resistance (R) of a rigid tube can be given by **Poiseuille's law** whereby

$$R = P/Q = (8 \times \text{viscosity} \times \text{length})/(r^4 \cdot \pi)$$

where Q = flow, r = radius, P = pressure drop.

In idealized conditions with laminar flow in a rigid tube, resistance is inversely proportional to the fourth power of the tube's radius. Reduction of the diameter of the arterial lumen is the most powerful determinant of resistance to flow. Normally blood viscosity is not an important factor except in severe **polycythemia** when the hematocrit rises above 55 percent.

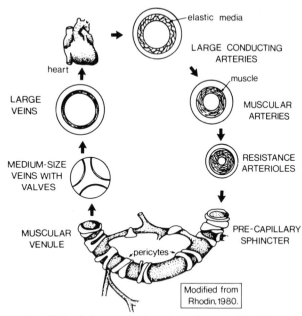

Fig. 17-1 Scheme of microcirculation, modified from Rhodin (1980). The major sites of adrenergic innervation are the small muscular arteries and the resistance arterioles; there is also some innervation of muscular and small venules. With permission from the author and the American Physiological Society.

Table 17-1

Vasoconstrictor and vasodilator influences on peripheral circulation

	Vasoconstrictors	Vasodilators
1. **Resistance arteriolar vessels**		
	Norepinephrine	Epinephrine
	Angiotensin II	Acetyl choline
	Vasopressin and	Prostaglandins
	related peptides	Histamine
		Bradykinin
		Metabolic dilators
2. **Precapillary sphincters**		
	Norepinephrine	Metabolic dilators:
	(? others as above)	Adenosine
		ATP
		Metabolites

In each organ the requirement for blood flow is met by autoregulation whereby, for example, the production of metabolites by exercising skeletal muscle causes arterial vasodilation and increases the blood flow. Similar autoregulation occurs in the heart and in the brain.

Peripheral vascular resistance

The major physiological effect of vasodilator therapy is to decrease peripheral vascular resistance. The basis for the calculation of systemic peripheral vascular resistance is the difference between the mean pressures in the aorta and in the right atrium, divided by the cardiac output. Two of these measurements can be obtained by Swan–Ganz catheterization and the mean arterial pressure calculated from the blood pressure. The systemic vascular resistance is frequently used in cardiological practice to monitor the vasoconstrictive effects of shock or of vasodilator therapy. Values for systemic vascular resistance of more than 1500 dynes.sec.cm^{-5} are probably abnormal, whereas values of pulmonary vascular resistance of more than 120 dynes.sec.cm^{-5} are probably abnormal.

Smooth Muscle Contraction Mechanism

Many of the events are similar to those already described in the cardiac contraction cycle: the entry of calcium, the (presumed) calcium-induced calcium release from the sarcoplasmic reticulum, the rise in cytosolic free calcium ion concentration, the interaction of calcium with the myosin ATPase, the subsequent uptake of calcium into the sarcoplasmic reticulum and the discharge of excess calcium via calcium exit channels as in the heart (Johansson, 1978).

Cyclic nucleotides and calmodulin

Three important differences between vascular smooth muscle and the myocardium are: (i) owing to the tonic **nature of the peripheral arteriolar contraction, there should be a sustained level of free ionized calcium or** another mechanism must come into play to sustain tone; (ii) owing to the lessened force of contraction that needs to be developed, the peak intracellular calcium concentration reached should be less; and (iii) there must be a major difference between heart and peripheral smooth muscle in response to the beta-receptor because **beta-stimulation causes the heart to contract and peripheral vessels to dilate**.

In peripheral vascular muscle, calcium ions also regulate the myosin–actin interaction as in myocardial cells. Yet the mechanism is quite different because troponin C is absent from the actin filaments of vascular smooth muscle cells. According to the **phosphorylation hypothesis** of Adelstein (1983), calcium ions interact with calmodulin to promote phosphorylation of the light chains of the myosin heads (Fig. 17-2). Whereas the role of such phosphorylation in the regulation of myosin ATPase activity in the heart is still speculative (see page 105), this step is now proposed as essential for the interaction of myosin and actin in vascular smooth muscle. Beta-adrenergic stimulation via cyclic AMP inhibits the phosphorylation of the myosin light chain, thereby decreasing the myosin ATPase activity and inhibiting contraction (Stephens and Kroeger, 1981). Whereas cyclic GMP is usually held to oppose the effects of cyclic AMP (see Fig. 6-8) in vascular smooth muscle these nucleotides both cause relaxation. Therefore both must decrease the myoplasmic calcium ion concentration. Cyclic GMP probably acts by inhibiting the inward calcium current (as in the sinus node); an accumulation of cyclic GMP may be the mechanism whereby nitrates and nitroprusside cause vasodilation. Cyclic AMP probably lowers the myoplasmic calcium by enhancing the uptake of calcium by the sarcoplasmic reticulum, without increasing calcium ion entry (Fig. 17-2).

VASCULAR SMOOTH MUSCLE

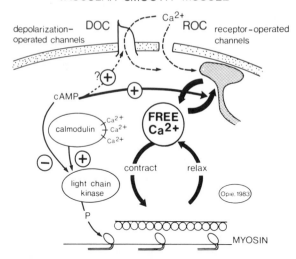

Fig. 17-2 Calcium entry in the vascular smooth muscle cell is complex and thought to proceed by at least two channels: the DOCs (depolarization-operated channels = PSC = potential sensitive channels) and the ROCs (receptor operated channels). The relatively small amounts of calcium entry into the vascular myocyte are thought to release much larger quantities of calcium from the sarcoplasmic reticulum. As the cytosolic calcium (Ca^{2+}) rises, calmodulin is activated to stimulate the activity of the light-chain kinase which in turn phosphorylates the myosin light-chain to enhance the activity of myosin ATPase. (see also Fig. 18-3)

Latch mechanism

Another major difference between the contractile mechanism in the heart and in vascular smooth muscle, is that vascular contraction is maintained for long periods with little use of ATP. The contractile mechanism has no ejection work to do as in the myocardium. Rather, contraction needs to be sustained to allow autovascular smooth muscle tone to have an effect in regulating the blood pressure. Murphy and Gerthoffer (1984) have described a "latch mechanism", whereby once myosin and actin are joined, they catch on to each other and fail to relax until a further signal is applied. At the end of a vasoconstrictor stimulus, when the calcium channels are no longer open, the continued uptake of calcium by the sarcoplasmic reticulum of the vascular smooth muscle then relaxes the muscle by two mechanisms:

first, the calcium–calmodulin complex is dissociated, and myosin is dephosphorylated by a phosphatase. Secondly, calcium leaves the unknown regulatory site on the latchbridges.

Calcium Channels in Smooth Muscle

In the heart the major mechanism for the entry of calcium is thought to be via the slow channel and dependent on depolarization. In the case of smooth muscle only part of the entry of calcium is mediated by depolarization (Fig. 17-2). Such **depolarization-operated channels** are found in smooth muscle as well as heart muscle. In smooth muscle, they have also been termed **potential sensitive channels** (Bolton, 1979). To maintain arterial tone, intermittent spontaneous autonomic nervous discharges are required. Such discharges could either directly operate the DOCs, or could intermittently release norepinephrine to activate **receptor-operated channels** (ROCs). Besides norepinephrine, serotonin and angiotensin also activate the ROCs. Both the depolarization and the receptor-operated channels enhance the entry of calcium ions, so that the powerful vasodilating effect of calcium-antagonists of the nifedipine group does not help to decide which type of channel is more important in maintaining peripheral vascular tone. The receptor-operated channels are sensitive to calcium-antagonists in only some of the vascular beds. The new calcium-antagonist nimodipine does not block the receptor-operated channels in the saphenous artery but does so in the basilar artery (Towart, 1981), thereby allowing regional cerebral vasodilation.

Phasic and tonic components

A general property of smooth muscle is that it has two components to contraction: phasic and tonic. It is the tonic component which is of most importance in peripheral vascular smooth muscle because it regulates peripheral vascular resistance. It is the tonic component which is sensitive to the norepinephrine and which responds to the calcium content of the extracellular fluid. Electrophysiological evidence stresses the role of the membrane potential in regulating vascular tone (Hermsmeyer et al., 1981). **Because a normal membrane potential is required for the operation of both types of calcium channels in vascular smooth muscle, it is not possible to say that** control of tone resides in a particular type of calcium channel.

Source of calcium for smooth muscle contraction

The heart stops beating within seconds of being deprived of external calcium, showing the dependence of contraction on the transmembrane flux of calcium. In the case of vascular smooth muscle, withdrawal of calcium is followed only slowly by contractile failure; hence internal calcium is able to maintain contracture for much longer than in the case of the heart. In some arteries this internal calcium may be the site on which norepinephrine can act without causing marked depolarizations by the ill-understood process of **pharmacomechanical coupling** (Somlyo and Somlyo, 1968). Thus norepinephrine can cause large arteries such as the aorta to contract even in the absence of external calcium (Droogmans et al., 1977). The longer the duration of exposure of the artery to the calcium-free solution, the feebler the contractions produced by norepinephrine. Hence pharmacomechanical coupling cannot be sustained for long in the absence of external calcium.

Norepinephrine can increase the cytosolic calcium ion concentration sufficiently to cause contraction of vascular smooth muscle either by the receptor operated channels, or by pharmacomechanical coupling. Because both processes need external calcium for a sustained effect of norepinephrine, it is simplest to hold a unitary hypothesis that norepinephrine primarily "opens" the receptor-operated channels.

Alpha- and Beta-adrenergic Control

The major vasoconstrictive response of vascular smooth muscle is to norepinephrine (Table 17-2). It is norepinephrine which regulates the rate of calcium entry. The source of this norepinephrine is both discharge from the adrenergic neuron and circulating norepinephrine. A reasonable hypothesis for the control of peripheral vascular tone is that norepinephrine acts on the vascular alpha-receptors to regulate the extent of calcium entry and hence the cytosolic calcium ion concentration, which in turn regulates smooth muscle tone in the resistance arteries and arterioles.

Table 17-2

Effects of catecholamines on blood vessels

1.	**Norepinephrine (noradrenaline)**
	(a) released from terminal neurons
	— vasoconstriction throughout vascular bed
	(b) circulating
	— vasoconstriction of cutaneous, splanchnic and renal beds
	— venoconstriction
2.	**Circulating epinephrine (adrenaline)**
	(a) predominant beta-2 vasodilatory effect
	— muscular arterioles (heart and skeletal muscle)
	(b) predominant alpha vasoconstrictor effect
	— other resistance vessels and veins

Autonomic innervation

It is especially the norepinephrine released from adrenergic nerve terminal neurons (or varicosities) that causes vasoconstriction (Fig. 17-3). Running along with the adrenergic fibers are the parasympathetic cholinergic fibers, which release the vasodilator acetyl choline. The vasodilator mechanism is probably the cholinergic inhibition of release of norepinephrine from the adrenergic nerve terminal neurons. Possibly acetyl choline first activates a muscarinic receptor, which hyperpolarizes the neuron to reduce the amount of norepinephrine released upon adrenergic stimulation.

There are two mechanisms which exist to modulate the effects of norepinephrine. First, norepinephrine stimulates not only the **postjunctional alpha-1 receptors** but the **prejunctional alpha-2 receptors** on the terminal varicosities; the latter receptors then inhibit further release of norepinephrine from the storage vesicles. Secondly, during a surge of catecholamine activity, circulating epinephrine and norepinephrine stimulate beta-receptors on the terminal neurons. Such prejunctional beta-receptors facilitate the release of norepinephrine. In contrast, the beta-receptors on the vascular wall (beta-2 subtype) cause vasodilation. In most vessels the beta-2 vasodilator receptors do not respond to sympathetic nervous stimulation but only to circulating epinephrine (Russell and Moran, 1980). Thus, when adrenergic activity is greatly increased, over-constriction can be countered by: (i) stimulation of prejunctional alpha-2 receptors to inhibit the release of norepinephrine; (ii) the

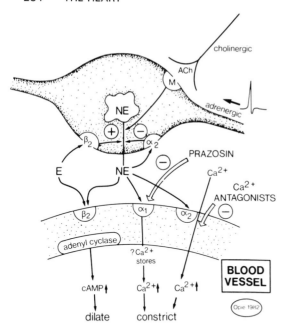

Fig. 17-3 Vascular smooth muscle receptors. Note the dilating effect of beta-2-stimulation and the constricting effect of alpha-stimulation. There are thought to be two alpha-receptors: the alpha-1 are inhibited by prazosin and the alpha-2 by calcium antagonists. The relation of these two types of alpha-receptors to the two calcium channels (DOCs and ROCs) shown in Fig. 17-2 remains an open question. Note that beta-adrenergic blockers may inhibit vasodilatory effects of cyclic AMP to allow unopposed alpha-adrenergic-mediated vasospasm (cold extremities, provocation of coronary artery spasm).

vasodilatory effects of epinephrine-mediated beta-2 vasodilation; and (iii) the activity of the cholinergic system. Nevertheless the overall effect will be vaso-constriction of the majority of arterioles and veins, except for vasodilation of the arterioles of the heart and skeletal muscle (Table 17-1). This response is ideally suited for the requirements of exercise (Chapter 14).

Prejunctional and postjunctional receptors

Besides the alpha-2 receptors, many other prejunctional receptors modulate the release of norepinephrine. For example, angiotensin and histamine increase norepinephrine release whereas it is decreased by vasodilatory prostaglandins. Epinephrine probably

promotes release of norepinephrine, which may be one mechanism whereby catecholamine beta-stimulation actually causes a rise rather than the expected fall of blood pressure. The classification of alpha-receptors has been made even more complex by the recent realization that some of the alpha-2 receptors are also situated on the vascular wall at a postjunctional site (Fig. 17-3). Van Meel et al. (1981) propose that it is here that the calcium-antagonist agents act to cause vasodilation. The relation between these vascular alpha-2 receptors and the receptor-operated channels is difficult to reconcile, yet both respond to calcium-antagonists. No simple hypothesis allows an easy marriage of the two concepts.

Renin, Serotonin and Prostaglandins

Besides the catecholamines, several endocrine factors play an important role in cardiovascular regulation. Within a few minutes of renal ischemia, or generalized fall of blood pressure, the kidneys secrete **renin** by a mechanism responsive to beta-stimulation. Renin in turn converts angiotensinogen into angiotensin I. Angiotensin II forms by the action of the converting enzyme, which is located largely in the endothelium of blood vessels in the lungs but also elsewhere. **Angiotensin II causes vigorous vasoconstriction by stimulating vascular receptors and also by increasing** the release of norepinephrine from terminal neurons. Another effect of angiotensin II is to release aldosterone. Fluid retention occurs, particularly in the presence of impaired renal function. The increased vascular volume predisposes to hypertension. **Aldosterone** indirectly helps to control the blood pressure by its effects on the extracellular volume. Its major effect is to increase the reabsorption of sodium from the renal tubules. This increases the volume of the extracellular fluid and the increase in blood volume **tends to elevate the arterial pressure, everything else being equal.** (see Figs. 22-5 and 22-6)

Vasoactive **kinins** are polypeptides which are normally inactive as kininogens, but when activated by an enzyme called kallikrein, are released and become powerful vasodilators. One such agent is **bradykinin** which increases blood flow and also decreases heart rate.

Serotonin (5-hydroxytryptamine) is present in large amounts in the platelets and in certain tissues in the intestine. Serotonin has complex effects which have been elucidated to some extent by the use of the serotonin antagonist **ketanserin**. When given to patients, ketanserin reduces blood pressure; in the presence of congestive heart failure it reduces the afterload to improve myocardial function. Serotonin therefore appears to be largely a vasoconstrictor.

Histamine acts through the H_1 and H_2 receptors to cause peripheral arterial and venous vasodilation. When released, as in allergic conditions, the combination of constriction of some vascular beds and dilation of others causes rapid failure of the circulation. At the same time large quantities of fluid leak through the capillaries (increased permeability resulting from histamine) to cause edema. A cardiac component (**cardiac anaphylaxis**) plays a role, as shown by the development of tachycardias, arrhythmias and pump failure. Clinical therapy is to give intravenous epinephrine urgently; how it is effective is not known. Beneficial effects may include bronchial dilation and a positive inotropic effect. The arrhythmias are experimentally antagonized by a combination of H_1 and H_2 blocking agents (see Table 19-2).

Prostaglandins are compounds with a long-chain cycle structure eventually derived from unsaturated fatty acids such as arachidonic and linoleic acids. The great number of different prostaglandins which exist, their wide range of biological activity and the major species differences make it difficult to ascribe to them an exact function. The prostaglandins with the most significance for cardiovascular function are: (i) **prostacyclin** (PGE_2), the major prostaglandin released from the heart which has vasodilatory and antithrombotic properties; and (ii) **thromboxane** A_2, a promotor of platelet aggregation and a vasoconstrictor which functions in opposition to prostacyclin. Both are continuously being formed and broken down, having very short half-lives. Despite the numerous agents regulating platelet function (Fig. 17-4), thus far the only generally accepted use is that of **aspirin** in (i) cerebrovascular disease with transient ischemic attacks; (ii) in unstable angina; and (iii) in combination with dipyridamole, to prevent occlusion of the grafting vein after coronary artery bypass surgery. Of the prostaglandins, only PGE_1 has an established therapeutic role — dilation of patent ductus arteriosus.

Leukotrienes are prostaglandin derivatives from arachidonic acid. They are released from white blood cells (leukocytes) and tissue macrophages to act as powerful vasoconstrictors. Some leukotrienes, however, also promote the formation of vasodilatory prostaglandins (Iacapino et al., 1983). Leukotrienes may perhaps play a role in a variety of clinical conditions such as coronary spasm, cardiovascular shock and histamine anaphylaxis. The "slow-reacting substance" of anaphylactic shock which mediates pulmonary vasoconstriction is now known to be a leukotriene (Piper, 1983).

Peripheral Vasodilators

Vasodilators are a complex category of agents acting on the peripheral circulation by multiple and diverse

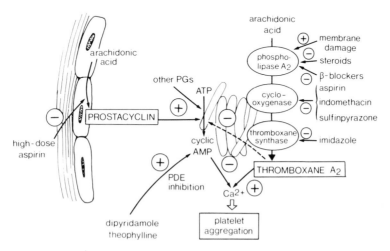

Fig. 17-4 Agents active on platelets. Two principal modes of action are: (i) altering the rate of formation of cyclic AMP which decreases the platelet calcium, and (ii) inhibition of the thromboxane pathway. PG = prostaglandin; PDE = phosphodiesterase.

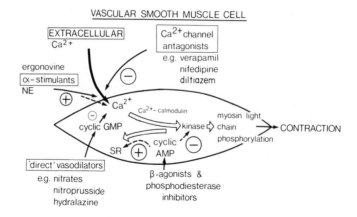

Fig. 17-5 Scheme for drug effects on vascular smooth muscle. Inhibition of calcium ion entry can be achieved by: (a) calcium channel antagonists such as nifedipine; (b) adenosine, resulting from inhibition of adenosine deaminase by dipyridamole; (c) alpha-blocking agents; (d) an increased intracellular cyclic GMP resulting from nitrates or nitroprusside. An increased cyclic AMP produced by beta-2-stimulants or phosphodiesterase inhibitors will cause vascular relaxation.

mechanisms (Fig. 17-5), among which are alpha-antagonism, calcium channel antagonism, beta-stimulation, inhibition of angiotensin formation and non-specific vasodilation by the nitrates, nitroprusside and hydralazine. Theoretically, vasodilators can act on different parts of the vascular tree—for example, nitrates act on the veins and large coronary arteries, but only slightly on the peripheral arterioles, whereas hydralazine acts on the peripheral arteries. Different calcium antagonists also have different sites of vasodilator activity. Thus verapamil acts chiefly on coronary arteries and only has milder effects on the peripheral arterioles, whereas nifedipine acts on both coronary arteries and peripheral arterioles. It is these different mechanisms and sites of action that allow for **selective regional vasodilation**, so that a venodilator allows reduction of the preload on the heart, an arteriolar dilator reduces the afterload and a coronary vasodilator relieves coronary spasm. The diseases for which vasodilators are indicated include congestive heart failure, arterial hypertension and vasospastic angina pectoris.

At a cellular level, vasodilators have different possible modes of action. Some inhibit the slow calcium channel in the vascular myocyte—such include the calcium antagonists, alpha-1-adrenergic antagonists, adenosine and agents increasing cyclic GMP. Of the agents enhancing cyclic GMP, some—such as acetyl choline—require an intact endothelium for their action (**endothelium-dependent relaxation**). Other vasodilators, such as the nitrates and nitro-

prusside, act independently of the endothelium to vasodilate (Rapoport et al., 1983). Hence nitrates should be—and are—vasodilators even in the presence of coronary artery disease. Other vasodilators decrease the phosphorylation of myosin by increasing tissue cyclic AMP levels; agents acting here include the beta-2-agonists, histamine and forskolin. A controversial and still unproven site of vasodilator action is by enhancing the dephosphorylation of myosin (Gerthoffer et al., 1984), theoretically a possible result of an increasing level of cyclic GMP (Rapoport et al., 1983).

Sodium Nitroprusside

Whereas the mechanism of most of the vasodilators listed in Table 17-2 is either known or can be guessed at with reasonable accuracy, chief speculation concerns the "direct-acting" agents—nitrates, nitroprusside, hydralazine, diazoxide and minoxidil. There are two important negative points: direct vasodilators act neither on the autonomic innervation nor primarily on the calcium channel. Nitroprusside and nitrates may indirectly inhibit the inward calcium current in the coronary arteries, but have none of the other properties of the true calcium antagonists.

A recent theory is that both nitroprusside and nitrates activate guanylate cyclase of coronary arterial smooth muscle to increase **tissue cyclic GMP** (Kukovetz et al., 1979), which presumably acts to

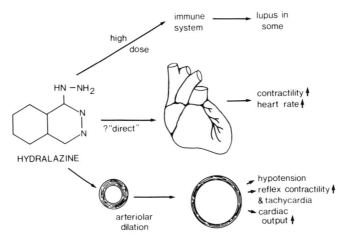

Fig. 17-6 Hydralazine achieves a reflex tachycardia and increase of cardiac output indirectly as a result of peripheral vasodilation. There may also be a direct cardiac effect. Prolonged use in high doses may produce a temporary lupus-like syndrome.

inhibit the slow, inward calcium current (Kohlhardt and Haap, 1978) or to alter protein phosphorylation (Rapoport et al., 1983). Nitroprusside seems to act as an "intracellular nitrate", so that once the molecule has crossed into the vascular smooth muscle cytosol, the same active nitric oxide molecule is formed with the same pharmacologic effects as in the case of nitrates.

Clinically, the major immediate effect of nitroprusside is to produce a very rapid hypotension; it can be used whenever rapid controlled reduction of blood pressure is required. Nitroprusside must be given intravenously; it is metabolized so rapidly that therapeutically required hypotension is reversible as soon as the infusion rate is reduced. A real danger is that when an infusion is suddenly stopped, there will be rebound of the arterial pressure due to compensatory mechanisms such as activation of the renin–angiotensin system invoked by the vasodilation (Packer et al., 1979).

Intravenous nitroprusside remains the **reference vasodilator for severe low-output left-sided heart failure** because it acts rapidly and has a balanced effect, dilating both arterioles and veins. Nitroprusside seems particularly useful for increasing left-ventricular stroke work in severe refractory heart failure caused by mitral or aortic valve incompetence. Because of the increased stroke volume there may be considerable hemodynamic improvement without much hypotension; but in general some hypotension accompanies and may limit the therapeutic effect of nitroprusside.

Theoretically all vasodilators are contra-indicated in severe mitral or aortic stenosis, both being essentially surgical problems. Nitroprusside is useful in selected patients with myocardial infarction and left ventricular failure. Here hemodynamic monitoring is required to keep the left ventricular filling pressure at an "optimal" value of 14–18 mmHg; in chronic congestive heart failure the filling pressure can be further reduced to the normal range without such monitoring (Franciosa et al., 1983). Other specific uses are in the control of dissecting aortic aneurysm and in hypertensive crises (especially those associated with left ventricular failure).

By dilating the small coronary arterioles, nitroprusside may drain away blood from the ischemic myocardium and thus put at risk patients with coronary artery disease (Mann et al., 1978). Hence nitroprusside should only be given to patients with acute myocardial infarction when hypertension needs carefully monitored reduction. In particular, excess hypotension must be avoided (Bodenheimer et al., 1981).

Hydralazine

The molecular mechanism whereby hydralazine vasodilates is unknown; a clue is that hydralazine hyperpolarizes the arterial wall, possibly at the same site as an adenosine receptor. Because depolarization is required for muscle contraction, hyperpolarization is

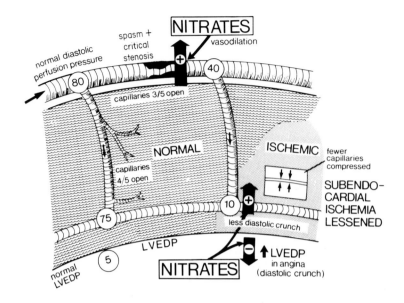

Fig. 17-7 When a patient with a critical stenosis exercises, subendocardial ischemia and temporary left ventricular failure accompany the onset of anginal pain. Alternatively, angina at rest can develop if there is super-added coronary spasm. Nitrates bring relief by increasing the diameter of large coronary arteries, by relaxing spasm, and chiefly by reducing left ventricular end-diastolic pressure (LVEDP). The numbers in circles are vascular pressures in mmHg. For evaluation of the importance of "diastolic crunch", see Parratt JR, Marshall RJ, Ledingham I McA (1980). J Physiol, Paris 76: 791–803. Modified from Parratt et al. (1980), with permission.

a vasodilatory influence (Kreye, 1981). Clinically, hydralazine is a powerful arteriolar vasodilator with virtually no venous effects. The rate of onset of its effects are slow, requiring up to 30–60 min; the dilator response also wanes slowly. The fall in the peripheral vascular resistance causes a marked compensatory reflex stimulation of the heart rate and hence of cardiac output so that arterial pressure falls less than expected (Fig. 17-7). In the therapy of low-output congestive heart failure it is logical to combine hydralazine (afterload reduction) with nitrates (preload reduction). When given to patients with cardiac failure hydralazine causes less tachycardia than in hypertensive subjects, possibly because the reflex arcs are dampened in congestive cardiac failure.

Hydralazine, usually in the form of dihydralazine, has been used parenterally in the therapy of acute severe hypertension; however delayed onset and long duration of effects make its use more difficult to control than alternatives such as sublingual nifedipine or intravenous nitroprusside or labetalol.

During prolonged therapy, tissue auto-antibodies may develop so that the patient's collagen tissue reacts abnormally with the production of joint pains and other features of the lupus syndrome. Hence the top dose is usually strictly limited to 200 mg daily, but in severe congestive heart failure very high doses may be used temporarily.

Because similar arteriolar dilation can be achieved by the calcium-antagonist nifedipine without as severe a reflex tachycardia, it follows that: (i) hydralazine is less and less the peripheral vasodilator of choice; (ii) hydralazine may have another stimulatory action besides acting purely by arteriolar dilation. One old proposal is that hydralazine evokes the release of histamine (Gershwin and Smith, 1967); a more recent proposal is that it acts as a beta-adrenergic stimulant to increase heart rate and cardiac output by a propranolol-sensitive mechanism (Khatri et al., 1977). Although the reflex tachycardia is usually unwanted, it may be used therapeutically in some patients with the sick sinus syndrome.

Endralazine is related structurally to hydralazine but metabolized differently so that it may be without hypersensitivity effects (lupus).

Other "Direct-acting" Vasodilators

Minoxidil and diazoxide, like hydralazine, have an unknown site of action. **Diazoxide** is chemically similar to thiazide diuretics (Rubin et al., 1962) yet it has a purely vasodilator effect without a diuretic effect (in contrast, the marked vasodilation causes salt and water retention by stimulation of aldosterone secretion). Like thiazide diuretics, diazoxide is potentially diabetogenic; this side-effect is caused in the case of diazoxide by an inhibitory effect on insulin release. In practice, diazoxide is now only used intravenously for hypertensive crises; when too much is given disastrous hypotension can cause cerebral underperfusion and stroke. **Minoxidil**, despite severe side-effects such as hirsuties and (possibly) pericardial disease, is sometimes used in patients with refractory hypertension because of its powerful vasodilating activity. A beta-adrenergic blocker should also be given concurrently to reduce reflex tachycardia, and a diuretic to avoid fluid retention (stimulation of aldosterone secretion follows vasodilation).

Alpha-1-adrenergic Blocking Agents

Prazosin

The binding of prazosin to the alpha-1-receptors (postsynaptic) is so highly specific that it is used as a reference point for radioligand binding studies. The failure to act on the presynaptic alpha-2-receptors means that the mechanisms inhibiting the release of norepinephrine are still active, which explains why prazosin only slightly increases the pulse rate in contrast to the "direct" acting vasodilators such as hydralazine. The site of action is the veins and peripheral arterioles; thus far there has been only equivocal evidence that prazosin also inhibits coronary vascular alpha-receptors. In congestive heart failure there is a major controversy: many studies have shown a fall-off in the effect of prazosin (tachyphylaxis) even after a few doses, so that the long-term effect is blunted and the chief remaining benefit is improved exercise tolerance. In one study prazosin was completely without effect after six months of therapy (Markham et al., 1983). Other studies argue that the phenomena of tachyphylaxis is exaggerated and that the effects of prazosin are long-lasting especially in the therapy of hypertension. All are agreed that the first dose of prazosin may have a very marked effect.

First-dose syncope may be due to the decrease in preload. It is especially likely when there is no left ventricular failure or when the patient is also receiving nitrates or potent diuretics. The absence of compensatory tachycardia may also play a role. Chronic postural dizziness is a less frequent side-effect. Retrograde ejaculation is an unusual and troublesome side-effect, common to alpha-1-blocking agents which relax the internal sphincter of the urethra.

Labetalol

This agent is a combined alpha–beta-blocker, with a more powerful effect on the beta- than on the alpha-receptors, the ratio being 7 : 1 when given orally (presumably the effect of liver metabolites) and 3 : 1 when given intravenously. The alpha-receptors involved are the alpha-1-vascular receptors, as in the case of prazosin. While the alpha-1 inhibitory effects may seem weak they are strong enough to ensure that the arterial pressures of hypertensive patients rapidly come down within minutes in response to intravenous labetalol, whereas the conventional beta-blockers take hours for their initial effect even when given intravenously. With oral dosing the added vasodilatory effect is much less, and not yet of added proven therapeutic benefit when compared with conventional beta-blockade. Because of its predominant beta-adrenergic inhibitory effects, labetalol may not be given to patients with congestive heart failure and is therefore primarily used as an antihypertensive agent.

Phenoxybenzamine

Phenoxybenzamine is a powerful alpha-blocking agent said to be inhibitory on both alpha-1 and alpha-2 receptors, but especially on the alpha-1 vascular receptors. It is used classically in the therapy of pheochromocytoma where excess alpha-activity results from increased norepinephrine produced by the tumor. Why is phenoxybenzamine used rather than prazosin? Possibly because it can be given both intravenously and orally. The onset of action of phenoxybenzamine is slow but the effects are long-lasting. Occasionally it is employed as an adjuvant in hypertension when its effects seem to be very similar to prazosin (Mulvihill-Wilson et al., 1983).

Phentolamine

Phentolamine is another powerful inhibitor of both alpha-1 and alpha-2 receptors so that complex effects can be expected. Alpha-1-blockade results in the expected vasodilation. Alpha-2 presynaptic blockade removes the "alpha-2-brake" on release of norepinephrine from the varicosities into the synaptic cleft. The vasoconstrictor effects of such released norepinephrine are inhibited by alpha-1-blockade, but increased inotropic and chronotropic effects result from beta-1 effects of norepinephrine. This spectrum of activity — vasodilation, inotropism and tachycardia — is not useful in the case of hypertension. When an intravenous vasodilator is required for congestive heart failure the complexity of the mode of action and the expense of phentolamine have generally ousted it in favor of sodium nitroprusside.

Indoramin

This is an alpha-1-adrenergic receptor vascular inhibitor, like prazosin, but with less venous effect. Therefore it is less suitable for congestive heart failure. Although used clinically as an antihypertensive agent, especially in the United Kingdom, it has antihistaminic and other complex effects which may explain why sedation is a side-effect.

Calcium Antagonists

From the point of view of peripheral vasodilation, the recently described interactions between the calcium antagonists and the vascular alpha-2-adrenergic receptors are important. Whereas an alpha-1 inhibitory effect is possessed chiefly by verapamil (high concentrations) but not by diltiazem or nifedipine, in the case of vascular alpha-2 receptors all three calcium antagonists are active. Nifedipine appears to be the most powerful peripheral dilator, followed by verapamil and then diltiazem. The use of these agents in the therapy of hypertension is increasing. In the case of severe left ventricular failure, it is especially nifedipine that is being assessed. (For details of calcium antagonists, see Chapter 18.)

Angiotensin-converting Enzyme Inhibitors

The activity of the renin–angiotensin system can be decreased by inhibition of the angiotensin-converting enzyme. **Captopril** acts as a vasodilator with a favorable hemodynamic effect when given to patients with chronic congestive heart failure. In hypertension captopril should be most effective when plasma renin is highest, as in renal artery stenosis. But captopril is also effective, alone or especially with diuretics or beta-blockers, in ordinary essential hypertension. Occasionally neutropenia or proteinuria occur as side-effects, especially at high doses of captopril. **Enalapril** is a new long-acting converting enzyme inhibitor which may have fewer side-effects (Cody et al., 1983), because of the absence of the sulfhydryl group in the molecule.

Other Vasodilator Agents

Beta-2-adrenergic agonists

Beta-2-agonists act on the vascular receptors to cause peripheral vasodilation. **Salbutamol**, an agent established in the therapy of bronchoconstriction, is now being evaluated intravenously or orally as a vasodilator in severe congestive heart failure. The classic beta-agonist, isoproterenol, will also have this effect and in addition has a direct cardiac inotropic and chronotropic effect; the danger of arrhythmogenesis usually prevents its use in congestive heart failure. Dobutamine may also owe part of its beneficial effect in the failing heart to peripheral vasodilation as a result of a spill-over effect on beta-2-receptors.

Ganglion-blocking agents such as trimethaphan have been used in carefully monitored patients with acute myocardial infarction to reduce arterial pressure and hence the infarct size. **Adrenergic-neuron-blocking** agents, such as guanethidine, are not employed in the therapy of chronic heart failure and are seldom tried in hypertension because of postural hypotension, impotence and interaction with centrally acting compounds which antagonize the hypotensive effects (tricyclic antidepressants, monoamine oxidase inhibitors, phenothiazine derivatives).

Furosemide when injected intravenously in standard doses can rapidly improve the severity of acute pulmonary edema, before the lung water volume changes. The probable mechanism of this early effect is venodilation, as also proposed for the thiazide diuretics.

Central alpha-2-stimulants (clonidine, methyldopa) have been used only in hypertension and not in heart failure. Central alpha-2 stimulation decreases peripheral alpha-vascular tone but these agents can have marked central sedative side-effects.

Nitrates and Other Coronary Vasodilators

Nitrates have been used for angina pectoris since 1867, when Lauder Brunton in Edinburgh, Scotland, successfully tried amyl nitrite to "lessen the arterial tension" in a patient with nocturnal angina. But in 1933 Sir Thomas Lewis held that the effect of amyl nitrite was probably due mainly to its powerful dilation of the coronary vessels, rather than to its effects in lowering the blood pressure. Emphasis swung back to the peripheral effect of nitrates when Gorlin, Brachfield and co-workers found that overall coronary blood flow was unchanged by nitroglycerin (Gorlin et al., 1959). Further support for a prime peripheral effect came with the observation that angina of effort was consistently precipitated by a certain value of the double product, heart rate × blood pressure, an index of the myocardial oxygen demand (Robinson, 1967).

Three newer observations again emphasize the cardiac effects of nitrates. First, in animal preparations nitrates can cause vasodilation in the ischemic zone. Secondly, in man coronary artery spasm may be a major factor in precipitating chest pain, even in some patients with angiographically proven coronary artery disease. Nitrates are very effective against vasospastic angina and angina at rest. Thirdly, direct angiographic measurements show that nitrates actually increase the diameter at the site of coronary artery stenosis (Lichtlen et al., 1984). But the peripheral hemodynamic effects of nitrates cannot be ignored. It is now clear that long-acting nitrates have long-lasting hemodynamic effects, reducing the afterload and especially the preload of the heart. Hence nitrates are now being used also to "unload" the heart in left ventricular failure and in selected cases of myocardial infarction.

Mechanism of action of nitrates

In relation to the oxygen supply to ischemic myocardium a distinction must be made between

ACTION OF NITRATES ON CIRCULATION

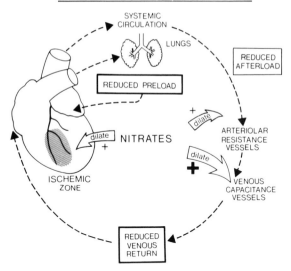

Fig. 17-8 Site of action of nitrates on the circulation. Note the prominent effect on venous capacitance vessels. From Opie LH (1980). Drugs and the Heart: II. Nitrates, Lancet 1981: 750–753, reprinted with permission from The Lancet.

anti-anginal and vasodilator properties. Nitrates redistribute blood flow along collateral channels and from epicardial to endocardial regions (Fig. 17-8). By reducing left ventricular end-diastolic pressure, nitrates increase the transmyocardial coronary arterial pressure gradient and facilitate subendocardial blood flow. Thus nitrates are "effective" vasodilators for angina, but dipyridamole and many other vasodilators are not and may increase angina by diverting blood from the ischemic area, creating a "coronary steal" effect.

Effects of nitrates on the oxygen demand are even more important than effects on the oxygen supply (Fig. 17-9). Nitrates increase the **venous capacitance**, causing pooling of blood in the peripheral veins and in the splanchnic vascular bed, resulting in a reduction in ventricular volume, which decreases the distension of the heart wall and reduces myocardial oxygen demand. The fall in arterial pressure will furthermore reduce myocardial oxygen demand, although this is accompanied by a reflex increase in heart rate. The latter effect increases myocardial oxygen demand but can be abolished by beta-adrenergic blockade. The beneficial effect of nitrates in congestive heart failure depends on venodilation.

One recent theory is that nitrates (like nitroprusside) act to increase **cyclic GMP** in vascular smooth muscle

(Kukovetz et al., 1979), thereby to inhibit calcium ion entry via the slow channel or to alter myosin phosphorylation (Rapoport et al., 1983). If nitrates and nitroprusside share the same molecular mechanism then it is not clear why nitrates dilate the major and nitroprussides the small coronary arterioles, nor why nitrates are chiefly venodilators whereas nitroprusside is a combined arteriolar and venodilator. An attraction of the cyclic GMP theory is that the development of partial tolerance to the effects of nitrates on the circulation is accompanied by impaired formation of cyclic GMP in the vascular myocyte (Keith et al., 1982). A less likely alternative theory is that nitrates help the formation of vasodilatory prostaglandins (Marcillio et al., 1980). Nitrates also differ in their site of action from adenosine, which acts on the small intramural vessels possessing the adenosine receptors that regulate most of the coronary resistance. Nitrates only increase coronary flow when the large coronary arteries are the site of vasoconstriction.

Nitrates for angina

Nitrates remain the basis of therapy for all forms of angina (Chapter 24), whether precipitated by effort or coronary spasm. In angina of effort sublingual short-acting nitrates can abort the attack. Both in angina at rest and in unstable angina, oral nitrates (both short-acting and long-acting) have long been used, but there is surprisingly little objective evidence of their efficacy. Recently intravenous nitrates have been shown to work (see Chapter 24). In Prinzmetal's angina at rest (see Fig. 24-5), caused by coronary artery spasm, nitroglycerin is given for acute attacks and long-acting nitrates for prophylaxis; combination with calcium antagonists (verapamil, diltiazem, nifedipine) is usual.

Long-acting nitrates

The "nitrate controversy" relates to the long-held opinion that long-acting nitrates have few truly long-lasting effects (Opie and Thadani, 1984). Long-acting nitrates are to some extent again back in favor because with high doses there are long-lasting hemodynamic effects both in congestive heart failure and coronary heart disease without failure, and because single doses of long-acting nitrates can confer longer protection against angina than can single doses of sublingual

nitroglycerin. The probable explanation is the formation of the long-acting hepatic metabolites, isosorbide 5-mononitrate and isosorbide 2-mononitrate. Mononitrates are now being developed as long-acting nitrates in their own right.

A different question is whether or not regular therapy with long-acting nitrates gives long-lasting protection against angina. In an important placebo-controlled study, exercise duration improved significantly for 6–8 hours after single oral doses of 15–120 mg isosorbide dinitrate, but for only 2 hours when the same doses were given repetitively four times daily (Thadani et al., 1982). Partial tolerance to the anti-anginal effects during sustained therapy developed despite higher plasma isosorbide dinitrate concentrations during sustained therapy than those of acute therapy. Thus the anti-anginal effects of long-term therapy with long-acting nitrates are attenuated; this issue remains highly controversial.

Left ventricular failure and myocardial infarction

Nitrates as long-acting preparations have also been assessed for the therapy of acute and chronic heart failure. Their dilating effects are more pronounced on veins than on arterioles, so they are best suited to patients with raised pulmonary wedge pressures and clinical features of pulmonary congestion. In acute pulmonary edema from various causes, including acute myocardial infarction, nitroglycerin can be strikingly effective. However, there is some risk of precipitous falls in blood pressure and unexpected tachycardia or bradycardia. In patients with acute myocardial infarction it would be safest to give nitrates only to those who have obvious left ventricular failure, although there is growing evidence that "infarct size" can be reduced by nitrates. For optimal hemodynamic control, intravenous nitrates are best. In severe congestive heart failure nitrates may be used as the sole vasodilator agent or may be added to afterload reduction by hydralazine or nifedipine. As in the case of prazosin or hydralazine, tolerance to the vasodilating agent may develop, requiring temporary discontinuation or interruption of therapy.

Other coronary vasodilators

The **calcium antagonists** (Chapter 18) are as effective as nitrates in causing coronary vasodilation. In patients with coronary artery stenosis the calcium antagonists have an additional vasodilatory effect to that of the nitrates (Lichtlen et al., 1984). Experimentally, the cellular site of action of calcium antagonists differs from that of nitrates, which helps to justify the frequent clinical practice of combining nitrates and calcium antagonists.

Phosphodiesterase inhibitors such as the methyl-xanthines have also been classified as coronary vasodilators and are sometimes still used for that purpose. Their complex additional effects on intra-cellular calcium fluxes have prevented general use of these agents for conditions such as angina pectoris. Furthermore, clinical trials have not shown any pronounced efficacy.

Coronary steal

It has been feared that nitroglycerin may, by its vasodilator effect on the large coronary vessels, "steal" blood from the diseased zone. It is more likely that the vasodilators of small-resistance vessels such as dipyridamole (which inhibits adenosine breakdown) can cause a coronary steal by opening up small arterioles throughout the myocardium, so that there is a relative lack of blood in the critical endocardial zone where the blood flow is most likely to be compromised in angina pectoris. Nitrates not only increase blood flow to the diseased parts of the myocardium but increase endocardial flow (Fig. 17-8).

Clinical Uses of Vasodilators

In all varieties of **angina** it is chiefly the nitrates and calcium antagonists that are used (frequently with beta-adrenergic blockers); these agents have well-documented effects on the coronary arteries which oppose the vasoconstrictive tendency of beta-blockade. In **congestive heart failure** specific load reduction can be aimed at the afterload by hydralazine or nifedipine, or at the preload by nitrates or furosemide, or at both by nitroprusside or prazosin. In **hypertension**, it is the agents with a prominent effect on the afterload that are used (hydralazine, nifedipine) as well as prazosin. The latter agent has combined pre- and afterload-reducing actions of which the preload effect is wanted in heart failure but not in hypertension. Careful introduction and titration of the dose progressively reduces the blood pressure and allows

autonomic reflexes to compensate for the reduced preload.

Summary

The peripheral vascular resistance is related to the radius of the blood vessel (being inversely proportional to the fourth power of the radius). The peripheral vascular resistance is chiefly regulated by the rate of release of norepinephrine from the sympathetic nerve endings, which in turn is subject to positive or negative neuromodulation. The postjunctional alpha-receptors are the major sites of norepinephrine-induced calcium entry into muscular smooth muscle. The chief mechanisms for vasodilators are: (i) vascular alpha-adrenergic blockade; (ii) calcium-antagonism; and (iii) "direct" vasodilation by agents such as hydralazine, nitrates and nitroprusside. The chief uses of peripheral vasodilators are in hypertension and in congestive heart failure. The chief coronary vasodilators are the nitrates and calcium antagonists. Both have additional sites of action on the peripheral circulation, nitrates acting on the preload and calcium antagonists on the afterload. Both categories of agents are used for all varieties of angina pectoris.

References

Adelstein RS (1983). Regulation of contractile proteins by phosphorylation. J Clin Invest 72: 1863–1866.

Bodenheimer MM, Ramanathan K, Banka VS, Helfant RH (1981). Effect of progressive pressure reduction with nitroprusside on acute myocardial infarction in humans. Determination of optimal afterload. Ann Int Med 94: 435–439.

Bolton TB (1979). Mechanism of action of transmitters and other substances on smooth muscle. Physiol Rev 59: 606–718.

Cody RJ, Covit AB, Schaer GL, Laragh JH (1983). Evaluation of a long-acting converting enzyme inhibitor (enalapril) for the treatment of chronic congestive heart failure. J Am Coll Cardiol 14: 1154–1159.

Droogmans G, Raeymaekers L, Casteels R (1977). Electro- and pharmaco-mechanical coupling in the smooth muscle cells of the rabbit ear artery. J Gen Physiol 70: 129–148.

Franciosa JA, Dunkman WB, Wilen M, Silverstein S (1983). "Optimal" left ventricular filling pressure during nitroprusside infusion for congestive heart failure. Am J Med 74: 457–464.

Gershwin ME, Smith NT (1967). Mode of action of hydralazine on guinea pig atria. Arch Int Pharm 170: 108–116.

Gerthoffer WT, Trevethick MA, Murphy RA (1984). Myosin phosphorylation and cyclic adenosine 3′,5′-monophosphate in relaxation of arterial smooth muscle by vasodilators. Circ Res 54: 83–89.

Gorlin R, Brachfeld N, MacLeod C, Bopp P (1959). Effect of nitroglycerin on coronary circulation in patients with coronary artery disease or increased left ventricular work. Circulation 19: 705–718.

Hermsmeyer K, Trapani A, Abel PW (1981). Membrane potential dependent tension in vascular muscle. In: Vasodilatation. Eds. PM Vanhoutte, I Leusen, pp 273–284, Raven Press, New York.

Iacopino VJ, Fitzpatrick TM, Ranwell RW, Rose JC, Kot PA (1983). Cardiovascular response to leukotriene C4 in the rat. J Pharm Exp Therap 227: 244–247.

Johansson B (1978). Processes involved in vascular smooth muscle contraction and relaxation. Circ Res 43: Suppl 1, 14–20.

Keith RA, Burkman AM, Sokoloski TD, Fertel RH (1982). Vascular tolerance to nitroglycerin and cyclic GMP generation in rat aortic smooth muscle. J Pharm Exp Therap 221: 525–531.

Khatri B, Lenera N, Noleogiacomo F, Freis ED (1977). Direct and reflex cardiostimulatory effect of hydralazine. Am J Cardiol 40: 38–42.

Kolhardt M, Haap K (1978). 8-Bromo-guanosine 3′,5′-monophosphate mimics the effect of acetyl choline on slow response action potential and contractile force in mammalian atrial myocardium. J Molec Cell Cardiol 10: 573–586.

Kreye VAW (1981). Role of the membrane potential in the function of vascular smooth muscle. In: Vasodilatation. Eds. PM Vanhoutte, I Leusen, pp 299–305, Raven Press, New York.

Kukovetz WR, Holzmann S, Wurm A, Poch G (1979). Evidence for cyclic GMP-mediated relaxant effects of nitro-compounds in coronary smooth muscle. Naunyn-Schiedeberg's Arch Pharmacol 310: 129–138.

Lichtlen PR, Engel H-J, Rafflenbeul W (1984). Calcium entry blockers, especially nifedipine, in angina of effort: possible mechanisms and clinical implications. In: Calcium Antagonists and Cardiovascular Disease, Ed. LH Opie, pp 221–236, Raven Press, New York.

Mann T, Cohn PF, Holman BL, Green LH, Markis JE, Phillips DA (1978). Effect of nitroprusside on regional myocardial blood flow in coronary artery disease. Results in 25 patients and comparison with nitroglycerin. Circulation 57: 732–738.

Marcillio E, Reid PR, Dubin N, Ghodgaonkar R, Pitt B (1980). Myocardial prostaglandin release by nitroglycerin and modification by indomethacin. Am J Cardiol 45: 53–57.

Markham RV, Corbett JR, Gilmore A, Pettinger WA, Firth BG (1983). Efficacy of prazosin in the management of chronic congestive heart failure: a 6-month randomized double-blind, placebo-controlled study. Am J Cardiol 51: 1346–1352.

Mulvihall-Wilson J, Gaffney FA, Pettinger WA, Blomqvist CG, Anderson S, Graham RM (1983). Hemodynamic and neuroendocrine responses to acute and chronic alpha-adrenergic blockade with prazosin and phenoxybenzamine. Circulation 67: 383–393.

Murphy RA, Gerthoffer WT (1984). Cell calcium and contractile system regulation in arterial smooth muscle. In: Calcium-Antagonists and Cardiovascular Diseases, Ed. LH Opie, pp 75–84, Raven Press, New York.

Opie LH, Thadani U (1984). Nitrates. In: Drugs for the Heart, Ed. LH Opie, pp 23–37, Grune & Stratton, Orlando, London and New York.

Packer M, Meller J, Medina N, Gorlin R, Herman MV (1979). Rebound hemodynamic events after the abrupt withdrawal of nitroprusside in patients with severe chronic heart failure. N Eng J Med 301: 1193–1197.

Piper PJ (1983). Pharmacology of leukotrienes. Brit Med Bull 39: 255–259.

Rapoport RM, Draznin MB, Murad F (1983). Endothelium-dependent relaxation in rat aorta may be mediated through cyclic GMP-dependent protein phosphorylation. Nature 306: 174–176.

Rhodin JAG (1980). Architecture of the vessel wall. In: Handbook of Physiology, Section 2, The Cardiovascular System, Vol II. Ed. Berne RM, pp 1–31, American Physiological Society, Bethesda, Maryland.

Robinson BF (1967). Relation of heart rate and systolic blood pressure to the onset of pain in angina pectoris. Circulation 35: 1073–1083.

Rubin AA, Roth FE, Taylor RM, Rosenkilde J (1962). Pharmacology of diazoxide, an antihypertensive non-diuretic benzothiadiazine. J Pharm Exp Therap 136: 344–352.

Russell MP, Moran NC (1980). Evidence for lack of innervation of beta-2 adrenoceptors in the blood vessels of the gracilis muscle of the dog. Circ Res 46: 344–352.

Somlyo AV, Somlyo AP (1968). Electromechanical and pharmacomechanical coupling in vascular smooth muscle. J Pharm Exp Therap 159: 129–145.

Stephens NL, Kroeger EA (1981). Calcium sequestration and relaxation of vascular smooth muscle. In: Vasodilatation. Eds PM Vanhoutte and I Leusen, pp 367–380, Raven Press, New York.

Thadani U, Fung HL, Darke AC, Parker JO (1982). Oral isosorbide dinitrate in angina pectoris. Comparison of duration of action and dose response relation during acute and sustained therapy. Am J Cardiol 49: 411–419.

Towart R (1981). The selective inhibition of serotonin-induced contractions of rabbit cerebral smooth muscle by calcium-antagonistic dihydropyridines. An investigation of the mechanism of action of nimodipine. Circ Res 48: 650–657.

Van Meel JCA, de Jonge A, Kalleman HO, Wilffert B, Timmermans PBMWM, van Zwieten PA (1981). Vascular smooth muscle contraction initiated by postsynaptic alpha$_2$-adrenoceptor activation is induced by an influx of extracellular calcium. Europ J Pharmacol 69: 205–208.

New References

Abshagen U (1985). Clinical Pharmacology and Antianginal Drugs. Springer-Verlag, Berlin.

Bühler FR, Bolli P (1985). Andrenoceptors, calcium and excitation-contraction coupling: Mechanisms and pharmacological interference (eds). J Cardiovasc Pharmacol 7 (Suppl 6): S3–S209.

Hathaway DR, Konicki MV, Coolican SA (1985). Phosphorylation of myosin light chain kinase from vascular smooth muscle by cAMP- and cGMP-dependent protein kinases. J Molec Cell Cardiol 17: 841–850.

Refsum H, Mjos OD (1985). Alpha-adrenoceptor blockers in cardiovascular disease. Churchhill Livingstone, Edinburgh.

Schröder H, Noack E, Müller R (1985). Evidence for a correlation between nitric oxide formation by cleavage of organic nitrates and activation of guanylate cyclase. J Molec Cell Cardiol 17: 931–934.

Serneri GC, McGiff JC, Paoletti R, Born GVR (1985). Platelets, prostaglandins and the cardiovascular system. Advances in Prostaglandin, Thromboxane and Leukotriene Research, Vol 13. Raven Press, New York.

Vanhoutte PM, Amery A (1985). Serotonergic mechanisms in the cardiovascular system (eds). J Cardiovasc Pharmacol 7 (Suppl 7): S2–S182.

Calcium Antagonists
(Slow Channel Blockers)

Calcium antagonist drugs can exert the most profound effects on the cardiovascular system by modifying the effects of calcium ion fluxes. Calcium ion fluxes control both myocardial contraction and the tone of vascular smooth muscle. Calcium ion fluxes contribute to the pacemaker current in the sinus node, to conduction of the impulse in the atrioventricular node and to the action potential plateau in atrial, Purkinje and ventricular fibers. Fortunately, the therapeutic effects of calcium antagonists are found in concentrations which inhibit vascular smooth muscle contraction (thereby causing coronary and peripheral vasodilation) or the atrioventricular node (in the case of verapamil and diltiazem) without exerting an undue negative inotropic effect. All three "first generation" agents (verapamil, diltiazem and nifedipine) are used in the treatment of angina of effort and angina at rest. An important additional practical point is that these three calcium antagonists act on different sites to produce clinically divergent effects—thus verapamil and diltiazem can inhibit supraventricular tachycardias with circuits through the atrioventricular node, while nifedipine acts more powerfully on the peripheral vasculature.

Basic Properties of
Calcium Antagonists

Besides their diversity of action, the major calcium antagonists (verapamil, nifedipine, diltiazem) do share common properties. All can, in the appropriate experimental conditions, have the following effects: (i) inhibition of contractile activity; (ii) inhibition of conduction through the atrioventricular node; (iii) inhibition of smooth muscle contraction. At an electrophysiological level, all these agents can decrease the entry of calcium ions by the slow channel as shown by voltage-clamp studies on myocardial tissue. They can all inhibit excitation–contraction coupling in smooth muscle and the slow responses provoked by cyclic AMP when the fast channel is blocked. All calcium antagonists also lessen myocardial necrosis caused by very high doses of catecholamines, and inhibit calcium-dependent reperfusion damage. The common denominator to all the above effects is inhibition of transmembrane calcium influx. It is for this reason that there are alternative names including calcium channel blockers (Table 18-1). In electrophysiological terms there is also true calcium antagonism as well as blockade, so that it is acceptable to use one of several terms for this category of agents (Lee and Tsien, 1983).

Electrophysiologically, it is the inhibition of the slow inward current that is now widely regarded as the critical property common to all calcium antagonists and explains one of the current names, viz. "calcium entry blocking agents".

The initial and classical calcium antagonist effect obtained by Fleckenstein (1971) was the decreased inotropic effect of verapamil, antagonized by the injection of calcium salts (Fig. 18-1). It is now known

Table 18-1

Alternative names for calcium antagonists

Name proposed	Point of emphasis
Ca^{2+}-antagonist	Reversal by Ca^{2+} of verapamil-induced cardiodepressant effect; allows for possible intracellular site of action in vascular smooth muscle. Defect: calcium fails to antagonize effect of verapamil on AV node.
Ca^{2+}-channel antagonist (or inhibitor or blocker)	Selective inhibition by these agents of the Ca^{2+}-dependent component of the cardiac action potential.
Ca^{2+}-entry antagonist	Allows for inhibition of calcium entry by channels not operated by depolarization.
Slow channel antagonist (or inhibitor or blocker)	Slow inward calcium channel also carries Na^+ ions in some experimental conditions (although $100 : 1$ preference for Ca^{2+}).

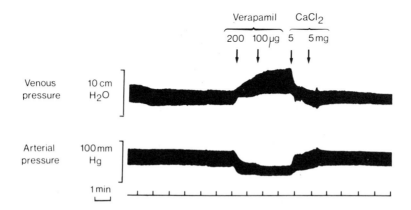

Fig. 18-1 The original experiment of Fleckenstein (1971) in which acute heart failure was produced in a guinea-pig by excess verapamil (about 10 times more than the usual clinical intravenous dose). Note that intravenous calcium salts antagonize the negative inotropic effect, hence the term "calcium antagonist" drug. Reproduced with permission.

that the tissue most sensitive to verapamil is not the myocardium but the atrioventricular node, and that therapeutic effects can be found at concentrations which have no effect on the sinus node nor on myocardial contractility; hence the effective use of verapamil in supraventricular tachycardias. Unexpectedly, the inhibitory effect on the atrioventricular node is only partially antagonized by an increased extracellular calcium (Harriman et al., 1979), whereas the inhibitory effect on the sinus node is not at all antagonized by calcium (Kolhardt et al., 1972). These differences argue for the concept of varying properties of the slow calcium channel in various tissue (myocardium vs atrioventricular node vs sinus node). Hence Nayler et al. (1984) propose that there are different types of calcium channels in different tissues—class I in the myocardium, class II in the vasculature and class III in nodal tissue. Alternatively, the same calcium channels in different tissues could

have different binding sites for the various drugs, or the drug-binding site interaction could vary. In rapidly firing atrial tissue such as that involved in re-entrant supraventricular tachycardias, the use-dependent qualities of verapamil and diltiazem may explain their greater efficacy over agents such as nifedipine which are not use-dependent (Lee and Tsien, 1983).

Membrane binding sites

Two types of sarcolemmal binding sites have been identified (Fig. 18-2). First, the dihydropyridine site should bind nifedipine but for technical reasons the related compound nitrendipine is usually used. Secondly, the other calcium channel antagonists such as verapamil and diltiazem bind to another spatially separated ("allosteric") site to modify the dihydropyridine site. Some indirect evidence suggests that the

HYPOTHESIS FOR Ca²⁺ ANTAGONISTS

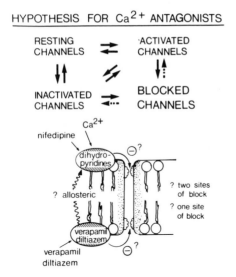

Fig. 18-2 Hypothesis for two types of sarcolemmal binding sites for calcium antagonist drugs, and their possible allosteric interaction. For details see text, Murphy et al. (1983), Dompert and Traber (1984) and Sperelakis (1984).

dihydropyridine site is located on the outer layer of the cell membrane, and the verapamil–diltiazem site on the inner layer (Hescheler et al., 1982). The dihydropyridine binding site may be near the calcium channel or part of it; it certainly interacts with the calcium channel because a new dihydropyridine with agonist properties mediates calcium influx (Schramm et al., 1983). Some investigators suggest that these drugs bind with different affinities to several populations of calcium channels; alternatively, the properties of one type of calcium channel may be regulated differently by allosteric influences — the latter idea resembles the modulated receptor hypothesis proposed for the sodium channel. Preferential binding of calcium antagonists to inactivated channels is suggested because they block inactivated cardiac calcium channels more than normal channels (Kanaya et al., 1983).

Structural–activity relationships

The verapamil group of calcium antagonists, structurally characterized by an aryl ring connected to an alkylamino or aralkylamino group, includes verapamil, diltiazem, cinnarizine and tiapamil (Meyer, 1983). The binding site for this group is sometimes identified by ³H-cinnarizine. Both verapamil and diltiazem have stereoselectivity. The second ("nifedipine") group of calcium antagonists, the 1,4 dihydropyridines, is completely different in structure from the verapamil group and includes nicardipine, nitrendipine, nimodipine, nisoldipine and felodipine. A third and very new type of calcium antagonist, KB-944, resembles diltiazem from the pharmacological point of view, but has an aralkyl phosphonate group.

The physiological significance of both types of binding sites is still in question. One view is that such binding sites do not identify the physiological active calcium channels, in contrast to the radiolabeled beta-adrenergic antagonists which specifically bind to the beta-receptor. Because blockade of the calcium current requires doses of dihydropyridines more than 100 times higher than those that bind to the sarcolemmal sites (Lee and Tsien, 1983), there may be a "step-up" amplification system at work. A second view is that the basic effect of all calcium antagonists is ultimately at the dihydropyridine site (Murphy et al., 1983) with agents binding on the "second" verapamil–diltiazem site acting on the dihydropyridine site by means of "allosteric" control.

Alpha-adrenergic receptors

The vascular postjunctional alpha-2-adrenergic receptors are seen increasingly as a major site of action of the calcium antagonists on vascular smooth muscle (Chapter 17). Such an interaction would explain why calcium antagonists rather than alpha-1-blocking agents lessen coronary spasm caused by adrenergic stimulation. In addition, some calcium antagonists (verapamil and diltiazem much more so than nifedipine) have a weak interaction with the alpha-1-adrenergic receptors. Possibly some of the high-dose effects of calcium antagonists against ischemic ventricular arrhythmias can be explained by this mechanism.

Sodium channels

Verapamil in the racemic form (*dl*) clinically used also inhibits the fast sodium channel in high doses. The (*d*) isomer is the more specific inhibitor of the calcium channel, while the (*l*) isomer has more of an effect on the sodium channel which explains its quinidine-like antiarrhythmic properties (Gloor and Urthaler, 1983).

Table 18-2

Relative effects of calcium antagonists in experimental preparations compared with therapeutic levels in man

	Verapamil	Nifedipine	Diltiazem
Therapeutic levels in man			
ng/mL	80–400	25–100	50–300
molecular weight	455	346	415
molar value	$2–8 \times 10^7$ M	$0.5–2 \times 10^7$ M	$1–7 \times 10^7$ M
protein binding	about 90%	about 95%	about 85%
molar value, corrected for protein binding	$2–8 \times 10^{-8}$ M	$0.3–1 \times 10^{-8}$ M	$1–5 \times 10^{-8}$ M
Usual oral dose	80–160 mg daily	10–20 mg daily	30–90 mg three times daily
Isolated coronary artery contraction			
50% inhibition	10^{-7} M	10^{-8} M	10^{-7} M
Myocardial depression			
40% depression of contractile force	5×10^{-6} M	5×10^{-7} M	5×10^{-4} M
Fast sodium current depression	10^{-4} M	no effect	10^{-4} M
Alpha-blockade, K_1 (myocardium)	5×10^{-7} M	4×10^{-6} M	7×10^{-6} M
Slowing of heart rate by 20%	10^{-6} M	10^{-5} M	10^{-8} M
Relative effect on AV node vs contractile force	6.5 : 1	1 : 1	20 : 1
Inhibition of enzyme release from infarcting myocardium	2×10^{-7} M	10^{-7} M	10^{-7} M
Inhibition of ventricular automaticity (ventricular fibrillation threshold in coronary ligated rat heart)	10^{-7} M	10^{-6} M	5×10^{-6} M

For data sources, see Singh and Opie (1984). In: Drugs for the Heart. Ed. LH Opie, pp 39–62, Grune & Stratton, Orlando, London and New York.

Diltiazem has similar sodium inhibitory effects, whereas nifedipine has little or no effect (Table 18-2).

Potassium channels

Another similarity of racemic verapamil to quinidine is in the inhibition of the repolarizing potassium current in the myocardium; this effect would tend to prolong the action potential duration in contrast to the shortening resulting from the inhibition of the slow inward current; hence there is little net effect of verapamil on the action potential duration. Of the various calcium antagonists it is nisoldipine which has no effect on the repolarizing current (Kass, 1983), and is from this point of view the "purest" of the various agents now available.

Vascular smooth muscle

In the myocardium it is clear that the major effect of the calcium antagonists is on the calcium channel and not on an intracellular site. In vascular smooth muscle, voltage-clamping is a difficult technique; hence proof of the effect on the slow inward current has been more difficult to obtain. The influx of $^{45}Ca^{2+}$ is not inhibited by verapamil, nifedipine or diltiazem (Church and Zsoter, 1980). Possibly an interaction with calmodulin may explain at least part of the inhibition of contraction of vascular smooth muscle by calcium antagonist drugs (Bostrom et al., 1981).

Autonomic effects

Calcium antagonists cause reflex sympathetic stimulation by peripheral vasodilation. Vagal inhibition is also withdrawn. Both effects are most marked in the case of nifedipine, and least in the case of diltiazem.

Calcium Antagonists versus Beta-adrenergic Receptor Blockade

At a cellular level there are marked differences between the effects of beta-adrenergic blockade and calcium

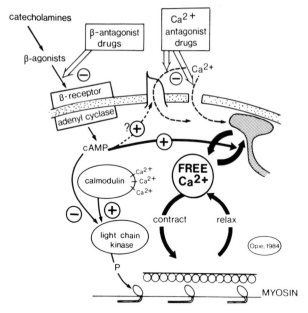

Fig. 18-3 Vascular smooth muscle. Contrasting cellular effects of calcium antagonists and beta-adrenergic receptor antagonist drugs. Calcium antagonists, by decreasing the cytosolic free calcium ion concentration in vascular smooth muscle, decrease calmodulin activity to decrease the activity of myosin light chain kinase. These processes lessen the phosphorylation of myosin light chain which is required for vascular smooth muscle contraction, so smooth muscle relaxes. Beta antagonists (i) allow a higher cytosolic calcium by decreasing uptake of calcium ions into the sarcoplasmic reticulum and (ii) lessen the inhibition by cyclic AMP of the phosphorylation of the myosin light chains. Both effects increase smooth muscle contraction. In addition, unopposed alpha-adrenergic mediated vascular spasm worsens the vasoconstrictive effect of beta-adrenergic antagonists.

antagonists on the vascular smooth muscle, where beta-blockade tends to vasoconstrict and calcium antagonists to relax. The probable explanation is that the beta-adrenergic receptor blockers act to reduce the formation of cyclic AMP within the vascular smooth muscle cell, which in turn inhibits the kinase required to phosphorylate the myosin light chains (Fig. 18-3). In the case of the myocardium, a common property is shared—that of reducing calcium influx by the slow channel. This the calcium antagonists do directly by "closing" the number of slow channels and the beta-antagonists indirectly, by decreasing the phosphorylation of the sarcolemmal protein which is hypothetically involved with slow channel control. In clinically

relevant doses, however, the chief calcium antagonist drugs have their therapeutic effect without a negative inotropic effect, whereas in the case of beta-adrenergic blockade, the negative inotropic effect is an integrated part of the anti-anginal mechanism.

Verapamil

Verapamil was introduced for angina pectoris as a calcium antagonist agent with vasodilator properties. More recently its major use has been for supraventricular tachycardias, especially re-entrant tachycardias involving the atrioventricular node. Even more recently, verapamil has been re-studied for its effects in angina of effort and angina at rest, where it is a remarkably effective agent.

Electrophysiological properties

Singh and Vaughan Williams (1972) established that high concentrations of verapamil could depress contractility while there was no inhibition of the fast sodium channel, thereby confirming that verapamil uncoupled excitation from contraction. They assigned verapamil to a new class of antiarrhythmic agents, class IV. Although verapamil had only minor effects on the ventricular action potential, it caused major changes in the action potential of the atrioventricular node (Landmark and Amlie, 1976), especially in the upper and middle nodal regions (Wit and Cranefield, 1974), where the slow inward current is a major component of the action potential.

By inhibiting slow channel-mediated conduction in the atrioventricular node, verapamil inhibits one limb of the re-entry circuit which is believed to underlie most paroxysmal supraventricular tachycardias. Increased atrioventricular block also explains the reduction of ventricular rate in atrial flutter and fibrillation. In contrast, verapamil has negligible effects on ventricular arrhythmias. Because of the effect of verapamil on the atrioventricular node, digitalis toxicity with AV nodal inhibition is an absolute contra-indication to rapid intravenous administration of verapamil.

Supraventricular arrhythmias

In paroxysmal supraventricular tachycardia an intravenous bolus of 5–10 mg restores sinus rhythm in 75 percent or more of cases (Singh and Roche, 1977) (see Fig. 23-4). Oral verapamil is also used to prevent attacks. In atrial fibrillation, whether or not previously treated with digitalis, intravenous verapamil reduces the ventricular rate with "regularization" in some cases (Khalsa and Olsson, 1979). Usually the benefits of inhibiting the tachycardia, which allows better ventricular filling, outweigh the disadvantages of the fall in blood pressure (vasodilation, negative inotropic effect). When there is co-existing myocardial disease, slow infusion or oral treatment (taking only 2 hours to act) is preferred to bolus infusion unless reduction of ventricular rate is urgent, when a low-dose bolus may be given. Clinical experience suggests that a bolus is more effective than an infusion for termination of supraventricular tachycardias.

In atrial flutter the block is increased; occasionally sinus rhythm is restored (especially in acute infarction), or the rhythm changes to atrial fibrillation. In acute atrial fibrillation an infusion allows control of the ventricular rate while oral verapamil or digoxin is taking effect (Fig. 18-4). In chronic atrial fibrillation, oral verapamil is frequently added to digoxin to achieve optimal control of ventricular rate. In the Wolff–Parkinson–White (WPW) syndrome, verapamil has no effects on the accessory pathway but

depresses the atrioventricular node and counters the reciprocating re-entry tachycardias. Verapamil does not work and may be harmful where there is atrial flutter or fibrillation with anterograde conduction down the anomalous bundle. In acute myocardial infarction, verapamil has been used with success in supraventricular tachyarrhythmias within the first 72 hours.

Negative inotropic effect and heart rate

A striking negative inotropic effect is seen in some experimental preparations, although seldom encountered with normal clinical doses (Table 18-2). Verapamil may cause very serious cardiodepression in diseased or beta-blocked hearts, especially when given rapidly intravenously; on the other hand, when given to patients with coronary artery disease without heart failure or conduction block, intravenous verapamil actually improves left ventricular performance, probably because of afterload reduction (Ferlinz et al., 1979). A new procedure to minimize the cardiodepressant effect of intravenous verapamil is to pretreat the patient with an intravenous calcium salt (Weiss et al., 1983).

It may be wondered why verapamil usually does not cause sinus bradycardia, despite depressing the automaticity of the sinus node. The usual explanation is that the peripheral vasodilating effect of verapamil probably leads to a reflex tachycardia, offsetting the direct bradycardia caused by sinoatrial depression and helping to maintain the cardiac output (Fig. 18-5). Yet even in beta-blocked patients, verapamil usually does not cause any major additive bradycardia. The explanation may be that the concentration required for an effect on the sinus node is lower than that needed for inhibition of excess rates of conduction through the AV node.

Other clinical indications

Besides inhibition of the atrioventricular node, verapamil is largely used for **angina** (Fig. 18-6). Verapamil is effective against angina of effort and very effective against coronary spasm, as in Prinzmetal's variant angina and some varieties of angina at rest. In **hypertrophic cardiomyopathy**, verapamil may be **more effective than beta-blockade (Kaltenbach et al., 1979). The response to verapamil is not uniform and**

ATRIAL FIBRILLATION/FLUTTER

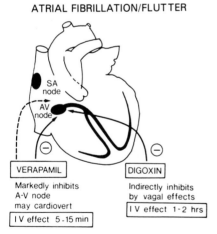

Fig. 18-4 Use of intravenous (IV) verapamil rapidly to inhibit atrioventricular (AV) nodal conduction in atrial flutter or fibrillation (see also Fig. 23-4). The resulting slowing of the ventricular rate is of considerable importance in patients with ischemic heart disease in whom tachycardia may precipitate angina. Even when given intravenously, digoxin takes longer for its vagal inhibitory effects to occur. Verapamil and digoxin inhibit the AV node by different, additive mechanisms.

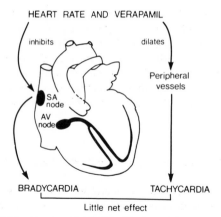

HEART RATE AND VERAPAMIL

inhibits   dilates

Peripheral
vessels

SA node
AV node

BRADYCARDIA   TACHYCARDIA

Little net effect

Fig. 18-5 Verapamil directly inhibits the sinoatrial (SA) node. Its indirect vasodilatory effect allows a compensatory reflex tachycardia with little net effect on the sinus rate (see Singh and Roche, 1977).

EFFECT OF CALCIUM ANTAGONISTS ON THE HEART

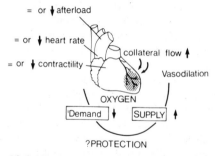

= or ↓ afterload

= or ↓ heart rate

collateral flow ↑

= or ↓ contractility

Vasodilation

OXYGEN

Demand ↓   SUPPLY ↑

?PROTECTION

Fig. 18-6 Possible modes of action of calcium antagonists on the ischemic myocardium. As a group, calcium antagonists act chiefly by improving the oxygen supply. Reduced oxygen demand is achieved by different mechanisms in the case of different agents.

cannot be predicted by acute hemodynamic studies. **In hypertension** verapamil is now becoming an established therapeutic agent; usually high doses are needed. Excess entry of calcium ions into cells may underlie the development of myocardial necrosis, hence calcium antagonist agents are being evaluated both experimentally (Yellon et al., 1983) and clinically for their potential effect in reducing **"infarct size"**.

Nifedipine

Nifedipine in some way resembles and in many ways differs from verapamil. As with verapamil, the original emphasis was on its coronary vasodilator properties, which explains its use in Prinzmetal's variant angina and other syndromes produced by coronary artery spasm. More recently its qualities as an unloading agent have been used in management of hypertension, acute pulmonary edema and angina of effort.

Electrophysiological properties

At a cellular level, nifedipine is a highly specific inhibitor of the myocardial slow inward current and acts without altering kinetics (Bayer et al., 1977). Unlike racemic verapamil, nifedipine has no effect on the fast sodium channel and little on the alpha-1-adrenergic receptors. The inhibition of the slow calcium channel appears to be maximal in the smooth muscle vascular wall, where nifedipine is 15 times more active than on cardiac muscle cells (Nayler and Poole-Wilson, 1981). On coronary smooth muscle the action of nifedipine is more powerful than that of verapamil (Himori et al., 1976). Although high concentrations of nifedipine can suppress conduction through the atrioventricular node of the dog, in the doses used for patients with angina pectoris or hypertension there is no clinically detected effect on the conduction system of the human heart (Rowland et al., 1979).

Angina pectoris

Besides its established efficacy in Prinzmetal's angina (Yasue et al., 1976), nifedipine is effective against angina of effort (de Ponti et al., 1979) and against pacing-induced angina (Lorell et al., 1981). Whereas nitrates do not benefit pacing-induced angina when given into the coronary arteries, nifedipine does so even when given as a very small dose (0.1 mg of a special intravenous preparation) which has no detectable peripheral effect (Kaltenbach et al., 1979). The dual mechanism is first by vasodilation of the coronary vessels and by widening of the stenotic site, and secondly by a favorable influence on myocardial metabolism. When given normally by the oral or sublingual route, afterload reduction is an important component of its mechanism (Engel and Lichtlen, 1981). Careful dose titration (for usual dose, see Table 18-2) is required to ensure that an excessive peripheral effect does not over-reduce blood pressure, thereby occasionally worsening angina of effort (Deanfield et al., 1983) and unstable angina.

Arterial vasodilation

Nifedipine consistently and rapidly reduces the arterial pressure (Fig. 18-7), acting by peripheral vasodilation. Some of its analogs may act preferentially on certain vascular beds so that, for example, a more specific cerebral vasodilating effect is possible (Towart, 1981). It is the afterload reducing effect which has led to the successful use of nifedipine in left-sided heart failure and acute pulmonary edema (Polese et al., 1979).

Thus nifedipine is a promising agent with few serious side-effects and useful in various disorders, especially angina (whether induced by spasm or effort) and hypertension. Because its major effect is to reduce the afterload nifedipine may be combined safely with beta-adrenergic blockade except in a few patients where additive hypotension presents a problem (Jee and Opie, 1984).

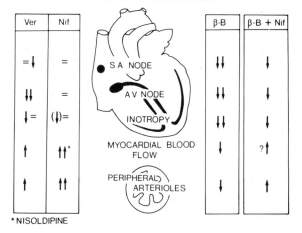

Ca^2 ANTAGONISTS VERSUS β-BLOCKADE

* NISOLDIPINE

Fig. 18-7 The major site of action of nifedipine (Nif) is the arteriolar vascular resistance, to cause peripheral and coronary vasodilation. These are the mechanisms of the beneficial effect in hypertension and angina pectoris. In congestive heart failure, afterload reduction may improve myocardial pump function. Verapamil (Ver) has similar though less marked vascular effect, with added depression of nodal tissue and a mild negative inotropic effect. These properties of calcium antagonists contrast with those of beta-adrenergic blockers (BB). The combination of nifedipine and beta-blockade reduces the negative inotropic and chronotropic effects of beta-blockade, and appears to improve peripheral blood flow. For clinical effects of calcium antagonists combined with beta-blockers see Chapter 24. From Jee and Opie (1984), with permission from Raven Press.

New dihydropyridines

Nitrendipine is about to be introduced as a long-acting vasodilator for the therapy of hypertension. **Nimodipine** is a potential cerebral vasodilator, while **nisoldipine** has both venous and arteriolar dilating effects. **Nicardipine** is primarily an arteriolar vasodilator. Of the dihydropyridines, nifedipine is likely to become the "gold-standard".

Diltiazem

Diltiazem is a newer agent than verapamil and nifedipine, having only recently become available clinically. Like these other agents diltiazem is very effective in Prinzmetal's angina and variant angina (Schroeder et al., 1982), and in angina of effort (for dose, see Table 18-2). The experimental sites of action are, however, somewhat different from the other two agents (Fig. 18-8). Diltiazem is also effective in arterial hypertension (Strauss et al., 1982) although not yet well tested. Its ability to inhibit the sinus node might account for part of the benefit in angina (Mitchell et al., 1982). Like other calcium antagonists, diltiazem protects against reperfusion damage and promotes recovery from ischemia (Sasayama et al., 1981). Preliminary reports show that it has a verapamil-like effect against re-entrant supraventricular arrhythmias (Fujimoto et al., 1981).

Experimentally it has remarkable effects in decreasing the severity of ischemia without causing myocardial depression, acting by a combination of

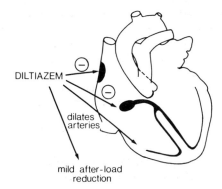

Fig. 18-8 Some of the proposed sites of action of diltiazem. Although the spectrum of experimental activity differs from that of verapamil and nifedipine (Table 18-2), in practice all three agents are effective against all types of angina pectoris.

coronary vasodilation, afterload reduction and "metabolic protection" (Hamm et al., 1982). Even in normal unsedated dogs, diltiazem causes less cardio-depression than either nifedipine or verapamil (Walsh et al., 1981). It might be concluded that diltiazem is less inhibitory on the myocardial calcium channels concerned with contractility and relatively more effective on the vascular calcium channels.

Other Calcium Antagonists

The class B calcium antagonists include perhexiline, prenylamine, and lidoflazine and bepridil. These agents have ancillary effects, making their true classification difficult. As a group, they have prominent sodium channel antagonist qualities and also interfere with the magnesium channel (Fleckenstein, 1984). Clinically class B agents are much less widely used than verapamil, diltiazem or nifedipine.

Prenylamine is of interest as it is an agent known to inhibit calmodulin in vascular smooth muscle. It also has many other complex effects such as inhibition of the fast channel and inhibition of the slow calcium channel. These diverse effects may explain its use as an anti-anginal agent (Winsor et al., 1971). Today it has largely been replaced by the standard calcium-antagonists.

Perhexiline has major side-effects (nervous system and liver) which limits its use for angina pectoris to those patients not responding to all other conventional agents.

Lidoflazine is an agent previously criticized by clinicians because it was feared that it caused "coronary steal". Now it is being used again for angina pectoris (Shapiro et al., 1982); like diltiazem it reduces heart rate. Lidoflazine may safely be combined with propranolol according to a preliminary report (Losardo et al., 1982).

Bepridil is a sodium–calcium blocker under evaluation for treating angina and arrhythmias (Narahara et al., 1984).

(For other new compounds, see Table 18-3).

Comparative Clinical Indications of Calcium Antagonists

Coronary artery spasm

As originally described by Prinzmetal, typical variant angina may occur at the site of an atheromatous lesion of a large coronary artery. Yasue (1984) showed a marked circadian rhythm in the susceptibility to coronary artery spasm, with most attacks occurring at night or in the early morning—possibly as a result of the high blood pH at night which in turn may induce an increase in the ionized serum calcium to provoke attacks. Calcium antagonists (including diltiazem, nifedipine, verapamil) all inhibit these attacks, whereas beta-blockade by propranolol is ineffective—and may be harmful (Hugenholtz et al., 1984). At present the best procedure for management of coronary artery spasm is the combination of nitrates and a calcium antagonist. Thus Conti et al. (1984) advise isosorbide dinitrate and nifedipine, each 10–30 mg 6-hourly.

Angina at rest

Besides being more effective than beta-adrenergic blockade in the therapy of variant angina, calcium antagonists may also be better therapy in some patients with angina at rest (Hugenholtz et al., 1984). Parodi et al. (1984) have shown that there is no benefit from beta-adrenergic blockade whereas calcium antagonism is very effective in some patients with angina at rest, especially when arterial spasm plays an important role. Spasm may contribute to the development of angina at rest, especially at night (Yasue, 1984). Hence calcium antagonists are now used increasingly with apparently beneficial effects: large-scale trials are presently comparing beta-adrenergic blockade with calcium antagonists in unstable angina at rest. The concept of spasm has been further extended to some patients with exercise-induced ST-elevation (Jee and Opie, 1984), in whom beta-adrenergic blockade is ineffective in contrast to calcium antagonists. A novel proposal is that varying degrees of spasm play a role in determining the different and variable levels of exercise which provoke angina in some patients.

Stable angina of effort

Initially it was thought that calcium antagonists lessened angina of effort by unloading the heart, as a result of peripheral vasodilation. Lichtlen et al. (1984) show two further important effects: an increase of post-stenotic coronary flow and actual relief of the spastic component of severe coronary obstruction, where the effects of nifedipine and nitrates appear to be additive. In the case of verapamil, a mild negative

Table 18-3

Some new calcium antagonists

	Comment
1. Dihydropyridines	
Nitrendipine	Specific arterial action; long duration of action; in use for hypertension, coronary spasm.
Nimodipine	Cerebrovascular dilator; in use for cerebral spasm, migraine, transient ischemic attacks.
Nisoldipine	Highly specific inhibitor of calcium current (Kass, 1983). Combined veno-arterial dilator. Being evaluated for congestive heart failure, hypertension.
Felodipine	May act on calmodulin (Bostrom et al., 1981); clinically similar to nitrendipine.
Nicardipine	Under evaluation for angina.
2. Verapamil-like	
Tiapamil	Similar to verapamil; also reduces heart rate.
3. Mixed agents	
Bepridil	Combined Na^+/Ca^{2+} blocker; being evaluated for angina and ventricular arrhythmias. **(Some risk of prolonged QT-interval)**

inotropic effect probably contributes to the anti-anginal effect. With diltiazem, a mild negative chronotropic effect may be a factor. As a group, calcium antagonists are at least as effective as beta-adrenergic blockers in patients with stable angina of effort and in some studies, calcium antagonists are more effective.

Arrhythmias

In supraventricular re-entrant arrhythmias, only verapamil has received a thorough testing; diltiazem may still emerge as an equally effective agent with possibly less risk of hemodynamic depression. In ventricular ischemic arrhythmias, slow response action potentials may be calcium-dependent and may initiate re-entrant ventricular arrhythmias (Sperelakis, 1984). Slow responses may already be inhibited in severely ischemic cells by marked acidosis, loss of ATP and by a very high extracellular K^+. Hence, even if slow responses were to play a role in ischemic ventricular fibrillation, then it may be expected that calcium antagonists would not be active against ventricular arrhythmias arising in severely ischemic tissue (Opie et al., 1984). Another reason for the ineffectiveness of calcium antagonists in ventricular ischemic arrhythmias is that the apparent slow action potentials in ischemic tissue may really be fast sodium channels whose activity is depressed (Chapter 23).

Hypertension

The marked effect of the calcium antagonist nifedipine on arterial vascular smooth muscle and the important role of calcium ions in the contractile mechanism of vascular smooth muscle, makes nifedipine an important antihypertensive agent (Rosendorff, 1984). Besides acute reduction of blood pressure, nifedipine has a sustained antihypertensive effect so that it can be used for apparently refractory hypertension with a satisfactory response (Opie and Jee, 1984). Part of the benefit of nifedipine may be in a capacity to promote salt and water excretion while leaving potassium excretion unchanged (Krebs, 1984). Hence there are expanding indications for nifedipine in hypertension suggesting that calcium antagonists as a group are well on the way to becoming a standard vasodilator therapy, displacing hydralazine. Calcium antagonists have fewer contra-indications than beta-adrenergic blockade (Table 18-4). Bühler et al. (1984) show a specific benefit of calcium antagonism by verapamil (and nifedipine) in elderly patients, in whom there is peripheral vasoconstriction dependent on calcium influx. The best response to verapamil appears to be in elderly patients with low plasma renin — the group which is least likely to respond to beta-adrenergic blockade. Calcium antagonists normalize blood pressure in at least one-third of patients with essential hypertension; in one trial nifedipine mono-therapy was uniformly effective over 24 hours provided that the dose was sufficiently high (Gould et al., 1982).

Future indications

Expanding indications for calcium antagonists are prophesied (Krebs, 1984). Cardiovascular indications currently under investigation include myocardial infarction, ventricular arrhythmias, congestive heart failure, pulmonary hypertension, cardioplegia, atherogenesis, hypertrophic cardiomyopathy, aortic insufficiency and cerebral stroke. In most cases the results are sufficiently promising to warrant further clinical exploration. In Raynaud's phenomenon, sublingual nifedipine usually gives rapid relief. Besides new indications there may be more "tissue-specific" calcium antagonists—for example, nimodipine acts more specifically on the cerebral circulation and nisoldipine resembles nifedipine but also acts on venous smooth muscle.

Side-effects of Calcium Antagonists

Initially the potential for severe side-effects with verapamil was stressed by reports of fatalities when intravenous verapamil was rapidly given to isolated patients with pre-existing atrioventricular inhibition through disease or beta-adrenergic blockade. Also the thrust of Fleckenstein's original experiments, defining myocardial depression as an inevitable consequence of calcium antagonism, led to reservations about the possible hazards of calcium antagonists as negative inotropic agents (Fig. 18-1). In particular, combination therapy using calcium antagonists and beta-adrenergic blockade was feared. While there still is some truth in these fears, it is now apparent that calcium antagonists when used correctly seldom induce serious side-effects.

In the case of **verapamil** contra-indications include: sick sinus syndrome, pre-existing AV-nodal disease, excess therapy with beta-adrenergic blockade or digitalis and significant myocardial depression. These apply particularly when intravenous verapamil is given rapidly in the therapy of supraventricular tachycardias. Another reservation is in the rarer type of Wolff–Parkinson–White syndrome with antegrade conduction through the bypass tract; here the risk is that atrial fibrillation can be conducted too rapidly to the ventricles with the possibility of ventricular

fibrillation. The fear is that verapamil may accelerate antegrade conduction by its inhibitory effect on the AV node. In the average patient with angina pectoris, verapamil therapy is probably as safe or safer than beta-adrenergic blockade. Two extreme reactions reported for beta-blockade—fatal bronchospasm and gangrene—have thus far not been found with verapamil, nor can they be expected. Cardiovascular collapse, occasionally found in patients with borderline heart failure given beta-adrenergic blockade, can be provoked when intravenous verapamil (Opie, 1980) is given incorrectly in the presence of overt cardiomegaly.

In the case of **nifedipine**, very few life-threatening adverse reactions have been found, probably because of the absence of clinical effects on the AV node, while the peripheral vasodilation presumably prevents overt heart failure from developing in patients with borderline failure. Nifedipine has caused excess hypotension or cardiovascular depression in a few seriously ill patients (Opie and White, 1980). In the vast majority of patients without serious pre-existing myocardial disease, nifedipine has been given with only a few side-effects such as facial flushing, ankle edema (mechanism unknown) and exaggeration of varicose veins. Sometimes lightheadedness or dizziness prevents continuation of nifedipine therapy. Although the powerful hypotensive effect of nifedipine could have been expected to cause frequent tachycardia and orthostatic hypotension, such effects are usually absent (Jee and Opie, 1984). No instance of exaggeration or precipitation of cerebrovascular symptoms have yet been reported, possibly because nifedipine may also act as a cerebral vasodilator (Bertel et al., 1983). The apparent provocation of angina pectoris, an unusual side-effect, can be avoided by careful dose-titration (Deanfield et al., 1983). Combination with beta-adrenergic blockade is usually safe and effective in the therapy of effort angina (Krikler et al., 1982).

The incidence of side-effects of **diltiazem** is remarkably low. In the United States the package insert claims that side-effects are similar to that of placebo, but lists nausea (3 percent), edema (2 percent), headache (2 percent) and heart block (0.4 percent). In contrast to nifedipine, flushing is rare. The inhibitory effect on the sinus node means that the sick sinus syndrome is a contra-indication and that combination therapy with beta-adrenergic blockade may cause excess bradycardia (Hung et al., 1983).

Two of the other (type B) calcium antagonists, prenylamine and lidoflazine, may prolong the QT-interval with potential for precipitation of atypical

Table 18-4

Comparative contra-indications of beta-blocking agents, verapamil, nifedipine and diltiazem

Contra-indications	Beta-blockade	Verapamil	Nifedipine	Diltiazem
Absolute				
Sinus bradycardia	+ +	0/ +	0	0/ +
Sick sinus syndrome	+ +	+	0	+
AV conduction effects	+	+ +	0	+
Digitalis toxicity with AV block[a]	+	+ +	0	+ +
Bronchospasm	+ +	0	0	0
Heart failure	+ +	+	0	+
Hypotension	+	+	+ +	+
Relative				
Digitalis without toxicity	Care	Care	0	Care
Beta-blockade	0	Care	Hypotension	Care
Verapamil therapy	Care	0	Hypotension	Hypotension AV block

[a]Contra-indication to rapid intravenous administration.
From Singh and Opie (1984). In: Drugs for the Heart. Ed. Opie LH, pp 39–62, Grune & Stratton, Orlando, London and New York.

ventricular tachycardia (Krikler and Curry, 1976); electrocardiograms should therefore be monitored during therapy with these agents.

Bearing in mind the very powerful cardiovascular effects of the calcium antagonist agents, the spectrum and severity of side-effects reported thus far is surprisingly reassuring and favorable when compared with beta-adrenergic blockade. In particular, the contra-indications to the use of calcium antagonists are fewer than those of beta-adrenergic blockers (Table 18-4). It remains appropriate to be careful and vigilant in the use of all calcium antagonists and to be sure that they are used when indicated in the appropriate dose and by the correct route.

Summary

The chief site of action of the calcium antagonist drugs is the slow calcium channel in two tissues: the atrioventricular node and vascular smooth muscle. The exact mode whereby these agents work is still unknown, but recently studies with radioligands suggest that the binding site for the dihydropyridines (such as nifedipine) is different from the site for the verapamil group (including diltiazem). In some way these agents "close" or "block" the calcium channels. Verapamil and diltiazem are both active against the calcium channel of the atrioventricular node whereas nifedipine in clinical doses is not; in contrast, nifedipine is more active on peripheral vascular arterial muscle, presumably inhibiting the calcium channel more strongly. An intracellular site of action of these agents on calmodulin in vascular smooth muscle cannot be excluded.

Clinically, the chief calcium antagonists (verapamil, nifedipine, diltiazem) constitute a powerful group of cardioactive agents with a spectrum of therapeutic actions rather similar to beta-adrenergic receptor blockade, being effective in angina of effort and rest, and hypertension. Critical differences are dependent on the individual properties of the calcium antagonists. Thus in clinical doses only verapamil and diltiazem are effective in inhibiting the AV node while the dihydropyridines such as nifedipine are only vaso-dilators. As a group, calcium antagonists cause vascular dilation and do not cause either bronchial or vascular constriction, in contrast to the potential of the beta-adrenergic receptor blocking agents.

References

Bayer R, Rodenkirchen R, Kaufmann R, Lee JH, Hennekes R (1977). The effect of nifedipine on contraction and monophasic action potential of isolated cat myocardium. Naunyn Schmiedeberg's Arch Pharm 301: 29–37.

Bertel O, Cohen D, Radu EW (1983). Nifedipine in hypertensive emergencies. Brit Med J 286: 19–21.

Bostrom SL, Ljung B, Mardh S, Forsen S, Thulin E (1981). Interaction of the antihypertensive drug felodipine with calmodulin. Nature 292: 777–778.

Bühler FR, Bolli P, Hulthen UL (1984). Calcium influx dependent vasoconstrictor mechanisms in essential hypertension. In: Calcium Antagonists and Cardiovascular Disease. Ed. LH Opie, pp 313–322, Raven Press, New York.

Church J, Zsoter TT (1980). Calcium antagonist drugs. Mechanism of action. Canad J Physiol Pharmacol 58: 254–264.

Conti CR, Hill JA, Feldman RL, Conti JB, Pepine CJ (1984). Comparison of nifedipine and nitrates: clinical and angiographic studies. In: Calcium Antagonists and Cardiovascular Disease. Ed. LH Opie, pp 269–275, Raven Press, New York.

Deanfield J, Wright C, Fox K (1983). Treatment of angina pectoris with nifedipine: importance of dose titration. Brit Med J 286: 1467–1470.

de Ponti C, Mauri F, Ciliberto GR, Caru B (1979). Comparative effects of nifedipine, verapamil, isosorbide dinitrate and propranolol on exercise-induced angina pectoris. Europ J Cardiol 10: 47–58.

Dompert WU, Traber J (1984). Binding sites for dihydropyridine calcium antagonists. In: Calcium Antagonists and Cardiovascular Disease. Ed. LH Opie, pp 175–179, Raven Press, New York.

Engel HJ, Lichtlen PR (1981). Beneficial enhancement of coronary blood flow by nifedipine. Comparison with nitroglycerin and beta blocking agents. Am J Med 71: 658–666.

Ferlinz J, Easthope JL, Aronow WS (1979). Effects of verapamil on myocardial performance in coronary disease. Circulation 59: 313–319.

Fleckenstein A (1971). Specific inhibitors and promoters of calcium action in the excitation–contraction coupling of heart muscle and their role in the prevention or production of myocardial lesions. In: Calcium and the Heart, Eds. P Harris, LH Opie, pp 135–188, Academic Press, London, Orlando and New York.

Fleckenstein A (1984). Calcium antagonism: history and prospects for a multifaceted pharmacodynamic principle. In: Calcium Antagonists and Cardiovascular Disease. Ed. LH Opie, pp 9–29, Raven Press, New York.

Fujimoto T, Peter T, Hahamoto H, Mandel WH (1981). Effects of diltiazem on conduction of premature impulses during acute myocardial ischemia and reperfusion. Am J Cardiol 48: 851–857.

Gloor HA, Urthaler F (1983). Differential effect of verapamil isomers on sinus node and AV junctional region. Am J Physiol 244: H80–H88.

Gould BA, Hornung RS, Mann S, Subramanian VB, Raftery EB (1982). Slow channel inhibitors verapamil and nifedipine in the management of hypertension. J Cardiovasc Pharm 4: S369–S373.

Hamm CW, Thandroyen FT, Opie LH (1982). Protective effects on isolated hearts with developing infarction: slow channel blockade by diltiazem versus beta-adrenoceptor antagonism by metoprolol. Am J Cardiol 50: 857–863.

Harriman RJ, Mangiardi LM, McAllister RG Jr, Surawicz B, Shabetai R, Kishida H (1979). Reversal of cardiovascular effects of verapamil by calcium and sodium: differences between electrophysiologic and hemodynamic responses. Circulation 16: 797–804.

Hescheler J, Pelzer D, Trube G, Trautwein W (1982). Does the organic calcium channel blocker D600 act from inside or outside on the cardiac cell membrane? Pflügers Arch 393: 287–291.

Himori N, Ono H, Taira N (1976). Simultaneous assessment of effects of coronary vasodilators on the coronary blood flow and the myocardial contractility by using the blood-perfused canine papillary muscle. Japanese J Pharm 26: 427–435.

Hugenholtz P, Verdouw PD, de Jong JW, Serruys TW (1984). Nifedipine for angina and acute myocardial ischemia. In: Calcium Antagonists and Cardiovascular Disease. Ed. LH Opie, pp 237–255, Raven Press, New York.

Hung J, Lamb IH, Connolly SJ, Jutzy KR, Goris ML, Schroeder JS (1983). The effect of diltiazem and propranolol, alone and in combination, on exercise performance and left ventricular function in patients with stable effort angina. Circulation 68: 560–567.

Jee LD, Opie LH (1984). Nifedipine for hypertension and angina pectoris: interactions during combination therapy. In: Calcium Antagonists and Cardiovascular Disease. Ed. LH Opie, pp 339–346, Raven Press, New York.

Kaltenbach M, Hopf R, Kober G, Bussmann WD, Keller M, Petersen Y (1979). Treatment of hypertrophic obstructive cardiomyopathy with verapamil. Brit Heart J 42: 35–42.

Kanaya S, Arlock P, Katzung BG, Hondeghem LM (1983). Diltiazem and verapamil preferentially block inactivated cardiac calcium channels. J Molec Cell Cardiol 15: 145–148.

Kass RS (1983). Nisoldipine: a new, more selective calcium current blocker in cardiac Purkinje fibers. J Pharmac Exp Therap 223: 446–456.

Khalsa A, Olsson SB (1979). Verapamil-induced ventricular regularity in atrial fibrillation. Acta Med Scand 205: 509–515.

Kolhardt M, Bauer B, Krause H, Fleckenstein A (1972). Differentiation of the transmembrane Na and Ca channels in mammalian cardiac fibers by the use of specific inhibitors. Pflügers Arch Physiol 335: 309–322.

Krebs R (1984). Calcium antagonists: new vistas in theoretical basis and clinical use. In: Calcium Antagonists and Cardiovascular Disease. Ed. LH Opie, pp 347–357, Raven Press, New York.

Krikler DM, Curry PUL (1976). Torsade de pointes, as atypical ventricular tachycardia. Brit Heart J 38: 117–120.

Krikler DM, Harris L, Rowland E (1982). Calcium channel blockers and beta blockers: advantages and disadvantages of combination therapy in chronic stable angina pectoris. Am Heart J 104: 702–708.

Landmark K, Amlie JP (1976). A study of the verapamil-induced changes in conductivity and refractoriness and monophasic action potentials of the dog heart in situ. Europ J Cardiol 4: 419–427.

Lee KS, Tsien RW (1983). Mechanism of calcium channel blockade by verapamil, D600, diltiazem and nitrendipine in single dialyzed heart cells. Nature 302: 790–794.

Lichtlen PR, Engel HJ, Rafflenbeul W (1984). Calcium entry blockers, especially nifedipine, in angina of effort: possible mechanisms and clinical implications. In: Calcium Antagonists and Cardiovascular Disease. Ed. LH Opie, pp 221–236, Raven Press, New York.

Lorell BH, Turi Z, Grossman W (1981). Modification of left ventricular response to pacing tachycardia by nifedipine in patients with coronary artery disease. Am J Med 71: 667–675.

Losardo A, Klein N, Willens H, Siegel L, Jentzer J, Kirschen N, Strom J, LeJemtel T, Sonnenblick E, Wexler J, Frishman W (1982). Lidoflazine and propranolol in stable angina pectoris: long-term safety and efficacy of combined calcium entry blocker beta-adrenergic blocker therapy (Abstract). Am J Cardiol 49: 930.

Meyer H (1983). Structural/activity relationships in calcium antagonists. In: Calcium Antagonists and Cardiovascular Disease. Ed. LH Opie, pp 165–173, Raven Press, New York.

Mitchell LB, Schroeder JS, Mason JW (1982). Comparative clinical electrophysiologic effects of diltiazem, verapamil and nifedipine: a review. Am J Cardiol 49: 629–635.

Murphy KMM, Gould RJ, Largent BL, Snyder SH (1983). A unitary mechanism of calcium antagonist drug action. Proc Natl Acad Sci 80: 860–864.

Narahara KA, Shapiro W, Weliky I, Park J (1984). Evaluation of bepridil, a new antianginal agent: clinical and hemodynamic alterations during the treatment of stable angina pectoris. Am J Cardiol 53: 29–34.

Nayler WG, Poole-Wilson P (1981). Calcium antagonists: definition and mode of action. Basic Res Cardiol 76: 1–15.

Nayler WG, Dillon JS, Daly MJ (1984). Cellular sites of action of calcium antagonists and beta-adrenoceptor blockers. In: Calcium Antagonists and Cardiovascular Disease. Ed. LH Opie, pp 181–191, Raven Press, New York.

Opie LH (1980). Calcium antagonists. In: Drugs and the Heart, pp 27–28, The Lancet, London.

Opie LH, Jee LD (1984). Nifedipine: expanding indications in hypertension. In: Calcium Antagonists and Cardiovascular Disease. Ed. LH Opie, pp 333–337, Raven Press, New York.

Opie LH, White DA (1980). Adverse interaction between nifedipine and beta-blockade. Brit Med J 281: 1462–1464.

Opie LH, Thandroyen FT, Muller CA, Hamm CW (1984). Calcium channel antagonists as antiarrhythmic agents: contrasting properties of verapamil and diltiazem versus nifedipine. In: Calcium Antagonists and Cardiovascular Disease. Ed. LH Opie, pp 303–311, Raven Press, New York.

Parodi O, Simonetti I, L'Abbate A, Maseri A (1984). Verapamil versus propranolol for angina at rest. Am J Cardiol 50: 923–928.

Polese A, Fiorentini C, Olivari MT, Guazzi MD (1979). Clinical use of a calcium antagonist agent (nifedipine) in acute pulmonary edema. Am J Med 66: 825–830.

Rosendorff C (1984). Calcium channel blockers and hypertension. In: Calcium Antagonists and Cardiovascular Disease. Ed. LH Opie, pp 323–331, Raven Press, New York.

Rowland E, Evans T, Krikler D (1979). Effect of nifedipine on atrioventricular conduction as compared with verapamil. Intracardiac electrophysiological study. Brit Heart J 42: 124–127.

Sasayama S, Takahashi M, Wakamura M, Ohyagi A, Yamamoto A, Shimade T, Kawai C (1981). Effect of diltiazem on pacing-induced ischemia in conscious dogs with coronary stenosis: improvement of postpacing deterioration of ischemic myocardial function. Am J Cardiol 48: 460–472.

Schramm M, Thomas G, Towart R, Franckowiak G (1983). Novel dihydropyridines with positive inotropic action through activation of Ca^{2+} channels. Nature 303: 535–537.

Schroeder JS, Lamb JH, Ginsburg R, Bristow MR, Hung J (1982). Diltiazem for long-term therapy of coronary arterial spasm. Am J Cardiol 49: 533–537.

Shapiro W, Narahara KA, Park J (1982). The effects of lidoflazine on exercise performance and thallium stress scintigraphy in patients with stable angina pectoris. Circulation 65: 1–43.

Singh BN, Roche AHG (1977). Effects of intravenous verapamil on hemodynamics in patients with heart disease. Am Heart J 94: 595–599.

Singh BN, Vaughan Williams EM (1972). A fourth class of antidysrhythmic action? Effect of verapamil on ouabain toxicity, on atrial and ventricular potentials and on other features of cardiac function. Cardiovasc Res 6: 109–119.

Sperelakis N (1984). Properties of calcium-dependent slow action potentials, and their possible role in arrhythmias. In: Calcium Antagonists and Cardiovascular Disease. Ed. LH Opie, pp 277–291, Raven Press, New York.

Strauss WE, McIntyre KM, Parasin AF, Shapiro W (1982). Safety and efficacy of diltiazem hydrochloride for the treatment of stable angina pectoris: report of a cooperative trial. Am J Cardiol 49: 560–566.

Towart R (1981). The selective inhibition of serotonin-induced contractions of rabbit cerebral vascular smooth muscle by calcium antagonistic dihydropyridines. An investigation of the mechanism of action of nimodipine. Circ Res 48: 650–657.

Walsh RA, Badke FR, O'Rourke RA (1981). Differential effects of systemic and intracoronary calcium channel blocking agents on global and regional left ventricular function in conscious dogs. Am Heart J 102: 341–350.

Weiss AT, Lewis BS, Hasin Y, Gotsman M (1983). The use of calcium with verapamil in the management of supraventricular arrhythmias. Int J Cardiol 4: 275–280.

Winsor T, Bleifer K, Cole S, Goldman IR, Karpman H, Oblath R, Stone S (1971). A double-blind, double cross-over trial of prenylamine in angina pectoris. Am Heart J 82: 43–54.

Wit AL, Cranefield PF (1974). Effect of verapamil on the sinoatrial and atrioventricular nodes of the rabbit and the mechanism by which it arrests re-entrant atrioventricular nodal tachycardia. Circ Res 35: 413–426.

Yasue H (1984). Coronary artery spasm and calcium ions. In: Calcium Antagonists and Cardiovascular Disease. Ed. LH Opie, pp 117–128, Raven Press, New York.

Yasue H, Touyama M, Kato H, Tanaka S, Akiyama F (1976). Prinzmetal's variant form of angina as a manifestation of alpha-adrenergic receptor-mediated coronary artery spasm: documentation by coronary arteriography. Am Heart J 91: 148–155.

Yellon DM, Hearse DJ, Maxwell MP, Chambers DE, Downey JM (1983). Sustained limitation of myocardial necrosis 24 hours after coronary artery occlusion: verapamil infusion in dogs with small myocardial infarcts. Am J Cardiol 51: 1409–1413.

New References

Glossmann H, Ferry DR, Goll A, Striessnig GJ, Schober M (1985). Calcium channels: basic properties as revealed by radioligand binding studies. J Cardiovasc Pharmacol 7 (Suppl 6) S20–S30.

Godfraind T (1986). Calcium entry blockade and excitation-contraction coupling in the cardiovascular system (with an attempt at pharmacological classification). Acta Pharmacol Toxicol, in press.

Green FJ, Farmer BB, Wiseman GL, Jose MJL, Watanabe AM (1985). Effect of membrane depolarization on binding of [³H] nitrendipine to rat cardiac myocytes. Circ Res 56: 576–585.

Nerbonne JM, Richard S, Nargeot J (1985). Calcium channels are 'unblocked' within a few milliseconds after photoremoval of nifedipine. J Molec Cell Cardiol 17: 511–515.

19 | Digitalis and Sympathomimetic Stimulants

Digitalis Glycosides

Whereas digitalis compounds have the advantage of both slowing the heart rate and stimulating the myocardial contractile force by inhibition of the sodium–potassium pump, sympathomimetic agents generally increase both rate and force of contraction by elevation of myocardial cyclic AMP (Fig. 19-1).

More than 200 years ago in 1775, the Scottish medical botanist William Withering discovered that the leaves of the foxglove, *Digitalis purpurea*, could benefit patients with dropsy (cardiac edema). Today the diuretic effect is explained by a positive inotropic

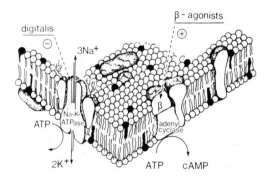

Fig. 19-1 Three-dimensional model of sarcolemma. Two commonly used positively inotropic procedures, digitalis and beta-adrenergic stimulation, act on two entirely different receptors although ultimately having a common site of action by increasing intracellular calcium.

effect on the failing heart. Digitalis compounds are still widely used for congestive heart failure, although if Withering had lived today he would have struggled to get his drug through the FDA because there are frequent toxic effects when incorrectly used. By 1933, three distinct properties of digitalis were well described: the positive inotropic effect, the inhibitory effect on atrioventricular conduction and the toxic side-effects. In that year Sir Thomas Lewis said that

> the most emphatic action of digitalis and its allies is in the case of auricular fibrillation. The use of drugs calculated to strengthen the heart beat is open to the theoretical objection that this would increase the work of the heart.   Lewis (1933)

Even today digitalis compounds are held to be most effective for patients with atrial fibrillation or with a combination of congestive cardiac failure and atrial fibrillation.

A critically important step was in 1953, with the discovery by Schatzmann that digitalis inhibited sodium transport in erythrocytes, a property which Skou (1957) could show was due to inhibition of the sodium pump. Schwartz et al. (1975) showed that the only glycosides which inhibited the sodium pump were those that had an inotropic effect, while the degree of binding of cardiac glycosides to the ATPase paralleled the clinical activity—glycosides with tighter binding were more effective. Thus the sodium pump is now universally regarded as the receptor for digitalis glycosides. The only point at issue is how this inhibition causes the increased availability of calcium within the myocyte to result in the positive inotropic effect which enhances cardiac muscle contractility.

The terms "digitalis" and "digitalis compounds" are used to designate the entire group of cardiac glycoside inotropic drugs. All digitalis drugs share an aglycone ring structure, wherein the pharmacological activity resides, combined with one to four molecules of sugar which modify the properties (Fig. 19-2). Digoxin is now the most widely used because its shorter half-life allows easier treatment of toxicity but digitoxin still has strong advocates.

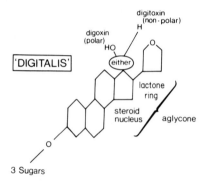

Fig. 19-2 Molecular structure of the "digitalis" compounds, digoxin or digitoxin. The term "digitalis" is used to include both the commonly used clinical preparations, digoxin and digitoxin, as well as other related compounds such as deslanoside (lanatoside C), ouabain and the original digitalis leaf preparation.

Inhibition of the Na⁺/K⁺-ATPase (sodium) pump

There is now widespread agreement that the sodium pump represents the tissue receptor for digitalis (Fig. 19-3). The binding is complex so that there is a change in the molecular configuration of the receptor site as digitalis binds to the receptor. Binding to the receptor is modified by the effects of sodium and potassium ions, which bind to ionic sites to alter the interaction of digitalis with the receptor. Intracellular sodium increases the binding of digitalis, whereas extracellular potassium decreases the binding. Thus both potassium and digitalis probably act on the external side of the catalytic subunit, where there are two potassium binding sites for each digitalis site. Because potassium can bind to the enzyme even when digitalis-binding

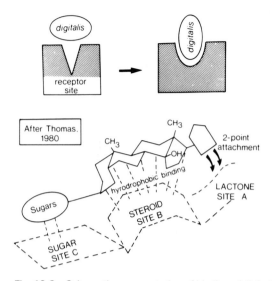

Fig. 19-3 Schematic representation of binding of digitalis to its receptor site. Note the change in the molecular configuration of receptor site as the digitalis–receptor complex forms. After Thomas et al. (1980). Circ Res Suppl 46: 167–172, with permission from the author and the American Heart Association.

sites are fully occupied, the sites for potassium and digitalis cannot be idential (Akera, 1981). Potassium inhibits both the rate of binding and slows dissociation; the greater effect on binding means that the overall affinity of the enzyme for digitalis is decreased by potassium ions. These inhibitory effects of potassium may explain why **hypokalemia** sensitizes the heart to the toxic effects of digitalis.

There are several proposals for the positive inotropic effects of digitalis (Fig. 19-4). The mechanism most commonly accepted is:

glycoside ⟶ inhibition of Na⁺ pump ⟶ less Na⁺ efflux ⟶ retention of Na⁺ ⟶ competition of Na⁺ with Ca²⁺ for the Na⁺/Ca²⁺ exchange mechanism on the sarcolemma ⟶ intracellular Ca²⁺ rises ⟶ inotropic effect

The second possibility is modified from the above and states that sodium displaces calcium from binding sites on the inner mitochondrial membrane. The third proposal is that the interaction of digitalis with its receptor actually allows more external calcium to cross the sarcolemma (Schwartz and Adams, 1980) and hence increases the availability of intracellular free calcium ions. However digitalis acts, the kinetic characteristics of its interaction with the receptor very

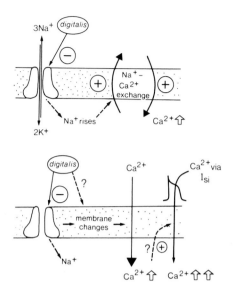

Autonomic influences

Digitalis has a **sympathomimetic** effect which probably facilitates the development of toxic arrhythmias. The site of this effect is central, near the floor of the 4th ventricle (Somberg and Smith, 1979). This sympathetic component could explain the reported beneficial effect of beta-blockade on digitalis-induced tachycardias (Fig. 19-5).

Whereas the sympathetic activation correlates with a toxic effect of digitalis, the **parasympathetic** (vagal) activation correlates with therapeutic effects—sinus bradycardia and AV nodal inhibition. Also in congestive heart failure the positive inotropic effect of digitalis leads to improved contractile function and less stimulation of the sympathetic system as heart failure ceases. An ill-understood direct depression of nodal tissue may account for those effects of digitalis still found even after vagal blockade (Gomes et al., 1981). Yet the effects of digitalis on the sinus node are sufficiently variable for the sick sinus syndrome not to be regarded as an absolute contra-indication to digitalis therapy.

Besides its clinical use as an inotropic agent, the other main indication for digitalis is to slow conduction through the **atrioventricular node** in atrial fibrillation and supraventricular tachycardias (Table 19-1). The inhibitory effect on the atrioventricular node depends on the degree of vagal tone, which varies from person to person (Kim et al., 1975).

Fig. 19-4 Two possible modes of action of digitalis in increasing the internal calcium ion concentration and thereby providing a positive inotropic stimulus. The proposed effect of internal calcium in enhancing the slow inward current (I_{si}) is shown only in the bottom panel for reasons of space. Note that inhibition of the pump, in the top panel, need only be partial. For details of proposed pump structure, see Fig. 4-2. Modified from Marcus et al. (1984). In: Drugs for the Heart, Ed. Opie LH, p 100, Grune & Stratton, Orlando, New York and London.

closely parallel the characteristics of the positive inotropic effect (Akera, 1981).

Other effects of digitalis on internal calcium

The inotropic effect of digitalis may sometimes be dissociated from its inhibition of the sodium pump, particularly at low concentrations (Lullman and Peters, 1979). Here there may be a direct interaction between digitalis and the sarcolemmal phospholipids, thereby releasing calcium from membrane-bound sites to increase internal calcium.

Another discrepancy is that the inotropic effect of digitalis may be marked albeit in circumstances where there is thought to be only a modest increase in internal calcium. The proposed explanation is that even a small increase in diastolic calcium could enhance calcium entry by stimulation of the slow inward current (Marban and Tsien, 1982).

NEURAL EFFECTS OF DIGITALIS

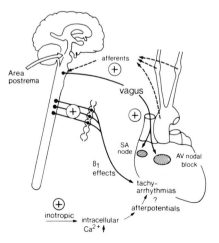

Fig. 19-5 Neural effects of digitalis are especially important in the generation of toxic arrhythmias.

Table 19-1

Digoxin: Summary of clinical use

1. **Proposed mechanism of action**
   Inotropic effect by inhibition of myocardial sodium pump
   AV nodal inhibition by stimulation of vagus (parasympathomimetic)

2. **Indications**
   Congestive heart failure (CHF) with atrial fibrillation
   Low-output congestive heart failure (with diuretics)
   Supraventricular tachycardias conducted through AV node (prophylaxis)
   Usually ineffective in high-output CHF including thyrotoxicosis
   Frequently ineffective during chronic therapy

3. **Contra-indications**
(i)	Absolute:	Hypertrophic obstructive cardiomyopathy
		WPW with antegrade conduction (see Fig. 23-15)
(ii)	Relative:	Sinus node depression (sick sinus syndrome; therapy with reserpine, methyldopa, beta-blockers, or diltiazem)
		AV nodal depression (heart block; therapy with clonidine, beta-blockers, verapamil or diltiazem)
		Old age; renal failure (reduce dose)

4. **Dosage**
(i)	Loading:	(if urgent) 0.75–1 mg, orally or intravenously; less in elderly or thin patients because of reduced muscle mass
(ii)	Steady state dose:	0.25 mg "standard" dose; range 0.06–0.75 mg, depending on renal function and serum K⁺
		Correct dose judged clinically and by blood level

   (Steady state dose: 0.25 mg "standard" dose; range 0.06–0.75 mg, depending on renal function and serum K^+)

5. **Therapeutic blood level**
   Usually 1–2 ng/mL on sample taken more than 6 hours after last digoxin dose; depends on serum K⁺ (Fig. 19-6) and other complex clinical factors (Marcus et al., 1984)

6. **Features of toxicity**
   (i)   Gastro-intestinal: anorexia, nausea, vomiting, diarrhea
   (ii) Neurologic: malaise, fatigue, confusion, facial pain, insomnia
   (iii) Cardiologic: palpitations, arrhythmias, aggravation of heart failure
   (iv) Confirmation by high blood level

Toxic effects

The molecular basis for digitalis toxicity is still ill-defined. In the case of arrhythmias factors include: (i) excess inhibition of the sodium–potassium pump so that intracellular calcium rises too much, to predispose to after-potentials and ventricular automaticity; (ii) a central neural stimulation of the adrenergic system to promote beta-adrenergic-mediated tachyarrhythmias; (iii) excess vagal stimulation so that there is too much inhibition of conduction through the atrioventricular node; thus the combination of an atrial tachyarrhythmia with marked heart block may be diagnostic of digitalis intoxication; and (iv) the effects of an associated diuretic-induced hypokalemia (Fig. 19-6).

Blood levels of digoxin and digitoxin can now be measured readily by immunoassay. The major points to emerge are that: (i) the usual therapeutic digoxin level is 1–2 ng/mL; (ii) there is a very narrow therapeutic–toxic margin; (iii) other drugs such as quinidine, verapamil (but not diltiazem), amiodarone and possibly nifedipine cause digitalis levels to rise; and (iv) hypokalemia sensitizes the heart to the possible toxic effects of any given blood level of digitalis (Fig. 19-6).

Digoxin is a compound which is excreted only by the kidneys (Fig. 19-7) and toxicity is more prone to develop in patients with poor renal function (renal failure; myxedema; severe congestive heart failure; elderly patients; drugs depressing renal function such as beta-blockers). In such patients, **digitoxin** (Fig. 19-8)

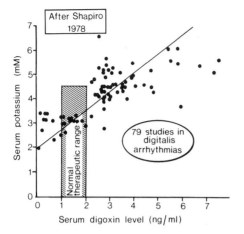

Fig. 19-6 As the serum potassium falls the heart is sensitized to the arrhythmias of digitalis toxicity. Conversely, as the serum potassium rises a higher serum digoxin level is tolerated. Modified from Shapiro (1978). Am J Cardiol 41: 852–859, with permission.

is the preferred therapeutic form of digitalis, because most of it is excreted by the gut (30 percent renal excretion). Its disadvantage is a very slow rate of elimination (half-life 6–7 days) so that if toxicity does develop, washout of the effects takes longer.

Despite the usefulness of blood-level assays the numerous factors influencing the therapeutic and toxic effects mean that it is not possible to extrapolate from blood levels to therapeutic or toxic effects without a careful clinical evaluation of the patient. For example, in patients with a high vagal tone the inhibitory effect of digitalis on the atrioventricular node will be found relatively easily; so also when the patient is receiving other inhibitors of the atrioventricular node such as verapamil or beta-adrenergic blockade.

Treatment of digitalis toxicity

Treatment of **digitalis arrhythmias** can be difficult. Basic therapy is to withdraw the drug and administer potassium salts (hypokalemia is usual) and to correct other plasma electrolyte changes. Ventricular ectopic beats may necessitate treatment with lidocaine, or with phenytoin if there is heart block. When digitalis toxicity causes atrial flutter, phenytoin is best avoided because of the danger of accelerated atrioventricular conduction. Procainamide is contra-indicated because it may increase conduction block. Quinidine may worsen digitalis toxicity by increasing the digoxin level, and if being taken it should be stopped. A new and very specialized approach for life-threatening toxicity employs the intravenous administration of fragments of digitalis antibodies.

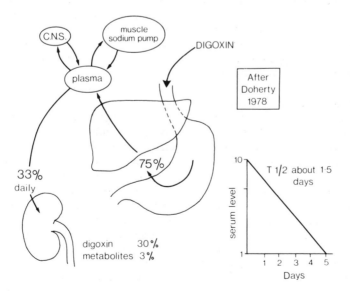

Fig. 19-7 Digoxin pharmacokinetics. In many patients a standard dose of 0.25 mg digoxin daily gives therapeutic blood levels (Fig. 19-8); in renal failure the dose must be reduced. For details see Marcus et al. (1983). Modified from Doherty et al. (1978). Prog Cardiovasc Dis 21: 141–158, with permission.

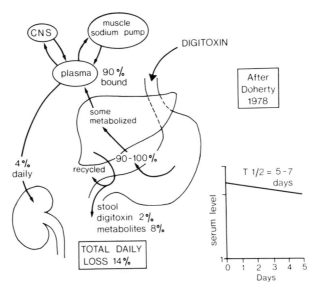

Fig. 19-8 Digitoxin pharmacokinetics. Note the following differences from digoxin (Fig. 19-7): (i) there is relatively little renal excretion, making it safer in renal failure; (ii) a high percentage is bound to plasma proteins so blood levels are much higher; (iii) the half-life is much longer so treatment of toxicity is more difficult than with digoxin. Modified from Doherty et al. (1978). Prog Cardiovasc Dis 21: 141–146.

Clinical indications for digitalis

The major indication for digitalis in 1984, as in 1933, is the combination of **congestive heart failure with atrial fibrillation** (Lewis, 1933; Marcus et al., 1984). Acute left-ventricular failure should be treated by load reduction before digitalis is considered. In valvular disease with acute failure, digitalization is conventionally the first line of treatment but patients with regurgitation may do better with vasodilators. Chronic **congestive failure with sinus rhythm**, failing a response to diuretics alone, is another customary indication, but there has been no proper comparison of digitalis with afterload reduction in such patients. Recent studies are in conflict about the effects of digitalis withdrawal in patients with grade III or IV heart failure (Taggart et al., 1983); therefore each patient needs individual assessment. Milder heart failure (grades I and II) is less likely to benefit from digitalization.

The types of failure responding best to acute digitalization are low-output states not caused by either valvular stenosis or chronic pericarditis; in high-output states including cor pulmonale, the response tends to be disappointing. Even in low-output failure chronic digitalis therapy is of disputed value and the old dictum "once on digitalis, always on digitalis" can no longer

be upheld. The usual rule now is to start with a diuretic; but some clinicians feel it is more logical to start with inotropic therapy. In old age, digoxin is frequently given when not needed and excessive fear of renal impairment may lead to under-dosage. Here blood digoxin levels are very useful. When a rapid positive inotropic effect is desired, then it must be considered that the peak inotropic effect with digoxin is delayed for about 4 hours (Fig. 19-8).

In **acute myocardial infarction** the arguments for and against digitalization are very complex. Hypoxia sensitizes the heart to digitalis, as does acute myocardial infarction (Lown et al., 1972). Hence digitalis is given only with care to patients with these conditions. Possible specific indications for cardiac glycoside in acute myocardial infarction may be: (i) to treat overt cardiac failure not responding to diuretics and oral vasodilators; (ii) to slow atrioventricular conduction when atrial fibrillation is accompanied by heart failure; and (iii) to counteract the cardiodepressant effects of beta-adrenergic blockade therapy (Vatner et al., 1978).

In the **post-infarct period** the early evidence is that digitalis therapy increases mortality (Moss et al., 1981). Yet digitalis is useful in specific clinical situations, as when there is limited exercise tolerance. Secondly,

Table 19-2

Digoxin: drug interactions and effects of concomitant diseases

1. **Increased blood level** for given dose with: quinidine, verapamil (not diltiazem), tiapamil, amiodarone, nifedipine (?) and diazepam

2. **Decreased blood levels:** dose not taken; malabsorption; drug interference by neomycin, kaolin-pectin

3. **Increased side-effects** with hypokalemia and/or hypomagnesemia (diuretics, chronic malabsorption) or other drugs suppressing nodal function (Table 19-1) or renal failure

4. **Increased sensitivity to usual dose** Hypercalcemia, myxedema, acute myocardial infarction, acute rheumatic carditis (danger of AV block), low body mass (lower loading dose)

5. **Decreased sensitivity to usual dose** Thyrotoxicosis

digitalis may sometimes have an antiarrhythmic effect, and not only in patients with cardiomegaly and/or heart failure. Thirdly, digitalis is used to counter the negative inotropic effect of beta-adrenergic blockade.

Digitalis: summary

Digitalis compounds bind to and inhibit the specific myocardial cell receptor, the sodium pump (the Na^+/K^+-ATPase). This inhibition is linked to an increase in the cytosolic calcium ion concentration so that an inotropic effect results. Digitalis compounds also have prominent neural effects, so that stimulation of the vagal nerve leads to sinus bradycardia and an important therapeutic effect — inhibition of conduction through the atrioventricular node. The ideal patient for digitalis therapy has a combination of heart failure and an atrial tachyarrhythmia such as atrial fibrillation. In patients with mild congestive heart failure the trend is away from automatic digitalization which is reserved for patients already receiving diuretics.

Sympathomimetic Inotropic Agents

The inotropic effect of naturally occurring catecholamines leads to their therapeutic use when the heart requires acute inotropic support by intravenous agents. Such catecholamines provide mixed alpha- and beta-stimulation and the latter gives combined chronotropic and inotropic effects. Yet an increased heart rate is frequently undesirable in the failing heart because the shortened period available for filling the ventricle in diastole limits the cardiac output. Hence more recently there has been the evolution of synthetic catecholamines with more specific inotropic properties.

Theoretically, the general properties of sympathomimetic agents are such that they benefit the failing heart by stimulating more than one receptor type. Thus beta-1-stimulation achieves an inotropic and chronotropic effect, beta-2-stimulation results in afterload reduction (peripheral vasodilation) and alpha-stimulation restores the blood pressure in hypotensive states. Unfortunately, the combined effect of the tachycardia (beta-1-effect) and the elevation in arterial pressure (alpha-effect) is to increase the myocardial oxygen demand. The ideal would be to have only the inotropic effect. Hence there has been a search for newer catecholamine-like agents with only positive inotropic effects that do not cause tachycardia and do not increase blood pressure.

Isoproterenol (Isoprenaline)

Isoproterenol acts on both cardiac beta-1- and peripheral beta-2-receptors. The $l(-)$ isomer is about 50 times more active than the $d(+)$ isomer (as in the case of the propranolol isomers). Isoproterenol must be given intravenously; it increases heart rate, contractility and cardiac output and decreases peripheral resistance. This apparently desirable spectrum of activity is seldom clinically useful because the myocardial oxygen consumption increases out of proportion to the increase in contractility, possibly because the non-specific beta-2-effect also increases lipolysis and hence the fatty acid component and oxygen-wastage. Similar metabolic changes added to increased tissue cyclic AMP may explain arrhythmia development. With current emphasis on limitation of ischemic damage, isoproterenol has gone out of favor. Hence the search for the newer catecholamines such as dopamine and dobutamine.

Dopamine

Dopamine (Fig. 19-9) is a naturally occurring catecholamine-like agent which must be given intravenously

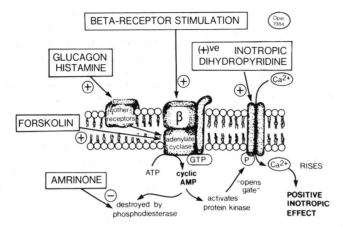

Fig. 19-9 Theoretical approaches to the development of new positively inotropic agents (other than digitalis). Note that the end result of all these agents is an increased cytosolic calcium ion concentration.

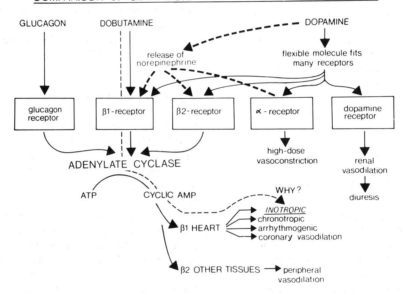

Fig. 19-10 Proposed receptor effects of glucagon, dobutamine and dopamine. Reproduced from Opie (1980) with permission from The Lancet.

and is used in the therapy of severe heart failure, cardiogenic shock and septic shock. Physiologically it is the precursor of norepinephrine. It has a considerable indirect sympathomimetic activity by releasing norepinephrine from the adrenergic nerve terminals; it may also inhibit the re-uptake into the nerve endings. Some dopamine is also broken down by the enzyme monoamine oxidase, so that patients receiving monoamine oxidase inhibitors can be very sensitive

to dopamine and need initial doses reduced to one-tenth. Part of the positive inotropic effect of dopamine is mediated by cyclic AMP (Fig. 19-10) whereas another component may be alpha-dependent and independent of cyclic AMP. Dopamine resembles dobutamine in having a relatively greater inotropic than chronotropic effect. The dopamine molecule has a "flexible" fit into multiple receptor sites, so that it directly stimulates both beta- and alpha-receptors.

Severe low-output heart failure may be complicated by decreased renal perfusion and renal failure. By stimulating dopamine receptors in the **renal vascular bed**, dopamine should specifically be able to promote renal blood flow and diuresis independently of effects in increasing the cardiac output; added therapy with furosemide potentiates the effect on urine flow. Another dopaminergic effect is that on hormone secretion, whereby glucagon and insulin rise while prolactin falls (Lorenzi et al., 1979). Theoretically the rise in insulin could contribute to the inotropic effect of dopamine. At high doses of dopamine (exceeding 20 μg/kg/min) the alpha-effects (probably mediated via norepinephrine) dominate and peripheral resistance rises with the danger that renal blood flow may fall. Hence in the therapy of severe congestive heart failure the dose should be strictly monitored; a combination of dopamine and another vasodilator therapy, such as nitroprusside or an alpha-blocker or dobutamine, should be better than increasing the dose of dopamine.

The major problem with the use of dopamine is that its complex molecular mechanism results in unpredictable effects. Like other catecholamines, dopamine given in high doses may provoke ventricular arrhythmias especially when there is an ischemic myocardium.

The cellular mechanism of **dopamine receptors** in general involve one of two receptors. First, formation of cyclic AMP occurs by the dopamine-sensitive adenyl cyclase (D_1) receptor which involves GTP as a molecule conferring an increased response. The D_1 receptor responds to apomorphine derivatives. The other subtype of dopamine receptors (D_2) act independently of adenylate cyclase and cyclic AMP; these receptors respond to the ergolines (Tsurata et al., 1981). This division of dopamine receptors has thus far found most application in the brain, where dopamine is an important neurotransmitter. In the heart, direct effects of dopamine on the beta- and alpha-receptors dominate.

Whatever the molecular mechanism involved, various catecholamines such as epinephrine, norepinephrine, dopamine and dobutamine all increase the oxygen demand by a similar extent for a given inotropic effect (Vasu et al., 1978).

Dobutamine

Dobutamine is a synthetic analog of dopamine with a different spectrum of interaction with beta-receptors; it must also be given intravenously. Dobutamine acts directly on beta-1-adrenergic receptors so as to cause a stronger inotropic than chronotropic effect (Jewitt et al., 1974). One explanation for such differential effects is by the postulate that there are two populations of beta-1-receptors—the inotropic and the chronotropic (Dreyer and Offermeier, 1975). This is a useful but unproven concept. Alternatively, beta-1-receptors in different regions of the myocardium could respond with varying sensitivity to dobutamine, so that the ventricles are more sensitive than atrial or sinus tissue (Tuttle et al., 1976).

Besides the cardiac effects, dobutamine in high doses has **effects on the circulation**. In the arterial circulation, both beta-2 and alpha-receptors are stimulated with the predominant effect being beta-2, thereby unloading the heart. On the venous capacitance bed, which contains 60–70 percent of the circulating blood volume, dobutamine has a vasoconstrictive effect which should increase the venous return (Fuchs et al., 1980). Although dobutamine does not dilate renal arteries, renal function may improve as a result of increased cardiac output.

In severe low-output congestive heart failure dobutamine is superior to dopamine (Leier et al., 1978). In selected cases of evolving myocardial infarction the relatively specific inotropic effect of dobutamine has been used without increasing infarct size or inducing arrhythmias (Gillespie et al., 1977). In experimental infarction dobutamine reduces infarct size, presumably because the increased myocardial oxygen demand is more than balanced by (i) improved coronary perfusion resulting from increased cardiac output; (ii) a coronary vasodilator effect; and (iii) a peripheral unloading effect. A recent indication for dobutamine is to reverse the effects of cardioselective beta-blockade in patients either with acute myocardial infarction or undergoing cardiac surgery (Waagstein et al., 1978).

Salbutamol (albuterol)

Salbutamol is a relatively selective beta-2-agonist widely used for the therapy of asthma (Fig. 19-9). In addition, salbutamol has apparent inotropic properties in congestive cardiac failure where it is one of the few sympathomimetic agents that can be given orally. When tested on isolated muscle there is no direct inotropic effect (Bourdillon et al., 1980). Rather, peripheral vasodilation unloads the heart; hence there is little increase in the myocardial oxygen demand despite an increased cardiac output (Timmis et al., 1979). An important metabolic side-effect is the pronounced fall in plasma potassium due to the stimulation of insulin release from the pancreas (Berend and Marlin, 1978); the hypokalemia theoretically could predispose to ischemic arrhythmias (Chapter 22). The cardiovascular effects of beta-2-stimulation by salbutamol are not entirely selective for smooth muscle and tachycardia can occur, especially at higher doses.

Other "-ols"

Other synthetic catecholamine molecules are being evaluated as possible direct or indirect inotropic agents. **Rimiterol** is very similar to salbutamol, being a beta-2-stimulant with a quicker onset of action (Stephens et al., 1978). **Metaproterenol** (orciprenaline) is structurally close to isoproterenol; it is chiefly a beta-2-stimulant though less specific than salbutamol. Frequently used as an intravenous bronchodilator, it has beta-1-stimulant qualities which may account for an increased heart rate and the arrhythmias sometimes caused (Senges et al., 1980). **Fenoterol** is closely related to metaproterenol and has similar cardiovascular effects (Tandon, 1980).

Sympathomimetic "-ines"

In general, many of the above agents could equally well have had names ending in -ine, because of their catecholamine nature; metaproterenol is called orciprenaline in Europe. **Terbutaline** is a beta-2-agonist similar to salbutamol in properties. Other sympathomimetic amines lack the catechol nucleus. Some of them act by release of norepinephrine from the terminal nerve endings. Hence these agents have beta-1-like effects on the heart and alpha-effects on the periphery. **Ephedrine** also has beta-2-stimulation with bronchodilation. Its main clinical use is for asthma, although also used in severe heart failure in combination with a vasodilator to avoid an alpha-mediated increase in peripheral resistance (Franciosa and Cohn, 1979).

Phenylephrine and **methoxamine** are alpha-agonists given parenterally, that have dominant alpha- and slight high-dose beta-effects. They basically stimulate the alpha-receptors and therefore vasoconstrict. They only have a slight capacity to release norepinephrine from the nerve terminals.

Intrinsic sympathomimetic activity (partial agonist activity)

Some beta-blocking agents such as pindolol, oxprenolol and acebutolol have the property of stimulating as well as inhibiting the beta-receptor, and are said to possess intrinsic sympathomimetic activity (ISA or PAA). A large degree of ISA should in theory protect against an excessive depressive effect of beta-blockade. On the other hand, ISA blunts the effect of beta-blockade in reducing an exercise-induced tachycardia. Compounds are now being evolved which have so much ISA that they act predominantly as positive inotropic beta-agonists while at the same time still slow down heart rate during exercise by virtue of the beta-blockade. This beneficial spectrum of properties theoretically resembles that of digitalis. Examples of such agents are **corwin** (Rousseau et al., 1983), prenalterol and pirbuterol.

Prenalterol in low doses has mild inotropic effects without increasing either heart rate or mean aortic pressure. It is also a coronary vasodilator acting on the large vessels by the beta-1-receptors (Vatner et al., 1982). At higher doses cardiac output increases even in patients with severe heart failure (Kirlin and Pitt, 1981) but there may be arrhythmias.

The inotropic effects of **pirbuterol** are blocked by metoprolol; hence beta-1-stimulation is the presumed mechanism (Ronne et al., 1981). Peripherally, pirbuterol induces vasodilation (beta-2-stimulation).

There are profound differences from the effects of isoproterenol on the heart, in that agents with ISA only slightly stimulate adenyl cyclase (despite occupying the beta-receptor) with only a small increase in tissue cyclic AMP (Fig. 19-11).

Synthetic vs natural catecholamines

Dopamine, dobutamine and salbutamol do not have the exact same spectrum of interaction with receptors as the natural catecholamines, norepinephrine and epinephrine (Table 19-3). As alpha-stimulation has a mild positive inotropic effect and a major peripheral vasoconstrictive effect, the effects of combined

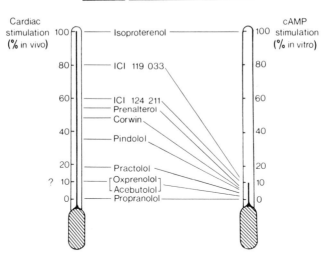

Fig. 19-11 Comparative effects of varying degrees of intrinsic sympathomimetic activity (ISA = partial agonist activity) on cardiac stimulation and on stimulation of tissue cyclic AMP. For details, see text. Modified from Main (1982). J Chem Tech Biotech 32: 617, with permission.

Table 19-3

Chief sites of action of sympathomimetic amines

Agent	Receptors stimulated
Norepinephrine (noradrenaline)	beta-1; vascular alpha
Epinephrine (adrenaline)	beta-1; some beta-2; vascular alpha
Isoproterenol (isoprenaline)	beta-1; beta-2
Dopamine	beta-1; some beta-2; high-dose vascular alpha; dopamine
Dobutamine	"Inotropic" beta-1; some beta-2
Salbutamol, rimiterol	beta-2
Pirbuterol	beta-2; some beta-1
Prenalterol	beta-1
Metaproterenol (orciprenaline)	beta-2; some beta-1
Ephedrine	NE release; beta-2
Phenylephrine, methoxamine	Vascular alpha

alpha- and beta-stimulation would be a markedly positive inotropic effect, tachycardia and (via systemic vasoconstriction) arterial hypertension. The dominant effect of such combined stimulation on the coronary system is not vasodilation, which is largely metabolically mediated with the added direct effect of beta-vasodilation. The sum of these effects is ideal for "flight or fight" reactions, but there are few clinical situations where such a group of effects is therapeutically desirable; hence the advantage of agents with more selective effects on renal vessels (dopamine) or inotropic receptors (dobutamine) or peripheral arteries (salbutamol).

Other Agents Stimulating Adenylate Cyclase

Glucagon, histamine and thyroid hormone can all interact with a membrane receptor (not the beta-adrenergic receptor) and stimulate formation of cyclic AMP (see Chapter 6). Glucagon is now seldom used as an inotropic agent (because of the side-effect of nausea) except to bypass the blocked beta-receptor in cases of overdosage with beta-blockers.

Histamine

H_2-receptors occur in the ventricles of many species, including man. They couple to adenylate cyclase to form cyclic AMP, thereby explaining the positive chronotropic and inotropic effects (Table 19-4). H_2-receptor stimulation could be the basis of a new class of inotropic agents (Fig. 19-9), of special potential in patients with "downgraded" beta-adrenergic receptors as are

Table 19-4

Effects of histamine on the heart

H$_1$-receptors mediate:
Peripheral vasodilation
Atrioventricular block
Indirect positive chronotropic effect (atropine-like
   side-effects)
Coronary vasoconstriction (in man)

H$_2$-receptors mediate:
Positive chronotropic effects
Positive inotropic effects
Peripheral vasodilation
Indirect coronary vasodilation (positive inotropic effect)
Direct coronary vasodilation
Ventricular arrhythmias

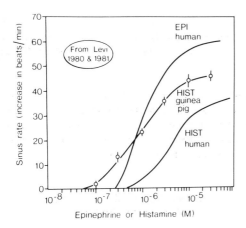

Fig. 19-12   In man, histamine is much less effective than epinephrine in increasing the heart rate. Data from Levi and Burke (1980). Europ J Pharmacol 62: 41–49, and Levi et al. (1981). Circ Res 49: 545–550, with permission.

found in severe congestive heart failure. Such agents are now receiving experimental evaluation.

A different question is the possible physiological role of endogenously produced histamine in cardiovascular regulation. It appears that the histamine concentration required to produce a chronotropic response in man is about 10^{-6} to 10^{-4} M (initial to maximal effects; Fig. 19-12). Beta-adrenergic agonists such as iso-proterenol start to increase the heart rate at lower concentrations. Thus the chronotropic effects of histamine are normally overshadowed by those of catecholamines. Histamine receptor blockade is likely

to be most active in extracardiac sites such as the gastro-intestinal tract where cimetidine and ranitidine are used in the therapy of peptic ulceration. Such therapy is usually without cardiac side-effects. There are occasional reports of cimetidine-induced sinus bradycardia especially after intravenous bolus injections, and in patients with the sick sinus syndrome.

Methylxanthines

Comparison with beta-adrenergic agonists

Phosphodiesterase inhibitors such as the methyl-xanthines also increase cardiac tissue cyclic AMP yet do not have the same effects as those of beta-adrenergic stimulation for several reasons (Table 19-5).

First, phosphodiesterase inhibition is a non-specific, non-selective process, and therefore also inhibits the phosphodiesterase for cyclic GMP. The simultaneous rise of cyclic GMP could counteract the inotropic effect of cyclic AMP (Argel et al., 1980). These conflicting effects may explain why such high doses of phosphodiesterase inhibitors (e.g. theophylline 2 μM) are required for an inotropic effect. Secondly, methylxanthines extend the active state of cardiac muscle so that the time to reach peak tension and the rate of relaxation are prolonged; catecholamines, in contrast, increase the rate both of contraction and of relaxation. The explanation is that methylxanthines interfere with both the uptake and release of calcium ions by the sarcoplasmic reticulum. The **calcium sequestering–blocking effect** can be overcome by the local anesthetic procaine and by a high stimulation frequency. Thirdly, catecholamines increase the heart rate, while methylxanthines tend to decrease the rate by vagal stimulation. A fourth difference between the two types of agents lies in the interaction with adenosine. Although methylxanthines should cause coronary vasodilation by allowing accumulation of cyclic AMP, a different interaction is that methylxanthines also compete with adenosine for the vascular adenosine receptor, so that adenosine no longer vasodilates. This is the proposed explanation for the inhibition of reactive hyperemia by methylxanthines.

With such complex effects (Table 19-5), it is not surprising that no methylxanthines are currently commercially promoted as inotropic agents.

Table 19-5

Beta-adrenergic stimulation vs phosphodiesterase inhibition by methylxanthines: effects on the heart

	Beta-stimulation	Phosphodiesterase inhibition by methylxanthine
Tissue cycle AMP	↑	↑
Tissue cyclic GMP	–	↑
Peak tension of contraction	+	+
Rate of contraction	faster	slower
Rate of relaxation	faster	slower
Ca^{2+} uptake by SR	↑	↓
Heart rate	↑	= or ↓ via vagus stimulation
Interaction with adenosine	Adenosine inhibits adenyl cyclase	Inhibition of adenosine receptor on vascular smooth muscle; inhibition of 5′ nucleotidase
Coronary dilation	+	+ but see above

SR = sarcoplasmic reticulum.

Table 19-6

Cardiovascular effects of methylxanthines

Site of action	Effect	End-result
Contractility[1,2]	Variable (species, dose)	Variable
	Increased time to peak tension	Slower contraction
	Increased peak tension	Stronger contraction
	Delayed relaxation	Contraction
Coronary arteries[3]	Dilation; possible vasoconstriction *in vivo*	Increased coronary blood flow; ? decrease also possible via adenosine
Enzymes[2,4]	Inhibition of phosphodiesterase Inhibition of 5′ nucleotidase	Increased cAMP and cGMP; ? decreased adenosine
Neuronal stores[5]	Release of catecholamines	Positive inotropy
Beta-receptors[5]	Sympathomimetic	Positive inotropy
Sarcoplasmic reticulum	Releases Ca^{2+}; inhibits uptake	Positive inotropy; delayed relaxation
Mitochondria[6]	Impaired Ca^{2+} uptake	Unknown
Sarcolemma[7,8]	Increased Ca^{2+} flux	Unknown
Action potential[9,10]	Papaverine inhibits sodium and calcium channels; caffeine differs	? negative inotropy; mixed effects

[1]Henderson et al. (1974). Cardiovasc Res 8: 162.
[2]Argel et al. (1980). J Molec Cell Cardiol 12: 939.
[3]Rutherford et al. (1981). Circulation 63: 378.
[4]Appleman et al. (1973). Adv Cycl Nucl Res 3: 65.
[5]Marcus et al. (1972). Am J Physiol 222: 1361.
[6]Blayney et al. (1978). Circ Res 43: 520.
[7]Nayler (1963). Am J Physiol 204: 969.
[8]Kavaler et al. (1978). Circ Res 42: 285.
[9]Schneider et al. (1975). J Molec Cell Cardiol 7: 867.
[10]Clusin WT (1983). Nature 301: 248.

Their major therapeutic use remains in the therapy of bronchial asthma. Yet

> Regardless of controversial claims and disappointing clinical results, the xanthines continue to be employed by some physicians in the treatment of coronary insufficiency.
> Ritchie (1975)

Papaverine (an isoquinolone derivative) is a much more powerful inhibitor of the cAMP phosphodiesterase than is theophylline; papaverine also inhibits the phosphodiesterase for cyclic GMP. That papaverine increases tissue cyclic AMP is well-established; that it increases contractility is not. High concentrations, such as 10^{-4} M, may in fact have a negative inotropic effect attributed to inhibition of calcium entry via the slow channel. Papaverine also has vasodilating properties which can best be accounted for by increased cyclic AMP levels in vascular tissue (Kukovetz et al., 1981).

Amrinone

Thus far the inotropic agents here discussed are either catecholamine-like or digitalis-like (Fig. 19-1); in either event a receptor is involved (the beta-receptor-adenylate cyclase system or the sodium pump) and the ultimate effect is an increased intracellular calcium ion concentration.

Amrinone, which has a bipyridine structure and is claimed to be effective even in patients who are fully digitalized, has a combination of positive inotropic and coronary vasodilator properties (Millard et al., 1980) that resembles the effects of catecholamines rather than of digitalis. Until recently it was believed that amrinone did not stimulate the formation of cyclic AMP in the heart; now it is known that amrinone is a phosphodiesterase inhibitor (Scholz, 1983). Thus the vasodilator effect is associated with a substantial increase in the level of cyclic AMP in vascular tissue (Meisheri et al., 1980). Amrinone might also act as a calcium ionophore, increasing the transfer of calcium across the cell membrane (Parker and Harper, 1980).

Clinically, amrinone has caused thrombocytopenia and other problems; **milrinone** is being assessed as an alternative.

Other Positively Inotropic Agents

Other experimental modes of inotropic action are being explored such as the positively inotropic dihydropyridines (Fig. 19-9) and ionophores. An example of the latter group is the agent veratrine which prevents inactivation of the fast sodium channel, thereby increasing the subsarcolemmal sodium pool with an end-result similar to digitalis (Barry et al., 1981). Monensin, another sodium ionophore, is a positive inotropic agent and coronary vasodilator. Another simple and relatively untried inotropic agent is elevation of the extracellular calcium level; this procedure avoids the "oxygen-wastage" caused by catecholamines (Levken and Semb, 1975) and requires evaluation in patients with acute myocardial ischemia. Forskolin "directly" stimulates adenylate cyclase to form intracellular cyclic AMP (Fig. 19-9). Of great promise is a new positively inotropic dihydropyridine, presumably acting on the "nitrendipine" site (Schramm et al., 1982).

Summary

Positively inotropic agents are all held to act by increasing the cytosolic calcium concentration, thereby in turn promoting interaction between actin and myosin. Digitalis compounds combine an inotropic effect with slowing of the heart. The mechanisms are an inhibition of the sodium pump and reflex vagal stimulation. The beta-adrenergic sympathomimetic agents increase cytosolic calcium indirectly by stimulating the formation of cyclic AMP which: (i) permits more calcium entry during the slow channel of the normal action potential and (ii) "preloads" the sarcoplasmic reticulum with more calcium by enhancing the uptake of calcium. Agents such as dobutamine have a more selective inotropic than chronotropic response. Such selectivity is a theoretical advantage in allowing better cardiac filling at a lower heart rate, thereby avoiding the tachycardia-induced component of the increased oxygen demand. An indirect positive inotropic effect can be obtained by peripheral vasodilation by relatively selective beta-2-stimulants such as salbutamol. Amrinone is a new positively inotropic agent, which probably acts by inhibiting phosphodiesterase, but there are clinical problems.

References

Akera T (1981). Effects of cardiac glycosides of Na^+, K^+-ATPase. In: Cardiac Glycosides, Part 1. Ed. K Greeff, pp 287–336, Springer-Verlag, Berlin.

Appleman MM, Thompson WJ, Russell TR (1973). Cyclic nucleotide phosphodiesterases. Adv Cyclic Nucl Res 3: 65–98.

Argel MI, Vittone L, Grassi AO, Chiappe LE, Chiappe GE, Cingolani HE (1980). Effect of phosphodiesterase inhibitors on heart contractile behavior, protein kinase activity and cyclic nucleotide levels. J Molec Cell Cardiol 12: 939–954.

Barry WH, Biedert S, Muira DS, Smith TW (1981). Changes in cellular Na^+, K^+ and Ca^{2+} contents, monovalent cation transport rate, and contractile state during washout of cardiac glycosides from cultured chick heart cells. Circ Res 49: 141–149.

Berend N, Marlin GE (1978). Characterization of beta-adrenoceptor subtype mediating the metabolic actions of salbutamol. Brit J Clin Pharm 5: 207–211.

Blayney L, Thomas H, Muir J, Henderson A (1978). Action of caffeine on calcium transport by isolated fractions of myofibrils, mitochondria and sarcoplasmic reticulum from rabbit heart. Circ Res 43: 520–526.

Bourdillon PDV, Dawson JR, Foale RA, Timmis AD, Poole-Wilson PA, Sutton GC (1980). Salbutamol in treatment of heart failure. Brit Heart J 43: 206–210.

Dreyer AC, Offermeier J (1975). Indications for the existence of two types of cardiac beta-adrenergic receptors. Pharm Res Comm 7: 151–161.

Franciosa JA, Cohn JN (1979). Hemodynamic effects of oral ephedrine given alone or combined with nitroprusside infusion in patients with severe left ventricular failure. Am J Cardiol 43: 79–85.

Fuchs RM, Rutlen DL, Powell WJ (1980). Effect of dobutamine on systemic capacity in the dog. Circ Res 46: 133–138.

Gillespie TA, Ambos HT, Sobel BE, Robert R (1977). Effects of dobutamine in patients with acute myocardial infarction. Am J Cardiol 39: 588–594.

Gomes JAC, Kang PS, El-Sherif N (1981). Effects of digitalis on the human sick sinus node after pharmacologic autonomic blockade. Am J Cardiol 48: 783–788.

Henderson AH, Brutsaert DL, Forman R, Sonnenblick EH (1974). Influence of caffeine on force development and force frequency relations in cat and rat heart muscle. Cardiovasc Res 8: 162–172.

Jewitt D, Birkhead J, Mitchell A, Dollery C (1974). Clinical cardiovascular pharmacology of dobutamine. A selective inotropic catecholamine. Lancet ii: 363–367.

Kavaler F, Anderson TW, Fisher VJ (1978). Sarcolemmal site of caffeine's inotropic action on ventricular muscle of the frog. Circ Res 42: 285–290.

Kim YI, Noble RJ, Zipes DR (1975). Dissociation of the inotropic effect of digitalis from its effect on atrioventricular conduction. Am J Cardiol 36: 459–467.

Kirlin PC, Pitt B (1981). Hemodynamic effects of intravenous prenalterol in severe heart failure. Am J Cardiol 47: 670–675.

Kukovetz WR, Poch G, Holzmann, S (1981). Cyclic nucleotides and relaxation of vascular smooth muscle. In: Vasodilatation. Eds PM Vanhoutte, I Leusen, pp 339–353, Raven Press, New York.

Leier CV, Heban PT, Huss P, Bush CA, Lewis RP (1978). Comparative systemic and regional hemodynamic effects of dopamine and dobutamine in patients with cardiomyopathic heart failure. Circulation 58: 466–475.

Levken J, Semb G (1975). Effect of dopamine and calcium on lipolysis and myocardial ischemic injury following acute coronary artery occlusion in the dog. Circ Res 34: 349–359.

Lewis T (1933). Diseases of the Heart, p 29, MacMillan, London.

Lorenzi M, Karam JH, Tsalikian E, Bohannon NV, Gerich JE, Forsham PH (1979). Dopamine during alpha- or beta-adrenergic blockade in man. J Clin Invest 63: 310–317.

Lown B, Klein MD, Barr I, Hagemeijer F, Kosowsky BD, Garrison H (1972). Sensitivity to digitalis drugs in acute myocardial infarction. Am J Cardiol 388–395.

Lullmann H, Peters T (1979). Action of cardiac glycosides on excitation–contraction coupling in heart muscle. Prog Pharmacol 2: 1–57.

Marban E, Tsien RW (1982). Enhancement of calcium current during digitalis inotropy in mammalian heart: positive feedback regulation by intracellular calcium? J Physiol (London) 329: 589–614.

Marcus FI, Opie LH, Sonnenblick FH (1984). Digitalis and sympathomimetic agents. In: Drugs for the Heart. Ed. Opie LH, pp 99–128, Grune & Stratton, Orlando, London and New York.

Marcus ML, Skelton CL, Grauer LE, Epstein SE (1972). Effects of theophylline on myocardial mechanics. Am J Physiol 22: 1361–1365.

Meisheri KD, Palmer RF, Van Breemen C (1980). The effects of amrinone on contractility, Ca^{2+} uptake and cAMP in smooth muscle. Europ J Pharm 61: 159–165.

Millard RW, Dube G, Grupp G, Grupp I, Alousi A, Schwartz A (1980). Direct vasodilator and positive inotropic actions of amrinone. J Molec Cell Cardiol 12: 647–652.

Moss AJ, Davis HT, Conrad DL, DeCamilla JJ, Odoroff CL (1981). Digitalis-associated cardiac mortality after myocardial infarction. Circulation 64: 1150–1155.

Nayler W (1963). Effect of ryanodine on cardiac muscle. Am J Physiol 204: 975–978.

Parker JC, Harper JR Jr (1980). Effects of amrinone, a cardiotonic drug, on calcium movements in dog erythrocytes. J Clin Invest 66: 254–269.

Podzuweit T, Dalby AJ, Cherry GW, Opie LH (1978). Cyclic AMP levels in ischemic and non-ischemic myocardium following coronary artery ligation: relation to ventricular fibrillation. J Molec Cell Cardiol 10: 81–94.

Ritchie JM (1975). Central nervous system stimulants. The xanthines. In: The Pharmacological Basis of Therapeutics, Eds Goodman and Gillman, pp 367–378, Macmillan Publications, New York.

Ronne O, Johnsson G, Lundborg P (1981). Interaction in healthy volunteers between prenalterol, a selective beta$_1$-adrenoceptor agonist, and metoprolol or propranolol. J Cardiovasc Pharm 3: 477–484.

Rousseau MF, Pouleur R, Vincent MF (1983). Effects of a cardioselective beta$_1$ partial agonist (corwin) on left ventricular function and myocardial metabolism in patients with previous myocardial infarction. Am J Cardiol 51: 1267–1274.

Rutherford JD, Vatner SF, Braunwald E (1981). Effects and mechanism of action of aminophylline on cardiac function and regional blood flow distribution in conscious dogs. Circulation 63: 378–387.

Scholz H (1983). Pharmacological actions of various inotropic agents. Europ Heart J 4: 161–172.

Schneider JA, Brooker G, Sperelakis N (1975). Papaverine blockade of an inward slow Ca^{2+} current in guinea pig heart. J Molec Cell Cardiol 7: 867–876.

Schramm M, Thomas G, Towart R, Franckowiak G (1983). Novel dihydropyridines with positive inotropic action through activation of Ca^{2+} channels. Nature 303: 535–537.

Schwartz A, Adams RJ (1980). Studies on the digitalis receptor. Circ Res 46: Suppl 1, 154–160.

Schwartz A, Lindenmayer GE, Allen JC (1975). The sodium-potassium adenosine triphosphatase: pharmacological, physiological and biochemical aspects. Pharmacol Rev 27: 3–134.

Senges J, Hennig E, Brachmann J, Pelzer D, Mizutani T, Kubler W (1980). Effects of orciprenaline on the sinoatrial and atrioventricular nodes in the presence of hypoxia. J Molec Cell Cardiol 12: 135–147.

Skou JC (1957). The influence of some cations on an adenosine triphosphatase from peripheral nerves. Biochim Biophys Acta 23: 394–401.

Somberg JC, Smith TW (1979). Localization of the neurally mediated arrhythmogenic properties of digitalis. Science 204: 321–323.

Stephens JD, Hayward RP, Ead H, Adams L, Spurrell RAJ (1978). Comparative peripheral and coronary haemodynamic effects of rimiterol and isoprenaline. Brit J Clin Pharm 6: 163–170.

Taggart AJ, Johnston GD, McDevitt DG (1983). Digoxin withdrawal after cardiac failure in patients with sinus rhythm. J Cardiovasc Pharm 5: 229–234.

Tandon MK (1980). Cardiopulmonary effects of fenoterol and salbutamol aerosols. Chest 77: 429–431.

Timmis AD, Strak SK, Chamberlain DA (1979). Haemodynamic effects of salbutamol in patients with acute myocardial infarction and severe left ventricular dysfunction. Brit Med J 2: 1101–1103.

Tsurata K, Frey EA, Grewe CW, Cote TE, Eskay RL, Kebabian JW (1981). Evidence that LY-141865 specifically stimulates the D-2 dopamine receptor. Nature 292: 463–465.

Tuttle RR, Hillman CC, Toomey RE (1976). Differential beta-adrenergic sensitivity of atrial and ventricular tissue assessed by chronotropic, inotropic, and cyclic AMP responses to isoprenaline and dobutamine. Cardiovasc Res 10: 452–458.

Vasu MA, O'Keefe DD, Kapellakis GZ, Vezeridis MP, Jacobs ML, Daggett WM, Powell WJ Jr (1978). Myocardial oxygen consumption: effects of epinephrine, isoproterenol, dopamine, norepinephrine and dobutamine. Am J Physiol 235: H237–H241.

Vatner SF, Baig H (1978). Comparison of the effects of ouabain and isoproterenol on ischemic myocardium of conscious dogs. Circulation 58: 654–662.

Vatner SF, Hintze TH, Macho P (1982). Regulation of large coronary arteries by beta-adrenergic mechanisms in the conscious dog. Circ Res 51: 56–66.

Waagstein F, Malek I, Hjalmarson AC (1978). The use of dobutamine in myocardial infarction for reversal of the cardiodepressive effect of metoprolol. Brit J Clin Pharm 5: 515–521.

New References

Chemnitius JM, Bing RJ (1985). Beta-1-adrenoceptor agonists with low adenylate cyclase activation – theoretical and clinical implications. Can J Cardiol 1: 186–190.

Fozzard HA, Sheets MF (1985). Cellular mechanism of action of cardiac glycosides. J Am Coll Cardiol 5: 10A–15A.

Lee CO, Abete P, Pecker M, Sonn JK, Vassale M (1985). Strophanthidin inotropy: role of intracellular sodium ion activity and sodium-calcium exchange. J Molec Cell Cardiol, in press.

Packer M, Medina N, Yushak M (1984). Hemodynamic and clinical limitations of long-term inotropic therapy with amrinone in patients with severe chronic heart failure. Circulation 70: 1038–1047.

Simonton CA, Chatterjee K, Cody RJ, Kubo SH, Leonard D, Daly P, Rutman H (1985). Milrinone in congestive heart failure: Acute and chronic hemodynamic and clinical evaluation. J Am Coll Cardiol 6: 453–459.

Surawicz B (1985). Factors affecting tolerance to digitalis. J Am Coll Cardiol 5: 69A–81A.

IV

Heart Disease: Pathophysiology and Pharmacological Therapy

20 Hypertension

One of the most common forms of a chronically increased work load on the heart is systemic arterial hypertension. The etiology of essential hypertension is unknown — some believe that in its early stages it is caused by an excess cardiac output, for example as the result of increased catecholamine stimulation. The increased cardiac output meets a peripheral resistance which is unable to relax adequately and the blood pressure goes up, at first intermittently and later in a sustained way. A reduced cardiac output is one mechanism whereby beta-adrenergic receptor blockade reduces blood pressure. In the later stages of hypertension the major defect appears to be an increased peripheral vascular resistance. In hypertension there is an increase of peripheral vascular resistance relative to the requirements of the body so that either the cardiac output must fall (which could cause tissue underperfusion) or the arterial pressure must rise. A decrease in the peripheral vascular resistance by vasodilation is one important mode of therapy of hypertension. Besides beta-adrenergic blockers and vasodilators, another important category of agents is the diuretics, which act in a largely unknown way to reduce blood pressure. Yet other agents act centrally or on the angiotensin–renin mechanism.

Evaluation of Hypertension

Sustained arterial hypertension results when vasoconstrictor influences on the peripheral resistance vessels chronically exceed the vasodilator influences.

In **essential hypertension** the cause is unknown, in contrast to those rather unusual patients with **secondary hypertension** in whom a single cause can be identified. For example, in patients with unilateral renal artery stenosis, or unilateral renal disease, the ischemic kidney puts forth renin which promotes the formation of angiotensin (Fig. 20-1). Sustained hypertension may cause cardiac hypertrophy which may progress the heart failure. Most deaths in severely hypertensive patients are from cerebrovascular accidents (strokes) or from renal failure (damage to renal blood vessels) or myocardial infarction. As the hypertension progresses, secondary irreversible vascular changes occur. Yet it must not be supposed that such a relentlessly progressive course is inevitable.

There is a **continuum of blood pressure** distribution from low to high throughout the population, so that the correct cut-off point for diagnosing hypertension is difficult to define. The commonly quoted value of 120/80 mmHg is indeed normal but the true question is what constitutes abnormality. A sustained level of over 140/90 mmHg in younger patients is generally accepted as abnormal, yet each possible antihypertensive therapy (except weight reduction and salt restriction) has its side-effects, so that different physicians set different levels for therapy, such as (for example) a value exceeding 160/100 mmHg (for a critical discussion, see Kaplan, 1981). Others suggest 95 mmHg as the cut-off point for drug therapy (page 285). In the elderly, higher values with controversial limits are required for therapy because the blood pressure normally increases with age and because the thickened arteriosclerotic arteries may not respond well to therapy.

Due to variable catecholamine discharge in response to emotions and environmental factors (such as cold), the arterial pressure can be highly variable so that care must be taken before deciding on therapy which will probably have to be life-long.

Systolic vs diastolic pressure

The systolic pressure is the highest pressure that can be measured and the diastolic is the lowest. These can readily be identified by the appearance and disappearance of arterial sounds with a sphygmomanometer (the **Korotkoff** sounds, after the Russian physiologist). The diastolic pressure is primarily determined by the amount of arteriolar vasoconstriction. The pulse pressure (difference between systolic and diastolic pressures) is determined mainly by the stroke volume and the elasticity of the aorta and arterial system. In particular the systolic pressure is labile in response to catecholamine stimulation as the stroke volume of the heart varies with altered catecholamine discharge to the myocardium. As vascular elasticity is lost with age, the systolic pressure may rise with age; such **systolic hypertension** was previously thought to be relatively harmless. However, the heart must work against both systolic and diastolic pressures and it is now known that both are important determinants of the severity of hypertension.

Mechanisms of Essential Hypertension

In the majority of patients with hypertension the cause is unknown (essential hypertension). In a minority, hypertension develops secondary to another cause, most frequently renal disease. The early descriptions of chronic glomerulonephritis by Bright included heart disease. The critical experiments were those of Goldblatt et al. (1934) who produced hypertension by unilateral renal ischemia, which activates the renin–angiotensin–aldosterone mechanism (Fig. 20-1).

Although the exact cause of essential hypertension is still not known, some of the mechanisms which have been proposed are as follows. First, links with renal disease led to the use of a salt-restricted diet, and diuretics for the therapy of hypertension. Even in the absence of renal disease, such procedures turned out to be beneficial, thereby establishing complex links between salt and blood pressure. Epidemiological surveys show that populations with a high salt intake are more prone to hypertension, but an individual may be hypertensive even though his salt intake is normal. A second type of mechanism for hypertension involves an increased adrenergic drive which could increase the blood pressure in several ways (Fig. 20-2), including an increased cardiac output and renin release from the kidney as a result of beta-adrenergic stimulation. Increased alpha-adrenergic stimulation could increase blood pressure by increasing peripheral

UNILATERAL RENAL ARTERY STENOSIS

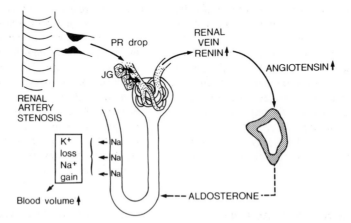

Fig. 20-1 Mechanisms responsible for hypertension in unilateral renal disease. This sequence stems from earlier work with unilateral renal ischemia, as induced in the Goldblatt kidney. Corrective arterial surgery (angioplasty) or balloon-dilation may be very effective in relieving unilateral renal artery stenosis. PR = arterial pressure; JG = juxtaglomerular apparatus, from which renin is formed.

CATECHOLAMINE MECHANISMS IN HYPERTENSION

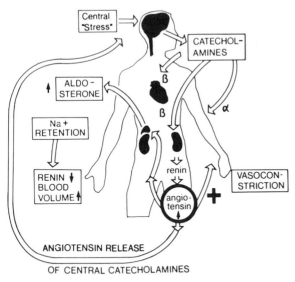

Fig. 20-2 Possible mechanisms whereby catecholamine stimulation plays a role in hypertension.

vasoconstriction. It is thought that adrenergic-mediated mechanisms are especially important in younger hypertensive subjects.

A third type of abnormality resides in the renin–angiotensin–aldosterone system which may predispose to hypertension by, for example, causing excessive renin release in response to beta-adrenergic stimulation or salt restriction. Additional hormonal factors may be involved, to explain the frequency with which hypertension is associated with obesity and the fall in blood pressure after weight reduction.

The common consequence of many of these mechanisms is an **increased peripheral vascular resistance**, mediated by at least two mechanisms: an enhanced influx of calcium ions into the smooth muscle cells of resistance arterioles, and enhanced alpha-adrenergic vasoconstriction (Buhler et al., 1984). Normally such an increased resistance would elevate blood pressure and depress cardiac output, which in turn would evoke a reflex to return the blood pressure to normal. Abnormalities of such reflexes, mediated by the baroreceptors, are therefore thought to play an important ancillary or perpetuating role in hypertension. Other genetic factors of importance might be a defect in the sodium–potassium exchange

mechanism of vascular smooth muscle cells, or other genetic imperfections of sodium or chloride regulation (Whitescraver et al., 1984).

Hypertension should probably be regarded as a multifactorial disease, with different mechanisms in operation in different individuals, in which a precipitating abnormality might trigger sustained elevation of blood pressure especially in a person with genetic imperfections of normal feedback mechanism.

Baroreflexes and Hypertension

To co-ordinate the circulation in different parts of the body requires the action of the autonomic nervous system and particularly its sympathetic branch. The **vasomotor center** at the base of the brain brings together signals from the body as a whole and then transmits afferent impulses through vasoconstrictor fibers to the blood vessels of the body. Some of the afferent stimuli going to the vasomotor center originate in the **baroreceptors** in the walls of the arch of the aorta and at the origin of the internal carotid artery (see Fig. 16-1). When the blood pressure increases these receptors are stimulated and the vasomotor center is inhibited so that there is peripheral vasodilation and the blood pressure drops back to normal. At the same time the heart rate slows (vagal effect). Abnormalities of the cardiovascular **baroreflexes** are thought to play a role in the development of hypertension. The baroreceptors which inhibit sympathetic activity, might not function normally when patients with borderline hypertension stand up. Therefore, there could be increased renin release from the kidneys and an increased peripheral vascular resistance. The increased peripheral resistance in hypertension might also develop in the peripheral venous system so that there is a large central blood volume with a shift of blood from the peripheral to the central venous capacitance system; the increased central blood volume may cause a greater stretch of cardiac receptors (Mark, 1983).

Similar vasodepressor reflexes also play a role in **other disease states**. In **carotid sinus hypersensitivity**, syncope may be caused by afferent stimuli originating in a carotid sinus rendered more sensitive by arteriosclerosis. The **Bezold–Jarish reflex** is another inhibitory reflex, originating in cardiac sensory receptors. The efferent arc (efferent = leading from) is conveyed by the vagus and results in a reflex bradycardia, vasodilation and hypotension. The afferent (leading to) arc of this reflex can be stimulated by inferoposterior myocardial ischemia and infarction, or by coronary arteriography. The reflex may be centrally set off in **vasovagal syncope** and by the central stimulating effect of digitalis.

Therapy of Hypertension

Diuretics

In hypertension there are multiple possible sites of therapeutic attack responding to the presumed multifactorial etiology (Fig. 20-3). Therapy with thiazide diuretics is still common "step-one" therapy for hypertension, with the subsequent introduction of other agents such as beta-adrenergic blockers and vasodilators (**step-care therapy**). How excess salt intake increases vascular reactivity and blood pressure is unclear. Some workers think that an aldosterone response evokes a diuresis in normal individuals whereas in genetically predisposed subjects the sodium excretion is delayed so that sodium accumulates with an increased intramuscular volume. Others emphasize the role of a sodium–potassium exchange mechanism, not the conventional sodium pump, which is sensitive to furosemide and not to digitalis; the mechanism may be abnormally sluggish in hypertension, to allow accumulation of sodium in vascular smooth muscle, with subsequent displacement of calcium from binding sites and vascular constriction. By acting on these

SITES OF ACTION OF ANTI- HYPERTENSIVE AGENTS

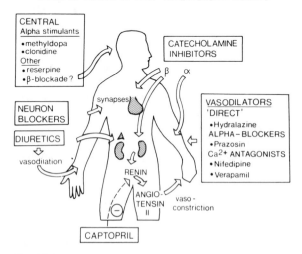

Fig. 20-3 Multiple possible therapeutic sites of attack in hypertension.

mechanisms or on others such as those regulating prostaglandin synthesis, diuretics can be efficient antihypertensive agents in mild to moderate hypertension, dropping the pressure by 5–10 mmHg. On the debit side, hypokalemia is a risk and long term therapy with thiazide diuretics may provoke diabetes, gout or impotence (unknown mechanism). Thus initial therapy with lower doses of thiazide diuretics such as 25 mg hydrochlorothiazide (to lessen side-effects) or beta-blockade is increasingly preferred.

Beta-adrenergic blockade

The mechanism whereby beta-adrenergic blockers decrease blood pressure is still not clear despite years of use. Several have been proposed: the fall of cardiac output; a central effect; inhibition of the formation of renin; and, most recently, inhibition of norepinephrine release by blockade of a prejunctional beta-adrenergic receptor. Each explanation fails to explain all the facts fully, so that most workers accept a multifactorial mechanism. What is important is that neither vascular sodium–potassium exchange nor the vascular contractile mechanism are affected. Thus beta-blockade can be added readily to therapy with diuretics and/or vasodilators in step-care therapy. Some "standard" doses are: propranolol 160–320 mg once daily of a long-acting preparation; nadolol 80–320 mg once daily; atenolol 50–100 mg once daily; and metoprolol 100–200 mg twice daily. Areas of concern are the frequent side-effects of beta-blockade which include fatigue (probably due to a low cardiac output), enhanced heart block and precipitation of cardiac failure (negative inotropic effect). Most serious of all potential side-effects is precipitation of severe bronchospasm, a risk which is lessened by the use of a cardioselective beta-blocker (see Fig. 16-9) in a low dose.

Alpha-adrenergic blockade

A recently favored theory is that the increased vascular resistance in hypertension is caused by an alpha-mediated vasoconstriction. For example, patients with essential hypertension have a more marked hypotensive response to prazosin (an alpha-1 postjunctional inhibitor) than do normotensive controls. In contrast, there is a similar response to the non-specific vasodilator sodium nitroprusside (Amann et al., 1981). The cause of the increased alpha-mediated vasoconstriction may either be an increased sensitivity of the vessels (hereditary factor) or increased adrenergic drive ("stress"). Hence prazosin is frequently used, with a low first dose (0.5 mg at night) to avoid first-dose syncope, increasing the dose step-wise up to 20 mg twice daily.

Calcium antagonists

First introduced for angina pectoris, compounds such as nifedipine, verapamil and diltiazem may yet come to have their major application in hypertension. Nitrendipine, a long-acting dihydropyridine, is currently under clinical evaluation. Besides reducing the afterload, calcium antagonists appear to have a significant diuretic effect.

Vasodilators

Besides vasodilators of known or reasonably well-understood mechanism of action—alpha-1-blockers, calcium-antagonists—there are compounds called "direct" vasodilators whose mode of action is not yet understood. Such are **hydralazine**, which is being used in the therapy of hypertension, but causes an unwanted **reflex tachycardia. Two agents are used only for severe hypertension—minoxidil (side-effect: hirsuties) and** diazoxide (side-effect: pancreatic damage).

Captopril, by inhibiting the renin-induced formation of angiotensin, is probably most effective when the circulating renin value is high (as in renal hyper-tension). Its defect is the development occasionally of severe immunologically based side-effects such as neutropenia or proteinuria, which are probably limited if the total daily dose is kept below 150 mg (in three divided doses). As with prazosin, the first dose should be low to avoid syncope (see page 311).

Agents acting on the sympathetic nervous system

As neurotransmission starts in the sympathetic nervous system it may be supposed that a decreased sym-pathetic discharge could be achieved by agents which act centrally. Clonidine and methyldopa stimulate central alpha-2-receptors (presynaptic) which activate an inhibitory system (possibly involving beta-endorphin and opiate receptors; Fig. 20-4) to reduce

CENTRAL EFFECTS OF CLONIDINE
AND METHYLDOPA

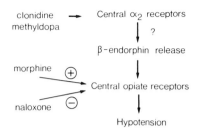

Fig. 20-4 Proposed central mechanisms of hypotensive action of clonidine and methyldopa.

peripheral sympathetic activity (Van Zwieten et al., 1983). Agents inhibiting ganglion transmissions such as guanethidine are no longer used. Agents depleting the terminal neurons of norepinephrine such as reserpine, cause a chemical sympathectomy and thereby decrease the rate of release of norepinephrine.

Several of these agents (clonidine, methyldopa, high-dose reserpine) can have sedation or depression as side-effects, presumably because the level of central awareness is decreased. In the case of clonidine a rebound hypertension may develop on sudden withdrawal (as when tablets run out). Lowering the dose of reserpine lessens side-effects while maintaining the hypotensive effect (Veterans Administration trial,

HYPERTENSION: SOME FACTORS GOVERNING
TREATMENT

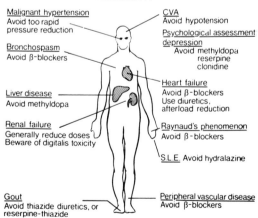

Fig. 20-5 Principles of choice of antihypertensive agent. Each patient needs individual assessment to avoid side-effects which might be harmful for them. SLE = systemic lupus erythematosus.

1982), because the peripheral effect is maintained even at the lower dose. While methyldopa is still widely used there is an increasing trend towards other agents which do not have prominent central side-effects; another of its defects is the occasional development of hepatitis or hemolytic anemia.

Combination therapy

Hypertension is frequently sufficiently severe to require a combination of agents, each acting through a different mechanism (Fig. 20-3). For example, a common combination is a diuretic, a beta-blocker and a vasodilator. Among vasodilators, prazosin or nifedipine are increasingly favored with hydralazine used less. Thereafter captopril is brought in. Powerful vasodilators with severe side-effects such as minoxidil are reserved for resistant cases. Centrally active agents such as reserpine, methyldopa and clonidine are all cheap and effective but limited by various side-effects. Of these, low-dose reserpine may be the safest. Apart from such generalizations, each patient needs individual assessment to avoid side-effects which might be harmful for that person (Fig. 20-5).

Step Care in Hypertension

Ideally the blood pressure should be normalized and kept so throughout the patient's life. This aim is frequently not achieved either because multiple therapy reduces compliance of the patient (too many tablets to take) or because drug side-effects prevent optimal doses from being used. The conventional approach at present is the use of diuretics, beta-blockade and then vasodilators in that order (Table 20-1). Strictly speaking each of these agents should be used one at a time before combination. Recently the approach to step-care therapy has undergone a change (Kaplan, 1983) with the realization that beta-blockade is logically the therapy of choice in younger patients where excess sympathetic drive appears to be more prominent. The demonstration that diuretic therapy has many unexpected side-effects such as impotence and loss of libido as well as the problems of electrolyte disturbances, together with the potential for serious diseases such as diabetes and gout, has lessened enthusiasm for diuretics as the first step. In several big trials in which diuretics have been used as first-

Table 20-1

Principles of therapy in hypertension

1. **Assessment** of severity of hypertension and of end-organ damage
2. Elimination of **secondary** causes, especially renal artery stenosis
3. **General measures**: weight reduction, salt restriction
4. **Decision to treat with drugs**: initiation of therapy if sustained diastolic exceeds 100 mmHg (high values in older age group, lower values in younger patients or those with end-organ damage)
5. **Initial therapy** with beta-adrenergic blockers or alpha-adrenergic blockers or diuretics
6. **Combination therapy** with two and thereafter three of the above agents
7. **Add** vasodilator—nifedipine (or hydralazine)
8. **Add** captopril (or replace vasodilator by captopril)
9. If financial considerations are important, start with low-dose **reserpine** instead of beta- or alpha-blocker
10. **Methyldopa** or **clonidine** may be used instead of reserpine with due care for prominent central side-effects such as drowsiness (other side-effects: methyldopa—liver dysfunction, hemolytic anemia; clonidine—withdrawal rebound hypertension)

step therapy, the blood pressure has been lowered and there has been a gratifying reduction in the incidence of some consequences of hypertension such as stroke without, however, decreasing the incidence of myocardial infarction. Possibly the diuretics in some way promote the development of vascular disease. Theoretically, diuretics are of most use in (i) elderly patients, where the renin levels are more likely to be low and where increasing the renin level may help to sensitize the patient to added beta-blockade; and (ii) in black patients, who are thought to be less sensitive to beta-blockers.

Whilst beta-blockade is increasingly becoming first-line therapy in other patients there can be major disadvantages. First, the lowered cardiac output may limit exercise performance which some younger patients find a serious inconvenience. Secondly, the blood lipids tend to develop an atherogenic pattern, especially with the use of non-selective blockers. For these reasons some clinicians are now exploring the use of alpha-1 blockers such as prazosin or even calcium-antagonists as first-line therapy. The latter might be of particular use in elderly patients (Bühler et al., 1984). The state of the art will be in flux until large-scale prospective trials, comparing a number of different potential first-line agents, become available. In the meantime it seems that there will be a trend away from diuretics, especially in the higher doses used in some combination tablets. A daily dose of a thiazide diuretic equivalent to 25 mg of hydrochlorothiazide should be effective, especially in combination with a beta-blocker or with low-dose reserpine, and higher doses of thiazide will in all probability only produce more complications.

New Principles in Therapy

Among the agents now being tested are (i) **ketanserin**, a serotonin antagonist and vasodilator; and (ii) synthetic vasodilatory **prostaglandins**. Conversely, **indomethacin** which is an inhibitor of the synthesis of prostaglandins (see Fig. 16-4) and widely used as an anti-inflammatory agent in arthritis, lessens the effect of many antihypertensives including beta-blockers, diuretics and captopril.

Non-pharmacological Therapy

In view of the problems and side-effects created by most types of drug therapy for hypertension, a reasonable first-line approach in patients with "mild hypertension" (e.g. diastolic values up to 95 mmHg) is a trial of non-drug therapy. Such measures include weight loss, restriction of dietary sodium chloride to 5 grams daily, modest low alcohol consumption and non-smoking.

Complications of Hypertension

The sole aim of therapy is not reduction of blood pressure. **End-organ damage** may include cardiac, renal and cerebral complications. Of these, control of the pressure by any therapy will reduce the incidence of strokes. The position with **cardiac complications** is less clear. Thus far no therapy has managed to bring down the incidence of coronary heart disease (possible exception: beta-adrenergic blockade). In the case of cardiac hypertrophy, the development of cardiomegaly does not necessarily mean a failing heart; the ejection fraction is frequently high–normal. Nevertheless the heart size should be reduced back to normal because early predominantly concentric hypertrophy may progress to cardiac dilation. A reasonable supposition would be that removal of wall stress by treatment of hypertension would cause regression of hypertrophy.

Yet in spontaneously hypertensive rats regression of hypertrophy depends on the type of therapy and not simply on the level of the blood pressure (Sher, 1983); adrenergic modifying agents such as methyldopa, reserpine and captopril (and probably beta-blockers) are more effective than vasodilators such as hydralazine or minoxidil. Diuretics, which may indirectly increase adrenergic activity, are also in the less effective group. In patients where the genesis of hypertension may differ from rats, several studies suggest that it is the level of pressure that matters more than the hypotensive agent used in determining regression of cardiac hypertrophy.

Renal failure is a dreaded complication of hypertension because, as it progresses, more and more of the renal arterioles are damaged till irreversible failure sets in; the kidney may in this process secrete excess amounts of renin to further elevate the pressure. Many claims have been made that certain specific beta-blockers or other agents are less likely to reduce renal blood flow and glomerular filtration than other agents. Thus far no advantage for any specific mode of therapy has been proven.

Malignant hypertension is diagnosed by the combination of an excessively high diastolic blood pressure, frequently above 140 mmHg, and papilledema. The cause is accelerated and the prognosis serious. Besides heart or renal failure, focal cerebral signs may develop (**hypertensive encephalopathy**). Traditionally the therapy has been with intravenous agents such as diazoxide or nitroprusside; now it is realized that an excessively rapid drop of blood pressure with these agents can precipitate cerebral hypoperfusion with infarction. A new relatively simple **and seemingly safe therapy is by sublingual nifedipine (Huysmans et al., 1983), which may avoid cerebral problems by being a cerebral vasodilator.**

Summary

An increased peripheral vascular resistance is important in hypertension, either as an initiating or perpetuating mechanism. In hypertension a common "step-care" approach is to use diuretics initially, followed by beta-adrenergic blockade and vasodilators. This rank order is now undergoing some revision as the long-term side-effects of diuretics are being evaluated.

References

Amann FW, Bolli P, Kiowski W, Bühler FR (1981). Enhanced alpha-adrenoceptor mediated vasoconstriction in essential hypertension. Hypertension 3: Suppl 1, 119–123.

Bühler FR, Bolli P, Hulthen UL (1984). Calcium-influx dependent vasoconstrictor mechanisms in essential hypertension. In Calcium-Antagonists and Cardiovascular Disease, Ed. LH Opie, pp 313–322, Raven Press, New York.

Goldblatt H, Lynch J, Hanzal RF, Summerville WW (1934). Studies on experimental hypertension. I. Production of persistent elevation of systolic blood pressure by means of renal ischemia. J Exp Med 59: 347–379.

Huysmans FTM, Sluiter HE, Thien TA, Koene RAP (1983). Acute treatment of hypertensive crisis with nifedipine. Brit J Clin Pharm 16: 725–727.

Kaplan NM (1981). Whom to treat: the dilemma of mild hypertension. Am Heart J 101: 867–870.

Kaplan NM (1983). New choices for initial drug therapy of hypertension. Am J Cardiol 51: 621–627.

Mark AL (1983). The Bezold–Jarish reflex revisited. Clinical implications of inhibitory reflexes originating in the heart. J Am Col Cardiol 1: 90–102.

Sher S (1983). Regression of cardiac hypertrophy — experimental animal model. Am J Med 75: 87–93.

Van Zwieten PA, Thoolen MJMC, Timmermans PBMWM (1983). The pharmacology of centrally acting antihypertensive agents. Brit J Clin Pharm 15: 455S–462S.

Veterans Administration (1982). Low doses vs standard dose of reserpine. A randomized, double-blind, multiclinical trial in patients taking chlorthalidone. J Am Med Assoc 248: 2471–2477.

Whitescarver SA, Ott CE, Jackson BA (1984). Salt-sensitive hypertension: contribution of chloride. Science 223: 1430–1432.

New References

Bühler FR, Bigger JT Jr (1985). Calcium antagonists and renin-angiotensin inhibitors for antihypertensive therapy (eds). J Cardiovasc Pharmacol 7 (Suppl 4): S1–S102.

Editorial (1985). Treatment of hypertension: the 1985 results. Lancet 2: 645–647.

Richards AM, Ikram H, Yandle TG, Nicholls MG, Webster MWI, Espiner EA (1985). Renal, haemodynamic, and hormonal effects of human alpha atrial natriuretic peptide in healthy volunteers. Lancet 1: 545–549.

21 Valvular Heart Disease and Cardiomyopathy

Congestive heart failure may develop in response to overload or myocardial disease (cardiomyopathy). Hypertensive heart disease is an example of pressure overload. Valvular heart disease (Table 21-1) provides examples of two types of overload—pressure and volume. Aortic stenosis is the classic example of

Table 21-1

Features of common valvular lesions

Lesion	Auscultation	Hemodynamics	Echocardiogram
Aortic stenosis	"Diamond-shaped" ejection murmur; soft A_2	Anacrotic pulse with slow rise; LV pressure increased; systolic pressure gradient from LV to aorta	Thick aortic valves with small orifice; concentric hypertrophy, later dilation and/or abnormal contractile function
Aortic regurgitation (= incompetence = insufficiency)	Early diastolic blowing murmur. May be "Austin Flint", murmur at apex resembling mitral stenosis (see page 292)	Low diastolic aortic pressure with collapsing pulse and hyperdynamic circulation. Angiographic reflex of dye from aorta into LV	Enlarged end-diastolic and later end-systolic volume; initially increased then poor systolic fractional shortening
Combined aortic lesions	Systolic and diastolic murmurs	Pulsus bisferiens; systolic pressure gradient; dye reflux in diastole	Combined features of above
Mitral stenosis	Mid-diastolic rumbling murmur with presystolic accentuation; may be opening snap, loud first sound. Atrial fibrillation frequent (no presystolic murmur)	High left atrial pressure with increased gradient to LV in diastole. Pulmonary hypertension in some. Low cardiac output	Normal systolic posterior valve movement replaced by anterior movement and concordance of movements of both valves; thickened valves; poor diastolic separation
Mitral regurgitation (= incompetence = insufficiency)	Pansystolic apical murmur; 3rd heart sound frequent	Wide pulse pressure, higher diastolic pressure than in AR. Angiographic systolic reflux of dye into left atrium	Enlarged left ventricle and left atrium with increased contractile activity
Mitral valve prolapse	Late apical systolic murmur; systolic click	Angiographic prolapse of valve	Abrupt posterior movement of posterior mitral leaflet in mid-systole

AORTIC VALVE DISEASE : ABNORMAL OXYGENATION

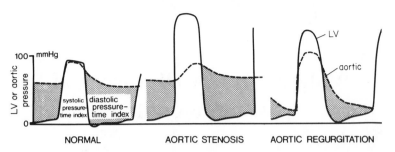

Fig. 21-1 Contrasting effects of pressure overload in aortic stenosis and volume overload in aortic regurgitation (= insufficiency). Potential mechanisms for anaerobic metabolism differ in aortic stenosis (increased systolic pressure and increased oxygen demand) from aortic regurgitation (reduced diastolic perfusion pressure with decreased oxygen supply). The diastolic pressure–time index reflects the oxygen supply and the systolic pressure–time index reflects the oxygen demand. LV = left ventricular pressure; aorta = aortic pressure.

pressure overload (Fig. 21-1), with aortic regurgitation and mitral regurgitation examples of volume overload. In addition, in aortic regurgitation there are the added effects of poor diastolic perfusion. In mitral stenosis there is neither pressure nor volume overload, but a markedly increased filling pressure is required to overcome the stenosis and thereby to maintain left ventricular filling. In some types of congenital heart disease there may be, in addition to the valvular lesions, the added problems of poor oxygen delivery because of systemic oxygen desaturation.

Models of Pressure and Volume Overload

Wollenberger (1949) was among the first to stress that a volume-overload could be tolerated much better than a pressure load (Fig. 21-2). Experimentally, when a volume load is applied to the heart by the production of a fistula, the sarcomere length increases to the optimum of 2.2 μm and stays there even when chronic dilation occurs (2.2 μm is the value near the apex of the length–tension curve of normal cardiac muscle; see Fig. 9-8). The mechanism of the dilation appears to be by a hypertrophy of myocardial cells in the longitudinal (circumferential) direction, with later "slippage" between adjacent fibers and fibrils accounting for the ultimate decrease in contractility.

In contrast, when an acute volume load is applied by acute aortic regurgitation the ventricle dilates little and the features are those of an elevated left atrial pressure (Morganroth et al., 1977).

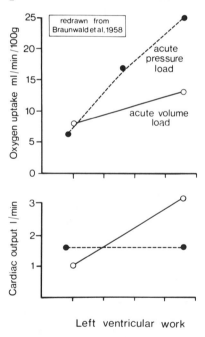

Fig. 21-2 An acute volume load will increase the preload and the cardiac output by the Starling mechanism and also increase myocardial oxygen uptake. An acute pressure load will increase the afterload and the oxygen uptake despite the fixed cardiac output. Here the increased oxygen uptake is used for synthesis of ATP required to overcome the pressure load. Redrawn from Braunwald et al. (1958). Am J Physiol 192: 148–156, with permission.

WALL STRESS : CHRONIC PRESSURE VS VOLUME LOAD

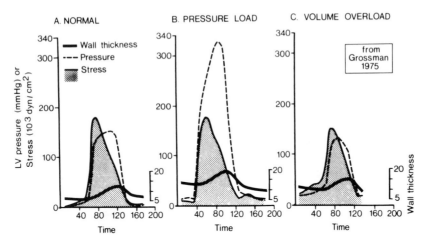

Fig. 21-3 These measurements made on patients by Grossman et al. (1975) show that in chronic aortic stenosis (middle panel), the increased wall thickness compensates for the increased left ventricular ejection pressure, so that wall stress increases little. During a chronic volume overload (right panel), the wall thickness and left ventricular pressure change little. Wall stress is therefore unchanged. From Grossman et al. (1975), with permission from J Clin Invest and the authors.

All such "volume models" are not typical of the usual patient with overload hypertrophy and failure, nor even of chronic aortic regurgitation where tension-induced hypertrophy may develop. In a pressure-overloaded heart (model: pulmonary artery constriction in the cat), the sarcomere lengths are also 2.2 μm — again the optimal values for normal muscle. At this stage there is no disengagement of the thick and thin filaments, although impaired cross-bridge function cannot be excluded. As the muscle mass increases (Fig. 21-3) a high systolic pressure can be maintained without loss of contractility. Thereafter the muscle develops defective contractile activity as an intrinsic defect rather than simply operating on the descending limb of the Frank–Starling curve. The decreased contractile activity may be correlated at a molecular level with decreased myosin ATPase activity (see page 302). Despite the decreased contractile activity the increased muscle mass allows maintenance of cardiac output at rest but not during exercise. This sequence is not inevitable. It is also proposed that if the initial load is not overly severe, or perhaps if applied gradually with adequate time for hypertrophy to occur, there may be an adequate adaptation to pressure overload without any depression of mechanical performance (see Fig. 15-4).

Hemodynamic Overload.
Concentric versus Eccentric Hypertrophy

Concentric hypertrophy is thought to be the result of an increased peak systolic tension producing a "parallel replication" of sarcomeres (Grossman et al., 1975). In contrast, a volume overload leads to increased diastolic tension which leads to a "series of replication" of sarcomeres with chamber enlargement and eccentric hypertrophy. The defect of this proposal is that true replication results in hyperplasia as opposed to hypertrophy; true hyperplasia is not thought to occur in the adult heart except in extreme conditions (Chapter 15). The analysis of Grossman could be modified to propose that the sarcomere undergoes "lateral" hypertrophy to become "fatter" in pressure overload, and "longitudinal" hypertrophy to become "longer" in volume overload. How the mechanical stimuli are transmitted to these sarcomere changes is not clarified.

An alternate view of concentric and eccentric hypertrophy was provided by Linzbach (1960) in a classic paper. He saw concentric hypertrophy as being the normal myocardial response until a critical limit was reached, when the hypertrophied heart outstripped its blood supply, whereupon degeneration and eccentric hypertrophy occurred. His views do not allow for the early eccentric hypertrophy in aortic regurgitation, when there is no evidence of anaerobic metabolism at rest (see later). Yet the idea of the hypertrophied myocardium outstripping its blood supply has stayed with cardiologists ever since Linzbach's paper.

Wall stress

In the early stage of compensatory hyperfunction, wall stress in systole is normalized by the concentric hypertrophy; diastolic wall thickness is also increased. Histologically, there is hypertrophy without degeneration (Ferrans, 1982; Table 1). It must not be presumed that a uniform process is occurring. Rather, during a severe pressure overload, some cells become hypertrophied and metabolically overactive while others suffer and degenerate. It is particularly the cells in the left ventricular endocardium where these divergent changes are most marked, presumably because it is there that the blood supply can most easily become defective in relation to the enhanced oxygen demand of the hypertrophied left ventricle (Hatt et al., 1982).

The pressure overloaded heart can stay in a stable state (Meerson stage 2; see Fig. 15-4) if the load is moderate and the histological signs of damage are minimal. If the load is severe then the consequences are: (i) histologic degeneration; (ii) impaired contractility; (iii) abnormal metabolic changes; and (iv) fibrosis. A combination of these factors leads to the "myocardial factor" so that even if the pressure load is relieved, the myocardium fails to recover adequately.

Degenerative changes

The most important change is disruption of the sarcomere structure, with lysis especially of the thick filaments (Ferrans, 1982). The remaining actin filaments are tangled and disorganized. The myofibril-free areas may be occupied by mitochondria or glycogen granules or by sarcoplasmic reticulum (both tubules and cisterns). A critical development is that of interstitial fibrosis, which is one factor preventing reversibility of function after surgical correction (Krayenbuehl et al., 1983).

The mechanism of these changes is ill-understood. Hatt et al. (1982) have described how a severe pressure-load can "exhaust" some cells while "stimulating" others, especially in the subendocardial zones. Focal loss of myosin suggests activation of proteases, but impaired synthesis is equally possible. Fibrosis can generally be seen as the end-result of ischemia or of non-specific damage. Vascular spasm is thought to play a role in some models; many disturbances of the microcirculation are found in patients (Strauer, 1983).

Impaired contractility

Hemodynamic and ultrastructural alterations have generally not been studied in the same preparations. Whether pressure hypertrophy can produce a stage of hypertrophy with a normal inotropic state is unclear. In extreme right ventricular hypertrophy produced by pulmonary artery banding, the cross-sectional area of the muscle fibers can double as the peak systolic pressure in the right ventricle doubles (Cooper et al., 1973). Even in the absence of hemodynamic failure, the force–velocity (= load–velocity) curves show depressed contractility (Fig. 22-1). When there is overt failure the curve is even more depressed (Spann et al., 1967).

Oxygen demand vs supply

The explanation for the depressed inotropic state may lie either in defective control of intracellular calcium ion movements by the damaged sarcoplasmic reticulum, and/or in the decreased myosin ATPase activity (see Chapter 22). An interesting finding in one model is an enhanced uptake of oxygen per gram of active tension developed, i.e. a variety of "oxygen-wastage". Here the cause is thought to be cytosolic calcium overload with enhanced uptake of calcium by the mitochondria, leading in turn to a stimulation of non-phosphorylating pathways of oxygen uptake (Cooper et al., 1973). The corresponding situation in patients may be "high stress hypertrophy" with an increased oxygen consumption per unit mass, despite impaired left ventricular function (Strauer, 1983). In compensated overload the coronary reserve is adequate; in the presence of heart failure it is not, so that there is a relative inadequacy of blood flow.

Volume overload

Volume overload can be caused not only by **regurgitant valve lesions**, but by **fistulae** and **shunts**—patent ductus arteriosus, atrial septal defect (right ventricular overload), arteriovenous fistulae and Paget's disease. A mild secondary volume overload can also result from states of chronic fluid retention as in chronic congestive heart failure. Volume overload should be distinguished from a number of potentially confusing conditions. A decreased circulation time with a normal circulating volume occurs in the **hyperkinetic states** of thyrotoxicosis and pregnancy. **High-output heart failure** is the combination of myocardial failure plus a state of peripheral vasodilation, including advanced thyrotoxicosis, cor pulmonale and arteriovenous fistulae.

In true volume overload the **pericardium** restrains left ventricular filling as the left ventricular filling pressure increases. Thus an acute volume overload has the degree of left ventricular dilation limited by the pericardium and the hemodynamic changes resemble those of constrictive pericarditis. In contrast, in chronic experimental volume overload the pericardium appears to exert no such restraining qualities, probably because its volume has increased either by stretching or by hypertrophy (LeWinter and Pavelec, 1982). Even after one week of volume overloading there is some hypertrophy of the pericardium (Wikman-Coffelt et al., 1979).

When volume-induced hypertrophy is fully developed in **atrial septal defect**, then contractility and myocardial oxygen consumption can still be normal (Cooper et al., 1973). If volume overload is progressive the chamber enlargement will produce a prolonged increase in the peak systolic wall tension and, eventually, an added element of pressure overload. Right ventricular failure develops from either pulmonary hypertension (chronic excess pulmonary blood flow) or from incomplete right ventricular emptying. These events typically do not complicate atrial septal defect until middle adult life.

Thus a "pure" volume overload can be well-tolerated for years, in contrast to pressure overload. These analyses of overload can now be extrapolated to the clinical pictures in aortic stenosis and regurgitation.

Aortic Stenosis

The stenosed aortic valve creates an increased impedance to left ventricular outflow so that the peak systolic pressure generated must rise to exceed that in the aorta. The increased intraventricular pressure leads to left ventricular hypertrophy, acting through the unknown stimulus discussed in Chapter 15, so that wall stress, originally increased, decreases to normal by the Laplace law (Fig. 21-3). The cause of the pressure overload is the abnormally stenosed aortic valve. The severity of the stenosis can be assessed in one of three ways: (i) clinical (features of left ventricular hypertrophy, syncope, angina pectoris, eventual left ventricular failure); (ii) pressure gradients across the aortic valve at catheterization, exceeding 50 mmHg; (iii) calculation of the aortic valve orifice size—valves below 0.8 cm^2 are associated with symptoms, whereas the normal size is $2.6–3 \text{ cm}^2$. The latter calculations are based on aortic valve flow, the pressure gradient across the valve and a number of coefficients (Rackley and Hood, 1976).

Characteristically, **syncope** is a symptom of severe aortic stenosis. The mechanism may be: (i) ischemia-induced ventricular arrhythmias; or (ii) severe slowing of the heart, as a result of ischemia or fibrosis of nodal tissue, or from vasodepressive reflexes akin to the Bezold–Jarish reflex (page 281); or (iii) exercise-provoked vasodilation (instead of the normal vasoconstrictor response) with an increased pressure gradient across the aortic valve and decreased coronary perfusion pressure. Angina pectoris is also characteristic, presumably the result of excess demand causing subendocardial ischemia on exercise (Fig. 21-1).

Therapy of aortic stenosis

The clinical course of aortic stenosis can stretch over many years with an average age of onset of about 60; once deterioration with syncope, angina or failure occurs, survival is usually only for a few years. Even in moderate and apparently compensated hypertrophy, when the ejection fraction is normal or high, there are changes in isovolumic contraction and in relaxation during exercise (Krayenbuehl et al., 1983), when the ejection fraction may fall (Fig. 21-4). The mechanism is, presumably, that the hypertrophied myocardium is subject to subendocardial ischemia. At that stage the myocardium will be increasingly fibrosed with degenerate changes.

Since the valve must be replaced, and no artificial valve is ideal, it must be established that the stenosis is critical (see above) before operating. As valves and surgical techniques improve,

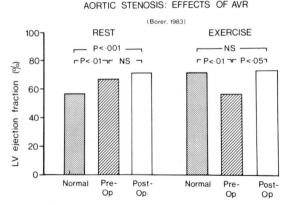

Fig. 21-4 Effect of aortic stenosis on ejection fraction at rest (left) and after exercise (right). Note there is an enhanced ejection fraction at rest, with a depressed value after exercise. The latter abnormality is improved by aortic valve replacement (AVR). From Borer et al. (1983). Am J Med 75: 38, with permission.

so will intervention become earlier. In patients treated medically, afterload reduction is avoided as it increases the pressure gradient across the valve.

Aortic Regurgitation
(= aortic incompetence
  = aortic insufficiency)

An **acute volume** load to the left ventricle, as when the aortic valve becomes acutely incompetent (bacterial endocarditis or acute rheumatic fever or rupture of the sinus of Valsalva) cannot distend the left ventricle much because of its normal compliance. The result is a severe increase in left atrial and pulmonary capillary wedge pressures. With a **chronic overload** as occurs in the ordinary type of aortic regurgitation (rheumatic or aortic dilation due to syphilis or hypertension), the left ventricle can dilate, probably by "slippage" of the fibers and by longitudinal hypertrophy. The end-diastolic volume is increased and the stroke volume rises by the Starling law. The effective stroke volume ejected into the aorta (total volume less regurgitant volume) is near normal. The increased diastolic volume means that the preload rises, and also the peak systolic wall stress is increased so that a measure of concentric hypertrophy may also occur, to keep wall tension within the normal range. Left ventricular work will be increased considerably due to the extra regurgitant

flow. This compensated situation can be maintained for many years; when deterioration sets in it can be sudden. As in the case of aortic stenosis, valve replacement will be undertaken earlier and earlier as techniques improve.

Because of the volume overload, the initial contractile tension is increased so that the maximal left ventricular pressure is reached earlier in systole. Because the pressure falls away in late systole the ejection phase is shortened. "Early systole is loaded, and late systole unloaded" (Wood, 1950). The low diastolic pressure is caused both by the incompetent valve and by peripheral vasodilation—the latter presumably is caused by marginal tissue oxygenation.

It is the combination of diastolic reflux and peripheral vasodilation that gives the characteristic hyperdynamic circulation. The aortic pressure rises rapidly and falls off rapidly to produce the characteristic peripheral signs (low diastolic blood pressure, collapsing pulse, pistol shot sounds). Regurgitant flow produces the early diastolic diminuendo murmur which may disappear in late diastole as aortic and left ventricular diastolic pressures equilibrate. A mitral-stenosis-like diastolic murmur, the **Austin Flint murmur**, occurs in the absence of mitral valve disease as the rapidly rising left ventricular diastolic pressure tends to push up the mitral valve at the same time that antegrade flow occurs from left atrium to ventricle; this explanation is the modern version of Austin Flint's idea of "relative" mitral stenosis as the left ventricle dilates. Frequently there is soft ejection systolic murmur as the left ventricle empties rapidly; the combined systolic and diastolic murmurs give a "to-and-fro" quality. A loud ejection murmur indicates accompanying organic aortic stenosis.

Diastolic perfusion

The fall-off in the aortic pressure in diastole means that the myocardium is poorly perfused and on the border of hypoxia (Fig. 21-3). However, an increase in systolic flow means that overall flow is normal, protecting the heart from anaerobic metabolism until the regurgitation is very severe (Falsetti et al., 1979). The normal nocturnal fall in blood pressure reduces perfusion further so that nocturnal angina may occur. Effort angina is not as common as might be expected, possibly because the already high end-diastolic pressure causes dyspnea before pain.

Valve replacement

In severe aortic regurgitation, therapy with vasodilators, diuretics and digitalis will not be effective. Surgical valve replacement is required. Generally there will be symptomatic and hemodynamic benefit. Cellular signs of irreversible changes are massive hypertrophy of fibers, much fibrosis and reduced activity of myosin ATPase and mitochondrial enzymes (Donaldson et al., 1982); such changes may be detected on a pre-operative endomyocardial **ventricular biopsy** using a biotome at the end of a catheter passed from the peripheral vessels into the ventricle. When such changes are present at the pre-operative or operative biopsy then cardiac function fails to recover adequately after operation.

At the other end of the spectrum is the problem of when to operate in patients with mild or minimal symptoms. Two common criteria are obtained on echocardiography: a left ventricular size which is too big at the end of systole (left ventricular **end-systolic dimension** exceeds 55 mm), or a left ventricle so poorly contractile that the **fractional shortening** with each systole is depressed below 25 percent. There can be large errors in the echocardiographic techniques (Fioretti et al., 1983) which nevertheless remain a useful guide. Another criterion is the fall in ejection fraction at rest and especially during exercise (Fig. 21-5). Logically it should be possible to detect the time when wall stress starts to rise as the left ventricular chamber dilates in excess of the amount of existing compensatory hypertrophy (see Laplace law, page 172). In patients treated medically, diuretics and digitalis are conventional; afterload reduction by prazosin or nifedipine is increasingly added for temporary support.

Combined aortic stenosis and regurgitation

When the slow rise of the pulse of stenosis is added to the fast rise and collapse of that of incompetence the typical **bisferiens pulse** ("double-bearing") is produced. The high velocity of blood passing through the stenosed aortic valve is thought to cause a dip in the aortic pressure with a secondary tidal wave which reflects to cause the second upstroke of the pulse. Here specific therapy is by aortic valve replacement.

Mitral Stenosis

The usual cause of mitral stenosis is chronic rheumatic heart disease. The usual consequence is a build up of pressure in the left atrium, with left ventricular function being limited by poor filling and, therefore, working on an unfavorable part of the Starling curve, near the origin. To restore normal filling requires surgical relief of stenosis. Ventricular filling may nevertheless remain near normal because of increased filling pressure. Filling falls with the onset of atrial fibrillation due to the absence of the left atrial booster, and due to the high ventricular response with inadequate filling time. Atrial fibrillation is, therefore, a prime cause of deterioration in mitral stenosis. It is predisposed to by left atrial enlargement and some fibrosis.

Therapy

Afterload reduction is contra-indicated because it will increase the pressure across the stenotic valve. Preload reduction may be tried with care so as not to reduce too much the elevated left atrial pressure required for normal filling of the left ventricle.

Splitting of the valve by closed valvotomy through the left atrium can give relief from pulmonary congestion, provided that the valve is both stenosed and pliable. If there is significant added mitral regurgitation or if the valve is calcified then mitral valve replacement is required.

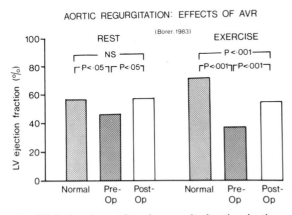

Fig. 21-5 In advanced aortic regurgitation the ejection fraction, depressed at rest, falls further with exercise. Aortic valve replacement (AVR) restores both changes towards normal. From Borer et al. (1983). Am J Med 75: 38, with permission.

If there is associated **atrial fibrillation** then digitalis can slow the ventricular response by inhibiting the atrioventricular node. If the ventricular response during exercise is too high then additional inhibition of the node may be achieved by verapamil, diltiazem, or beta-adrenergic blockade. In mitral stenosis in sinus rhythm "prophylactic digitalization" is sometimes used to avoid the possible harmful effects of the sudden onset of atrial fibrillation. This procedure is of unproven value.

Anticoagulation may be required in patients with mitral valve disease (including regurgitation) when the combination of atrial fibrillation, marked left atrial enlargement and previous embolic episodes warns that the risk of thrombo-embolism is high. When cardioversion is required in patients with atrial fibrillation, the risk of an embolus is increased so that, if possible, anticoagulation is undertaken for 1–3 weeks prior to elective cardioversion.

Mitral Regurgitation
(= mitral incompetence
= mitral insufficiency)

There are many causes of mitral regurgitation: rheumatic fever, ruptured chordae tendinae (myocardial infarction) or a chronically dilated left ventricle. As in aortic regurgitation the stroke volume is enhanced and monitored by an enlarged left ventricle. Unlike aortic regurgitation the aortic diastolic pressure is maintained. The peak left ventricular systolic pressure is relieved as the regurgitant flow empties into the left atrium so that left ventricular end-diastolic pressure and volume rise far less than in aortic regurgitation (Braunwald, 1969). The volume load in the virtual absence of a pressure load causes little increase in the myocardial oxygen demand so that the hemodynamic situation can be tolerated for many years, without features of myocardial ischemia. The ejection fraction and end-systolic volume are kept correspondingly; when the latter is near normal, surgical valve replacement is more likely to be successful.

Eventually the volume load produces chamber enlargement with an increase of systolic tension and hypertrophy, which normalizes the tension. The enhanced back pressure into the left atrium tends to cause pulmonary venous hypertension and left atrial enlargement. When atrial fibrillation occurs it is not as serious as in mitral stenosis because there is less problem with filling the ventricle.

Medical therapy includes diuretics, digitalis, afterload reduction, and anticoagulation in some patients with atrial fibrillation. The timing of mitral valve replacement is difficult. In principle, the aim is to intervene at the earliest signs that the heart is going into failure.

Billowing Valve Syndrome
(= Barlow's syndrome = midsystolic click–murmur syndrome = floppy mitral valve = ballooned mitral valve)

The billowing valve syndrome is a common condition usually caused by some inherent abnormality of the mitral valve such as hereditary myxomatous degeneration. Because it is frequently an isolated abnormality, and because mitral regurgitation is so well tolerated, this condition is frequently asymptomatic.

The prognosis is good from the hemodynamic point of view but it is the associated arrhythmias which cause most problems. The origin of associated arrhythmias is difficult to understand, but may lie in the unexpectedly dense innervation of the mitral valve and its capacity to produce after-depolarizations (Chapter 23). Alternatively, an enhanced sympathetic tone caused by an associated anxiety may be at fault: the arrhythmias respond well to therapy with beta-blockade.

Fallot's Tetralogy

The most frequent example of cyanotic congenital heart disease, Fallot's tetralogy is characterized by four abnormalities: pulmonary stenosis, right ventricular hypertrophy, an over-riding aorta and a ventricular septal defect. Most important are the pulmonary stenosis (which increases right ventricular wall tension to produce right ventricular hypertrophy) and a ventricular septal defect so high that the aorta hangs over it. The pulmonary stenosis (valve too stenosed to make an opening sound) causes right ventricular hypertrophy which generates enough pressure to empty in part directly into the aorta to explain the cyanosis. The poor blood flow through the pulmonary artery may be compensated for by bronchial collaterals or an accompanying patent ductus arteriosus. The great American pediatric cardiologist Taussig (a colleague of Dr Richard Bing at the Johns Hopkins Hospital) found that cases with a patent ductus did better than those without, so that an artificial ductus (Blalock operation) was for long the standard therapy. Now specific surgical correction of the defects and stenosis is undertaken if possible. Cyanotic spells occur when an increased right-to-left shunt decreases pulmonary blood flow to critical levels; the cause is thought to be an adrenergic-mediated increase in the degree of outflow obstruction to the right ventricle which then shunts blood to the aorta and diminishes flow to the lungs. Relief is by the knee–chest position (increasing arterial vascular resistance) or by beta-blockade which appears to decrease right ventricular contractility (Cumming and Carr, 1967).

Myocardial Disease

The previous sections have described how an initially normal myocardium responds to a pressure or volume load by hypertrophy and eventual failure. In contrast are the diseases where there is a primary myocardial defect (cardiomyopathy). Such cardiomyopathies (Table 21-2) include an apparently heterogeneous group of conditions wherein myocardial function is disturbed by the fibrosis of chronic ischemic heart disease or by a variety of metabolic or endocrine disturbances; the etiology of others is ill-understood and "idiopathic". Some clinicians limit the term cardiomyopathy to the idiopathic variety. From the functional point of view the three varieties of cardiomyopathies are: (i) dilated (or congestive) where a dilated heart is usually associated with symptoms of congestive heart failure; (ii) hypertrophic, where there is very prominent left ventricular hypertrophy (Fig. 21-6) sometimes especially involving the interventricular septum; and (iii) restrictive, where the myocardium is infiltrated and venous filling is restricted.

Dilated or congestive cardiomyopathy

In congestive cardiomyopathy the cause may be idiopathic or else secondary to pregnancy, alcoholism, hypertension, diabetes, ischemic heart disease and various myocardial infections especially viral myocarditis. In the idiopathic variety there is no good evidence for a primary metabolic cause, but once the disease is established there are non-specific metabolic

Table 21-2

Classification of cardiomyopathy

By clinical characteristics
1. Dilated or congestive cardiomyopathy
2. Hypertrophic cardiomyopathy
3. Restrictive cardiomyopathy

By etiology
1. Toxic–metabolic
    Alcoholic heart disease
    Nutritional heart disease
    Cobalt
    Adriamycin
    Excess catecholamines
2. Endocrine
    Thyrotoxicosis
    Myxedema
    Acromegaly
    Diabetes mellitus
3. Infective
    Myocarditis, acute and chronic
4. Extra-cardiac disease
    Uremia
    Anemia
    Hepatic failure
    Carcinoid heart disease
5. Infiltrations
    Amyloid
    Iron
    Carcinoidosis

changes such as loss of cardiac enzymes and focal fibrosis. As implied by the name, the clinical picture is that of congestive heart failure with gallop rhythm; mitral regurgitation secondary to left ventricular dilation leads to an added volume load. Left ventricular dilation and impaired contractility can be shown by echocardiographic or radionuclide studies.

Hypertrophic cardiomyopathy

Hypertrophic cardiomyopathy has a multiplicity of synonyms, including idiopathic hypertrophic subaortic stenosis (IHSS) and asymmetrical septal hypertrophy (ASH). If there is outflow tract obstruction then one name is hypertrophic obstructive cardiomyopathy (HOCUM); if not, hypertrophic non-obstructive cardiomyopathy. It is a condition with several "characteristic" features, none of which are absolutely specific. Asymmetrical septal hypertrophy, myocardial fiber disarray and systolic anterior motion of the mitral

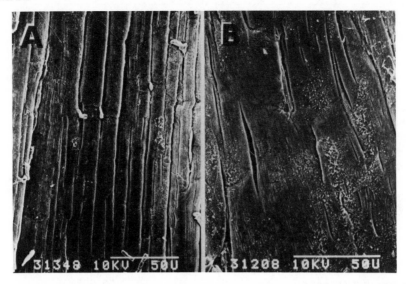

Fig. 21-6 Effects of severe cardiomyopathy with marked left ventricular hypertrophy on myocardial fiber size, shown by scanning electron microscopy. On the left, normal human heart. On the right, heart with severe cardiomyopathy. The fiber diameter has increased by about 3–4 fold. Bar: 50 μm. From Izumi et al. (1984). J Molec Cell Cardiol 16: 452, with permission.

valve have all been reported in other conditions, and the subaortic septal hypertrophy may or may not be present. The symptoms are equally varied, ranging from an asymptomatic person with abnormal signs to near-incapacity from angina pectoris (excess oxygen demand), dyspnea and syncope (as in aortic stenosis). Objectively, the presence of localized septal hypertrophy causing outflow obstruction is important; when present the signs include: left ventricular hypertrophy, an ejection murmur like that of aortic stenosis, echocardiographic features of asymmetrical septal hypertrophy (septal to free wall ratio exceeding 1.3 : 1), narrowing of the outflow tract and systolic anterior motion of the mitral valve (SAM). An abnormal apical impulse, caused by a late systolic bulge as the obstruction develops, is shown well on an apexcardiogram. At angiography the left ventricular cavity is small and systolic ejection vigorous. Diastolic relaxation is impaired; in some ways the hypertrophic myocardium behaves like a calcium overloaded heart (vigorous contraction, impaired relaxation). Therapy is aimed at reducing the hypercontractile state (to prevent further hypertrophy) by either beta-adrenergic blockade or calcium-antagonists. Although the basic condition is usually genetic in origin, similar pathological changes can be provoked in animal models giving clues that the genetic defect acts via altered metabolism of proteins to result in the cardiomyopathy.

Restrictive cardiomyopathy

Among the causes of a restrictive cardiomyopathy are infiltrations of the myocardium itself by a variety of metabolic causes, including fibrosis, amyloidosis and iron-storage disease. Myocardial **fibrosis** is a relatively non-specific end-result of a wide number of different insults to the heart, including infarction, infection, alcohol and nutritional damage by severe beri-beri. The common factor is probably chronically impaired metabolism of the muscle fibers, some of which undergo atrophy to be replaced by fibrosis.

Clinically, restricted filling causes an increased jugular venous pulse; during deep inspiration as the intrathoracic pressure falls, the venous return increases but the right ventricle cannot distend sufficiently so there is inspiratory swelling of the neck veins (**Kussmaul's sign**, also found in constrictive pericarditis). The systolic function is normal, as shown by echocardiography or radionuclide studies, the heart volume is small and impaired ventricular expansion in diastole means that after an initial abrupt fall (early diastolic ventricular suction enhanced for unknown reasons), the ventricular pressure rises due to poor relaxation to cause the characteristic dip and plateau pattern (**"square-root"** sign, also found in constrictive pericarditis). Restrictive heart disease is frequently due to metabolic infiltrations such as **amyloidosis** or iron overload. Clinically, the differential diagnosis between restrictive cardiomyopathy and constrictive pericarditis can be very difficult.

Cardiomyopathy: principles of therapy

In hypertrophic cardiomyopathy, surgical removal of a localized obstructive septal hypertrophy may relieve the outflow tract gradient. Otherwise the appropriate therapy is to "rest" the hypercontractile myocardium by using high-dose propranolol (up to 480 mg per day), but watching for heart failure and excess bradycardia. Digitalis is contra-indicated unless there is atrial fibrillation and cardiac failure. Verapamil also improves symptoms and decreases the outflow gradient and improves diastolic function; side-effects must be guarded against: sinoatrial or atrioventricular nodal dysfunction and heart failure. Another therapy with favorable results on initial evaluation is the combination of propranolol and nifedipine.

The arrhythmias of hypertrophic cardiomyopathy usually do not respond to conventional antiarrhythmic agents. Amiodarone is used increasingly, with due care for its serious side-effects.

In congestive cardiomyopathy the basic therapy is that of congestive heart failure (Chapter 22). Beta-adrenergic blockade, normally contra-indicated in congestive heart failure, has been used by some workers with apparent benefit. The presumed explanation of this controversial therapy is (i) the beneficial effects of slowing the heart rate, thereby improving ventricular filling, and (ii) a reversal of the harmful effects of excess circulating catecholamines, which are thought to "down-grade" the cardiac beta-receptors.

Metabolic Heart Disease

Alcoholic cardiomyopathy

The association of chronic alcoholism and cardiac disease was probably first described by Evans (1961). Shortly thereafter alcoholic cardiomyopathy (Ferrans et al., 1965) was delineated as a separate entity. More recently, latent heart disease has been uncovered in chronic alcoholics with liver disease but without overt clinical evidence of heart disease. Alcohol (ethyl alcohol) is itself not metabolized by the myocardium. The cardiomyopathy may be the result of a combination of factors: toxic effects of metabolites (Langer and Sobel, 1983), indirect effects of acetaldehyde

produced in the liver and associated nutritional defects such as thiamine or protein deficiency. The origin of alcoholic ventricular arrhythmias, including the "holiday heart", is obscure. Experimentally, chronic alcohol intake can also cause perivascular fibrosis, which could help explain the myocardial infarction found in some alcoholics in the absence of classical coronary artery disease.

Beri-beri heart disease

Beri-beri heart disease is caused either by direct dietary lack of thiamine, as in oriental or African populations, or by dietary deficiencies associated with chronic alcoholism. There are two major components to beri-beri: the myocardial lesion and peripheral vaso-dilation. The former gives a low-output picture, the latter a high cardiac output. Both respond to thiamine but the peripheral vasodilation is least well understood; possibly there are changes in the vascular sympathetic neurons caused by thiamine deficiency. Myocardial failure is usually explained by the requirement for thiamine pyrophosphate of enzymes involving oxidative decarboxylation, especially pyruvate dehydrogenation (see Fig. 10-9) and the decarboxylation of alpha-ketoglutarate, which explains the low oxygen uptake. Decreased activity of transketolase, an enzyme of the pentose shunt, is found in blood cells and helps in diagnosis.

Cardiac cachexia

Some patients with chronic valvular heart disease develop a state of severe cachexia. Experimentally, cardiac cachexia results from the production of severe, untreated mitral stenosis in dogs despite an apparently enhanced appetite (Segar et al., 1971). Gastrointestinal loss of nutrients probably plays an important role.

Potassium deficiency

Experimentally, the cardiomyopathy of chronic potassium deficiency is characterized by severe impairment of mechanical function, moderate changes in mitochondrial function and by a relative increase in the oxygen uptake. Myocytes become smaller in size and some undergo myofibril degeneration; such changes are reversible with potassium repletion (Sarkar and Levine, 1979). In patients, chronic hypokalemia can be found in some patients with chronic laxative abuse, chronic diuretic therapy for congestive heart failure and in severe potassium-losing nephropathy. Whereas the characteristic electrocardiographic features of hypokelemia are well-organized, a causal relationship to a cardiomyopathy in patients has not yet been established. Rather, hypokalemia is an established risk factor for arrhythmias (Chapter 22).

Gross obesity

In very obese subjects there may develop a cardiomegaly which is not due to fat infiltration, nor can it be explained by the frequently associated systemic hypertension alone. Such cardiomegaly can occur in the absence of any associated hypoventilation caused by the Pickwickian syndrome. The cardiomegaly could reflect the chronic load of the heart caused by the excess work of perfusing the excess adipose tissue, because congestive failure and cardiomegaly can both respond to weight reduction.

Toxic cardiomyopathy

Adriamycin (= **doxorubicin**) or **daunorubicin** are antitumor agents. When given in a large initial dose they can cause acute left ventricular failure, which is probably caused by a low cytosolic calcium, because experimentally the failure responds to digitalis, isoproterenol and a high perfusion calcium concentration. Much more important clinically is the cardiomyopathy that can result from chronic administration especially in a high dose. The mechanism is ill-understood, but may include formation of lipid peroxides, mitochondrial changes and effects on DNA.

Catecholamine cardiomyopathy is an experimental entity, although it may have a clinical counterpart in some patients given chronic high-dose beta-agonist therapy for chronic asthma, or in pheochromocytoma. The mechanism is in part chronic calcium overload, but sarcolemma permeability is also increased and there are many other complex changes, including altered rates of protein synthesis.

Endocrine Heart Disease

Thyrotoxicosis

In certain specific types of congestive heart failure there is an identifiable, non-mechanical cause in the form of endocrine or diabetic heart disease. In severe and chronic thyrotoxicosis there may develop congestive heart failure of the "high-output" type because increased **heat production** leads to peripheral vasodilation and an increased cardiac output.

The **hyperdynamic hypersympathetic circulation** is probably in part the result of increased beta-adrenergic receptor numbers and also in part decreased number of muscarinic cholinergic receptors (Watanabe et al., 1982). A second factor is the peripheral vasodilation, causing a reflex tachycardia. A third factor is of particular interest, namely the possibility that thyroid hormone, by changing the expression of the genes for myosin isoenzymes, is able to promote the synthesis of a myosin with an increased ATPase activity. The result would be enhanced myocardial contractility. This mechanism has been found in experimental animals, but has not yet been established in man.

A difficult problem can arise in the **therapy** of thyrotoxic heart disease. In thyrotoxicosis, beta-adrenergic blockade is increasingly used as adjuvant therapy to antithyroid drugs or radiotherapeutic ablation of the thyroid gland, with the aim of diminishing the tachycardia and other unwanted sympathomimetic factors such as tremor. Yet if there should be thyrotoxic heart failure, beta-adrenergic blockade may be harmful. Clinically, some of the features of the hyperkinetic circulation of thyrotoxicosis resemble those of heart failure: tachycardia, a third heart sound and a modest elevation of the jugular venous pressure. If there is doubt in differentiating between the physiological hyperkinetic circulation and pathological heart failure, measurement of the ejection fraction should be undertaken before beta-adrenergic blockade is given.

Myxedema heart disease

In hypothyroid patients, symptoms and signs of heart failure may develop. Although the occurrence of a true myxedema heart disease has been questioned, the coexistence of a serum lactate dehydrogenase pattern indicating myocardial damage, together with electrocardiographic and radiological abnormalities, is positive evidence. Experimentally, there are decreased values for contractility, myosin ATPase activity and the rate of calcium uptake by the sarcoplasmic reticulum (Suko, 1973). There is also a general decrease of sarcolemmal-associated proteins such as the beta- and alpha-adrenergic receptors, the sodium pump and adenyl cyclase (Smith et al., 1978).

Clinically, the bradycardia is striking but does not wholly explain the reduced cardiac output because the stroke volume falls. As in skeletal muscle, the relaxation time is prolonged in cardiac muscle when indirectly assessed by movements of the apex of the heart (Manns et al., 1976). Therapy is by careful replacement of thyroid hormone; there may be associated artery disease.

Acromegalic heart disease

The occasional development of giant hearts over 1000 grams in weight stresses the possible extent of cardiac enlargement in acromegaly. However, in the "average" case of acromegaly the heart merely shares in the general splanchnomegaly. Echocardiography has allowed non-invasive measurements of left ventricular wall dimensions and motion in patients with acromegaly. Cardiomegaly is frequently asymptomatic (Matter et al., 1979). Acromegaly may be accompanied by diabetes mellitus or hypertension, both of which predispose to cardiomegaly and coronary artery disease. Therefore the role of the abnormalities of growth hormone is not always clear. Experimentally, growth hormone has anabolic effects including stimulation of the synthesis of both mRNA and tRNA. Eventually, with continued administration of growth hormone, a cardiomegaly results which can be reversed by hypophysectomy.

Diabetes mellitus

Defects in ventricular contraction in animal models (Fein et al., 1980) can be explained in part by the decreased activity of myosin ATPase associated with a changed pattern of myosin isoenzymes (Dillman, 1980). Dogs with chronic diabetes have impaired myocardial mechanics so that left ventricular end-diastolic pressure rises during volume-loading. The cause is increased ventricular stiffness which in turn is thought to be due to enhanced formation of glycosylated proteins and collagen. The importance of insulin for normal protein synthesis and transport of sugar and amino acids into the cell, argues for a specific diabetic cardiomyopathy. Yet many patients with diabetes will have non-specific and mixed forms of heart disease which could result from accelerated coronary atherosclerosis, associated hypertension or diabetic renal disease. Diabetic autonomic neuropathy explains the abnormal response to procedures stimulating vagal reflexes such as the Valsalva maneuver, which fails to slow the heart rate (unaltered RR interval on the electrocardiogram).

Summary

Valvular heart disease exemplifies the contrasting effects of pressure and volume overload. In aortic stenosis the left ventricle undergoes concentric hypertrophy (cellular mechanism still not known) which is able to reduce the otherwise abnormally high wall tension by Laplace's law. The penalty the myocardium must pay is abnormal susceptibility to ischemia caused by excess demand (and inadequate blood flow), with syncope and angina. In chronic aortic regurgitation the primary defect is a volume overload. The left ventricle enlarges (slippage and/or longitudinal hypertrophy), initially to produce an eccentric hypertrophy. As the wall tension also rises, some pressure hypertrophy also occurs to help revert systolic wall tension to normal. The penalty paid for the valve lesion is poor diastolic perfusion which predisposes to ischemia. Both diastolic reflex and peripheral vasodilation account for the characteristic hemodynamic changes.

In mitral stenosis there is neither pressure nor volume load; the problem is a poorly filling left ventricle with a low cardiac output. Compensation is by an increased left atrial filling pressure. The penalty to pay is by (i) left atrial enlargement, which predisposes to atrial fibrillation and further impairment of left ventricular filling; and (ii) increased pulmonary venous pressure and symptoms of venous engorgement.

In mitral regurgitation the volume load enters the left atrium in systole so that systolic wall tension is kept low. A volume load is well tolerated and the condition can be symptomatically silent for years. In the billowing mitral valve syndrome the degree of regurgitation is less, because the anterior cusp of the mitral valve only starts to balloon as systole develops.

References

Braunwald E (1969). Mitral regurgitation: physiological, clinical and surgical considerations. N Engl J Med 281: 425–433.

Constant J (1976). Bedside Cardiology, 2nd Edition, Little Brown, Boston.

Cooper G, Puga FJ, Zujko KJ, Harrison CE, Coleman HN (1973). Normal myocardial function and energetics in volume-overload hypertrophy in the cat. Circ Res 32: 140–148.

Cumming G, Carr WE (1967). Hemodynamic effects of propranolol in patients with Fallot's tetralogy. Am Heart J 74: 29–36.

Dillman WH (1980). Diabetes mellitus induces changes in cardiac myosin of the rat. Diabetes 29: 579–582.

Donaldson RM, Florio R, Rickards AF, Bennett JG, Yscoub M, Rodd DN, Olsen E (1982). Irreversible morphological changes contributing to depressed cardiac function after surgery with chronic aortic regurgitation. Brit Heart J 48: 589–597.

Evans W (1961). Alcoholic cardiomyopathy. Am Heart J 61: 556–567.

Falsetti HL, Carroll RJ, Cramer JA (1979). Total and regional myocardial blood flow in aortic regurgitation. Am Heart J 97: 485–493.

Fein FS, Korstein LD, Strobeck JE, Capasso JM, Sonnenblick EH (1980). Altered myocardial mechanics in diabetic rats. Circ Res 47: 922–933.

Ferrans VJ (1982). Human cardiac hypertrophy: structural aspects. Europ Heart J 3: Suppl A, 15–27.

Ferrans VJ, Hibbs RC, Weilbaecher DG, Black WC, Walsh JJ, Burch GE (1965). Alcoholic cardiomyopathy: a histochemical study. Am Heart J 69: 748–765.

Fioretti P, Roelandt J, Bos RJ, Meltzer RS, Van Hoogenhuijze D, Serruys PW, Nauta J, Hugenholtz PG (1983). Echocardiography in chronic aortic insufficiency. Is valve replacement too late when left ventricular end-systolic dimension reaches 55 mm? Circulation 67: 216–221.

Grossman W, Jones D, McLaurin L (1975). Wall stress and patterns of hypertrophy in the human left ventricle. J Clin Invest 56: 56–64.

Hatt PY, Cluzeaud F, Perennec J (1982). Left ventricular hypertrophy—experimental aspects. Europ Heart J 3: Suppl A, 9–14.

Krayenbuehl HP, Hess OM, Schneider J, Turina M (1983). Physiologic or pathologic hypertrophy. Europ Heart J 4: Suppl A, 29–34.

Langer LG, Sobel BE (1983). Myocardial metabolites of ethanol. Circ Res 52: 479–482.

LeWinter MM, Pavelec R (1982). Influence of the pericardium on left ventricular end-diastolic pressure-segment relation during early and later stages of experimental chronic volume overload in dogs. Circ Res 50: 501–509.

Linzbach AJ (1960). Heart failure from the point of view of quantitative anatomy. Am J Cardiol 5: 370–382.

Manns JJ, Shepherd AMM, Crooks J, Adamson DB (1976). Measurement of cardiac muscle relaxation in hypothyroidism. Brit Med J 1: 1366–1368.

Matter HM, Boyd MJ, Jenkins JS (1979). Heart size and function in acromegaly. Brit Heart J 41: 697–701.

Morganroth J, Perloff JK, Zeldis SM, Dunkman WB (1977). Acute severe aortic regurgitation. Ann Int Med 87: 223–232.

Rackley CE, Hood WP Jr (1976). Aortic valve disease. In: Clinical Cardiovascular Physiology. Ed. H Levine, pp 493–521, Grune & Stratton, Orlando, New York and London.

Ross J Jr, Sonnenblick EH, Taylor RR, Spotnitz HM, Covell JW (1971). Diastolic geometry and sarcomere lengths in the chronically dilated canine left ventricle. Circ Res 28: 49–61.

Sarkar K, Levine DZ (1979). Repair of the myocardial lesion during potassium repletion of kaliopenic rats: an ultrastructural study. J Molec Cell Cardiol 11: 1165–1172.

Segar WE, Novrak LP, Hawe A, Rastelli GC, Zehr J (1971). Body composition in mitral cachexia. Am Heart J 82: 371–376.

Smith RM, Osborne-White WS, King RA (1978). Changes in the sarcolemma of the hypothyroid heart. Biochem Biophys Res Comm 80: 715–721.

Spann JF, Buccino RA, Sonnenblick EH, Braunwald E (1967). Contractile state of cardiac muscle obtained from cats with experimentally produced ventricular hypertrophy and heart failure. Circ Res 21: 341–354.

Strauer BE (1983). Left ventricular dynamics, energetics and coronary hemodynamics in hypertrophic heart disease. Europ Heart J 4: Suppl A, 137–142.

Suko J (1973). The calcium pump of cardiac sarcoplasmic reticulum. Functional alterations at different levels of thyroid state in rabbits. J Physiol (London) 228: 563–582.

Watanabe AM, Jones LR, Manalan AS, Besch HR (1982). Cardiac autonomic receptors. Circ Res 50: 161–174.

Wikman-Coffelt J, Parmley WW, Mason DT (1979). The cardiac hypertrophy process. Analyses of factors determining pathological vs physiological development. Circ Res 45: 697–707.

Wollenberger A (1949). The energy metabolism of the failing heart and the metabolic action of cardiac glycosides. Pharmacol Rev 1: 311–352.

Wood P (1950). Disease of the Heart and Circulation. 2nd Edition, p 295, Eyre and Spottiswoode, London.

Congestive Heart Failure

The clinical picture of congestive heart failure is an admixture of three separate components—first, there is impaired contractile behavior of the heart with decreased force development and shortening of the contractile elements, so that the myocardium is on a lower Frank–Starling curve than normal. Secondly, as a result of the decreased inotropic state, a greater filling pressure is associated with the same stroke volume so that features of pulmonary congestion and increased venous pressure develop; there is also a decreased cardiac output (in the usual type of low-output failure) so that peripheral perfusion is impaired and muscular fatigue develops. Thirdly, there are important neurohumoral changes in the periphery— the sympathetic tone is increased, the renin–angiotensin system is activated and there is fluid retention with peripheral congestion and edema. Most of the available therapy depends on either (i) inotropic agents or (ii) unloading agents or (iii) agents reversing neurohumoral abnormalities.

Causes of Congestive Heart Failure

How does the inotropic state of the myocardium become impaired? First, frequently as a result of long-continued overwork—the myocardium having adapted to either a pressure or volume load, first successfully and then unsuccessfully. The mechanical demand on the myocardium exceeds the "supply" of contractile work which is a useful adaptation of the supply versus demand idea. Secondly, the amount of myocardial tissue available for contractile purposes

can be reduced as a result of a cardiomyopathy, which in turn could be congestive, hypertrophic, or restrictive. Similar or related conditions are caused by various metabolic, nutritional, endocrine or toxic diseases (Table 22-1). Thirdly, the availability of contractile force can be reduced by ischemia, acting in a complex way as outlined in Chapter 24.

Table 22-1

Causes of congestive heart failure

1. Excessive pressure load
aortic stenosis
arterial hypertension
2. Excessive volume load
aortic or mitral regurgitation
high-output states (thyrotoxicosis)
some types of congenital heart disease
3. Impaired LV filling
tight mitral stenosis
restrictive cardiomyopathy
constrictive pericarditis
4. Primary myocardial disease
hypertrophic obstructive cardiomyopathy
hypertrophic non-obstructive cardiomyopathy
dilated cardiomyopathy
myocarditis
metabolic heart disease
endocrine heart disease

Is There a Biochemical Defect?

A biochemical defect in the failing heart has been suspected since at least 1913, when Clark found that the hypodynamic frog's heart "loses its power of combining with calcium". Since then studies too numerous to analyze have delineated defects in oxidative phosphorylation, high-energy phosphate metabolism, calcium ion movements, contractile proteins, protein synthesis and breakdown, and in catecholamine metabolism. It is apparent that there is no unifying hypothesis to explain divergent findings. Much of the confusion arises because models of congestive heart failure differ from each other and from the situation in real life, where congestive failure is the end-product of numerous different chronic processes such as ischemic heart disease, valvular heart disease, hypertension, cardiomyopathy and high-output states such as thyrotoxicosis.

Added to any "basic" defect which could vary according to the type of heart failure would be the distortion and destruction of sarcomere structure by undue stretching in congestive failure. The consequences could well include decreased ATPase activity, decreased contractility of isolated myofibrils, decreased utilization of high-energy phosphate compounds and heart failure with normal, or near normal, levels of high-energy phosphate compounds.

The early hope that there would be a unitary molecular explanation for congestive heart failure (or that heart failure could simply be classified into defects of ATP generation or of ATP utilization) has not been supported. There is no firm evidence that the final common path in congestive heart failure is decreased availability of energy for cellular integrity and function. Rather it seems that each type of experimental failure involves different mechanisms and that the final end-result is compounded of the earlier "specific" changes together with added "non-specific" changes resulting from molecular stretch and distortion. Biochemical studies of particular interest can be analyzed as follows.

Oxygen uptake

As long as no reasonable consensus can be reached on basic observations such as the oxygen uptake of the muscle and the state of mitochondria in congestive heart failure, it would be fair to conclude that any such abnormalities found are not the basic defect in congestive failure. From the clinical point of view, no therapy has been evolved based on correcting possible defects of mitochondrial metabolism. Rather, the major clinical problem relates to the increased oxygen uptake (relative to the mechanical function) required by the large dilated heart, and the benefits obtained by changing the position of the heart on the Frank–Starling curve by altering either preload or afterload. From the practical point of view, a defect in energy production does not seem fundamental to congestive heart failure.

Myosin ATPase activity

Decreased intrinsic contractility in advanced heart failure should therefore reflect decreased energy utilization. There could be either abnormal myocardial proteins with normal calcium ion movements or abnormal interaction of calcium ions with normal proteins (or combinations of these changes). Increasing attention is being paid to the links between the contractile state of the myocardium and the myosin ATPase activity. The hypothesis has been postulated and probably proven that abnormal myosin isoenzymes are formed in congestive heart failure (Lompre et al., 1979). The decreased ATPase values and depressed mechanical function are seen as beneficial "compensatory" changes by Alpert and Mulieri (1982), so that high-pressure low-speed work is more easily managed by the hypertrophied, failing heart in contrast to its poor ability to cope with the high-volume load created temporarily by exercise.

The decreased myosin ATPase activity in the failing, overloaded heart stands in contrast to the enhanced ATPase activity of the thyrotoxic heart (Litten et al., 1982), which can be accounted for by yet other abnormalities of the patterns of myosin isoenzymes. Now the myocardium is adapted to the hyperkinetic circulation where a large volume of blood must be emptied rapidly against a relatively normal pressure. There are thus interesting biochemical links between the clinical condition of "low output failure" where decreased myosin ATPase activity and a decreased maximal velocity of contraction would be expected, and "high output failure" where the myosin ATPase and the rate of contraction are expected to be high.

Calcium cycles in heart failure

The sarcoplasmic reticulum of the failing heart is unable to accumulate calcium normally. Is this a fundamental defect? A particularly attractive suggestion is that abnormalities of excitation–contraction coupling occur in the hypertrophied cell as a simple consequence of altered geometry with a decreased surface to volume ratio (Kaufmann et al., 1971). Thus there is decreased calcium uptake per unit surface area. The fundamental defect remains the hypertrophy of the heart.

Other membrane defects

Not surprisingly, several changes in activities of membrane-associated enzymes have been reported. Adenylate cyclase activity is decreased as is the activity of the sodium–potassium pump. While a generalized membrane defect may exist in severe heart failure (Dhalla, 1976) there is as yet no evidence that such a defect is primary or fundamental.

Human hearts

Most of the above results are based on experimental aortic or pulmonary stenosis in animals. Such overloading does not increase the heart weight by more than about 50 percent, whereas in human heart hypertrophy, the heart may enlarge by 200–300 percent. In man, shifts of isoenzyme pattern (from V_1 to V_3; see Fig. 15-6) do not seem to occur. There must be another explanation for decreased myosin ATPase activity (Mercadier et al., 1983), which falls abruptly when the heart weight exceeds a critical value of 500 g (Leclerq and Swynghedauw, 1976). This "critical value" is reminiscent of the concept that above a similar critical mass the capillary supply is outstripped (Linzbach, 1960) and myocytes increase in number as well as size (page 289).

Consequences of Congestive Heart Failure

The basis of abnormalities of the mechanical properties of the myocardium was laid more than 20 years ago by Sonnenblick's group, who studied isolated papillary muscles from cats with right ventricular hypertrophy (secondary to pulmonary stenosis). Both the length–tension and force–velocity relationships are depressed (Fig. 22-1). These findings are the exact opposite of those evoked by an increased inotropic state resulting from catecholamine stimulation. Hence the intrinsic inotropic state of the failing myocardium

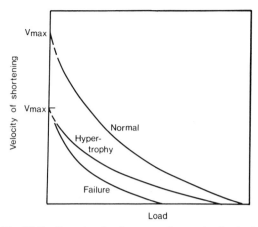

Fig. 22-1 Hypertrophy decreases the maximal velocity of shortening (V_{max}), probably by shifts of myosin ATPase isoenzyme activity (see Fig. 15-6) in animals. In man a different unknown mechanism is at work. In failure, both V_{max} and P_o are decreased (see Fig. 13-9). With permission from Swynghedauw and Delcayre (1982). Pathobiol Ann 12: 137–183.

is depressed. The reason why the myocardium is defective is probably multiple; the simple idea of overstretch of the sarcomere may now be discarded and "slippage" may be the explanation. For whatever reason, when the myocardium is stretched over a long period it dilates, in contrast to the failure to dilate during an acute stretch as in acute aortic regurgitation. Besides the ultrastructural changes already described, the decrease in myosin ATPase activity and changes in calcium metabolism, a further important change is the loss of catecholamines in the myocardium (Table 22-2). Paradoxically, this may be associated with increased circulating catecholamines. Possibly part of the increased circulating catecholamines may be derived from myocardial stores.

Catecholamines and receptors

The myocardial tissue content of norepinephrine is low, not only because of loss into the circulation but also because there is decreased synthesis and uptake in the terminal neurons (Maurer et al., 1981), with a block of the normal conversion of dopamine to norepinephrine (Pierpont et al., 1983). In extreme congestive heart failure, Harrison's group has found that the beta-receptor population is very low (Bristow et al., 1982). Hence there can be no response to

Table 22-2

Compensatory mechanisms in congestive heart failure

Compensation	Mechanism	Advantages	Disadvantage
Tachycardia	? Baroceptor-mediated	Helps to maintain cardiac output as stroke volume falls	MVO_2 increased
Arteriolar vasoconstriction	(i) **Adrenergic drive increased** (ii) Renin–angiotensin (iii) Vascular Na^+ increased	Helps to maintain blood pressure	Cardiac output decreased
Heart volume increased	? Fiber slippage Mitral regurgitation	Helps to maintain stroke volume by Starling mechanism	MVO_2 increased No increase in CO Risk of focal necrosis
Myosin ATPase activity reduced	Unknown. Altered isoenzymes in animal experiments	High pressure, low speed work more easily achieved	Slower rate of contraction, decreased inotropic state
Catecholamine depletion of heart	Unknown. ?Decreased uptake and synthesis	None	May contribute to decreased inotropic state

MVO_2 = myocardial oxygen uptake; CO = cardiac output.

stimulation by beta-agonists. Thus the myocardium cannot respond by an enhanced inotropic stimulation, despite the increased circulating catecholamines. The sustained response to histamine suggests a new therapeutic approach by histamine-2-receptor stimulation. The explanation for the depletion of beta-adrenergic receptors may be an extreme example of "down-grading" of the receptors in response to prolonged stimulation. It is not thought that impairment of beta-receptor response is a primary defect in the failing heart. A logical therapy, being carefully tested in severe congestive cardiomyopathy, is the addition of very low dose beta-blockade which is thought to oppose the harmful effects of excess adrenergic stimulation on the beta-receptors of the heart.

Neurohumoral changes

An important consequence of the usual type of severe cardiac failure is a low cardiac output. To maintain arterial pressure in such circumstances requires that the peripheral vascular resistance should rise; this adaptive change is achieved by a combination of alpha-catecholamine stimulation and an increased circulating angiotensin. Elevated levels of angiotensin II may be the cause of a troublesome hyponatremia, secondary to a stimulation of the thirst center and release of antidiuretic hormone. A third vasoconstrictive factor is increased arteriolar vascular stiffness, possibly related to sodium and water retention.

Not all the neurohumoral changes are vasoconstrictive. Rather there may be a balance between vasoconstrictive and vasodilator stimuli (such as the prostaglandins). The latter concept leads to the further suggestion that anti-inflammatory drugs such as indomethacin, which inhibit prostaglandin synthesis, should not be used in patients with congestive heart failure (Dzau et al., 1984).

Zelis and Flaim (1981) propose a progression of events as the severity of congestive heart failure increases. (i) There is a low level of alpha-stimulation which redistributes blood within muscle, so that more blood is available to exercising than to inactive muscle, and within the kidney, so that there is sodium retention, which activates the renin–angiotensin system. (ii) The increased circulating angiotensin maintains the arterial perfusion pressure; in a dog model the use of angiotensin blockade at different stages has suggested that activation of the renin–angiotensin system is only sustained during severe or uncompensated heart failure. (iii) Increased vascular stiffness impairs the normal metabolically induced vasodilation mechanisms, contributes to an increased peripheral vascular resistance and causes muscular ischemia. (iv) High-level alpha-stimulation results from the reduced skeletal muscle oxygen tension.

The theme common to the above changes is an increased peripheral vascular resistance. The responses to alpha-receptor stimulation and to angiotensin stimulation can be understood in terms of the molecular mechanisms of smooth muscle contraction (Chapter 17).

Reflex changes

Changes in baroreceptor responsiveness may also explain some of the events in congestive heart failure. There is a failure to increase the heart rate in heart failure in response to normal stimuli and in response to vasoconstriction. The normal decrease of parasympathetic tone during exercise does not occur in congestive heart failure. This may explain the exaggerated reflex forearm vasoconstrictor responses during exercise in patients with heart failure. Inflation of the left atrium with a balloon causes an increase in urinary flow (a similar mechanism accounts for the diuresis associated with supraventricular tachycardias). However, in heart failure this diuresis does not occur despite the increase in atrial pressure. The proposed explanation is that reflex control of the renal vascular bed is impaired; for example, sodium restriction and diuretics normally increase renin activity and angiotensin levels whereas renin and angiotensin fall in patients with heart failure (Mark, 1983).

The Critical Limit of Failing Myocardium

First, the ventricle may dilate to the limit of the Starling curve. This adaptation is limited by the heart volume which in turn is limited by the connective tissue, the degree of slippage and the degree of tension development. As dilation increases, tension rises by the Laplace law. Secondly, as the beta-receptor density falls in extreme heart failure the inotropic effect of circulating catecholamines is diminished and the processes of adaptation fail. As myocardial norepinephrine is depleted there is less stimulation of those beta-receptors more accessible to the sympathetic neurons than to circulating catecholamines.

Next, the anatomical mass of the heart may become so large that a limit is reached. Linzbach (1960) originally proposed that the myocardium could outstrip its blood supply. The idea that the blood supply is "outstripped" has recently been revived. In the early stages of hypertrophy the vascular supply lags behind the degree of hypertrophy of the cell so that there is a relative ischemia in certain circumstances. Later on the vascular supply appears to "catch up". Later again, as the hypertrophy becomes more extreme and possibly as wall tension rises abnormally, the oxygen supply is once again impaired in relation to the demand, especially in the subendocardial layers

(Unverfeth et al., 1983). Because coronary artery disease is not part of the clinical picture, this relative lack of oxygen leads not to angina nor myocardial infarction, but to a diffuse lack of oxygen which in turn causes focal ischemia. This sequence may account for the development of focal fibrosis and necrosis, worse in the subendocardial zone. Alternatively, focal arterial spasm may occur at this stage, with similar effects.

All of these critical events mean that the myocardium reaches its "limit" so that fibrosis formation occurs, contractility decreases and wall tension rises further. In advanced heart failure the myocardium is as fibrosed as a cirrhotic liver and its compliance is lost. (This analogy was made by Sonnenblick.)

Compliance of ventricles

In the normal myocardium, distension by a volume load leads to an increased pressure. If the pressure–volume relationship is normal then the compliance (an index of stiffness) is normal. If there is fibrosis or myocardial infarction then compliance is lost — in technical terms, the modulus of elasticity is increased. The decreased compliance leads to a decreased distension of the myocardium so that an increase of volume greatly increases intraluminal pressure. The result is that the wall tension rises more than expected and the oxygen demand increases correspondingly; the demand outstrips the supply. Loss of compliance is therefore one factor leading to deterioration of the situation of the heart on the Frank-Starling curve (Fig. 13-14).

Starling Curve in Heart Failure

A useful way of looking at the inotropic state of the left ventricle in heart failure is McMichael's diagram, since elaborated by many others (Figs 1-7, 22-2). The cause of the downward limb is probably the greatly increased impedance or afterload, so that myocardial performance is now afterload-dependent. A downward slope once entered, an increase of filling pressure can only lead to an unchanged or even falling stroke volume, because the heart size has reached its limit and because the myocardial contractile state is so low. Either an inotropic drug or an unloading agent can move the heart to a more favorable curve, so that either (i) the same stroke volume is achieved with fewer congestive symptoms or (ii) the stroke volume is

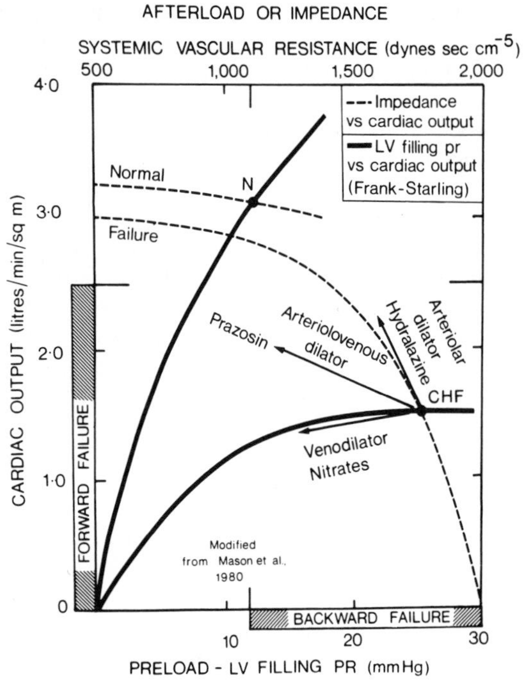

AFTERLOAD OR IMPEDANCE

SYSTEMIC VASCULAR RESISTANCE (dynes sec cm^{-5})

Fig. 22-2 In the normal heart (point N), CO (cardiac output) is regulated principally by changes in preload; alterations in impedance are of minor importance. In contrast, in congestive heart failure (CHF), CO is regulated principally by changes in impedance; alterations in preload are of minor importance (depressed Frank–Starling curve). In CHF the pure arteriolar dilator, hydralazine, raises lowered CO markedly with mild decline of elevated LVEDP (left ventricular end-diastolic pressure = LV filling pr). The balanced arteriovenous dilator, prazosin, raises lowered CO and decreases elevated LVEDP considerably. The pure venodilator, sublingual nitroglycerin, decreases elevated LVEDP markedly with little or no improvement of lowered CO. From Mason et al. (1980). Arch Int Med 140: 1578, with permission.

actually increased so that "forward failure" also improves. An important point is that the myocardium of advanced heart failure may be so severely damaged (like the cirrhotic liver) that therapy is aimed at a periphery (Fig. 22-3) and only a limited positive inotropic response can be expected.

Diuretic Therapy

Combined with digitalis, diuretic agents are standard therapy for heart failure (Table 22-3). Diuretics stop the reabsorption of chloride and sodium by the renal tubules, the most powerful ones (such as furosemide, 40–120 mg daily) acting on the loop. As a result, there is enhanced loss of sodium and water and the circulating blood volume (increased in congestive heart failure) falls, thereby unloading the heart. Sometimes, too, potassium is lost so that the blood level needs monitoring; an additional potassium-retaining diuretic such as amiloride or triamterene is frequently given, or else conventional oral potassium supplements. Diuretics are also thought to have a venodilator effect, which is most marked in the case of furosemide, thereby also relieving the preload by another mechanism. It is of interest that digitalis was first described by Withering as a diuretic; recently its renal effect has been re-examined. Digitalis stops sodium transport from urine to blood by inhibiting the sodium pump of the tubules, and thereby theoretically has some added diuretic effect in experimental doses.

Inotropic Therapy

The chief effect of an inotropic agent is to alter the contractile state of the myocardium. Positively inotropic agents are used for heart failure, negative ones for angina pectoris, to relieve the oxygen demand. The various agents used for a positive inotropic effect are: (i) digitalis glycosides; (ii) sympathomimetic agents; and (iii) phosphodiesterase inhibitors. All these inotropic agents ultimately act by increasing the cytosolic calcium ion concentration. This simple hypothesis, first emphasized by Nayler in 1967, has stood the test of time. Digitalis increases the cytosolic calcium by inhibition of the sodium pump; the sympathomimetic agents act by stimulation of adenylate cyclase with formation of cyclic AMP which "opens" the calcium channels; while phosphodiesterase inhibitors indirectly raise the cyclic AMP. Other newer and as yet clinically untested agents act in novel ways (Fig. 19-9). Amrinone is a phosphodiesterase inhibitor but might also act on calcium influx (page 274).

Inotropic therapy, if successful, can decrease the heart size to allow better operation of the Starling curve. But in a severely damaged myocardium increased cytosolic calcium predisposes to calcium overload and can be dangerous. Thus there must be care not to "flog the failing heart".

TREATMENT OF "INTRACTABLE" HEART-FAILURE

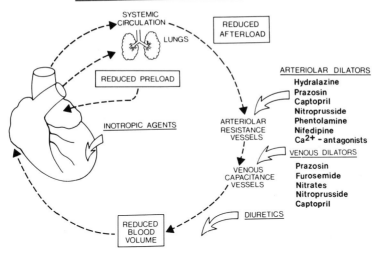

Fig. 22-3 Sites of action of agents acting on afterload or preload to relieve severe congestive heart failure. From Opie and Harrison (1984). In: Drugs for the Heart. Ed. LH Opie, Grune & Stratton, Orlando, London and New York.

Table 22-3

Principles of therapy of congestive heart failure

1. **General principles**
   (a) Relief of underlying condition. Valve replacement or valvotomy; therapy of hypertension
   (b) Relief of associated or aggravating conditions. Anemia, atrial fibrillation, pulmonary or systemic emboli
   (c) Relief of edema. Diuretic therapy
2. **Inotropic therapy**
   —digitalis
   —intravenous dopamine or dobutamine
   —amrinone and other experimental agents
3. **Relief of excessive preload**
   —diuretics including furosemide
   —vasodilators (nitrates and others)
4. **Reduction of afterload**
   —hydralazine
   —nifedipine
5. **Combined pre- and afterload reduction**
   —prazosin
   —captopril or enalapril
6. **Inhibition of renin–angiotensin system**
   —captopril
   —enalapril
7. **Reduction of heart rate**
   —digitalis
   —alanidine (Table 5-2)

Digitalis

Many positively inotropic agents have important additional effects. Digitalis stimulates the vagus to slow the heart and to allow better diastolic filling. It also has a vasoconstrictive effect (presumably as a result of inhibition of the sodium pump in vascular smooth muscle with a rise of vascular cytosolic calcium) which can, to some extent, counter its inotropic and bradycardiac effect. Thus when digitalis is given to a non-failing heart, the cardiac output may actually decrease. The latter sequence is an argument against what is known as prophylactic digitalization, which is sometimes used when it is suspected that heart failure may develop.

In chronic congestive heart failure the inotropic effect of digitalis is lessened and may sometimes be lost—possibly because sarcolemmal changes alter the binding sites or because the myocardium is so damaged that the number of functioning cells which can respond to inotropic stimulation is limited.

In left ventricular failure of acute myocardial infarction, inotropic therapy by digitalis is used less and less in the early stages because (i) better control of the inotropic state can be achieved by intravenous dopamine or dobutamine; (ii) positive inotropic agents must be used with care because of the risk of increasing ischemic damage; hence vasodilators such as nitroprusside are used first or in combination with an inotropic agent such as dobutamine.

In hypertension with left ventricular failure, unloading is now more logical therapy than inotropic stimulation.

Sympathomimetic agents

Sympathomimetic agents are most effective in cases where the beta-adrenoreceptor is still fully responsive. Sympathomimetic agents are generally not active given orally. The two agents used most are **dopamine** and **dobutamine**; both are given intravenously and are especially successful when the myocardium fails acutely, as in acute myocardial infarction or postoperatively (Chapter 19). In severe chronic congestive heart failure where beta-receptor response is lost, **amrinone**, an inhibitor of phosphodiesterase (page 274), may have a limited role; during its use possible thrombocytopenia must be monitored.

Unloading Agents

Lately the very logical concept has gained ground that instead of flogging the failing heart one should reduce the load on it by means of vasodilators (Table 22-4). The afterload, the preload, or both can be reduced. Relief of congestive failure by pharmacological reduction of preload was reported by Burch (1956). The concept of afterload reduction (Fig. 22-2) is already well-established in the therapy of systemic hypertension and has now come to be applied in several other conditions — severe congestive heart failure, especially when caused by hypertension, ischemic heart disease, cardiomyopathy or aortic or

Table 22-4

Indications for vasodilator therapy in heart failure

When conventional therapy is inadequate for:
1. Severe congestive heart failure
   — cardiomyopathy
   — ischemic heart disease
   — valvular regurgitation
2. Acute myocardial infarction with left ventricular failure[a]
3. Hypertension with left ventricular failure[a]

[a]In these conditions, vasodilator therapy is used increasingly before or together with digoxin or other inotropic agents.

mitral incompetence; and acute myocardial infarction with failure or shock. Gould et al. (1969) and Majid et al. (1971) argued that the reflex vasoconstriction of severe pump failure was excessive, that such constriction was alpha-mediated and that alpha-blockade with phentolamine should improve severe heart failure — it did. Today vasodilators are widely used as adjuvants in the therapy of heart failure. But the major indication for afterload reduction is still hypertension, for which all vasodilators have been used except (i) nitrates, which are primarily reducers of the preload, and (ii) the beta-adrenergic agonists, which have a direct inotropic effect which is undesirable for the overactive hypertrophied heart in hypertension.

Afterload

The aim of vasodilator therapy is to reduce the resistance to blood flow through the aorta. In clinical terms this is the **aortic impedance** or the aortic pressure divided by the aortic flow at the same time. This clinical concept of impedance, although widely used, has no counterpart in the physical sciences and, strictly speaking, is an inappropriate term (O'Rourke, 1982). As the impedance increases and the afterload rises, the performance of the failing myocardium is increasingly limited (Fig. 22-2). The afterload is now no longer appropriately matched to the inotropic state — this is called "**afterload mismatch**" (Ross, 1976). Hence reduction of peripheral arteriolar resistance will not only reduce blood pressure, but increase cardiac output. According to Laplace's law, the tension on the walls of a thin-walled sphere equals intraluminal pressure × radius. Wall tension is one of the major determinants of the myocardial oxygen uptake (Fig. 13-5). Reduction of the afterload (or the preload) is followed by a decrease in the myocardial oxygen uptake, with probable benefit to the subendocardial zones which may develop chronic ischemia (Unverfeth et al., 1983). Another reason for reducing the afterload is to "redirect" the work of the myocardium. Thus the amount of work put into overcoming wall stress is decreased while that put into producing cardiac output is increased. Taking the simplified approximation (page 169):

work = systolic aortic pressure × cardiac output

it is apparent that afterload reduction will decrease aortic pressure and increase cardiac output, without altering the total work performed.

Preload

Preload is the left ventricular filling pressure, which is raised in left heart failure. It can be measured indirectly by insertion of a Swan–Ganz flotation catheter via the right heart into the pulmonary capillary bed to obtain the "wedge" pressure (see Fig. 1-10). Normally as the preload increases, so does the peak left ventricular systolic pressure and the stroke volume rise (ascending limb of the Starling curve). But in diseased hearts the increase in stroke volume is much less than normal, and the stroke volume may even fall as the filling pressure rises (the controversial descending limb of the curve). Increasing the initial fiber length, a reflection of the preload, should increase the inotropic state (page 182). Hence there is a "**preload reserve**" (Ross, 1976) which initially compensates for the afterload mismatch. Beyond a certain point there is no further increase in fiber length and any additional increase in the preload simply means that the wall stress increases without a corresponding rise in the stroke volume. Hence the filling pressure should be reduced to an optimal value which may help to compensate for the decreased inotropic state without provoking excess wall stress on the ventricle.

Sites of vasodilation

The effect of peripheral vasodilators on the heart can be seen by their influence on the Starling curve obtained from patients (Fig. 22-4). Three types of response can be found. First, pure venous dilation achieved by nitrates keeps the cardiac output unchanged; the loop diuretic furosemide has a similar effect. Reduction of the excess preload to optimal values reduces the wall stress and maintains the cardiac output. (In normal subjects, a reduction of left ventricular filling pressure would result in a reduction of cardiac output.) In contrast, in the second response, hydralazine or nifedipine give pure arteriolar dilation which increases the cardiac output for any given filling pressure. Thirdly, combined venous and arteriolar dilation by nitroprusside or prazosin gives effects intermediate between those of nitrates and of hydralazine. Increasing the cardiac output relieves features of forward failure such as fatigue and poor renal perfusion (Pierpont et al., 1980), whereas decreasing the left ventricular end-diastolic pressure relieves the symptoms of dyspnea. Therefore it is possible to select

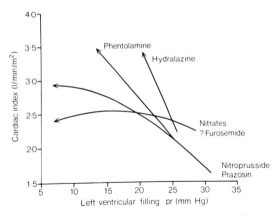

Fig. 22-4 Comparative effects of various vasodilators on left ventricular filling pressure (wedge-pressure) and cardiac index in patients with severe left ventricular failure. Drawn from combined data in the literature; for data sources see Opie and Harrison (1984). In: Drugs for the Heart, Ed LH Opie, pp 129–151, Grune & Stratton, Orlando, London and New York. Note the apparent inotropic effects of hydralazine and phentolamine.

the agent required according to the patient's symptoms (Fig. 22-2). The major drawback to vasodilator therapy has been the rather frequent development of tolerance (Chapter 17) so that increasing doses are required or the agent becomes ineffective. For example, with hydralazine the maximal daily dose for hypertension is usually 200 mg; for congestive failure this may rise to 800 mg. Only captopril is relatively free of the defect of tolerance, which may develop in about 15 percent of patients (Packer, 1983).

Vasodilator plus inotropic therapy

Load reduction has not been used customarily in the therapy of congestive heart failure until after optimal doses of diuretics and digitalis. Now clinicians increasingly are starting to add captopril or other vasodilators early in the treatment of congestive heart failure. The danger is that excessive load reduction may cause hypotension with poor perfusion of heart, kidney or brain. Hence the combination of vasodilator and inotropic therapy is appealing. Besides the combination with digitalis, an intravenous vasodilator such as nitroprusside may be combined with an intravenous inotropic agent such as dobutamine in the case of acute severe failure.

Heart rate

Vasodilators alter in their effects on hypertension and heart failure. In hypertension the general effects are tachycardia, sodium and fluid retention, as well as a fall in blood pressure. Interestingly, the tachycardia may be found even in beta-blocked patients, suggesting that some vasodilators have direct pharmacological effects on heart rate (Mroczek et al., 1976). In heart failure, vasodilators improve cardiac output thereby promoting diuresis (Pierpont et al., 1980) and tending to maintain the blood pressure; there may be unexpectedly little extra tachycardia because relief of failure reduces the heart rate.

Valvular heart disease

When congestive heart failure is caused by valvular heart disease the place of load reduction depends on the lesion. Stenosis is essentially a plumbing problem and should be relieved surgically; afterload reduction could worsen aortic stenosis by increasing the pressure gradient. Thus abrupt arterial vasodilation by nifedipine can lead to acute pulmonary edema in aortic stenosis, while nitrates in mitral stenosis may remove the high venous filling pressure required to push the blood past a severely stenosed valve. The general rule is thus that load reduction is most effective for valvular

regurgitation and least effective, or contra-indicated, for valvular stenosis.

Renin–Angiotensin–Aldosterone System

In the presence of heart failure, activation of the renin–angiotensin–aldosterone system by increasing levels of angiotensin may be likely to contribute to the systemic vasoconstriction of congestive heart failure **(Cohn and Levine, 1982). Captopril is thought to act primarily by inhibition of the angiotensin-converting** enzyme, reducing serum concentrations of angiotensin II and thereby peripheral vasoconstriction (Figs 22-5 and 22-6). In patients with congestive heart failure this

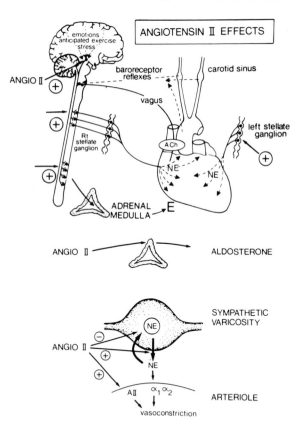

Fig. 22-6 Multiple sites of action of angiotensin II (= angio II), including central adrenergic activation, facilitation of ganglionic transmission, release of aldosterone from the adrenal medulla, release of norepinephrine (NE) from terminal sympathetic varicosities with inhibition of re-uptake and direct stimulation of vascular angiotensin II receptors. The major net effect is powerful vasoconstriction.

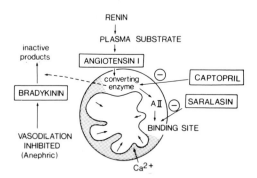

Fig. 22-5 Site of action of captopril on the converting enzyme (found especially in pulmonary vascular bed), thereby reducing formation of angiotensin II (AII). Another possible factor is the decreased breakdown of the vasodilator, bradykinin. The latter mechanism is thought to account for an effect of captopril detected even in anephric patients. Saralasin is a receptor antagonist which, by interacting with the same vascular binding site as angiotensin II, causes vasodilation. Saralasin is not in clinical use.

decrease in systemic vascular resistance improves cardiac output and decreases filling pressures. An additional mechanism of benefit is by inhibition of the angiotensin-stimulated release of aldosterone from the adrenal medulla. Sustained hemodynamic improvement in heart failure with captopril is documented, with tolerance developing in only about 15 percent of patients. The response may be gradual. Another angiotensin-converting enzyme inhibitor, **enalapril**, has a different molecular structure which may lessen immunologically based side-effects. It is likely that this class of drugs will become an important addition to the therapeutic armamentarium of heart failure. Because captopril tends to increase the serum potassium, combination with potassium-retaining diuretics such as triamterene or amiloride should be avoided. Neutropenia and renal toxicity are rare side-effects of high-dose captopril. A recently emphasized problem is first-dose hypotension, avoided either by giving a very low first dose (up to 6.25 mg; dose thereafter up to 12.5–50 mg three times daily) or by omitting diuretic therapy before introducing captopril or by avoiding captopril if the serum sodium is low.

Congestive Heart Failure: Present Trends in Therapy

With so many possible sites of therapeutic intervention, the ideal "step-care" therapy of congestive heart failure is undergoing reappraisal with earlier reliance on vasodilators and/or captopril (Gersh et al., 1984). Yet despite newer agents (particularly the vasodilators), the long-term prognosis of congestive heart failure remains poor, unless a reversible cause such as valvular heart disease is present. The usual policy is to initiate treatment with diuretics, salt restriction and then digitalis before proceeding to vasodilators — this may change with time. The role of digitalis remains contentious, particularly in the light of some evidence that this may adversely affect prognosis in certain patients (post-myocardial infarction survivors). To some extent scepticism about the sustained inotropic activity of digitalis has been resolved by recent data confirming a beneficial long-term action on cardiac performance, although this effect is not readily transferred into patient benefit (page 266). While there is insufficient current evidence to deny digitalis to patients with objective signs of congestive heart failure (especially after diuretics have been used), there is also not enough evidence to assume that digitalis will maintain its beneficial effect.

Alternative inotropic agents to digitalis have not yet established themselves (see Fig. 19-9). Orally active beta-2-stimulants such as salbutamol are being tried, with intravenous agents of the amrinone group being kept in reserve.

There is ample documentation of the acute hemodynamic and symptomatic benefits of vasodilator therapy. In the chronic management of congestive heart failure the long-term benefit is not known. A major question, as yet unanswered, is the role of **vasodilators in early or mild heart failure and their possible place as first-choice drugs in selected patients.**[*]

Choice of vasodilator

Optimal use of vasodilators requires that they be tailored to the hemodynamic status of the individual. Ideally, this requires invasive monitoring with its associated demands on skilled personnel and with economic caveats (Gersh et al., 1984). Certainly the patient with severe intractable heart failure warrants this approach. Those patients with predominantly elevated filling pressures require long-acting nitrates. If the systemic vascular resistance is also elevated, hydralazine or nifedipine may be added. Patients with relatively normal filling pressures but low cardiac output and elevated systemic vascular resistance may respond best to hydralazine or nifedipine. Prazosin should be ideal for combined "backward" and "forward" failure. Tachyphylaxis is a problem with prazosin, hydralazine and nitrates, but may be overcome by higher doses or intermittently stopping therapy for a few days. Tachyphylaxis has not yet been found with nifedipine, but overall experience is very limited. In the case of prazosin, excess diuresis and hypovolemia predispose to tachyphylaxis. In practice, when tachyphylaxis to prazosin develops a change to captopril is seen increasingly as the best solution — especially if fluid retention persists despite diuretic therapy. In severely ill patients intravenous nitroprusside with dopamine or dobutamine may be necessary. Heart failure due to valvular heart disease (especially mitral and aortic regurgitation), responds to vasodilators, which are used primarily as a temporizing measure prior to surgery.

In patients with mild heart failure, recourse to invasive monitoring is less desirable and impractical. Vasodilator therapy in these patients must be tailored

---

[*]Section modified from Gersh et al (1984) with permission.

to the clinical presentation. In those without clinical or radiographic evidence of left ventricular failure or pulmonary congestion, it is crucial to avoid excessive preload reduction; this may precipitously reduce filling pressures and cardiac output. Two other useful rules are (Opie and Harrison, 1984): not to decrease the systolic blood pressure by more than 5 mmHg (unless there is hypertension) nor to drop the systolic pressure below 90 mmHg. In such circumstances inotropic therapy is preferable.

Summary

In congestive heart failure the primary problem is myocardial failure, either secondary to overwork **(pressure or volume overload) or due to energy deprivation (ischemic heart disease) or due to actual** disease of the myocardium (cardiomyopathy). The inotropic state of the myocardium is depressed and it functions on a "lower" Starling curve. Secondary hemodynamic effects are those of blood pressure (of the lungs) and forward failure (low output). Therapy is by improving the inotropic state (digitalis), which may be difficult to achieve in the end-state "cirrhotic" heart, or by use of unloading agents (including diuretics). Either the preload can be reduced or the afterload or both. The neurohumoral abnormalities in congestive heart failure can be tackled at source by use of the converting enzyme inhibitor captopril.

References

Alpert NR, Mulieri LA (1982). Increased myothermal economy of isometric force generation in compensated cardiac hypertrophy induced by pulmonary artery constriction in the rabbit. Circ Res 50: 491–500.

Bristow MR, Ginsburg R, Minobe W, Cubicciotti RS, Sageman WS, Lurie K, Billingham ME, Harrison DC, Stinson EB (1982). Decreased catecholamine sensitivity and beta-adrenergic receptor density in failing human hearts. New Engl J Med 307: 205–221.

Burch GE (1956). Evidence for increased venous tone in chronic congestive heart failure. Arch Int Med 98: 750–766.

Clark AJ (1913). The action of ions and lipids upon the frog's heart. J Physiol (London) 47: 66–107.

Cohn JN, Levine TB (1982). Angiotensin-converting enzyme inhibition in congestive heart failure: the concept. Am J Cardiol 49: 1480–1483.

Dhalla NJ (1976). Involvement of membrane systems in heart failure due to intracellular calcium overload and deficiency. J Molec Cell Cardiol 8: 661–667.

Dzau VJ, Packer M, Lilly LS, Swartz SL, Hollenberg NK, Williams GH (1984). Prostaglandins in severe congestive heart failure. New Engl J Med 310: 347–352.

Gersh BJ, Opie LH, Kaplan NM (1984). Which drugs for which disease? In: Drugs for the Heart. Ed. LH Opie, pp. 153–191, Grune & Stratton, Orlando, London and New York.

Gould L, Zahir M, Ethinger S (1969). Phentolamine and cardiovascular performance. Brit Heart J 31: 154–162.

Kaufmann RL, Homburger H, Wirth H (1971). Disorder in excitation–contraction coupling of cardiac muscle from cats with experimentally produced right ventricular hypertrophy. Circ Res 28: 346–357.

Leclerq JF, Swynghedauw B (1976). Myofibrillar ATPase, DNA and hydroxyproline content of human hypertrophied heart. Europ J Clin Invest 6: 27–33.

Linzbach AJ (1960). Heart failure from the point of view of quantitative anatomy. Am J Cardiol 5: 370–382.

Litten RZ, Martin BJ, Low RB, Alpert NR (1982). Altered myosin isoenzyme patterns from pressure-overloaded and thyrotoxic hypertrophied rabbit hearts. Circ Res 50: 856–864.

Lompre AM, Schwartz K, D'Albis A, Lacombe G, Thiem NV, Swynghedauw B (1979). Myosin isoenzymes redistribution in chronic heart overloading. Nature 282: 105–107.

Majid PA, Sharma B, Taylor SH (1971). Phentolamine for vasodilator treatment of severe heart failure. Lancet ii: 719–724.

Mark AL (1983). The Bezold–Jarisch reflex revisited: clinical implications of inhibiting reflexes originating in the heart. J Am Coll Cardiol 1: 90–102.

Maurer W, Tschada R, Manthey J, Ablasser A, Kubler W (1981). Catecholamines in patients with heart failure. In: Catecholamines and the Heart. Eds. W Delius, E Gerlach, H Grobecker, W Kubler, pp 236–246, Springer-Verlag, Berlin.

Mercadier JJ, Bouveret P, Gorza L, Schiaffino S, Clark WA, Zak R, Swynghedauw B, Schwartz K (1983). Myosin isoenzymes in normal and hypertrophied human ventricular myocardium. Circ Res 53: 52–62.

Mroczek WJ, Lee WR, Davidov ME, Finnerty FA (1976). Vasodilator administration in the presence of beta-adrenergic blockade. Circulation 53: 985–988.

Nayler WG (1965). The inotropic action of delta-aldosterone on papillary muscles isolated from monkeys. J Pharm Exp Therap 148: 215–217.

Nayler WG (1967). Calcium exchange in cardiac muscle: a basic mechanism of drug action. Am Heart J 73: 379–394.

Opie LH, Harrison DC (1984). Vasodilating drugs. In: Drugs for the Heart. Ed. LH Opie, pp 129–151, Grune & Stratton, Orlando, London and New York.

O'Rourke MF (1982). Vascular impedance in studies of arterial and cardiac function. Physiol Rev 62: 570–623.

Packer M (1983). Vasodilators and inotropic therapy for severe chronic heart failure: passion and skepticism. J Am Coll Cardiol 2: 841—852.

Pierpont GL, Brown DC, Franciosa JA, Cohn JN (1980). Effect of hydralazine on renal failure in patients with congestive heart failure. Circulation 61: 323–327.

Pierpont GL, Francis GS, DeMaster EG, Levine TB, Bolman RM, Cohn JN (1983). Elevated left ventricular myocardial dopamine in preterminal idiopathic dilated cardiomyopathy. Am J Cardiol 52: 1033–1035.

Ross JR, Jr (1976). Afterload mismatch and preload reserve: a conceptual framework for the analysis of ventricular function. Prog Cardiovasc Dis 18: 255–264.

Unverfeth DV, Magorien RD, Lewis RP, Leier CV (1983). The role of subendocardial ischemia in perpetrating myocardial failure in patients with non-ischemic congestive cardiomyopathy. Am Heart J 105: 175–179.

Williams FJ Jr, Mathew B, Hern DL, Potter RD, Deiss WP Jr (1983). Myocardial hydroxyproline and mechanical response to prolonged pressure loading followed by unloading in the cat. J Clin Invest 72: 1910–1917.

Zelis R, Flaim SF (1981). Hemodynamic effects of vasodilator drugs. In: Vasodilation, Eds. PM Vanhoutte, I Leusen, pp 441–449, Raven Press, New York.

New References

Bayliss J, Norell MS, Canepa-Anson R, Reid C, Poole-Wilson P, Sutton G (1985). Clinical importance of the renin-angiotensin system in chronic heart failure: double-blind comparison of captopril and prazosin. Brit Med J 290: 1861–1865.

Edwards CRW, Padfield PL (1985). Angiotensin-converting enzyme inhibitors: past, present, and bright future. Lancet 1: 30–34.

Franciosa JA, Wilen MM, Jordan RA (1985). Effects of enalapril, a new angiotensin-converting enzyme inhibitor, in a controlled trial in heart failure. J Am Coll Cardiol 5: 101–107.

Haber E (1984). Renin inhibitors. New Engl J Med 311: 1631–1633.

Moser M, Zanchetti A (1985). Angiotensin converting enzyme inhibition in clinical practice. J Cardiovasc Pharmacol 7 (Supp 1): S2–S147.

Packer M, Medina N, Yushak M (1984). Relation between serum sodium concentration and the hemodynamic and clinical responses to converting enzyme inhibition with captopril in severe heart failure. J Am Coll Cardiol 3: 1035–1043.

Arrhythmias and Antiarrhythmic Agents

A useful practical classification of arrhythmias (= abnormal heart rhythm = dysrhythmias) is according to their origin, i.e. supraventricular or ventricular. Supraventricular arrhythmias may, in turn, be divided into those like supraventricular tachycardia, where an anatomical or functional re-entry circuit is at work, and atrial fibrillation where there is some form of chronic atrial disease. Ventricular arrhythmias are frequently ischemic in origin and complex in genesis (Fig. 23-1). This chapter will concentrate on tachy-arrhythmias; heart block and related conditions are discussed with the conduction system (Chapter 5).

Common Arrhythmias

Atrial ectopic beats

The most common arrhythmia is the ectopic beat (ectopic = out of place, Greek) which is almost a physiological event when the heart "drops a beat" in response to excitement (Fig. 23-2). Normally harmless, such ectopics may initiate supraventricular tachy-cardias in those predisposed by physiological or anatomical pathways for re-entry circuits. The mechanisms whereby ectopic beats develop are still not understood; probably they originate when potentially automatic tissue, normally suppressed by the sinus node, is provoked into firing by a variety of factors including beta-adrenergic stimulation.

Ectopic beats can only develop when the sodium channel opens in response to the initiating stimulus. During the **refractory period** (Fig. 23-3) an early electrical stimulus cannot evoke any response, because repolarization is not sufficiently far advanced to regain the voltage range in which the sodium channel can operate. In the **relative refractory period**, towards the end of the action potential, the voltage is sufficiently negative to allow some sodium channels to open in response to an appropriate voltage stimulus. The rate of depolarization of such an ectopic beat is slower than normal, because only some of the sodium channels open. As a result fewer calcium channels open and the action potential duration is decreased (Fig. 23-3).

Supraventricular tachycardias

Supraventricular arrhythmias are those originating in the atria, including the atrioventricular node. A common variety occurring particularly in the younger age groups is a **paroxysmal supraventricular tachycardia** (tachycardia = fast heart, Greek) in which the atria and ventricles beat very rapidly and regularly (150–250 beats/min) so that ventricular filling may become impaired. At the higher atrial rates, atrioventricular block may develop (Fig. 23-2).

In **atrial flutter** the atrial rate is so rapid (250–350 f waves/min) that atrioventricular block must develop. In **atrial fibrillation** there are many small wavelets of excitation traversing the atria, originating (it is thought) from multiple re-entry cycles or from

ARRHYTHMOGENIC MECHANISMS

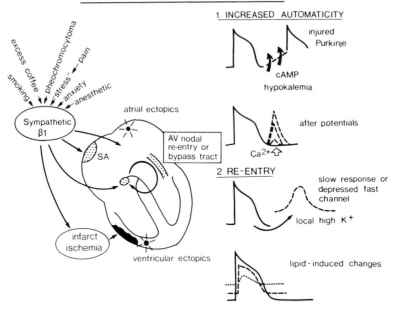

Fig. 23-1 Basic arrhythmogenic mechanisms. Sympathetic stimulation can provoke ectopic beats or, in the presence of re-entry circuits, a tachycardia. Supraventricular tachycardias are frequently based on AV nodal re-entry or the existence of a bypass tract. Ventricular tachycardias are often based on the existence of an infarcted or ischemic zone in which the cellular mechanisms may include the development of slow responses or depressed fast channels or lipid-induced changes. Other arrhythmias are the result of increased automaticity, the cellular mechanisms of which include spontaneous depolarization developing in otherwise non-automatic fibers, or the development of after-potentials.

multifocal ectopic beats; the word "fibrillation" is derived from the Latin "fibril" (= a small fiber); the contractions of the atria are no longer co-ordinated but it seems as if many small fibers are contracting separately. Only some of the numerous atrial beats are transmitted at irregular intervals through the filter of the atrioventricular node to the ventricles, which characteristically have a "chaotic" rhythm.

Ventricular arrhythmias

Numerous alternative names exist for **ventricular ectopic beats** or VEB (= ventricular ectopic activity = ventricular extrasystole = ventricular premature beat; abbreviated as VEA or VES or VPB). The **vulnerable period** occurs during the relative refractory period (Fig. 23-3), when it is normally difficult to provoke atrial or ventricular ectopic beats. The fact that ectopics do occur and can provoke either atrial or ventricular fibrillation suggests that part of the myocardium in the region of the ectopic focus has

already recovered normal excitability; thus there is electrical **inhomogeneity** which predisposes to an abnormality called re-entry (see next section). The ventricular ectopic beats most feared are those with many different forms on the electrocardiogram, which may reflect a multifocal origin; those which occur frequently; and the early ectopics which occur in the vulnerable period on the apex of the T wave (**R-on-T ectopics**, Fig. 23-2) with greater risk of precipitating ventricular fibrillation. In patients with acute myocardial infarction such **warning arrhythmias** are regarded by some authorities as an indication for vigorous antiarrhythmic therapy, because it is feared that they may herald the onset of **ventricular tachycardia** (three or more ventricular ectopic beats occurring regularly and at a rapid rate), which may in turn degenerate into ventricular fibrillation. In reality it now seems that ventricular fibrillation of unexpected onset may occur sufficiently frequently to question the relationship between warning arrhythmias and ventricular fibrillation.

Whereas atrial fibrillation can be withstood by the

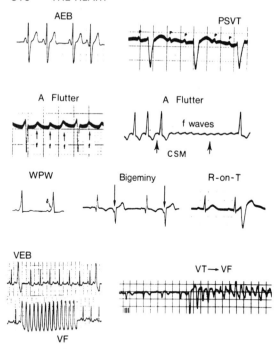

Fig. 23-2 Examples of some common arrhythmias. AEB = atrial ectopic beat. VEB = ventricular ectopic beat. PSVT = paroxysmal supraventricular nodal tachycardia. AFI = atrial flutter. CSM = carotid sinus massage. VT = ventricular tachycardia. VF = ventricular fibrillation. WPW = Wolff–Parkinson–White syndrome with characteristic delta wave and short PR interval. Bigeminy = coupled ventricular ectopic beats in digitalis toxicity. R-on-T = ventricular ectopic beat occurring on apex of T wave in vulnerable period. By permission of D Dubin (1974). Rapid Interpretation of EKG's, Cover Publishing Co, Tampa, Florida; FL Meijler et al. (1975). Electrocardiography for Intensive Care Units, Excerpta Medica, Amsterdam; and L Schamroth (1982). An Introduction to Electrocardiography, Blackwells, Oxford.

MODELS OF ECTOPIC ACTIVITIES

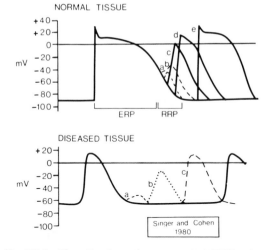

Fig. 23-3 The effective refractory period (ERP) exists until repolarization decreases the voltage enough to allow the sodium channel to open again in response to an artificial stimulus. During the relative refractory period (RRP), impulses can form, but the maximum rate of depolarization of the new impulses will be less than normal (i.e. the sodium channel does not open fully). As full depolarization is regained, progressively more normal action potentials are formed. Modified from Singer and Cohen (Fig. 9-7 in Mandel WJ, Cardiac Arrhythmias, Lippincott, 1980), with permission. In normal tissue, the RRP corresponds to the vulnerable period (R-on-T ectopics, see Fig. 23-2).

(For nodal disease and conduction disturbances see Chapter 5.)

Mechanisms of Supraventricular Arrhythmias

Supraventricular tachycardia

The majority of supraventricular tachycardias has a twofold mechanism: an initiating ectopic beat and a re-entry pathway in the atrioventricular node (**atrioventricular nodal re-entrant tachycardia**). The proposal is that there are two functioning pathways (**dual nodal pathways**: alpha and beta paths), one slower in conduction than the other (Fig. 23-4). In the usual type, an appropriately timed atrial ectopic impulse may enter the slow beta pathway in the normal direction and then travel up the fast alpha pathway. The latter is no longer in the

heart because the atrioventricular node "filters" the number of ectopic impulses reaching the ventricles, in **ventricular fibrillation** the numerous re-entry wavelets leave the ventricle unable to respond by an orderly contraction so that pump failure results; death is inevitable unless **defibrillation** is applied by passing through the heart a direct current strong enough to obliterate all the ectopic wavelets and to allow the normal sinus rhythm to resume. Direct current **cardioversion**, using much weaker energy, is now also used extensively in an attempt to revert supraventricular tachycardia or atrial fibrillation of recent onset to sinus rhythm should drug treatment fail.

AV NODAL RE-ENTRY TACHYCARDIA

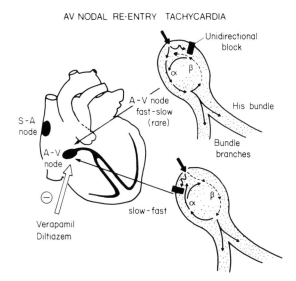

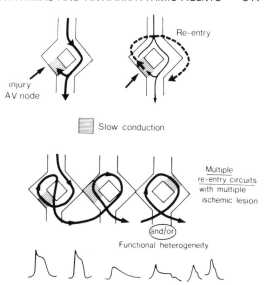

Fig. 23-4 In the common type of atrioventricular (AV) nodal re-entry tachycardia there is retrograde conduction along the fast fibers and normally directed conduction along the slow fibers of the node (slow–fast type). Unidirectional block is invoked to explain why the normal impulse cannot travel down the fast pathway. Less commonly, the direction is reversed and resembles antegrade conduction through a bypass tract. The major therapeutic site of action of the calcium antagonists verapamil and diltiazem in supraventricular tachycardias is inhibition of conduction through the slow fibers of the AV node. In addition to verapamil, agents such as quinidine and disopyramide may inhibit the conduction through the fast fibers. The differentiation between slow and fast fibers is functional, not anatomical.

Fig. 23-5 Model for formation of the re-entry circuit. When the conducted impulse reaches a zone of injury, conduction becomes slowed by formation of the type of action potential shown in diseased tissue in Fig. 23-3. The slow rate of conduction delays the impulse until the refractory period of the normal impulse has passed, so that re-entry is possible. The bottom panel shows how multiple re-entry circuits could form from multiple ischemic injuries or from the abnormal action potentials (possibly caused by focal glycolytic abnormalities or accumulation of lysophosphoglycerides) so that heterogeneity of function results.

refractory period either because the normal impulse passed over some time ago, or because a **unidirectional block** acts like a one way valve only to allow retrograde conduction (Fig. 23-4). From the fast pathway the impulse may now re-enter the slow pathway. Repetitive **re-entry** of this nature causes a sustained tachycardia. A similar general model for re-entry also applies to ventricular muscle when ischemic injury provokes localized slow conduction (Fig. 23-5).

Beta-adrenergic stimuli predispose to re-entry by enhancing the rate of conduction down the slow pathway. Conversely, many patients with supraventricular tachycardia have a re-entry circuit involving vagal-sensitive fibers in the atrioventricular node. Inhibition of the atrioventricular node can be achieved by stimulation of efferent links of the reflex arc by

baroreceptors, e.g. a brief Valsalva maneuver or unilateral carotid massage, or the diving reflex, induced by immersing the face in cold water (eyeball pressure is best avoided because there may be glaucoma).

In the less common type of nodal re-entry the ectopic impulse travels up the slow pathway in the opposite direction to normal to re-enter the fast pathway in the antegrade direction.

In the unusual condition of **paroxysmal reciprocating sinus tachycardia**, re-entry occurs through the sinus node and not the atrioventricular node. The principles of formation of the re-entry pathway remain the same.

Bypass tract and
AV reciprocating tachycardias

When there is an anatomical bypass tract, another type of re-entry circuit is possible. In this condition — the

Wolff–Parkinson–White syndrome—a ventricular ectopic impulse can travel back up the bypass tract, arriving late enough for the normal forward conducting impulse to have passed (bypass tract no longer refractory). Such **retrograde conduction** allows the impulse to enter the atrioventricular node, thereby establishing a re-entry circuit involving the node, the bypass tract, the atrium and the ventricle or the His–Purkinje system (AV reciprocating tachycardia). In a minority of patients with this syndrome there are attacks of atrial fibrillation. The atrial impulses pass forward at an accelerated rate along the bypass tract (**anterograde** or **antegrade conduction**) to the ventricles, with danger of ventricular tachycardia and fibrillation. Antegrade conduction also occurs during sinus rhythm, so that part of the atrial impulse arrives more rapidly than normal at the ventricles by the bypass tract, thereby causing a characteristic hump on the upstroke of the QRS complex (delta-wave, Fig. 23-2).

Atrial flutter

The mechanism of atrial flutter is controversial: either repetitive firing of an ectopic focus or a re-entry circuit may be responsible. In patients, comparisons of the cycle length in spontaneous and electrically induced atrial flutter have been made (Disertori et al., 1983); the pattern of spread favors a re-entry cycle. Thus the early circus movement theory proposed by Sir Thomas Lewis (1920) is supported. It is true that Prinzmetal et al. (1950) used high speed cinematography to prove that an irritable focus could cause atrial flutter, but their experimental model need not have corresponded closely to the human disease.

Electrocardiographically, the **flutter waves** (Fig. 23-2) of atrial activity beat regularly at rates of about 250–350/min, usually close to 300. The normal atrioventricular node cannot conduct impulses much faster than an atrial rate of 200/min, so that block results. Frequently an atrial rate of about 300/min results in a ventricular rate of about 150/min (2 : 1 block). Thus a fixed ventricular rate of 120–170/min should lead to suspicion of atrial flutter with block or a supraventricular tachycardia with 1 : 1 conduction. Usually atrial flutter occurs with organic heart disease and the fast ventricular rate may cause symptoms such as angina or syncope. When atrioventricular nodal disease is also present the degree of block may be higher (4 : 1 or even 8 : 1; note usual progression in multiples of 2). With a 2 : 1 block one of the atrial complexes may fall on the QRS complex so that the diagnosis is in doubt until carotid sinus stimulation increases the degree of block by enhancing vagal tone.

Atrial fibrillation

In atrial fibrillation there frequently is a chronic predisposing disease damaging the atria, such as ischemic heart disease, hypertension, mitral stenosis or thyrotoxicosis. The initial event is either an early atrial beat in the atrial vulnerable period or an increased rate of atrial flutter (Killip and Gault, 1965). The wave front of depolarization undergoes fractionation because of numerous inhomogeneities, so that multiple wave fronts form with the characteristic loss of P wave on the electrocardiogram. Only recently has it been recognized that there are effects of atrial fibrillation, other than those on the heart rhythm. First, the "atrial booster" effect of atrial contraction is lost which itself may contribute to decreased ventricular function. Secondly, the fibrillation causes the atria to become stiffer than normal, and increases the oxygen demand and the atrial blood flow (McHale et al., 1983). The proposal is that the additional atrial metabolic demands lead to atrial ischemia and fibrosis, thereby converting episodes of acute fibrillation into chronically sustained atrial fibrillation (White et al., 1982).

Ventricular Automaticity

There are three main proposals for the mechanisms underlying the development of ventricular arrhythmias. First, automaticity may develop in otherwise non-automatic tissue. Secondly, there may be a re-entry circuit. Thirdly, abnormalities of repolarization associated with the prolonged QT interval may develop into atypical ventricular tachycardia. Two proposed mechanisms for the origin of ventricular ectopic beats are (i) the development of phase 4 depolarization in Purkinje or myocardial fibers and (ii) delayed afterdepolarization.

Automaticity in Purkinje fibers

Purkinje fibers, normally quiescent, can develop phase 4 depolarization (as in ischemia) when partially depolarized, so that the threshold for firing is more easily reached. A pacemaker current, I_f, can be invoked experimentally and is now known to be sensitive to inhibition by lidocaine and quinidine (Carmeleit and Saikawa, 1982). The voltage range at which this current operates is about -65 to -55 mV (Chapter 5), explaining why partial depolarization caused by ischemia predisposes to automaticity in Purkinje fibers.

Hypokalemia (e.g. $K^+ = 2.7$ mM) increases phase 4 depolarization whereas a high normal level (5.4 mM) decreases phase 4 depolarization. If the potassium level is sufficiently high then catecholamine stimulation, which normally also evokes phase 4 depolarization in Purkinje fibers, becomes ineffective. When cyclic AMP is introduced by iontophoresis into spontaneously active cardiac Purkinje fibers there is a shortened action potential and a steeper rate of phase 4 depolarization, in keeping with catecholamine effects. Catecholamine stimulation and a low external level of potassium should be a potent arrhythmogenic combination. Acute myocardial infarction in man is characterized by acute liberation of catecholamines, which are known to decrease arterial blood potassium. In addition, some patients with acute infarction will have been given diuretic therapy, a frequent cause of hypokalemia. Patients with hypokalemia at the time of onset of myocardial infarction have a greater incidence of ventricular arrhythmias, including ventricular fibrillation (Dyckner et al., 1975).

Much less well understood is the development of automaticity in normal ventricular cells, where phase 4 depolarization is provoked with much greater difficulty than in Purkinje fibers.

Delayed after-depolarization

Ventricular myocardium can also develop automatic activity in specified experimental conditions which cause delayed after-depolarizations (DADs) or **after-potentials**. Normally ventricular cells have a flat phase 4 with no spontaneous depolarization. Delayed depolarizations are abnormal oscillations found in ventricular or Purkinje cells in certain abnormal circumstances, including digitalis poisoning and micro-injection of cyclic AMP in the cell (Fig. 23-6). The factor common to these two stimuli is the increase in cytosolic calcium ion concentration, which induces a transient diastolic inward current (I_{ti}), probably by promoting sodium–calcium exchange (Clusin et al.,

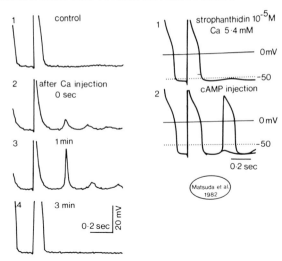

Fig. 23-6 Provocation of transient diastolic depolarizations by intracellular injections of calcium ions (left) or by the combination of a high concentration of a digitalis glycoside (right). Such depolarizations appear to underlie the development of digitalis-induced automaticity; their role in other circumstances is still conjectural. Modified from Matsuda et al. (1982). Circ Res 51: 142, with permission from the author and the American Heart Association.

1983). Delayed after-depolarization tends to be a cyclical event with a series of ever smaller waves, which probably reflect calcium ion oscillations in the cytosol because there are accompanying after-contractions. Depletion of calcium from the sarcoplasmic reticulum can stop the development of the after-depolarizations. The current causing the repetitive after-depolarizations is activated ("switched on") by an increased intracellular calcium. Therefore verapamil and a low external calcium both inhibit the phenomenon. Tetrodotoxin and lidocaine, inhibitors of the sodium channel, also inhibit this current probably by reducing internal calcium as internal sodium falls (Eisner et al., 1983). Delayed after-depolarizations are thought to underlie the development of ventricular automaticity during **digitalis poisoning** (Fig. 23-2); interestingly, such digitalis arrhythmias respond to therapy with either lidocaine (sodium antagonist) or verapamil (calcium antagonist).

In ventricular muscle, delayed after-depolarizations can lead to **triggered automaticity**, and hence play a role in converting a focus of automaticity into a sustained ventricular arrhythmia—as originally proposed by Cranefield. This sequence seems most likely to occur when there is prior inhibition of the sodium pump by digitalis or by a low external potassium concentration. In Purkinje fibers delayed after-depolarizations can develop even at normal external potassium levels and theoretically be a cause of automaticity even in the absence of excess digitalis. Hence after-depolarizations are suspected of contributing to some of the ventricular arrhythmias of acute myocardial infarction (El-Sherif et al., 1983).

Ventricular Re-entry Circuits

Ventricular re-entry circuits may develop whenever there is electrical inhomogeneity of the myocardium, which in turn reflects the focal ionic and metabolic abnormalities that cause slow conduction in one limb of a re-entry circuit (Fig. 23-5). Slow conduction is achieved by inhibition of the fast channel with residual slow channel activity, resulting from ischemic or other injury to the conduction tissue. These conditions predispose to the development of re-entry which when rapid and regular is one cause of ventricular tachycardia (the other being a rapidly firing automatic focus). In acute ischemic damage heterogeneous areas of slow conduction can cause **micro re-entry circuits**

which are thought to underlie the development of ventricular fibrillation. The five major theories to explain slow conduction in ischemic tissue are, first, the effect of localized hyperkalemia and partial depolarization. Secondly, the development of slow responses in completely depolarized tissue may occur when the tissue content of cyclic AMP rises. Thirdly, residual fast channel activity may explain why some apparently slow responses are sensitive to fast channel inhibitors. Fourthly, disturbed metabolism of lipids and calcium may directly affect the action potential. Fifthly, electrical coupling between cells may be disrupted.

Potassium and depolarization

In the early 1950s Harris (1954) found increasing coronary venous potassium values during the onset of arrhythmias after coronary arterial ligation. Since then there has been increasing evidence of links between potassium and arrhythmogenesis. The mechanism whereby potassium loss promotes very early arrhythmias after coronary ligation cannot be merely

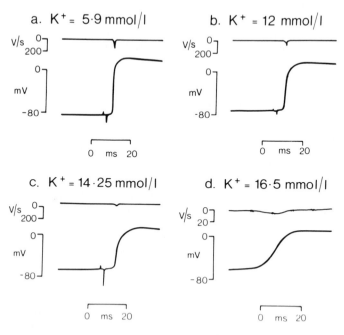

Fig. 23-7 Effect of hyperkalemia on upstroke velocity ($dV/dt = \dot{V}_{max}$) of the action potential. There is progressive unmasking of an apparently slow response, which is in reality depressed fast channel activity. Inhibition of the fast response explains the use of a high external potassium in cardioplegia. For details see Opie et al. (1979). Reproduced with permission from the American Journal of Cardiology.

depletion of cell potassium, which requires 2–4 hours to become evident. Hyperkalemia, as found in coronary venous blood very early after coronary occlusion, may play a more important role (Fig. 23-7). Theoretical considerations show that when the cell is depolarized to values less negative than − 50 mV, the rapid inward current is inactivated and the resting potential approaches the threshold potential for the slow inward current. The intravenous or intra-arterial infusion of potassium salts rapidly produces ectopic activity possibly by promoting automaticity in Purkinje fibers. Eventually ventricular fibrillation develops, even in otherwise normal hearts.

Cyclic AMP and slow responses

When myocardial cells are completely depolarized, as can happen when the extracellular potassium level rises to 18 mM and higher (Hirche et al., 1980), then the cells become inexcitable. Now added beta-adrenergic stimulation can invoke a slow response action potential (Fig. 23-8). Other factors elevating cyclic AMP such as phosphodiesterase inhibition or exposure to dibutyryl cyclic AMP have a similar effect, as does intracellular introduction of cyclic AMP by micro-iontophoresis (Vogel and Sperelakis, 1981). Because this phenomenon is prevented by calcium antagonists and a low external calcium ion concentration, it is also

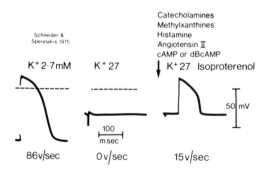

Fig. 23-8 The development of the slow response. In fibers depolarized by hyperkalemia, agents increasing intracellular cyclic AMP such as catecholamines, methyl-xanthines or histamine can provoke slow-response action potentials provided that the electrical stimulation is continued. One theory for ventricular arrhythmia development is that slow responses contribute to delayed conduction and to the development of re-entry circuits. v/sec = volts per second. dBcAMP = dibutyryl cyclic AMP. Modified from Schneider and Sperelakis (1975) with permission.

reasonable to hold that cyclic AMP promotes the "opening" of the calcium channels (see also Chapter 4). Cyclic AMP rises in ischemic tissue in early experimental myocardial infarction, as does the extracellular potassium (Opie et al., 1979). Yet there is no direct proof that slow responses are involved in the early ventricular arrhythmias of developing myocardial infarction; indirect evidence favoring this possibility is that slowed conduction is accelerated by the calcium antagonist diltiazem which delays the onset of ventricular fibrillation (Clusin et al., 1984a) and that high concentrations of calcium antagonists protect the ischemic heart against electrically induced ventricular fibrillation (Thandroyen, 1982).

Apart from slow responses, cyclic AMP may be the intracellular messenger of other effects of beta-adrenergic stimulation: enhanced phase 4 depolarization of nodal and Purkinje tissue and the development of delayed afterdepolarizations (see previous discussion).

Residual fast channel activity

In some models, apparently slow responses are sensitive to the sodium channel inhibitor tetrodotoxin (Arita et al., 1983), suggesting that the real nature of the action potential depends on residual fast channel activity, as found during progressive hyperkalemia (Fig. 23-7). The practical implication is that fast channel inhibitors such as lidocaine could be therapeutically effective.

Shortening and lengthening of action potential duration

In ischemia, accumulation of lysophosphoglycerides (see Fig. 10-22) could induce a variety of abnormalities of the action potential with narrowing in some cells and lengthening in others (Corr et al., 1982). These membrane-active agents may predispose to slow conduction by depressing most of the components of the membrane currents (Clarkson and Ten Eick, 1983). The real problem is whether or not the intracellular concentrations of free lysophosphoglycerides reached in ischemia are high enough to provoke ventricular arrhythmias in this way. The action potential duration is shortened by inhibitors of glycolysis such as iodoacetate, lactate and pyruvate, free fatty acids and acidosis (Opie et al., 1979). The proposal is that ATP made by glycolysis has a special role in maintenance of the action potential duration—as supported by the effects of direct intracellular injection of ATP (Taniguichi et al., 1983). Such metabolic changes can be highly focal (Russell, 1982). During acute myocardial ischemia the shortening of the action potential duration can be related to the inhibition of glycolysis in zones with very low blood flow (Russell, 1982) or to an increased cytosolic calcium concentration (page 95; Clusin et al., 1984b). By these mechanisms, focal metabolic changes may produce localized abnormalities of conduction. Variations in the action potential duration between ischemic and non-ischemic cells, and between sites with different severities of ischemia produce the critical differences in the refractory state of the myocardium that explain dispersion of refractoriness (Kuo et al., 1983).

Impaired intercellular conduction

Conduction between cells normally proceeds by the gap or nexus junctions (see Fig. 2-5). Two changes found in ischemia, an increased intracellular calcium ion activity and a decreased pH (acidosis), can uncouple intercellular conduction to block conduction and to predispose to arrhythmias (De Mello, 1982).

Prolonged QT-syndrome

Besides inducing phase 4 depolarization, hypokalemia (or hypomagnesemia) can also prolong the QT-interval by interfering with the repolarizing potassium current. Especially dangerous is the combination of diuretic-induced hypokalemia with antiarrhythmic drugs which may also prolong the QT-interval such as quinidine, disopyramide, amiodarone and sotalol (Moss and Schwartz, 1982). The type of ventricular arrhythmia resulting is characteristically that with QRS complexes which widen and narrow, called *torsade de pointes* (twisting of the points) or atypical ventricular tachycardia; the danger is ventricular fibrillation. The mechanism is complex and may include: (i) differential changes in refractoriness in different parts of the myocardium; (ii) the development of **early after-depolarizations** or "**humps**" as found in patients when right ventricular action potentials are recorded by suction electrodes (Bonatti et al., 1983). The interpretation of such humps is still controversial. What is clear is that they are quite different from

delayed afterdepolarizations (see page 319). First, the humps occur before the end of complete repolarization, whereas the delayed afterdepolarizations occur well thereafter (Fig. 23-5). Secondly, the humps disappear as the heart rate rises, explaining why a bradycardia predisposes to the development of *torsade de pointes* and why tachycardia induced by pacing or isoproterenol is effective in the therapy of that condition. In contrast, a tachycardia exaggerates true delayed afterdepolarizations, perhaps because the rapid repetitive opening of the calcium channel overloads the cell with calcium. Thirdly, humps do not develop into automatic activity as do delayed afterdepolarizations. The cellular mechanisms causing the humps are unknown; a reduced conductance for postassium increases the humps and brings out the U-wave of the surface electrocardiogram (Bonatti et al., 1983). Thus the humps may be the intracardiac counterpart of the U-wave, and may be related to an abnormal potassium current.

In a few patients there is a congenital prolongation of the QT-syndrome (**long QT-syndrome**). The danger is again ventricular tachycardia. Excess activity of the left stellate ganglion is proposed as the underlying cause (Crampton, 1979). The therapy is either by beta-adrenergic blockade or by unilateral stellate ganglion-ectomy.

It may be difficult to understand why certain antiarrhythmic agents such as amiodarone have a widened action potential duration as the basis of their antiarrhythmic effect, whereas QT prolongation which reflects a prolonged action potential duration actually predisposes to ventricular arrhythmias. The proposed explanation is that amiodarone "equalizes" the action potential duration throughout the heart, whereas in the long QT syndrome there are heterogeneities of the action potential duration which cannot be equalized in this way. It is these heterogeneities which predispose to the arrhythmias.

Development of Ventricular Arrhythmias in Acute Myocardial Infarction

Four processes are currently held to be basic to the genesis of such cardiac arrhythmias: (i) increased automaticity; (ii) slowing of conduction in specific areas of the heart with resultant re-entry and re-excitation; (iii) variable shortening or lengthening of the refractory period with an increased dispersion of refractoriness between the ischemic and non-ischemic zones; and (iv) delayed after-depolarizations (as a possible cause of automaticity). Increased dispersion of refractoriness to conduction between the ischemic and the non-ischemic zones sets the stage for re-entrant arrhythmias (Levites et al., 1975). Unidirectional abnormalities of conduction between ischemic and non-ischemic zones have been recorded as have areas of localized fibrillation that can, it is thought, spread from the ischemic to the non-ischemic zone.

The actual initiating ectopic beat may arise in the non-ischemic zone, and then pass through a zone with a shortened action potential duration, thereby producing different refractory states in different zones of the heart (**dispersion of refractoriness**; Kuo et al., 1983). Purkinje fibers of the infarcted zone may be another source of arrhythmias. Impulses originating in surviving Purkinje fibers have a reduced diastolic potential and a decreased action potential amplitude as well as a decreased upstroke velocity (Friedman et al., 1973) and hence resemble the slow response. The action potential duration can be extraordinarily prolonged. Purkinje fibers can be the site of origin both of slowly conducted normal impulses and also of ectopic foci.

Apart from the differential rate of involvement of epicardium and endocardium in some models, and the superior survival of Purkinje fibers, the persistence of a variable collateral circulation introduces further metabolic and histologic inhomogeneity. Changes in receptor density (such as increased numbers of alpha-adrenergic receptors), hypokalemia and other general metabolic disturbances may all play a role. It seems likely that there is no unique causal event to link metabolic changes and ischemic arrhythmias but rather that a variety of factors, each arrhythmogenic in certain specific experimental conditions, could be interacting in the very complex situation in patients with acute myocardial infarction (Opie et al., 1979). Such multiple mechanisms may explain the difficulties frequently encountered in treating the ventricular arrhythmias of acute infarction.

Classification of Antiarrhythmic Drugs

Antiarrhythmic agents, currently divided into four classes (Table 23-1), should be active on two of the major factors provoking arrhythmias: automaticity and re-entry circuits. The development of ectopic beats depends on opening of the fast channel even if it does not open as rapidly as normal. Therefore it may be anticipated that the sodium channel inhibitors (Class I, Fig. 23-9) are potentially antiarrhythmic agents. A critical feature is that these agents act preferentially on partially inactivated sodium channels so that they inhibit ectopic beats arising (i) in the relative refractory **or vulnerable period, and (ii) in partially depolarized (ischemic) tissue. Thus Class I antiarrhythmics preferentially inhibit abnormal depolarizations.**

Beta-adrenergic stimulation enhances automaticity by several mechanisms. First, phase 4 depolarization in Purkinje fibers is stimulated. Secondly, delayed

Table 23-1

Classification of antiarrhythmic agents

Class	Drugs
I. Membrane-stabilizing agents	A. Quinidine and quinidine-like agents (major effect, inhibition of fast Na^+ channel; repolarization also lengthened): quinidine, procainamide, disopyramide
	B. Lidocaine and lidocaine-like agents (complex effects including fast channel inhibition); lidocaine, phenytoin, mexiletine, tocainide, aprindine. (Amiodarone also belongs here)
	C. Other membrane stabilizing agents which have differential effects on **ventricular muscle and Purkinje fibers: encainide, lorcainide, flecainide, cibenzoline, propafenone**
II. Beta-blocking agents	Propranolol and all other beta-blockers
III. Agents widening action-potential duration (as major effect)	Amiodarone, bretylium Investigational: sotalol, N-acetyl-procainamide, melperone
IV. Calcium antagonist agents	Verapamil, diltiazem

From Singh, Opie and Marcus (1984). In: Drugs for the Heart, Ed. LH Opie, Grune & Stratton, Orlando, New York and London.

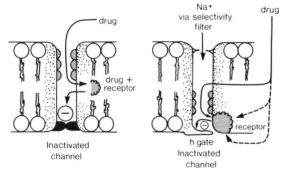

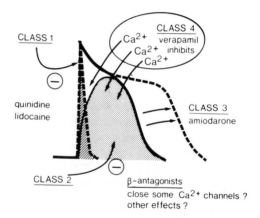

Fig. 23-9 Two models for effects of Class I anti-arrhythmic agents on the sodium channel. On the left the drug enters the lipid bilayer via an "open" channel, to bind to a receptor site, thereafter keeping the channel in the inactivated state according to the modulated-receptor hypothesis (also see Fig. 4-3). On the right, a selectivity filter limits the size of molecules entering to between 0.3 and 0.5 nm (3–5 Angstrom) so that the drug molecule must reach the receptor by lipophilic pathways or from the inside of the channel. (See Armstrong CM (1981). Physiol Rev 61: 644–683.)

Fig. 23-10 Proposed effects of various antiarrhythmic agents on the cardiac action potential, and the currents on which they are thought to act.

from the inactivation gate ("h" gate) which "shuts" the channel (Hauswrith and Singh, 1979; Fig. 23-9).

Kinetics of receptor for Class I agents

According to the **modulated receptor hypothesis** of Hondeghem and Katzung (1977), quinidine and lidocaine can interact with the sodium channel in any one of its three states: resting, open or inactivated (see Fig. 4-3). Rate constants for the association and dissociation of the binding of quinidine and lidocaine with each of these states have been proposed, from which it can be predicted that they largely reach the receptor site through the "open" channel using a hydrophilic route. It is the occupancy of the receptor site which "closes" the inactivation gate or keeps the inactivation gates shut longer than normal to prolong the refractory period. The molecules leave the receptor site to regain the extracellular space by dissociation which occurs largely when the "m" gates are open. To a lesser extent the molecules can reach or leave the receptor site by "lateral" diffusion through the bilipid membranes. It is the increasing number of drug-associated non-conducting channels that accounts for the inhibition of the fast sodium current. The state of the channel modulates these interactions. Lidocaine in particular preferentially interacts with the inactivated state, as found in partially depolarized tissue in which there are thought to be a greater number of inactivated sodium channels; lidocaine blocks the channel by binding one-to-one (Bean et al., 1983). Preferential binding of lidocaine to inactivated,

after-depolarizations are provoked. Thirdly, the slow response may develop in completely depolarized cells. One or more of these mechanisms may be inhibited by beta-adrenergic blocking agents which constitute Class II antiarrhythmic agents.

Re-entry circuits develop when there are differences in the rate of conduction down two limbs of a potential circuit. Drugs prolonging the duration of the refractory period—Class III agents—may inhibit conduction through one limb of the circuit besides inhibiting ectopic formation. Other re-entry circuits involve the AV node or part of it, in which case inhibition of the calcium channel of the node by Class IV agents is antiarrhythmic.

Sodium Channel Inhibitors
(Class I agents)

Both quinidine and lidocaine (= lignocaine) inhibit the fast phase by interacting with the **sodium channels** of the sarcolemma (Fig. 23-10). Previous doubts about this interaction have been resolved by voltage-clamp studies (Lee et al., 1981). Many models have been proposed; a recent one is based on the Hodgkin–Huxley proposal that the activation gates (three "m" gates) which "open" the sodium channel are different closed channels rather than to open channels explains why ectopic beats arising in damaged or ischemic tissue are inhibited in preference to the normal impulse. Quinidine on the other hand is prone to interact with the sodium channel over a broad range of membrane potentials, so that there is less preferential effect on depolarized cells. Quinidine therefore has a more powerful inhibition of the upstroke velocity of the normal action potential (Fig. 23-11).

This model resembles closely that proposed for the interaction of local anesthetic agents, such as cocaine, with nervous tissue (Hille, 1977) so that quinidine and lidocaine are sometimes referred to as **local anesthetic agents** even though quinidine itself is not so used. An alternative name for this property is **membrane stabilization**. Stabilization of electrical activity occurs at therapeutic concentrations; higher levels are required to cause true stabilization, so that, for example, hemolysis in erythrocytes is inhibited.

Molecular properties

The "molecular size" hypothesis of Courtney (1980) ascribes some of the differences between quinidine and lidocaine to different molecular properties, including molecular weight and state of charge. The lidocaine molecule is considerably smaller than that of quinidine, so that it can enter or leave its binding site on the sodium channel very much more rapidly than can quinidine. Quinidine is seen as a "long-memory" drug which should result in a prolonged depression of conduction by its prolonged action on the sodium channel. The slower moving quinidine molecule is more likely to enter the sodium channel when it is open, so that an increased heart rate increases its inhibition of the channel (Weld et al., 1982); this is the **use-dependent** (= **frequency-dependent**) effect. The model predicts that there are no absolute differences between lidocaine and quinidine; rather quinidine occupies one extreme of a scale by its very large molecular size. On the other hand benzocaine is a local anesthetic with a lower molecular weight than lidocaine (Sanchez-Chapula et al., 1983) and is so mobile that it can enter nervous tissue even when the sodium channel is not open.

Lidocaine is particularly effective against certain high-rate tachycardias with a re-entry circuit of an appropriate cycle length (Man and Dresel, 1979). The smaller more mobile lidocaine molecule not only arrives more rapidly at the receptor site, but leaves

more rapidly. Thus there is a shorter half-time of recovery of the sodium channel to normal, so that the "h" inactivation gate reopens more readily to end the lidocaine effect (Sanchez-Chapula et al., 1983).

Effects on action potential duration

Lidocaine shortens the action potential duration whereas quinidine lengthens it (Fig. 23-11). The explanation may be that quinidine also inhibits the potassium current causing delayed rectification, thereby delaying repolarization. In the past, lidocaine has also been thought to act on this potassium current. Now voltage-clamp studies have shown that lidocaine virtually only affects the sodium current (besides the pacemaker current of Purkinje tissue; Bean et al., 1983). Shortening of the action potential plateau by lidocaine may result from blocking the contribution of the background sodium current (Colatsky, 1982). This effect of lidocaine should promote arrhythmias by shortening the refractory period. In reality, the

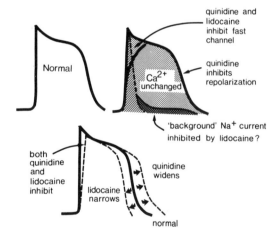

Fig. 23-11 Both quinidine and lidocaine inhibit the fast sodium channel. The effect on upstroke velocity is much exaggerated for diagrammatic purposes. Lidocaine maximally inhibits the fast channel when it is in the inactivated state, as found in ischemic tissue. Lidocaine promotes repolarization to narrow the action potential duration, possibly through inhibition of a "background" sodium current. In contrast, quinidine readily inhibits the sodium channel in its open state, hence explaining the more marked inhibition of the upstroke velocity of the action potential. Quinidine also prolongs action potential duration, possibly by inhibition of the repolarizing K^+ current.

powerful depressant effect on excitability in the ischemic zone converts zones of partial block into total block, inhibiting re-entry circuits (Cardinal et al., 1981) as they travel through the ischemic zone.

Optical isomers

Thus in the case of quinidine there are two major proposals for its antiarrhythmic actions: inhibition of the sodium channel and prolongation of the action potential duration. Light may be shed on which mechanism is of major importance by comparing the electrophysiological effect of quinidine with its optical isomer, quinine (Mirro et al., 1981). Quinine inhibits the upstroke velocity and shortens the action potential duration; it is not thought to be as effective an antiarrhythmic as quinidine.

Atrial vs ventricular effects

Lidocaine is relatively ineffective against atrial arrhythmias, despite depressing the upstroke velocity of the atrial action potential at least as much as that of the ventricles (Singh and Vaughan Williams, 1971). The explanation for this is not known but may lie in the duration of the action potential which is shorter in atrial tissue so that lidocaine has less possibility of inhibiting the "background" sodium current (Fig. 23-11). Another factor may be that atrial arrhythmias seldom involve ischemically induced zones of slow conduction upon which lidocaine acts preferentially. Quinidine is active against both atrial and ventricular arrhythmias, and also against those involving the conduction tissue such as that of the bypass tract and the fast limb of dual AV nodal pathways. There may be an additional biochemical explanation for these differences. Agents active against atrial arrhythmias (such as quinidine, disopyramide and procainamide) have a non-specific anti-adrenergic effect on atrial tissue; lidocaine has no such effect (Mirro, 1981).

Quinidine and Related Agents (Class IA)

Despite the common site of action of quinidine and lidocaine on the sodium channel, numerous differences (Tables 23-2 and 23-3) justify separate classification of quinidine (Class IA) and lidocaine (Class IB). An important recent proposal is that class IA agents predominantly inhibit "open" sodium channels, whereas class IB agents act chiefly on inactive, closed channels (Courtney, 1983). The side-effects of quinidine are serious enough to outweigh its substantial advantages in the view of many physicians. Quinidine is now used only in selected patients, usually with recurrent, chronic supraventricular or ventricular arrhythmias, where it is frequently able to inhibit the ectopic beats that fire re-entry circuits. In contrast to lidocaine, quinidine is used against supraventricular arrhythmias including those that involve the bypass tract. Quinidine inhibits peripheral alpha-adrenergic receptors so that there is a risk of hypotension with intravenous administration. It also inhibits cholinergic receptors to cause tachycardia. An idiosyncratic reaction may cause cardiovascular collapse. The most feared complication is undue widening of the QRS and QT intervals (Fig. 23-9). Quinidine inhibits the speed at which the electrical impulse spreads through the ventricles to provide zones of potential electrical instability, and sometimes, to cause a type of atypical ventricular tachycardia (*torsade de pointes*) which explains some cases of **quinidine syncope**. In others quinidine may increase blood digoxin to toxic levels.

Other quinidine-like agents

Disopyramide is a compound structurally quite unlike quinidine, yet with many similar properties, including the feared widening of the QRS and QT intervals with the risk of atypical ventricular tachycardias (Meltzer et al., 1978). Its interaction with the muscarinic cholinergic receptors is more powerful so that side-effects include paralysis of accommodation, constipation and urinary retention. When given intravenously it too can cause hypotension. Even when given orally, left ventricular failure can develop especially in compromised ventricles (Podrid et al., 1980). On the other hand, gastro-intestinal irritation is less frequent than with quinidine and there is no interaction with digitalis. The choice between disopyramide and quinidine may be based on the side-effects that are more easily tolerated by a particular person.

Procainamide is structurally different from both quinidine and disopyramide; yet it is also active against both atrial and ventricular ectopic beats. Interaction with muscarinic receptors is less than quinidine, and risk of hypotension is decreased when given intravenously. Hence procainamide is one of the intravenous agents used when lidocaine fails in patients

Table 23-2

Comparison of electrophysiological effects of quinidine and lidocaine

	Quinidine	Lidocaine
Electrophysiological		
Depression of upstroke velocity	+ +	+
Action potential duration	Widened	Shortened
Conduction through Purkinje system	Delayed	0
QRS interval	Prolonged	0
QT interval	Prolonged	0
Effects on currents		
Fast inward sodium current	↓	↓
"Background sodium current"	0	↓
Pacemaker Purkinje current	↓	↓
Rectifying K^+ current	Inhibited	0
Sodium channel binding		
Inactivated state, "closed channels"	+ / −	+ +
Activated state, "open channels"	+ +	+ / −
Molecular properties		
Size	"Large"	"Small"
Lipid solubility	Moderate	Moderate
Local anesthetic on nerve	No	Yes

0 = no effect; ↓ = reduction of current; + = effect indicated.
The advice of Professor E. Carmeliet, Leuven, Belgium, and Dr K Courtney, Palo Alto, California, is gratefully acknowledged.

Table 23-3

Comparison of clinical effects of quinidine and lidocaine

	Quinidine	Lidocaine
Antiarrhythmic spectrum		
Atrial arrhythmias: initiating ectopic	+	0
Circus tachycardia through AV node	0	0
WPW: retrograde/anterograde[a]	+	0
Ventricular tachycardia	+	+
Ventricular fibrillation, prophylaxis	0, ±	+
Receptor interaction		
Muscarinic receptors	Anticholinergic	None
Alpha-receptors (vascular)	Inhibition	None
Hemodynamic effects		
Myocardial depression	Marked	Little/none
Idiosyncrasy (collapse)	Needs test dose	None
Precipitation of arrhythmias		
Torsade de pointes	+	0
Ventricular fibrillation	? +	0
Average dose	1.2–2 g daily orally	75–100 mg IV then 2–4 mg/min infusion
Therapeutic level	about 10^{-4} M = 2.3–5.0 μg/mL	about 10^{-5} M = 1.4–6.0 μg/mL

0 = no effect; + = effect indicated.
[a]Inhibitory effect on bypass tract in Wolff–Parkinson–White syndrome with retrograde re-entrant arrhythmias, or with anterograde conduction (Fig. 23-4).

with acute myocardial infarction (Burton et al., 1976). Chronic use of oral procainamide is limited by the short half-life and the rare side-effect of lupus erythematosus. Although the QRS and QT intervals may lengthen, there is less effect than with quinidine. There is less risk of lupus with N-acetyl-procainamide (NAPA), a derivative of procainamide; the problem is that good initial responses may yield to recurrent arrhythmias during long-term therapy (Kluger et al., 1981).

Lidocaine and Related Agents (Class IB)

Lidocaine (= lignocaine) is probably the most widely used agent for the ventricular arrhythmias of acute myocardial infarction. As ventricular fibrillation frequently cannot be predicted, increasingly more clinicians hold the view that all patients with acute infarction should receive lidocaine as soon as possible after the onset of symptoms (DeSilva et al., 1981), starting with an intravenous bolus (about 75 mg) in the pre-hospital phase and continuing an intravenous infusion (2–4 mg/min) at a rate designed to maintain an adequate blood level (Fig. 23-12). Other clinicians only give lidocaine if warning arrhythmias appear so

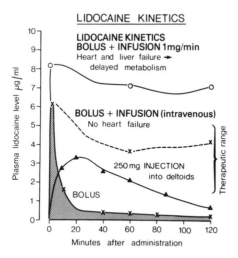

LIDOCAINE KINETICS

LIDOCAINE KINETICS
BOLUS + INFUSION 1mg/min
Heart and liver failure →
delayed metabolism

BOLUS + INFUSION (intravenous)
No heart failure

250 mg INJECTION into deltoids

BOLUS

Therapeutic range

Plasma lidocaine level μg/ml

Minutes after administration

Fig. 23-12 Lidocaine kinetics. To achieve and to maintain an adequate blood level of lidocaine requires an initial bolus or intramuscular injection followed by an infusion. For an intramuscular injection to give sustained high blood levels may require a dose of 400 mg. Note that in the presence of cardiac or liver failure, delayed metabolism increases the blood level with danger of toxic effects.

as to avoid central nervous system side-effects if the infusion is not carefully controlled. Lidocaine is metabolized so rapidly in the liver by a first-pass effect that it is ineffective when given orally. Administration by repetitive intravenous bolus injections or by prolonged infusion is required; many possible different regimens exist (Harrison, 1978). Intramuscular lidocaine is used especially by general practitioners called to a patient with suspected infarction; for this procedure to be effective in preventing early ventricular fibrillation a dose of 400 mg is required (Koster and Dunning, 1983).

Like quinidine, lidocaine more effectively inhibits sodium channels which are already partially blocked by potassium; the effect is very marked in the case of lidocaine so it is sometimes difficult to detect lidocaine effects on normal ventricular action potentials. This selectivity allows a more marked action of lidocaine on the ischemic zones of the myocardium (Gerstenblith et al., 1978), where it acts to prevent the fragmentation of wavefronts into multiple micro-re-entry circuits characteristic of ventricular fibrillation (Cardinal et al., 1981). A new proposal is that lidocaine inhibits after-depolarizations (page 319).

Clinical advantages of lidocaine are (i) the absence of any major hemodynamic depressant side-effects; (ii) no interaction with the muscarinic receptor; and (iii) very infrequent prolongation of the QRS or QT intervals. These qualities make lidocaine a relatively safe agent. The chief disadvantage is the high rate of first-pass metabolism in the liver so that lidocaine must be given intravenously and the dose decreased when liver blood flow is low, as in severe cardiac failure or during therapy with beta-adrenergic receptor blocking agents or during cimetidine therapy (Feely et al., 1982). Its side-effects are largely confined to the central nervous system.

Lidocaine-like agents

Mexiletine and **tocainide** both have properties similar to those of lidocaine, while being orally active because of changes in molecular structure from that of lidocaine. Hence they are more resistant to hepatic "first-pass" metabolism. Both are being used in the control of chronic arrhythmias following myocardial infarction; in neither case is there yet a proven reduction in sudden death. Both agents have central nervous system side-effects. An advantage is that they may initially be given intravenously in acute myocardial infarction, to be followed by oral therapy with the same agents. **Phenytoin** is still used specifically in digitalis intoxication, because of earlier work showing that it may enhance depressed AV nodal conduction. Phenytoin may also centrally depress the adrenergic system, thought to be activated in digitalis toxicity. Electrophysiologically, inhibition of the fast current by phenytoin has similarities to the effect of lidocaine (Sanchez-Chapula and Josephson, 1983). In addition phenytoin depresses the slow calcium current in Purkinje fibers (Scheuer and Kass, 1983), which could theoretically help to inhibit after-depolarizations developing as a result of digitalis-induced calcium overload.

Class IC Agents

Many new agents (see Table 23-1) are at present undergoing clinical and experimental evaluation. It is convenient to categorize these agents as Class IC agents: ecainide, flecainide, lorcainide, indecainide, propafenone, pirmenolol and cibenzoline. The main action of these compounds is to depress the upstroke velocity of phase 0 of the action potential and, as in the case of all Class I agents, they lengthen the time-dependent refractoriness. They also exert a differential effect on repolarization in Purkinje fibers (produce shortening) and ventricular muscle (lengthening). They are all potent antiarrhythmic agents but as a class all have QRS prolongation which is a major disadvantage. Their clinical utility is likely to be largely in the control of ventricular tachyarrhythmias. For example, a large co-operative study suggests that flecainide is superior to quinidine (Flecainide–Quinidine Research Group, 1983), although the QRS widening is more marked with flecainide which is potentially more harmful from this point of view. Propafenone particularly is widely used in Europe, where it is regarded as a safe and very effective drug. It has multiple sites of action including some beta-blocking effect, so that true classification of this drug is difficult.

Class II Agents:
Beta-adrenergic Receptor Antagonists

Beta-adrenergic receptor blockade is used especially for inappropriate or unwanted sinus tachycardia, paroxysmal atrial tachycardia provoked by emotion

and exercise, in chronic ventricular arrhythmias when heart failure is absent, in the arrhythmias of pheochromocytoma (combined with alpha-adrenergic receptor blockade to avoid hypertensive crises), in the hereditary prolonged QT syndrome and in the arrhythmias of mitral valve prolapse. This class of drug is exceptionally useful in the treatment of the unusual patient who has minimal or no heart disease but has exercise-induced ventricular premature beats or ventricular tachycardia. In acute myocardial infarction the cardiodepressant effects argue against designation of beta-blockers as the antiarrhythmic agents of choice, but in appropriate dosage and in patients without manifest heart failure these compounds are used increasingly for the control of supraventricular tachyarrhythmias, for the prevention of ventricular arrhythmias including ventricular fibrillation and to limit "infarct size". The common denominator to many of these indications is increased sympathetic beta-adrenergic activity. At a cellular level, occupancy of the beta-adrenergic receptors and decreased formation of cyclic AMP seems a probable mechanism involved in the antiarrhythmic effects.

In recent years, beta-adrenergic receptor blockers have drawn considerable attention as agents which, when given prophylactically to survivors of acute myocardial infarction, may reduce the incidence of sudden death in the first year or two after the acute event. Whether the beneficial effect is related to a primary antiarrhythmic action or whether it arises as a secondary consequence of lessened ischemia is not completely certain. In experimental animals chronic administration of these agents may lead to significant lengthening of the action potential duration, although in man QT lengthening is variable or absent. The possible significance of this weak Class III action in man is difficult to evaluate. In the case of sotalol, it is now reasonably certain that the acute lengthening of the action potential duration is a property that is independent of beta-adrenergic blockade and may constitute a major (Class III) antiarrhythmic mechanism for the control of a variety of cardiac arrhythmias.*

Class III Agents:
Amiodarone, Bretylium and Sotalol

It is becoming increasingly clear that Class III compounds are likely to emerge as the most significant ones for the control of cardiac arrhythmias. There are

*Section extracted from Singh et al. (1984), with permission.

several reasons for this. First, by inhibiting the repolarizing potassium currents they increase refractoriness without reducing conduction velocity in most tissues. Secondly, they have the ability to lessen heterogeneity in refractoriness and excitability in the heart. Thirdly, they have a low arrhythmogenic potential. Fourthly, as a group they have little or no negative inotropic activity. Fifthly, potency exceeds that of other antiarrhythmic compounds especially in the so-called refractory cardiac arrhythmias. Despite these common features, Class III agents are structurally and pharmacokinetically, as well as electrophysiologically, heterogeneous — and neither their antiarrhythmic effects nor their clinical indications are interchangeable. The best studied are amiodarone, bretylium and sotalol; other agents under development include N-acetyl-procainamide (NAPA). Whether sotalol truly has antiarrhythmic properties different from other beta-blockers seems likely (Rizos et al., 1984).*

Amiodarone

Besides prolonging the action potential duration and increasing the refractory period (Class III activity), amiodarone has a powerful lidocaine-like inhibitory effect on the sodium channel (Class I activity; Mason et al., 1981). Amiodarone also reduces accumulation of the proposed arrhythmogenic agent, cyclic AMP, in ischemic tissue (Lubbe et al., 1979). It may also have calcium antagonist properties, thereby explaining the bradycardia and vasodilator effects (it was first used in Europe as an anti-anginal agent). Clinically, it has three remarkable properties: efficacy against many arrhythmias including ventricular fibrillation and supraventricular or ventricular arrhythmias resistant to other agents (Bexton and Camm, 1982); a wide safety margin, including safety in the presence of severe congestive heart failure; and tissue accumulation, so that the effect continues for 10–45 days after the last dose. The therapeutic action of amiodarone takes several days to develop, unless it is given intravenously or in very high oral dose. When given to animals it is still active when the heart is isolated, indicating firm binding to cardiac receptors.

The main drawback of amiodarone lies in side-effects such as the development of corneal microdeposits and pulmonary fibrosis (Sobel and Rakita, 1982). The corneal deposits are reversible, and serious subjective visual impairment has not yet been reported. Photosensitivity and gastro-intestinal irritation occur

frequently (Ward et al., 1980). Amiodarone contains iodine and has structural similarities to thyroxine. Altered thyroid function (Melmed et al., 1981) may cause hypothyroidism or hyperthyroidism. Side-effects may be reduced by keeping the dose as low as possible. Once daily or even once weekly dosage and the prolonged therapeutic effect (weeks) are unusual advantages.

Bretylium tosylate

Bretylium tosylate is reputedly effective against ventricular fibrillation refractory to lidocaine and multiple direct current (DC) shocks (Holder et al., 1977). It may be used in other ventricular arrhythmias resistant to standard parenteral therapy such as lidocaine or procainamide (Heissenbuttel and Bigger, 1979). The mechanism of the antifibrillatory action is controversial. It has Class III activity in both Purkinje fibers and ventricular muscle (Heissenbuttel and Bigger, 1979). Bretylium has adrenergic-neuron-blocking properties (Fig. 23-9): it accumulates in sympathetic ganglia, depresses the release of norepinephrine and produces a chemical sympathectomy in repeated high doses. Initial sympathomimetic effects (transient hypertension and increased arrhythmias) probably result from transient discharge of norepinephrine from adrenergic postganglion terminals.

Class IV:
Slow Calcium Channel Inhibitors

Verapamil, the prototype Class IV agents, selectively inhibits the slow channels which are largely selective for calcium ions. It has a powerful inhibitory effect on the atrioventricular node where the action potential has little fast channel activity and is largely a reflection of slow calcium channel activity. The effect of verapamil on the atrioventricular node is found at concentrations which do not depress muscular contraction, so that verapamil is now the agent of choice for supraventricular paroxysmal tachycardias with circus re-entry pathways through the atrioventricular node. A single bolus of intravenous verapamil (5–10 mg over 1–2 min) will revert the majority of such arrhythmias to normal (Singh et al., 1978). In diseased hearts, or in patients already treated by a beta-adrenergic receptor blocking drug, the potential of verapamil for myocardial depression can be dangerous.

*Section modified from Singh et al. (1984), with permission.

Pretreatment with intravenous calcium can lessen myocardial depression while not preventing the beneficial effect on the AV node (Weiss et al., 1983).

Verapamil is also used to inhibit the flow of impulses from atria to ventricles in atrial flutter or fibrillation; in the latter condition it may be added to digoxin therapy to give better control of the ventricular response. Verapamil, like quinidine, enhances the blood digoxin level so that adjustment of the digoxin dose is required.

Diltiazem resembles verapamil in being a calcium antagonist with inhibitory properties on the atrioventricular node. It can also be used intravenously against paroxysmal supraventricular tachycardia.

Therapy of Arrhythmias

An urgent indication for therapy is **supraventricular paroxysmal tachycardia** (Table 23-4). Conduction

through the atrioventricular node is slowed firstly by physiologically increasing vagal activity by carotid sinus massage or other procedures. Previously elevation of arterial pressure by the alpha-stimulant methoxamine was used cautiously to stimulate vagal activity by elevating the arterial pressure by 20–40 mmHg. Cholinesterase inhibition by edrophonium may also be used. Today the advent of verapamil has made these procedures outdated (Table 23-4). Quinidine-like agents can also be used to inhibit conduction through the fast path; only disopyramide and not quinidine can be given intravenously. Their vagolytic effect may provoke re-entry, and disopyramide is negatively inotropic. Verapamil remains the drug of choice. When re-entry occurs through the sinus node, verapamil can also depress conduction by acting on the slow calcium channel.

Digitalis compounds and beta-adrenergic receptor antagonists also inhibit the AV node—the former by enhanced vagal tone and the latter by decreasing

Table 23-4

Agents used for supraventricular arrhythmias

Condition	Agent	Mode of action	Comment
Sinus bradycardia	IV atropine	Vagal inhibition	When hypotension accompanies bradycardia in acute infarction
Sinus tachycardia	Beta-blockade	Inhibition of pacemaker current	When symptomatic in anxiety or in thyrotoxicosis
Paroxysmal supra-ventricular tachycardia	1. Physiological carotid sinus massage	Vagal stimulation	Simple self-therapy but may not work
	2. Verapamil (or diltiazem) or beta-blockade	Inhibition of AV node	For acute therapy and prophylaxis
	3. Disopyramide or oral quinidine	Inhibition of fast fibers of AV node	For acute therapy and prophylaxis
	4. Digoxin	Vagal stimulation	For prophylaxis
Atrial flutter Acute therapy	IV verapamil (or diltiazem)	Inhibits AV node	Digoxin or beta-blockade also used
Prophylaxis	Quinidine or disopyramide (or diltiazem)	Inhibits initiating ectopic	
Atrial fibrillation to control ventricular response	Verapamil (or diltiazem) or digoxin or both Beta-blockade sometimes added to digoxin	Inhibition of AV node	For acute response IV verapamil preferable; for heart failure, digoxin preferable
Atrial fibrillation Prophylaxis pre- and post-cardioversion	Quinidine	Stops initiating ectopic	Disopyramide should also be effective

Note: (i) Electrical cardioversion may be used in serious supraventricular arrhythmias of recent onset either preferentially or after drug therapy.

(ii) Diltiazem is still being evaluated for antiarrhythmic effect (not yet FDA-approved).

IV = intravenous; AV = atrioventricular; beta-blockade = beta-adrenergic receptor blockade.

sympathetic nervous system effects on the node. Verapamil and the beta-adrenergic receptor antagonists both inhibit calcium channels so that in clinical practice the effects of the two agents are additive. In patients with very severe recurrent supraventricular tachycardias all three agents (verapamil, digitalis, beta-adrenergic receptor antagonists) may be required to inhibit the ventricular response. Here care is required to monitor possible interactions (verapamil and digitalis; verapamil and beta-adrenergic receptor antagonists).

In **atrial flutter** or **fibrillation**, block of the atrioventricular node can be induced by various inhibitors (verapamil, digitalis or beta-adrenergic receptor blockade) each of which acts by a different mechanism to reduce the ventricular response rate. There is an additive effect of these three agents. The aim is to achieve an acceptably slow ventricular response (Fig. 23-13) without inducing high degree AV block. Of these compounds, beta-adrenergic receptor antagonists are now becoming less popular because of their major additional effect in decreasing contractility. In patients not on digitalis, therapy may include digitalization or verapamil to slow the conduction through the atrioventricular node. Digitalis is the agent of choice when there is also left ventricular failure. In others verapamil is used increasingly especially in combination with digitalis (watching blood digoxin levels). Other drugs of the quinidine-type are sometimes used to prevent the ectopic beats that fire the re-entrant circuits which initiate the arrhythmias. Yet there is a danger that quinidine may slow the flutter rate sufficiently to remove the block and to allow an undesired fast conduction to the ventricles. Hence quinidine is usually combined with digitalis (again, watching blood digoxin levels). In patients with **digitalis toxicity**, atrial flutter with block is one of the most common arrhythmias found; the treatment is to withdraw digitalis and sometimes to give an extremely low dose of verapamil (0.0001 mg/kg/min) which is increased cautiously while watching the ventricular rate.

In the **Wolff–Parkinson–White syndrome** agents which prolong the QRS interval also prolong conduction through the bypass tract. Hence quinidine, disopyramide, aprindine and Class IC agents are all used to inhibit both antegrade and retrograde conduction (Fig. 23-14). Alternatively verapamil can be used to inhibit the re-entry circuit as it passes through the AV node (Fig. 23-14). As the direction of conduction cannot be predicted in advance, agents of choice are those inhibiting the bypass tract in both directions (Fig. 23-15). The initiating ectopic beat can be either atrial or ventricular; quinidine-like agents are active against both sites (Table 23-5). In refractory cases, amiodarone is specifically effective.

Sometimes digoxin or verapamil or beta-adrenergic blockade can accelerate antegrade conduction presumably because inhibition of the atrioventricular node diverts more impulses to the bypass tract. In addition, digitalis shortens the refractory period of the bypass tract. To test whether or not such dangerous antegrade

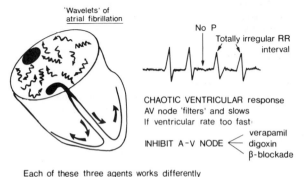

Fig. 23-13 Mechanisms of action of drugs used therapeutically in atrial fibrillation to control the ventricular rate.

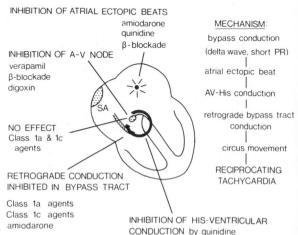

Fig. 23-14 Mode of action of drugs in the Wolff–Parkinson–White syndrome in which conduction occurs retrogradely along the bypass tract.

WPW: ANTEROGRADE CONDUCTION IN ATRIAL
FIBRILLATION OR FLUTTER

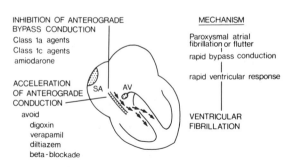

Fig. 23-15 Mode of action of drugs in the Wolff–Parkinson–White syndrome with antegrade (= anterograde) conduction. Note the major differences between the common type in which conduction occurs retrogradely along the bypass tract (Fig. 23-14), in comparison with the dangers of antegrade (anterograde) conduction down the bypass tract toward the ventricle. In the latter case agents inhibiting the AV node are potentially harmful.

conduction can occur, and whether or not drugs such as verapamil which inhibit the node are really undesirable, electrophysiological studies are required. The appropriate electrical stimuli can provoke conduction along the bypass tract in either direction; the test is repeated after administration of the drug.

In **acute myocardial infarction** therapy against life-threatening ventricular arrhythmias is initiated with intravenous lidocaine (if the patient is not yet receiving it) before resorting to other intravenous agents such as procainamide, mexiletine, lorcainide and tocainide (Table 23-6). Procainamide has been well-tested in this setting (Burton et al., 1976). In severe cases intravenous bretylium is used. Hemodynamically depressing agents such as quinidine and disopyramide are best avoided.

Serious **paroxysmal ventricular arrhythmias** may occur in otherwise apparently healthy patients or in survivors of acute infarction. Monitoring the effects of drug therapy requires a **Holter monitor**. The patient carries with him a small portable ECG machine with a high-fidelity recording system for periods of 24–72 hours. Another modern approach is to provoke the arrhythmias deliberately by programmed electrical stimulation (next section) to test which agents act acutely before embarking on chronic therapy. Yet there is concern about the reproducibility of the laboratory results in the clinical setting and so therapy frequently remains "hit-and-miss", with first one agent being tried and then another. The most effective prophylactic oral agent is probably amiodarone, but numerous side-effects make its use a very specialized procedure.

Acute therapy of *torsade de pointes* is by iso-proterenol or cardiac pacing, both of which could act

Table 23-5

Agents used for Wolff–Parkinson–White syndrome

Type	Agent	Mode of action	Comment
Retrograde conduction through AV node	1. Verapamil (or diltiazem)	Inhibits AV node	Usually effective, can be given IV
	2. Quinidine, disopyramide, procainamide, aprindine and related compounds	Inhibit bypass tract	Not as safe as verapamil for IV use
	3. Amiodarone	Inhibits bypass tract	Amiodarone has serious and complex side-effects
	4. Digoxin	Inhibits AV node; see below	Being replaced by verapamil
	5. Beta-blockers	Inhibit AV node	Being replaced by verapamil
Antegrade (= anterograde) through bypass tract	1. Quinidine, disopyramide, procainamide, aprindine	Inhibit bypass tract	Usually effective for conduction both ways
	2. Digoxin, verapamil, diltiazem, beta-blockade	No effect or may accelerate conduction	Potentially dangerous; avoid

Note: Surgical incision of bypass tract is increasingly used in refractory cases, especially if there is antegrade conduction. IV = intravenous; AV = atrioventricular; beta-blockade = beta-adrenergic receptor blockade.

Table 23-6

Agents used for ventricular arrhythmias

Conduction	Agent	Proposed mode of action	Comment
Ventricular tachycardia, acute therapy	1. Lidocaine	Fast channel inhibition; also narrowing of action potential duration	Standard agent for prophylaxis and treatment in acute myocardial infarction
	2. IV procainamide	Fast channel inhibition	Possibly agent of second choice; well-tested
	3. IV newer Class IC agents	As above	Still being evaluated
	4. Lidocaine-like agents, IV mexiletine, IV tocainide	As above	Lidocaine-like agents less cardiodepressant than quinidine-like agents; unlikely to work if lidocaine fails
	5. IV disopyramide	As above	Danger of myocardial depression; best avoided
	6. IV bretylium	Action potential widened	Cholinergic side-effects; complex agent; some catecholamine depletion; reduced release of NE
Ventricular tachycardia, chronic prophylaxis	1. All above agents (except lidocaine)	Fast channel inhibition	"Hit and miss" procedure unless programmed stimulation used
	2. Quinidine	Fast channel inhibition	Relatively safe orally; risk of QRS widening
	3. Amiodarone	Action potential widened; fast channel inhibition	Very effective; numerous side-effects
	4. Class IC agents	Fast channel inhibition	Under evaluation, may have pro-arrhythmic effects
Ventricular fibrillation, prophylaxis	1. IV lidocaine	Fast channel inhibition	For acute myocardial infarction
	2. Chronic beta-blockade	? inhibits excess adrenergic drive at start of myocardial infarction	Post-myocardial infarction follow-up

IV = intravenous; NE = norepinephrine = noradrenaline.
For doses, see Singh et al. (1984).

by shortening the action potential duration and preventing the formation of "humps" (see page 322). Intravenous magnesium is safer (Tzivoni et al., 1984); it seems to work even when the serum magnesium level is normal.

Whether or not **asymptomatic ventricular arrhythmias** such as chronic stable ectopic beats need therapy is not known, especially because most antiarrhythmic agents paradoxically can provoke arrhythmias (Velebit et al., 1982). An increasing tendency is to treat post-infarct patients more vigorously than others, but reduction of sudden death has only been shown for beta-adrenergic receptor blocking agents.

Programmed Electrical Stimulation

A major step forward in understanding tachycardias has been the introduction of programmed electrical stimulation. A coronary sinus catheter is inserted with multiple electrocardiographic recording sites to record the patterns of passage of an artificially introduced electrical stimulus (Fig. 5-10). The mechanism is clarified in about 95 percent of patients with a supraventricular tachycardia (dual atrioventricular nodal path or bypass tract). In patients with a bypass tract, electrical induction of atrial fibrillation can allow measurements of the maximal rate of antegrade conduction to the ventricles, and the possible adverse effect of digoxin or verapamil thereon. Thus those patients likely to respond well to drug therapy (Class IA or IC drugs) can be separated from those requiring surgical division of the tract at open-heart surgery. In patients with ventricular tachycardias, programmed stimulation can provoke the arrhythmia in the laboratory to help select the best antiarrhythmic drug for that patient. An apparent exception is in the case of amiodarone where the drug is more successful than anticipated from the results of acute programmed testing.

Summary

The four basic principles of antiarrhythmic therapy are: (i) inhibition of the fast sodium channel by quinidine or lidocaine or related compounds; (ii) beta-adrenergic receptor antagonism; (iii) inhibition of repolarization by amiodarone; and (iv) inhibition of the slow calcium channel in the atrioventricular node by verapamil or diltiazem. In each case the potential benefit to be achieved must be balanced against the possible side-effects, which are probably least with lidocaine. The chief advances have been quinidine, the first agent discovered; lidocaine, the agent most widely used in acute myocardial infarction but limited to intravenous use; beta-adrenergic receptor blockade, which is increasingly used as prophylaxis both in the early stages of acute infarction and especially post-infarct; amiodarone, perhaps the most potent agent against all types of arrhythmias but also with potentially serious side-effects; and verapamil, the prototype calcium antagonist agent.

References

Arita M, Kiyosue T, Aomine M, Imanishi S (1983). Nature of "residual fast channel" dependent action potentials and slow conduction in guinea pig ventricular muscle and its modification by isoproterenol. Am J Cardiol 51: 1433–1440.

Armstrong CM (1981). Sodium channels and gating currents. Physiol Rev 61: 644–683.

Bean BP, Cohen CJ, Tsien R (1983). Lidocaine block of cardiac sodium channels. J Gen Physiol 81: 613–642.

Bexton RS, Camm AJ (1982). Drugs with a class III anti-arrhythmic action. Pharmac Therap 17: 315–355.

Bonatti V, Rolli A, Botti G (1983). Recording of monophasic action potentials of the right ventricle in long QT syndromes complicated by severe ventricular arrhythmias. Europ Heart J 4: 168–179.

Burton JR, Mathew T, Armstrong PW (1976). Comparative effects of lidocaine and procainamide on acutely impaired hemodynamics. Am J Med 61: 215–220.

Cardinal R, Janse MJ, Eeden van I, Werner G, D'Alnoncourt CN, Durrer D (1981). The effects of lidocaine on intra-cellular and extracellular potentials, activations and ventricular arrhythmias during acute regional ischemia in the isolated porcine heart. Circ Res 49: 792–806.

Carmeleit E, Saikawa T (1982). Shortening of the action potential and reduction of pacemaker activity by lidocaine, quinidine and procainamide in sheep cardiac Purkinje fibers. Circ Res 50: 257–272.

Clarkson CW, Ten Eich RE (1983). On the mechanism of lysophosphatidylcholine-induced depolarization of cat ventricular myocardium. Circ Res 52: 543–556.

Clusin WT, Fischmeister R, DeHaan RL (1983). Caffeine-induced current in embryonic heart cells: time course and voltage dependence. Am J Physiol 245: H528–H532.

Clusin WT, Buchbinder M, Ellis AK, Kernoff RS, Giacomini JC, Harrison DC (1984a). Reduction of ischemic de-polarization by the calcium channel blocker diltiazem. Circ Res 54: 10–20.

Clusin WT, Buchbinder M, Bristow MR, Harrison DC (1984b). Evidence for a role of calcium in the genesis of early ischemic cardiac arrhythmias. In: Calcium-Antagonists and Cardiovascular Disease. Ed. LH Opie, pp 293–302, Raven Press, New York.

Colatsky TJ (1982). Mechanisms of action of lidocaine and quinidine on action potential duration in rabbit cardiac Purkinje fibers. An effect on steady state sodium currents? Circ Res 50: 17–27.

Corr PB, Gross RW, Sobel BE (1982). Arrhythmogenic amphiphilic lipids and the myocardial cell membrane. J Molec Cell Cardiol 14: 619–626.

Courtney KR (1980). Interval-dependent effects of small antiarrhythmic drugs on excitability of guinea-pig myocardium. J Molec Cell Cardiol 12: 1273–1286.

Courtney KR (1983). Inactive versus open channel blocking of cardiac sodium channels. Biophys J 41: 76.

Crampton R (1979). Preeminence of the left stellate ganglion in the long Q-T syndrome. Circulation 59: 769–778.

De Mello WC (1982). Intercellular communication in cardiac muscle. Circ Res 51: 1–9.

DeSilva RA, Lown B, Hennekens CH, Casscells S (1981). Lignocaine prophylaxis in acute myocardial infarction: an evaluation of randomized trials. Lancet ii: 855–858.

Disertori M, Inama G, Vergara G, Guarnerio M, Del Favero A, Furlanello F (1983). Evidence of a reentry circuit in the common type of atrial flutter in man. Circulation 67: 434–440.

Dyckner T, Helmers C, Lundman T (1975). Initial serum potassium level in relation to early complications and prognosis in patients with acute myocardial infarction. Acta Med Scand 197: 207–210.

Eisner DA, Lederer WJ, Sher S (1983). The role of intracellular sodium activity in the antiarrhythmic action of local anaesthetics in sheep Purkinje fibres. J Physiol Lond 340: 239–257.

El-Sherif N, Gough WB, Zeiler RH, Mehra R (1983). Triggered ventricular rhythms in 1-day-old myocardial infarction in the dog. Circ Res 52: 566–579.

Feely J, Wilkinson GR, McAllister CB, Wood AJJ (1982). Increased toxicity and reduced clearance of lidocaine by cimetidine. Ann Int Med 96: 592–594.

Flecainide–Quinidine Research Group (1983). Flecainide versus quinidine for treatment of chronic ventricular arrhythmias. A multicenter clinical trial. Circulation 67: 1117–1123.

Friedman I, Moravec J, Reichart E, Hatt PY (1973). Subacute myocardial hypoxia in the rat. An electron microscopic study of the left ventricular myocardium. J Molec Cell Cardiol 5: 125–132.

Gerstenblith G, Scherlag BJ, Hope RR, Lazzara R (1978). Effect of lidocaine on conduction in the ischemic His–Purkinje system. Am J Cardiol 42: 587–591.

Harris AS, Bisteni A, Russell RA, Brigham JC, Firestone JE (1954). Excitatory factors in ventricular tachycardia resulting from myocardial ischemia: potassium a major excitant. Science 119: 200–203.

Harrison DC (1978). Should lidocaine be administered routinely to all patients after acute myocardial infarction? Circulation 58: 581–584.

Hauswrith O, Singh BN (1979). Ionic mechanisms in heart muscle in relation to the genesis and the pharmacological control of cardiac arrhythmias. Pharm Rev 30: 5–63.

Heissenbuttel RH, Bigger JT Jr (1979). New drugs: bretylium tosylate: a newly available antiarrhythmic drug for ventricular arrhythmias. Ann Int Med 91: 229–238.

Hille B (1977). Local anesthetics: hydrophilic and hydrophobic pathways for the drug–receptor reaction. J Gen Physiol 69: 497–515.

Hirche HJ, Franz C, Bos L, Bissig R, Lang R, Schramm M (1980). Myocardial extracellular K^+ and H^+ increase and noradrenaline release as possible causes of early arrhythmias following acute coronary artery occlusion in pigs. J Molec Cell Cardiol 12: 579–593.

Holder DA, Sniderman AD, Fraser G, Fallen EL (1977). Experience with bretylium tosylate by a hospital cardiac arrest team. Circulation 55: 541–544.

Hondeghem LM, Katzung BG (1977). Time and voltage dependent interactions of antiarrhythmic drugs with cardiac sodium channels. Biochim Biophys Acta 472: 373–398.

Killip T, Gault JH (1965). Mode of onset of atrial fibrillation. Am Heart J 70: 172–179.

Kluger J, Leech S, Reidenberg MM, Lloyd V, Drayer DE (1981). Long-term antiarrhythmic therapy with acetyl-procainamide. Am J Cardiol 48: 1124–1132.

Koster RW, Dunning AJ (1983). Pre-hospital prevention of ventricular fibrillation in acute myocardial infarction. Circulation 68: Suppl III, 275.

Kuo CS, Munakata K, Reddy CP, Surawicz B (1983).

Characteristics and possible mechanism of ventricular arrhythmia dependent on dispersion of action potential durations. Circulation 67: 1356–1367.

Lee KS, Hume JR, Giles W, Brown AM (1981). Sodium current depression by lidocaine and quinidine in isolated ventricular cells. Nature 291: 325–327.

Levites R, Banka VS, Helfant RH (1975). Electrophysiological effects of coronary occlusion and reperfusion. Observations of dispersion of refractoriness and ventricular automaticity. Circulation 52: 760–765.

Lewis T, Feil HS, Stroud WD (1920). Observations upon flutter and fibrillation. II. Nature of auricular flutter. Heart 7: 191–245.

Lubbe WF, McFadyen ML, Muller CA, Worthington M, Opie LH (1979). Protective action of amiodarone against ventricular fibrillation in the isolated perfused rat heart. Am J Cardiol 43: 533–540.

McHale PA, Rembert JC, Greenfield JC (1983). Effect of atrial fibrillation on atrial blood flow in conscious dogs. Am J Cardiol 51: 1722–1727.

Man RYK, Dresel IPE (1979). A specific effect of lidocaine and tocainide on ventricular conduction of midrange extrasystoles. J Cardiovasc Pharm 1: 329–342.

Mason JW, Hondeghem LM, Katzung BG (1981). Amiodarone blocks inactivated cardiac action potentials. Pflügers Arch 396: 79–81.

Melmed S, Nademanee K, Reed AW, Hendrickson JA, Singh B, Hershman JL (1981). Hyperthyroxinemia with bradycardia and normal thyrotropin secretion after chronic amiodarone administration. J Clin Endocrinol Metab 53: 997–1001.

Meltzer RS, Robert EW, McMorrow M, Martin RP (1978). Atypical ventricular tachycardia as a manifestation of disopyramide toxicity. Am J Cardiol 42: 1049–1056.

Mirro MJ (1981). Effects of quinidine, procainamide and disopyramide on automaticity and cyclic AMP content of guinea pig atria. J Molec Cell Cardiol 13: 641–653.

Mirro MJ, Watanabe AM, Bailey JC (1981). Electrophysiological effects of the optimal isomers of disopyramide and aprindine in the dog. Circ Res 48: 867–874.

Moss AJ, Schwartz PJ (1982). Delayed repolarization (QT or QTU prolongation) and malignant ventricular arrhythmias. Mod Concepts Cardiovasc Dis 51: 85–90.

Opie LH, Nathan D, Lubbe WF (1979). Biochemical aspects of arrhythmogenesis and ventricular fibrillation. Am J Cardiol 43: 131–148.

Podrid PJ, Schoeneberger A, Lown B (1980). Congestive heart failure caused by oral disopyramide. N Engl J Med 302: 614–617.

Prinzmetal M, Corday E, Brill IC, Sellers AL, Oblath RW, Flieg WA, Kruger HE (1950). Mechanism of auricular arrhythmias. Circulation 1: 241–245.

Rizos I, Senges J, Jauernig R, Lengfelder W, Czygan E, Brachman J, Kübler W (1984). Differential effects of sotalol and metoprolol on induction of paroxysmal supraventricular tachycardia. Am J Cardiol 53: 1022–1027.

Russell DC (1982). Early ventricular arrhythmias: relationship of electrophysiology to blood flow and metabolism. In: Early Arrhythmias Resulting from Myocardial Ischaemia. Ed. JR Parratt, pp 37–56, Macmillan, London.

Sanchez-Chapula J, Josephson I (1983). Effect of phenytoin on the sodium current in isolated rat ventricular cells. J Molec Cell Cardiol 15: 515–522.

Sanchez-Chapula J, Tsuda Y, Josephson IR (1983). Voltage and use-dependent effects of lidocaine on sodium current in rat single ventricular cells. Circ Res 52: 557–565.

Scheuer T, Kass RS (1983). Phenytoin reduces calcium current in cardiac Purkinje fiber. Circ Res 53: 16–23.

Schneider JA, Sperelakis N (1975). Slow Ca^{2+} and Na^+ responses induced by isoproterenol and methylxanthines in isolated perfused guinea pig hearts exposed to elevated K^+. J Molec Cell Cardiol 7: 249–273.

Singh BN, Vaughan Williams EM (1971). Effects of altering potassium concentration on the action of lidocaine and diphenylhydantoin on rabbit atrial and ventricular muscle. Circ Res 29: 286–295.

Singh BN, Ellrodt G, Peter CT (1978). Verapamil: a review of its pharmacological properties and therapeutic use. Drugs 15: 169–197.

Singh BN, Opie LH, Marcus IF (1984). Antiarrhythmic drugs. In: Drugs for the Heart, Ed. LH Opie, pp 65–98, Grune & Stratton, Orlando, New York and London.

Sobel SM, Rakita L (1982). Pneumonitis and pulmonary fibrosis associated with amiodarone therapy: a possible complication of a new antiarrhythmic drug. Circulation 65: 819–824.

Taniguchi J, Noma A, Irisawa H (1983). Modification of cardiac action potential by intracellular injection of adenosine triphosphate and related substances in guinea pig single ventricular cells. Circ Res 53: 131–139.

Thandroyen FT (1982). Protective action of calcium channel antagonist agents against ventricular fibrillation in the isolated perfused rat heart. J Molec Cell Cardiol 14: 21–32.

Tzivoni D, Keren A, Cohen AM, Loebel H, Zahavi I, Chenzbraun A, Stern S (1984). Magnesium therapy for torsades de pointes. Am J Cardiol 53: 528–530.

Velebit V, Podrid P, Lown B, Cohen BH, Graboys TB (1982). Aggravation and provocation of ventricular arrhythmias by antiarrhythmic drugs. Circulation 65: 886–894.

Vogel S, Sperelakis N (1981). Induction of slow action potentials by microiontophoresis of cyclic AMP into heart cells. J Molec Cell Cardiol 13: 51–64.

Ward DE, Camm AJ, Spurrell RAJ (1980). Clinical anti-arrhythmic effects of amiodarone in patients with resistant paroxysmal tachycardias. Brit Heart J 44: 91–95.

Weiss AT, Lewis BS, Halon DA, Hasin Y, Gotsman MS (1983). Use of calcium with verapamil in the management of supraventricular arrhythmias. Int J Cardiol 4: 275–280.

Weld FM, Coromilas J, Rottman JN, Bigger JT Jr (1982). Mechanisms of quinidine-induced depression of maximum upstroke velocity in bovine cardiac Purkinje fibers. Circ Res 50: 369–376.

White CW, Kerber RE, Weiss HR, Marcus ML (1982). The effects of atrial fibrillation on atrial pressure-volume and flow relationships. Circ Res 51: 205–215.

New References

Clarkson CW, Hondeghem LM (1985). Evidence for a specific receptor site for lidocaine, quinidine, and bupivacaine associated with cardiac sodium channels in guinea-pig ventricular myocardium. Circ Res 56: 496–506.

Ferrier GR, Moffat MP, Lukas A (1985). Possible mechanisms of ventricular arrhythmias elicited by ischemia followed by reperfusion. Studies on isolated canine ventricular tissues. Cir Res 56: 184–194.

Fozzard HA, January CT, Makielski JC (1985). New studies of the excitatory sodium currents in heart muscle. Circ Res 56: 475–485.

Hondeghem LM, Katzung BG (1984). Mechanism of action of antiarrhythmic drugs. In: Physiology and Pathophysiology of the Heart. Ed. N Sperelakis, pp 459–476, Nijhoff, Boston.

Riemersma RA, Dart AM (1985). Adrenergic mechanisms in ischemic and reperfusion arrhythmias. J Cardiovasc Pharmacol 7 (Suppl 5): S2–S85.

Roden DM, Hoffman BF (1985). Action potential prolongation and induction of abnormal automaticity by low quinidine concentrations in canine Purkinje fibers. Relationship to potassium and cycle length. Circ Res 56: 857–867.

Schwartz PJ, Vanoli E, Zaza A, Zuanetti G (1985). The effect of antiarrhythmic drugs on life-threatening arrhythmias induced by the interaction between acute myocardial ischemia and sympathetic hyperactivity. Am Heart J 109: 937–948.

Torres V, Flowers D, Somberg JC (1985). The arrhythmogenicity of antiarrhythmic agents. Am Heart J 109: 1090–1097.

Angina Pectoris

"Ischemia" means too little blood; myocardial ischemia exists when there is a reduction of coronary flow sufficiently severe that the supply of oxygen to the myocardium is inadequate for the oxygen demands of the tissue. Myocardial ischemia is initially reversible. Prolonged ischemia causes irreversible changes with the development of cell death and necrosis or myocardial infarction. The clinical correlates of these experimental situations are reversible angina pectoris and irreversible acute myocardial infarction. In the vast majority of patients with these conditions there is advanced coronary arterial disease, either diffuse or localized. Angina pectoris ("pain of the chest", Latin) is a clinical condition in which an acute attack of a characteristic constricting chest pain is provoked by exercise and relieved by rest (**angina of effort**) or occurs spontaneously at rest (**angina at rest**). Sometimes angina may become progressively more severe (**unstable angina**) and develop into myocardial infarction (**pre-infarction angina**).

Oxygen Balance in the Ischemic Zone

A useful hypothesis is that angina pectoris can be caused whenever the myocardial oxygen demand exceeds the supply to cause myocardial ischemia (Fig. 24-1). Factors likely to precipitate angina of effort are all those that increase the oxygen demand, in the face of a supply limited by coronary artery disease. During exercise it is the increase of heart rate and blood pressure which consistently precipitate effort angina at a constant double product, while an increase of

heart rate (together with some rise of blood pressure) is probably the major factor in emotion-provoked angina. A role of catecholamine-induced "oxygen-wastage" has not been defined, nor has it been

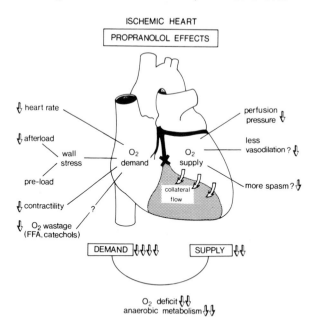

Fig. 24-1 Effects of beta-blockers such as propranolol on the ischemic heart. Beta-blockers have a beneficial effect on the ischemic myocardium, unless the preload rises substantially as in left heart failure, by predominantly reducing the oxygen demand. Modified from Opie LH (1980). Drugs and the Heart. I. Beta-blocking agents. Lancet i: 693–698 (with permission from the Lancet).

Table 24-1

Principles of therapy of angina pectoris

1. **Reduction of oxygen demand**
   — reduce heart rate by beta-blockade
   — reduce afterload by beta-blockade, calcium
     antagonists and control of hypertension
   — reduce metabolic demand by calcium antagonists,
     beta-blockade
   — reduce preload by nitrates

2. **Increase oxygen supply**
   — coronary vasodilators (calcium antagonists,
     nitrates)
   — promote growth of collaterals (? exercise)
   — change anatomy of coronary disease (coronary
     bypass grafting, angioplasty, laser techniques)

searched for, apart from a specific experimental situation where low-dose catecholamine infusion given to patients with coronary artery disease was able to evoke an increased oxygen uptake independently of hemodynamic changes (Simonsen and Kjekshus, 1978).

The metabolic effects of experimental ischemia are well-understood. The occurrence of lactate production during anginal attacks produced by pacing (see Fig. 11-14) or during attacks of Prinzmetal's angina shows that angina is accompanied by **anaerobic glycolysis** (see Fig. 10-11). There is no reason to believe that the basic metabolic patterns found in human myocardial ischemia differ in any way from those in animal preparations. The release of inorganic phosphate and potassium proves that there is breakdown of high-energy phosphates and loss of potassium from ischemic cells in humans as in animals.

Ischemic Pump Failure

Because clinical emphasis usually falls on the chest pain or electrocardiographic features of angina pectoris, it is less well appreciated that angina is a reversible form of acute heart failure precipitated by ischemia.

Ischemic contractile failure

Many theories have been advanced for the contractile failure that occurs rapidly in ischemia. The two basic

mechanisms advanced relate to either (i) the effects of poor oxygen delivery or (ii) the accumulation of intermediates. The first mechanism results in depletion of high-energy phosphate compounds, including ATP and creatine phosphate. Many experiments have shown that contractile failure occurs before there is a major depletion of ATP probably because of the buffer function of creatine phosphate. Such data cast doubt on the solitary role of a lack of ATP in contractile failure. Nonetheless, very careful repetitive measurements in very early ischemia show that there is some fall of ATP within the first 10 sec of severe ischemia, and preceding the start of contractile failure at about 10 sec (Hearse, 1979). The amount of fall of ATP is not enough to account for contractile failure, but a reconciliatory hypothesis is that ATP falls in a ''contractile'' compartment to cause early pump failure. If this were so there should be an early impairment of diastolic relaxation (Bricknell et al., 1981), as confirmed by echocardiography.

The hypothesis of most historical interest is that the accumulation of products of ischemia cause pump failure. Tennant (1935) thought that early contractile failure could be related to a build-up of lactate ions. Katz and Hecht (1969) expanded this hypothesis in an influential editorial which proposed that an intracellular acidosis decreased contractility because protons displaced calcium from binding sites on the thin filaments. A very similar proposal stresses the role of retention of carbon dioxide, also acting by the production of an intracellular acidosis (Cobbe and Poole-Wilson, 1980).

A new idea was the further proposal of Kübler and Katz (1977) that the build-up of inorganic phosphate (released from ATP and creatine phosphate) deprived the cytosol of calcium by forming calcium phosphate. Whatever the mechanism (and it seems that an intracellular acidosis is as good a proposal as any), the important point is that marked contractile failure and metabolic changes can occur within 10–120 sec of the onset of severe ischemia. When contractile failure is very severe the ischemic myocardium not only fails to contract but actually bulges in systole. The disastrous consequences of contractile failure for the patient with angina pectoris can now be understood.

Reversible heart failure

A prominent feature of an anginal attack is the development of acute shortness of breath, usually at the same time as the chest pain. Hemodynamic measurements show that characteristic features of acute left ventricular failure are present, such as an increased left ventricular end-diastolic pressure and decreased indices of contractility. There is venous vascular engorgement, explaining the dyspnea. The increased pressure within the left ventricle together with the decreased coronary perfusion pressure, cause compression of the subendocardial tissue with severe ischemia (Fig. 17-6). Unless the pressure is taken off by relief of the anginal attack there is danger of the "advancing wave front" phenomenon and the development of myocardial infarction (Fig. 12-8). Such acute relief of the anginal attack can be achieved either by decreasing the oxygen demand (the patient rests) or by increasing the blood supply (calcium antagonists) or by nitrates, which achieve both aims. Beta-adrenergic blockers, while preventing attacks of angina of effort, do not act quickly enough to be used for relief of acute attacks.

Exercise Testing

Exercise testing has become a standard procedure in the assessment of patients with ischemic heart disease and in the diagnosis of doubtful angina. The basis of this acute test is the increased myocardial oxygen consumption caused by exercise and attributed to the increased myocardial oxygen uptake. Thus during acute exercise the product of the heart rate and the blood pressure (**"double product"**) correlates well with the coronary blood flow and the myocardial oxygen consumption. Conversely, the beneficial effects of beta-adrenergic blockade in patients with angina pectoris can largely be explained by a decreased double-product.

The limiting factor for maximal exercise in normal subjects is not settled. Whereas abrupt sprinting without warm-up may cause transient myocardial ischemia (page 193), maximal response to graded exercise is not limited by myocardial ischemia but by factors such as skeletal muscle fatigue and/or dyspnea.

In subjects with coronary artery disease it is the development of myocardial ischemia that is usually rate-limiting. During exercise, myocardial ischemia can be detected in several ways: subjectively, by the development of an anginal-like pain, and objectively, by the consequences of ischemia such as electro-cardiographic ST-segment displacement (next section), arrhythmias, a fall of cardiac output with a drop in blood pressure and fatigue, abnormal patterns in radioscintigrams, or by detection of anaerobic metabolism in coronary sinus blood. The electro-cardiographic features of ischemia are basically deflections of the TQ-ST segment, and the reflection of potassium loss from the newly ischemic cells during exercise (Fig. 24-2). Since exercise-induced ischemia is usually subendocardial and diffuse, ST-depression is a classic sign of coronary artery disease.

The Electrocardiogram in Exercise Stress Testing

Because angina pectoris is a subjective symptom of variable occurrence, the effect of any given therapy is difficult to assess. Hence **effort testing**, using the changes in the electrocardiogram as one end-point, has become a standard procedure in the assessment, diagnosis and therapy of angina pectoris. The typical electrocardiographic changes in angina of effort are a characteristic depression of the ST-segment at the time of onset of chest pain. The origin of this current of injury is best understood by taking as example a localized zone of transmural ischemia, which produces ST-elevation rather than the depression characteristic of angina of effort.

Current of injury

During ischemia a current of injury develops as the negative transmembrane potential found in diastole decreases and becomes more positive than the surrounding normal tissue (Fig. 24-2). Therefore, in diastole the current flows from ischemic to normal tissue. **If an electrode were to be placed directly on the ischemic zone (epicardial electrode), then the current** flowing away from the ischemic zone would produce diastolic (ST) depression. The net effect is that of elevating the ST-segment relative to the rest of the complex (**ST-elevation**). Ischemia also decreases the amplitude of the action potential and shortens the action potential duration (possibly by causing a deficiency of ATP, page 322), so that the ischemic zone is less negative in systole than is the normal myocardium. Hence, in systole, current flows from the normal myocardium to the ischemic zone and some true ST-elevation is produced to add to the apparent elevation (produced by the diastolic, K^+-induced current). Exact measurement of the isoelectric line (Fig. 24-2) in patients can be made by a direct-current magnetocardiogram, which shows that about 70 percent of the ST-change is explained by diastolic currents and a lesser component by systolic currents (Cohen et al., 1983).

Potassium ion loss from ischemic cells is the most probable cause of the TQ–ST deflections. Topical application to the epicardium or intracoronary infusion of hyperkalemic solutions provoke changes very similar to those of acute ischemia. The loss of only 1 percent of cellular potassium, raising the extracellular potassium from 4.0 to 9.6 mM, can markedly decrease the resting membrane potential and the action potential duration (Holland and Brooks, 1977). Assuming that potassium movements are the major (although probably not the only) factor explaining the early ST-deviation, the very rapid loss of potassium within seconds of the onset of ischemia needs explanation. Such a rate of loss of potassium could be explained by complete inhibition of all active inward transport of potassium, with continued outward flux, as a result of ischemic inhibition of the sodium pump. It seems unlikely that ischemia inhibits the pump so rapidly, so Kleber (1984) has proposed that potassium ions may be lost in a non-specific way, in response to the formation of weak acids formed during anaerobic metabolism.

ST-depression

The above events explain the origin of the apparent ST-segment elevation in transmural ischemia or in epicardial ischemia, as found in early transmural myocardial infarction or Prinzmetal's variant angina. When only the subendocardial zone is rendered ischemic, then the direction of current flow is away from the electrode so that there is apparent ST-depression, as in subendocardial ischemia during effort angina or in the early stages of subendocardial myocardial infarction (see Fig. 25-8).

ST-deviations basically reflect extracellular potassium ion accumulation, which in turn reflects ischemic injury. As yet no studies have tightly correlated the degree of ST-deviations to the magnitude of extracellular potassium accumulation and to the severity of myocardial ischemia. Furthermore, there are complex geometric factors which influence how a flow of current is recorded by an electrode (the solid angle theorem of Holland and Brooks). So at best, measurements of early ST-segment elevation in the early stages of developing infarction, while the myocardium is still ischemic, will give only an approximation of the severity of ischemia. In contrast, ischemic ST-segment depression during

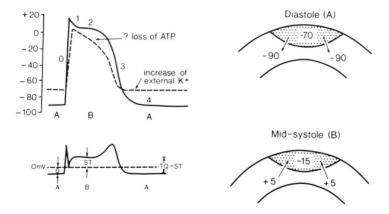

Fig. 24-2 Mechanism of generation of ST-segment shifts as found in ECG of patients with an anginal attack or during early developing infarction. **Top left:** Effect of ischemia (broken curve) in comparison with normal action potential showing phases 0–4. The two major changes are diastolic depolarization (due to ischemic loss of potassium and a rise of external K+) and shortening of the action potential duration (possibly due to ATP loss). **Bottom left:** Electrocardiogram recorded by an electrode directly in contact with the ischemic tissue. The T-Q segment is located below the isoelectric line (broken) and the S-T segment above. Together these changes constitute "ST-elevation" on the surface ECG. On the right, the arrows indicate the current flow (positive to negative) at the boundary. In angina of effort, the ischemic zone is predominantly subendocardial so that the surface electrodes show ST-depression on exercise (similar to panel B, Fig. 25-8). In transmural ischemia or infarction, there is apparent ST-segment elevation (panel A, Fig. 25-8). Modified from Holland and Brooks (1977). Am J Cardiol 40: 110, with permission.

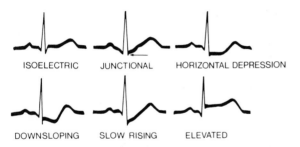

ISOELECTRIC   JUNCTIONAL   HORIZONTAL DEPRESSION

DOWNSLOPING   SLOW RISING   ELEVATED

Fig. 24-3 Various end-points of the electrocardiogram in effort-testing. A positive test is shown by ST-segment depression, which must be a horizontal or down-sloping depression of at least 1 mm (preferably 2 mm) below the isoelectric J-point and persisting for 80 msec thereafter. Depression of the J-point alone with a rapid rise in the ST-segment (J-point depression) may occur normally with exercise. The slow rising pattern correlates with ischemic heart disease but there is a high incidence of false positives. ST-segment elevation probably represents a severe degree of myocardial ischemia or a left ventricular aneurysm. From Heger JW, Niemann JT, Boman KG, Criley JM (1982). Cardiology for the House Officer, p 44, Williams and Wilkins, Baltimore, with permission.

effort testing is a reliable end-point (Fig. 24-3). Generally a depression of 1–2 mm of the ST-segment is required for a positive effort test. With 2 mm depression there are fewer false positives. Only about two-thirds of patients with coronary artery disease have a positive effort test, and sometimes features other than ST-depression are the end-point (chest pain, blood pressure fall, arrhythmias, fatigue). Hence other procedures for stress testing (radionuclide) are frequently undertaken.

In the rare phenomenon of **exercise-induced ST-elevation** (Fig. 24-3), severe transmural ischemia is the result of either exercise-induced coronary artery spasm, or of the effects of exercise superimposed on a critical coronary artery stenosis. In general, the prognosis is much worse when ST-elevation rather than depression is induced by exercise.

T wave and ischemia

Particularly confusing is the difference between metabolic ischemia, characterized by ST-segment deviation (as argued) and the "ischemia" of the electrocardiologist, which also includes an inverted T wave (see Fig. 25-7). It is true that an acute, inverted T wave may be a manifestation of true metabolic ischemia, as may lesser T-wave changes, which reflect variations in the rate of repolarization throughout the myocardium and variations in the action potential duration (shortened by ischemia). However, a permanently inverted T wave usually does not indicate true metabolic ischemia; rather, ischemia has probably progressed to fibrosis so that the epicardium is repolarized differently from the endocardium.

Cardiac pain vs ST-deviation

Taking ST-deviation on the electrocardiogram as an indirect index of transfer of potassium ions from within to without the cells (Fig. 24-2), leads to the conclusion that there are numerous episodes of silent ischemia in patients with angina pectoris. Such episodes may occur independently of effort, and presumably reflect the effect of spontaneous variations in the caliber of the coronary arteries in the presence of borderline myocardial ischemia and in the absence of factors which increase oxygen demand, such as exercise or emotion.

That such "attacks" of ST-deviation are genuinely related to silent myocardial ischemia is also suggested by the finding that therapy of angina with either beta-blockade or calcium-antagonists reduces the incidence both of episodes of ST-deviation and of chest pain (Lynch et al., 1980). Presumably the "ST-attacks" are not of sufficient duration to cause subjectively perceived ischemia as pain. The mechanism of cardiac ischemic pain remains ill-understood. Lewis's "P" factor is still not identified, but could include release of vasoactive substances such as bradykinin, histamine or serotonin from ischemic heart cells.

Radionuclide Stress Testing

Initially **potassium-43** (^{43}K) was the radionuclide used to assess myocardial perfusion by external imaging with a gamma camera. An area of decreased radioactivity ("cold spot") results from either exercise-induced ischemia or from established myocardial infarction because the coronary flow to such areas is reduced, particularly during exercise, when flow to the non-ischemic myocardium increases. In the case of infarction the myocardial uptake of potassium is further reduced because the tissue is dead. While there is a high degree of accuracy in the detection of anterior or lateral ischemia or infarction, imaging of inferior lesions is much more difficult. A technical limitation of ^{43}K is the long half-life (22 hours) and the added beta-emission which gives an increased radiation dose to the patient. Therefore, the more recent analogs of potassium such as rubidium and especially thallium have been introduced and used extensively.

Thallium-201 (^{201}Tl) is cleared from blood nearly as rapidly as ^{43}K, so it is equally useful for exercise stress testing and equally unsuited for repetitive measurements of myocardial perfusion. In addition, ^{201}Tl concentrates in the myocardium more than either potassium or rubidium. The uptake of thallium by the myocardium is dependent on the same sodium–potassium pump (Na^+/K^+-ATPase) that transports potassium, but thallium binds ten times more avidly at two sites instead of one site for potassium. This difference may explain the delayed clearance compared with ^{43}K.

The myocardial distribution of ^{201}Tl is the result of two processes. The initial distribution reflects the distribution of the coronary blood flow to the various zones of the myocardium. The second phase of redistribution reflects actual uptake by the myocardial cells. In underperfused but potentially viable zones both the uptake and washout of ^{201}Tl is slow, so that in time the levels of radioactivity in the normal and ischemic zones tend to equalize. In infarcted, scarred myocardium the tissue cannot take up ^{201}Tl; hence no equalization can occur. These differences can be useful in distinguishing the potential viability of poorly contracting myocardial segments (Rozanski et al., 1981). Very recently a new use for ^{201}Tl has been in detecting improved myocardial perfusion following intracoronary thrombolysis.

The non-metabolizable tracer **xenon-133** (^{133}Xe) can be injected into a coronary artery and the rate of washout found in a localized zone of the heart used to derive the regional myocardial blood flow. A precordial crystal scintillation camera records the rate of washout of xenon and the myocardial blood flow is calculated from a number of mathematical assumptions. In patients with angina pectoris, zones of decreased blood flow can sometimes be found at rest, but more frequently after the oxygen demand has been increased by atrial pacing. Nitrates increase regional myocardial blood flow in ischemic zones by improving the diameter of the stenotic artery. Calcium antagonists such as nifedipine have similar and additive effects (Lichtlen et al., 1984).

Regional Wall Motion Abnormalities

Because the ischemic myocardium suffers from contractile failure, systolic wall thickening is decreased. In the past, quantitative ventricular angiography was required to assess regional wall motion. Such regional abnormalities can now be detected non-invasively by echocardiography, which detects wall thinning and localizes the impairment of contractile activity. Hypokinetic or dyskinetic areas (see Fig. 25-7) can also be shown by gated radionuclide angiography. In true effort angina such defects are evident only during the increased heart rate of atrial pacing or exercise, whereas in chronic ischemic heart disease abnormal wall motion may be found at rest.

Therapeutic Modification of Oxygen Balance in Effort Angina

Metabolic manipulation in angina

Some workers have administered glucose–insulin–potassium to achieve a large extraction of glucose in the hope of a possible metabolic benefit in angina pectoris. The results of these studies can at best be described as conflicting. The explanation probably lies in the short duration of angina pectoris, usually only a matter of minutes; during this period anaerobic glycolysis derives from glycogen and not circulating glucose. Pharmacological measures such as nitrates, beta-adrenergic blockade and calcium antagonists are much more powerful and effective than substrate-manipulation in the therapy of angina pectoris.

Table 24-2

Proposed step-care for angina of effort

1. Nitrates, short- or long-acting, given intermittently as needed to control pain
2. Intermittent nitrates plus beta-adrenergic blocker
   or
3. Intermittent nitrates plus calcium antagonist
4. Beta-blocker + calcium antagonist + intermittent nitrates
5. Sometimes beta-blocker + calcium antagonist + constant (prophylactic) long-acting nitrates
6. Failure to respond to medical therapy or left main stem lesion requires bypass surgery

An alternative to steps 2–5: Replace intermittent nitrates by prophylactic long-acting nitrates in above plan (danger of nitrate tolerance).

Nitrates

Nitrates were the first agents to be used in the therapy of effort angina. Their mode of action in effort angina is still controversial, but probably the major effect in effort angina is as a venodilator which reduces the preload so abruptly built up by the anginal attack (Fig. 17-6). At a cellular level the mode of action is poorly understood (page 236). A puzzling problem is why other coronary vasodilators such as dipyridamole are not active against angina. It might be supposed that adenosine, being a powerful physiological vasodilator, could be stimulated to form in increased amounts by inhibiting adenosine deaminase by dipyridamole. Adenosine dilates the small and medium-sized coronary arteries; nitrates dilate large coronary arteries, thereby presumably increasing the driving force and the perfusion pressure. It is also the preload reduction which distinguishes nitrate therapy (effective) from inhibition of adenosine deaminase (ineffective).

Sublingual nitroglycerin remains the basic initial therapy in anginal attacks. When angina starts the patient should rest in the sitting position (standing promotes syncope, lying enhances venous return and heart work) and take sublingual nitroglycerin (0.3–0.6 mg) every 3 min until the pain goes or a maximum 4–5 tablets have been taken. Nitrates are more effective if taken before the expected onset of the pain. In some patients nitrates are less effective than anticipated due to tachycardia; then combined treatment with beta-blockade should give better results.

Beta-adrenergic receptor blockade

The effect of beta-agonists on the beta-receptor can be antagonized by the beta-adrenergic receptor blockers which benefit angina by decreasing the demand side of the equation (heart rate falls, blood pressure down, contractility decreased). It is true that coronary flow also falls because the perfusion pressure falls. Yet the demand falls more than the supply, so that the ultimate metabolic effect is decreased ischemic damage (Fig. 24-1). Conventional therapy is by propranolol, 80 mg twice daily, with increases in dose sometimes obtaining a better result. In the correct doses all beta blockers seem equally effective. Tachycardia and reduction of exercise-induced tachycardia are important determinants of the response to treatment and the dose of propranolol is usually adjusted to secure a resting heart rate of 55–60 beats/min,

and more importantly, an exercise heart rate of less than 100–110 beats/min. In patients with angina pectoris who have abnormal left ventricular function at rest, beta-blockade decreases the incidence of angina but may lessen exercise tolerance. The addition of anti-failure therapy (digitalis and diuretics) can then prevent this deterioration in exercise tolerance and reverse the cardiac enlargement induced by beta-blockers. Side-effects and contra-indications require careful clinical attention (page 227).

Calcium antagonists

The major calcium antagonists have been used successfully in angina of effort (page 254; Fig. 18-6). The different agents have different mechanisms of benefit: diltiazem somewhat slows the heart rate and mildly reduces the afterload; verapamil has a negative inotropic effect with added afterload reduction; while nifedipine acts chiefly by afterload reduction. Theoretically, where one agent fails another might be more useful. Which of the three agents the clinician might use will depend on his familiarity with the agent and the presence of associated clinical features. For example, co-existing sick sinus disease, atrioventricular conduction impairment, moderate or more ventricular dysfunction, or co-existing hypertension, might make nifedipine preferable to diltiazem or verapamil. On the other hand, when supraventricular tachycardia is part of the clinical picture, either verapamil or diltiazem is preferred. Each agent has its own advantages. Potential side-effects are also important (Chapter 18); diltiazem is probably least likely to bother the patient.*

Combination therapy

Beta-blockade is often combined with **nitrates** in the therapy of angina. Both beta-blockers and nitrates decrease oxygen demand and nitrates may also increase oxygen supply. Beta-blockade cancels the tachycardiac effect of nitrates but does not reduce the hypotensive effect. Beta-blockade tends to increase heart size, nitrates to decrease it. Anginal patients on beta-blockers are better able to withstand pacing-stress when nitroglycerin is added (Shang and Pepine, 1978). Patients already receiving beta-blockade respond no less well than do others to the addition of nitroglycerin (Fox et al., 1977). Whether the combination of iso-sorbide dinitrate and beta-blockade is more effective

*Parts of this paragraph are extracted from Singh and Opie (1984), with permission.

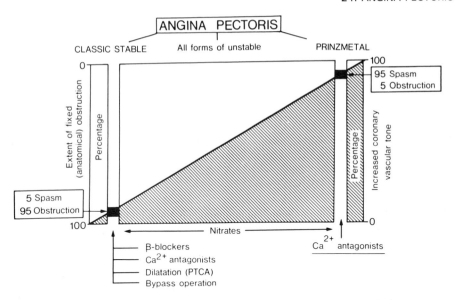

Fig. 24-4 Proposed therapeutic approach to angina pectoris. In classic stable angina of effort (left side), fixed anatomical stenosis (see Fig. 12-6) plays a major role and beta-adrenergic blockers act to improve the oxygen balance (Fig. 24-1). It is in this group that percutaneous transluminal coronary angioplasty (PTCA) and coronary bypass operations may be most effective. Calcium antagonists were initially used chiefly for angina of spasm (Prinzmetal, Fig. 24-6); now they have increasingly become early therapy even in angina of effort. Modified from Hugenholtz et al. (1984). In: Calcium Antagonists and Cardiovascular Disease, Ed. LH Opie, pp 237–256, Raven Press, New York.

than either drug alone is not well documented, although such combination therapy is often prescribed.

Beta-blockade remains the conventional cornerstone of long-term therapy of angina pectoris, whereas sublingual preparations of nitrates are the cornerstone of acute pain relief. Some patients with angina pectoris respond adequately to long-acting nitrates alone. Combination therapy with beta-blockers and long-acting nitrates, however, is often prescribed and has the practical advantages already outlined. Over a prolonged period, increasing doses of nitrates may be required to maintain therapeutic effects. Some clinicians are switching to long-term therapy with beta-blockers combined not with the long-acting nitrates, but with **calcium antagonists** (Lynch et al., 1980) which do not seem to cause tolerance. Here the safest combination may be with nifedipine, where beta-blockade can counter some of the vasodilatory side-effects of nifedipine (Krikler et al., 1982). Long-term combination of verapamil with beta-blockade is also very effective despite the theoretical risk of added negative inotropic and dromotropic effects (Weiner et al., 1983). Diltiazem may also be safely combined with beta-blockade unless there are unwanted additive negative chronotropic or dromotropic effects (Hung

et al., 1983). In practice, verapamil, nifedipine and diltiazem may each be safely combined with beta-blockade in the therapy of hemodynamically stable patients with chronic effort angina (Subramanian, 1983).

Step-care therapy in effort angina

Medical therapy of angina is at present undergoing a significant change (Fig. 24-4). This results from the demonstration of the role of coronary artery spasm in the pathogenesis of transient myocardial ischemia. Attention must therefore be focused not only on attempts to reduce myocardial oxygen demand, but also to increase the oxygen supply. The arrival of the calcium antagonists and long-acting nitrate preparations as coronary vasodilators is thus timely. The question arises regarding the nature of "step-care" therapy of angina. Most clinicians still resort to short-term nitrates as first-line therapy for most forms of angina, yet it is now somewhat controversial whether the next "step" is beta-blockade or calcium antagonism. For most patients with chronic stable angina, the choice between these agents is unresolved and likely to remain so in the future. Calcium antagonists have fewer serious side-effects and may be safer. Combinations of calcium antagonists and beta-blockade are being used increasingly with each other and with nitrates, because each has a basically different effect in relieving angina pectoris. For patients who have angina combined with chronic obstructive airways disease, peripheral vascular disease or diabetes mellitus or other contra-indications to beta-blockade, calcium antagonists are clearly superior. As tolerance has been reported with nitrates but not with calcium antagonists, it would seem rational to consider using prolonged therapy with calcium antagonists for chronic vasodilator therapy with added intermittent nitrates for additional pain relief. In practice, intermittent nitrates (long- or short-acting) are still "step-one".*

Angina at Rest

Because of some differences in the pathophysiology between effort angina and angina at rest, the latter merits separate consideration. When the patient experiences anginal pain at rest, myocardial ischemia cannot be relieved by stopping exercise (because there is none) and the risk is that prolonged subendocardial ischemia may advance to infarction. A number of potential vicious circles operate, including a secondary increase in sympathetic drive and the left ventricular "crunch" mechanism (Fig. 24-5). Angina at rest is not a uniform entity—it may vary from a mixed picture where both oxygen supply and demand are altered to include the situation where only the oxygen supply is decreased.

The mechanisms decreasing oxygen supply may include coronary artery spasm, the presence of critical arterial stenosis, arterial thrombosis or platelet aggregation. Multiple mechanisms mean that multiple therapeutic approaches may be needed. Different severities of disease mean that some patients respond well to bed rest and drug therapy, whereas others go on to early bypass grafting.

Special attention is now given to the role of **coronary artery spasm** in angina at rest. Initially spasm was defined as the cause of **Prinzmetal's variant angina** (Fig. 24-6). More recently, Maseri and co-workers (1978) have shown that spasm may play a more important role than suspected in the "average" case of unstable angina at rest. It seems that atheromatous damage to the vascular endothelium may sensitize the arteries to various autonomic nervous influences causing the spasm. Spasm may also contribute to exercise-induced angina, either indirectly as when exercise is undertaken in the cold, or sometimes exercise can directly provoke spasm. To test if a patient

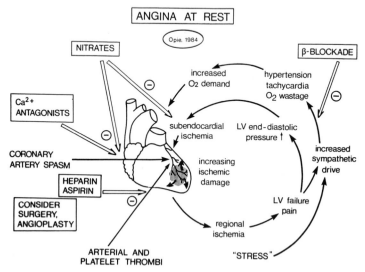

Fig. 24-5 Hypothetical events during angina at rest, supposing that the initial event is coronary artery spasm or another temporary obstruction such as arterial thrombosis or platelet thrombosis. Beta-adrenergic blockade will not relieve (and may aggravate) coronary spasm, although it will relieve secondary hypertension and tachycardia. From Opie LH (1983). Drugs for the Heart, American Edition, Grune & Stratton, p 9, with permission.

*This paragraph is extracted from Singh and Opie (1984), with permission.

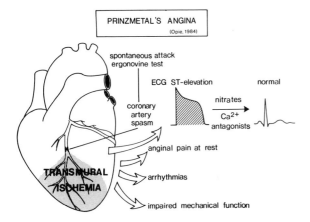

Fig. 24-6 In Prinzmetal's angina there is severe spasm of one of the large coronary arteries, producing transmural ischemia and ST-segment elevation. This contrasts with the ST-segment depression typical of the subendocardial ischemia found in effort angina. Spasm can be relieved by nitrates or calcium antagonists.

is abnormally sensitive to vasoconstrictor influences, the response to cold (reflex vasoconstriction of coronary arteries) or to **ergonovine** may be employed. A small dose of ergonovine, an alpha-receptor stimulant, can cause angina in susceptible individuals when given under careful monitoring.

Spasm may be enhanced by beta-adrenergic blockade, leaving unopposed alpha activity to cause vasoconstriction which may be mediated by alpha-2 receptors (Heusch and Deussen, 1983). Alpha-2 receptors are thought to "open" the calcium channels which respond to calcium antagonists (Fig. 17-3); these observations would explain why only the calcium antagonists and not alpha-1 antagonists such as prazosin are used in the therapy of angina caused by spasm. Thus far agents for direct blockade of the alpha-2 coronary receptors have not been clinically available (other than calcium antagonists).

Normal coronary vasoreactivity is enhanced by alkalosis which enhances vasoconstriction so that it has the opposite effect to an intracellular acidosis. Added vasoconstrictive elements are provided by a variety of factors — alpha-adrenergic stimulation, histamine H_1 receptor stimulation and possibly thromboxane. Whatever the mechanism, the spasm is usually promptly relieved by vasodilation by nitrates or calcium-antagonists.

Unstable angina

Strictly speaking, unstable angina is a condition in which the pattern of anginal attacks is changing. The term could, for example, be applied to worsening effort angina. In reality, unstable angina usually includes episodes of angina at rest and carries the implied connotation of myocardial infarction (pre-infarction angina). Therefore the therapeutic plan in unstable angina is usually similar to that in angina at rest. However, the closer unstable angina becomes to myocardial infarction, the stronger the rationale for the use of beta-blockade.

General therapy in angina at rest

The common clinical practice of giving nasal oxygen is supported by the observation that nitrates may cause arterial hypoxemia. Anticoagulants (heparin) and antiplatelet agents are also given, but the critical clinical trials have been missing. A recent trial in 1266 men with unstable angina showed a protective effect of buffered aspirin in a dose of 324 mg daily (Lewis et al., 1983).

Nitrates

Short-acting and long-acting nitrates are both used widely in angina at rest and unstable angina, but there has been little objective evidence of their efficacy. Recently spontaneous ST-deviations on the electrocardiogram have been used to assess the benefits of nitrates and other agents. In patients with repetitive episodes of angina at rest, infusion of isosorbide dinitrate 1.2–5.0 mg/hour relieves pain and reduces the incidence of ischemic episodes (Distante et al., 1979), with few side-effects. Intravenous nitroglycerin 100–200 µg/min with a combination of oral isosorbide dinitrate (20–60 mg) and nitropaste (0.5–2 inches) reduced repetitive attacks of resting angina to a similar extent, but did not abolish the ischemic episodes completely (Curfman et al., 1983). In Prinzmetal's angina at rest caused by coronary artery spasm, nitroglycerin is given for acute attacks and long-acting nitrates for prophylaxis; combination with calcium antagonists is usual.

Beta-blockade for angina at rest

Beta-blockade is used widely in **unstable angina**, angina at rest and threatened infarction, but is usually ineffective when coronary spasm is the cause. Fischl and co-workers tried beta-blockade in twenty patients with angina at rest and threatened infarction (Fischl et al., 1973). None had experienced complete relief of pain with nitrates, and hypertension and tachycardia commonly accompanied the pain. Propranolol was given in a starting dose of 20 mg orally and was stepped up every 4 hours until the pain was controlled or the heart rate was below 60 beats/min. The average dose of propranolol was 170 mg/day. Seventeen patients had prompt relief of pain. In seven patients with clinical left ventricular failure at the time of their pain, heart failure was lessened by beta-blockade.

In **Prinzmetal's variant angina**, beta-blockade is ineffective and may even be harmful, probably because of unopposed alpha-tone in the large coronary arteries. Such arguments favor the use of nitrates and/or calcium antagonists in angina at rest with short-lived attacks of chest pain; in such patients propranolol is ineffective (Parodi et al., 1982). The apparent contradiction between the latter study and that of Fischl et al. (1973), both dealing with angina at rest, may be explained as follows. First, Fischl's patients probably did not have prominent vasospasm because the pain did not respond fully to nitrates; secondly, the attacks of pain were long enough to cause a secondary tachycardia and hypertension which propranolol could inhibit (Fig. 24-4).

Calcium antagonists for angina at rest

For angina at rest, Parodi et al. (1979) found that 80-mg doses of verapamil every 4 hours, followed by 80 mg 3–5 times a day, were effective in pain relief and correcting ST-segment deviations. Similarly nifedipine and diltiazem have also been used effectively in the control of unstable angina. In Prinzmetal's variant angina, each of the three agents is successful. For example, verapamil (average dose: 450 mg/day 3–4 divided doses) and nifedipine (average dose: 70 mg/day 3–4 divided doses) are equipotent; the side-effects with nifedipine are somewhat more and more likely to limit the dose (Winniford et al., 1982).

Alpha-1-blockers for angina at rest

Prazosin has not been effective in the therapy of unstable angina, probably because it is the alpha-2 receptors rather than the alpha-1 receptors which are involved in coronary artery spasm.

Choice of therapy for angina at rest

High-dose oral or transcutaneous nitrates are usually the initial therapy in angina at rest, with the addition of calcium antagonists if coronary vasospasm is suspected. Beta-blockade may be added instead of calcium antagonists if there is reactive hypertension or tachycardia. Generally combinations of oral agents are used first before going on to intravenous nitrates or intravenous calcium antagonists.

Recent trials have suggested that the calcium antagonists are at least as effective as beta-blockers, and in some instances preferable, in the therapy of unstable angina and angina at rest. There is a new trend to emphasize calcium antagonists rather than beta-blockade. Documentation of coronary vasospasm in some patients with rest angina reinforces the use of calcium antagonists as primary agents in this setting, particularly if anginal pain is accompanied by ST-segment elevation or if there are repetitive short-lived attacks of pain. Calcium antagonists may be used synergistically with beta-blocking agents and with high-dose nitrates; careful attention to the development of side-effects is mandatory.

Coronary artery bypass surgery

The indications for coronary artery bypass surgery have expanded widely with refinements in techniques and improved results. The results of current trials will probably clarify the role of bypass surgery in specific sub-sets of patients with coronary artery disease, and this in turn may modify the approaches to drug therapy. Coronary artery surgery is used increasingly in patients with angina at rest, once they have passed the acute attack, and once coronary angiography has established that the lesions are amenable to surgery. The type and severity of coronary artery disease and the adequacy of left ventricular function are two important factors in determining whether or not patients are suitable for surgical intervention. Percutaneous transluminal coronary angioplasty (PTCA) appears to be a promising alternative to surgery in certain patients but requires further evaluation.

Summary

In angina pectoris there is failure of the normal oxygen balance of the myocardium so that anaerobic metabolism develops. It may be caused either by an increased demand (effort angina) or by a decreased supply (angina of coronary spasm or vasospastic angina). An extreme example of the latter mechanism is Prinzmetal's angina where there is severe transmural myocardial ischemia caused by severe coronary spasm. In effort angina, exercise stress testing with electro-cardiographic or radionuclide techniques is used widely in diagnosis and in assessing the severity of the disease. Therapeutic procedures to relieve angina include those decreasing the oxygen demand (beta-adrenergic blockade), and those relieving the increased preload resulting from acute ischemic contractile failure (nitrates). The calcium-antagonists act in part by afterload reduction (nifedipine), reduced heart rate (diltiazem), a negative inotropic effect (verapamil) and especially by combinations of mechanisms. In the case of angina caused by coronary spasm, beta-adrenergic blockade will not benefit and may harm. Here the appropriate therapy is by coronary vasodilation (nitrates or calcium-antagonists).

References

Bricknell OL, Daries PS, Opie LH (1981). A relationship between adenosine triphosphate, glycolysis and ischaemia contracture in the isolated rat heart. J Molec Cell Cardiol 13: 941–945.

Cobbe SM, Poole-Wilson PA (1980). The time of onset and severity of acidosis in myocardial ischemia. J Molec Cell Cardiol 12: 745–760.

Cohen D, Saxard P, Rifkin RD, Lepeschkin E, Strauss WE (1983). Magnetic measurement of S-T and T-Q segment shifts in humans. Exercise-induced S-T segment depression. Circ Res 53: 274–279.

Curfman GD, Heinsimer JA, Lozner EC (1983). Intravenous nitroglycerin in the treatment of spontaneous angina pectoris. A prospective, randomized trial. Circulation 67: 276–282.

Distante A, Maseri A, Servi S (1979). Management of vasospastic angina at rest with continuous infusion of isosorbide dinitrate. A double-blind cross-over study in a coronary care unit. Am J Cardiol 44: 533–539.

Fischl SJ, Herman MW, Gorlin R (1973). The intermediate coronary syndrome. Clinical, angiographic and therapeutic aspects. N Engl J Med 288: 1193–1198.

Fox K, Dyett JF, Portal RW, Aber CP (1977). The combined clinical and hemodynamic effects of trinitrin and propranolol. Europ J Cardiol 5: 507–515.

Hearse DJ (1979). Oxygen deprivation and early myocardial contractile failure: a reassessment of the possible role of adenosine triphosphate. Am J Cardiol 44: 1115–1121.

Heusch G, Deussen A (1983). The effects of cardiac sympathetic nerve stimulation on perfusion of stenotic coronary arteries in the dog. Circ Res 53: 8–15.

Holland RP, Brooks H (1977). TQ-ST segment mapping: Critical review and analysis of current concepts. Am J Cardiol 40: 110–129.

Hung J, Lamb IH, Connolly SJ, Jutzy KR, Goris ML, Schroeder JS (1983). The effect of diltiazem and propranolol, alone and in combination, on exercise performance and left ventricular function in patients with stable effort angina. Circulation 68: 560–567.

Katz AM, Hecht HH (1969). The early "pump" failure of the ischemic heart. Am J Med 47: 497–502.

Kleber AG (1984). Extracellular potassium accumulation in acute myocardial ischemia. J Molec Cell Cardiol 16: 389–394.

Krikler DM, Harris L, Rowland E (1982). Calcium channel blockers and beta blockers: advantages and disadvantages of combination therapy in chronic stable angina pectoris. Am Heart J 104: 702–708.

Kübler W, Katz AM (1977). Mechanism of early "pump" failure of the ischemic heart: possible role of adenosine triphosphate depletion and inorganic phosphate accumulation. Am J Cardiol 40: 467–471.

Lewis HD Jr, Davis JW, Archibald DG (1983). Protective effects of aspirin against acute myocardial infarction and death in men with unstable angina. N Engl J Med 309: 396–403.

Lichtlen PR, Engel H-J, Raffenbeul W (1984). Calcium entry blockers, especially nifedipine in angina of effort. In: Calcium Antagonists and Cardiovascular Disease, Ed. LH Opie, pp 221–236, Raven Press, New York.

Lynch P, Dargie H, Krikler S, Krikler D (1980). Objective assessment of antianginal treatment: a double-blind comparison of propranolol, nifedipine and their combination. Brit Med J 281: 184–187.

Maseri A, Severi S, Denes M, Labbate A, Chierchia S, Marzilli M, Ballestra AM, Parodi O, Biagini A (1978). Variant angina — one aspect of a continuous spectrum of vasospastic myocardial ischemia — pathogenetic mechanisms, estimated incidence and clinical and coronary arteriographic findings in 138 patients. Am J Cardiol 42: 1019–1035.

Parodi O, Maseri A, Simonetti I (1979). Management of unstable angina at rest by verapamil. A double-blind cross-over study in the coronary care unit. Brit Heart J 41: 146–174.

Parodi O, Simonetti I, L'Abbate A (1982). Verapamil versus propranolol for angina at rest. Am J Cardiol 50: 923–928.

Rozanski A, Berman DS, Gray R, Levy R, Raymond M, Maddahi J, Panteleo N, Waxman AD, Swan HJC, Matloff J (1981). Use of thallium-201 redistribution scintigraphy in the preoperative differentiation of reversible and non-reversible myocardial asynergy. Circulation 64: 936–944.

Shang ST Jr, Pepine CJ (1978). Coronary and myocardial metabolic effects of combined glyceryl trinitrate and propranolol administration. Brit Heart J 40: 1221–1228.

Simonsen S, Kjekshus JK (1978). The effect of free fatty acids on myocardial oxygen consumption during atrial pacing and catecholamine infusion in man. Circulation 58: 485–471.

Singh BN, Opie LH (1984). Calcium antagonists. In: Drugs for the Heart. American Edition, pp 39–64, Grune & Stratton, Orlando, New York and London.

Subramanian BV (1983). Calcium Antagonists in Chronic Stable Angina Pectoris, pp 217–229, Excerpta Medica, Amsterdam.

Tennant R (1935). Factors concerned in the arrest of contraction in an ischemic myocardial area. Am J Physiol 113: 677–682.

Weiner DA, McCabe CH, Cutler SS, Creager MA, Ryan TJ, Klein MD (1983). Efficacy and safety of verapamil in patients with angina pectoris after 1 year of continuous, high-dose therapy. Am J Cardiol 51: 1251–1255.

Winniford MD, Johnson SM, Mauritson DR (1982). Verapamil therapy for Prinzmetal's variant angina: comparison with placebo and nifedipine. Am J Cardiol 50: 913–918.

New References

Fozzard HA, Makielski JC (1985). The electrophysiology of acute myocardial ischemia. Ann Rev Med 36: 275–284.

Henry PD (1984). Coronary artery spasm. In: Physiology and Pathophysiology of the Heart. Ed. N Sperelakis, pp 819–833, Nijhoff, Boston.

Passamani E, Davis KB, Gillispie MJ, Killip T (1985). A randomized trial of coronary artery bypass surgery. Survival of patients with a low ejection fraction. New Engl J Med 312: 1665–1671.

Tolins M, Weir EK, Chesler E, Pierpont GL (1984). "Maximal" drug therapy is not necessarily optimal in chronic angina pectoris. J Am Coll Cardiol 3: 1051–1057.

25 | Myocardial Infarction

Whereas angina pectoris is essentially a complex clinical situation with no really appropriate animal model, myocardial infarction is readily produced by sustained coronary artery occlusion. Infarction is ischemia that has reached the point of irreversibility. In principle, any model of sustained ischemia will result in myocardial cell death or necrosis. Although a pathologist will only diagnose myocardial infarction in the presence of cellular necrosis, a clinical diagnosis is frequently made in the early hours or even minutes when there is probably myocardial ischemia or a mixture of ischemic, dying and dead cells. Hence the most appropriate clinical description of this important state is "developing" or "impending" myocardial infarction.

Ischemia vs Infarction

In the case of ischemia, different models produce different end-results. **Regional ischemia** produced by coronary artery occlusion will eventually develop into myocardial infarction; this evolving process corresponds quite well to the early stages of developing infarction in man. The juxtaposition of ischemic and non-ischemic tissue leads to the existence of the controversial **border zone**, where steep metabolic gradients may be responsible for arrhythmogenesis. The severity of this type of ischemia will be determined by the extent to which the collateral circulation penetrates the ischemic zone from the non-ischemic tissue. Patterns of metabolism in developing infarction are very complex, depending not only on the effects

of lack of oxygen and poor washout of metabolites, but also on the extent of the collateral circulation. The existence of the collateral circulation is variable, depending on the species, being high in dogs and low in pigs. There is much variation from patient to patient which is one of the factors underlying the extreme clinical variability of acute myocardial infarction. In the ischemic zone a variable number of cells are supplied by the collateral circulation and are still surviving by normal oxidative metabolism. Yet the zone as a whole is dying.

Global ischemia results when the whole heart is deprived of its blood supply, so that the heart as a whole stops its mechanical work. Global ischemia is one method of producing cardioplegia, when it is called **ischemic arrest**. This method is no longer used because the contractile arrest is caused by depletion of ATP which in turn limits viability upon reperfusion. **Cold cardioplegic arrest** of the heart followed by aortic cross-clamping also causes global ischemia in which the rate of decline of ATP is sufficiently slowed by hypothermia to allow recovery on reperfusion (Fig. 25-1). Such global ischemia produces total anoxia within 20 sec at 15°C and is also called **anoxic arrest**. Unexpectedly, the ischemia may not be total because there is a low rate of non-coronary collateral blood supply, originating from the mediastinal and bronchial vessels to reach the myocardium by pericardial connections. The non-coronary collateral flow may reach 10 percent of the normal flow in children with cyanotic heart disease or when the heart is hypertrophied; otherwise such flow is estimated at about 3 percent or less of normal. Thus, the real pattern of

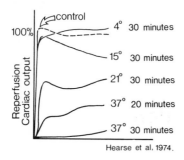

Fig. 25-1 Global or "surgical" ischemia results when the aorta is cross-clamped. Redrawn from Hearse et al. (1974). Circ Res 35: 450, with permission from the author and the American Heart Association. Note markedly protective effect of hypothermia. Cardioplegia, for example by a high potassium solution, gives added protection.

metabolism in surgically arrested hearts is not simply that of total, global ischemia; rather there is some washout by the collateral flow.

Anatomical heterogeneity in ischemia

The varying pattern of the collateral blood flow in regional ischemia causes cellular heterogeneity, resulting in a mixture of living and dying and dead cells in the zone of developing infarction. Not even global ischemia results in homogenous ischemia, because microzones of total ischemia develop with consequent total tissue anoxia (Steenbergen et al., 1977). Photographs of the surface fluorescence, which reflects the formation of $NADH_2$, can be used to show that such heterogeneous zones of total ischemia lie side-by-side with tissue which is much better perfused. The cause of this "microheterogeneity" may be in different degrees of patency of adjacent capillary beds. Heterogeneity, on a much larger scale (macroheterogeneity), in the transverse section of the heart also occurs so that subendocardial ischemia is more severe than subepicardial ischemia. Further anatomical macroheterogeneity may originate in the different reactions of atria, ventricles and the conduction system to anoxia and ischemia. The atria and the conduction system have higher glycogen values which may explain their resistance to oxygen deprivation.

Metabolic heterogeneity in ischemia

An important point, frequently not appreciated, is that coronary artery occlusion causes a region of myocardium with a predominantly ischemic metabolism producing lactate, yet with some features of oxidation metabolism. This apparent contra-indication may arise as follows. As long as there is some blood flow to the ischemic zone, some oxygen is delivered. Because the mitochondria require very little oxygen, that oxygen is sufficient to permit oxidative production of ATP in those mitochondria to which the oxygen can penetrate. Other mitochondria in the ischemic zone will receive no oxygen at all, because of the microheterogeneity of the ischemic process. Cells with such anoxic mitochondria will produce lactate by anaerobic metabolism. For lactate produced by anaerobic cells to wash out and be detected in coronary venous blood requires diffusion along a concentration gradient from an anoxic area to a perfused area.

Initial Events in
Acute Myocardial Infarction

Animal models of myocardial infarction have generally used either: (i) acute occlusion by ligature of otherwise healthy coronary arteries, or (ii) massive injections of catecholamines. The former procedure produces transmural myocardial infarction and the latter procedure causes subendocardial infarction. The ideal model would be spontaneously occurring severe coronary atherosclerosis; superimposed thereon would be the triggering event, which is still unknown. In those patients with a sudden arrhythmic death, probably due to ventricular fibrillation, the initial event does not appear to be an occlusive thrombus although usually there is advanced coronary artery disease. In contrast, in those patients presenting with the classical features of early acute myocardial infarction, the initial event is likely to be a thrombosis, as shown by the current practice of early angiography prior to revascularization. Despite the defects of the various animal models, very early lesions both in animals and in man have a variable and possibly predominant element of reversibility (ischemia) with eventual irreversiblity (infarction, see Fig. 25-2).

Vascular factors in ischemia

Traditionally, arterial obstruction has been the event initiating ischemia of sufficient severity to lead to acute myocardial infarction, and mechanical block has been regarded as the most important cause of vascular

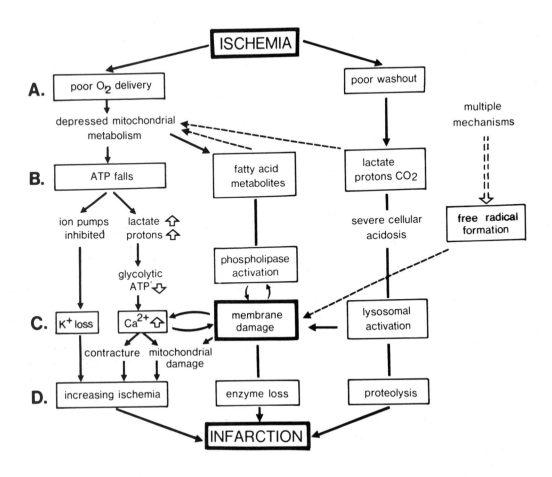

Fig. 25-2 Proposed metabolic mechanisms whereby ischemia can produce infarction. Panel A shows the two major effects of ischemia, namely poor O_2 delivery (hypoxia) and poor washout of metabolites. Panel B proposes that depressed mitochondrial metabolism results in decreased production of ATP and accumulation of fatty acid metabolites which are normally metabolized in the mitochondria. Anaerobic metabolism causes accumulation of lactate and protons (the latter from breakdown of ATP) and continued residual respiration causes accumulation of CO_2. Panel C proposes that decreased production of glycolytic ATP (a result of accumulation of lactate and/or protons) results in calcium accumulation. Release of norepinephrine (NE) from storage granules may explain an increased cyclic AMP in early ischemia and enhanced Ca^{2+} entry. Inhibition of ion pumps by lack of ATP and by inhibition of fatty acid metabolites, results in sodium and water retention, and cell swelling. Fatty acid metabolites also probably cause membrane damage, which may result from lysosomal activation as a result of a severe cellular acidosis or possibly as a result of other mechanisms such as ATP depletion. Panel D proposes that the final events leading up to infarction may be: increasing ischemia caused by ischemic contracture and cell swelling, enzyme loss from membrane damage, and proteolysis from lysosomal activation. Modified from Opie LH (1980). Am Heart J 100: 355–372, with permission.

obstruction. The true initial event may be thrombosis, embolism, formation of platelet aggregates, plaque rupture, a thrombus on a pre-existing plaque or coronary spasm. The occlusive theory may well be correct in the majority of patients with acute infarction, as shown by very early angiography in preparation for introducing thrombolytic agents into the occluded coronary artery. That coronary occlusion could cause reflex vasospasm through an adrenergic mechanism was suggested by Grayson in 1966. Now, after a long interval, the phenomenon has been re-analyzed (Gorman and Sparks, 1982). The probable explanation is that subtotal ischemia produced by severe stenosis of the left anterior descending coronary artery causes a progressive vasoconstriction, apparently mediated by alpha-adrenergic activity and triggered by unknown stimuli. Experimentally, the degree of collateral circulation influences the extent and severity of the infarction process: in the presence of a well-developed collateral circulation, coronary occlusion may have no effects.

That hemodynamic factors can influence the myocardial oxygen uptake is firmly established. That they could influence the progression from ischemia to infarction depends on the hypothesis that there is a balance between the oxygen supply and demand of the ischemic zone, which can be tipped in either direction with consequent sparing or increased injury to those critically jeopardized or vulnerable cells, with either their ultimate survival or necrosis. This point of view calls for (i) the existence of a zone of intermediate blood supply, (ii) a collateral blood supply to the severely ischemic tissue, and (iii) the persistence of some contractile activity in the ischemic zone.

Catecholamines

Much evidence has supported the concept that catecholamines can exaggerate the degree of myocardial ischemia and extend "infarct size". Beta-adrenergic catecholamines appear to be harmful to the ischemic myocardium and the mechanisms involved may include (i) an increased heart rate and contractility; (ii) an increased arterial blood pressure; (iii) increased circulating free fatty acids; (iv) the effects of increased intracellular cyclic AMP level, which may enhance the entry of calcium ions into ischemic myocardial cells; and (v) an increased sarcolemmal permeability.

Mechanism of Irreversible Injury

The basic processes involved in the transition from ischemia to infarction include the sustained effects both of poor oxygen delivery and of poor washout of metabolites (Fig. 25-3). The former process depletes the ischemic myocardium of ATP and activates anaerobic metabolism to produce lactate and protons. Impaired mitochondrial metabolism leads to intra-

cellular accumulation of lipid metabolites which may further inhibit ATP transfer and help promote membrane disruption. Poor washout results in the accumulation of lactate, protons and $NADH_2$ which conjointly inhibit anaerobic glycolysis; protons and accumulated CO_2 cause a severe intracellular acidosis and (probably) activation of lysosomal enzymes which damage the membranes and destroy the cellular proteins. Calcium ions accumulate as a result of several mechanisms and probably promote the development of heart cell necrosis.

ATP depletion

The overall events in the transition of ischemia to infarction are very complex and cannot simply be related to depletion of ATP (see page 149). Rather depletion of ATP should be seen as a marker of (i) the severity of the ischemic process; (ii) a depressed rate of anaerobic glycolysis in severely ischemic tissue caused by an accumulation of glycolytic end-products; (iii) inhibited lipid metabolism with accumulation of intermediates such as intracellular free fatty acids, and long-chain derivatives such as acyl CoA and acyl carnitine, with inhibition of mitochondrial metabolism; and (iv) an accumulation of intracellular calcium with ischemic contracture and utilization of ATP. All these processes contribute to damage to the cell membranes (sarcolemma, mitochondria, sarcoplasmic reticulum) which is seen as a critical event in irreversible damage (Jennings and Reimer, 1981). A rough guide is: ATP depletion below about 25 percent is an indirect marker of cells destined to

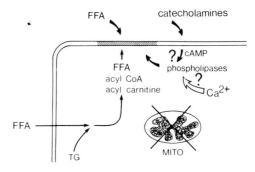

Fig. 25-3 Possible mechanisms of early membrane damage in developing infarction. FFA = free fatty acids; TG = triglyceride; acyl CoA = long chain acyl co-enzyme A; MITO = mitochondria.

necrosis, and below 10 percent is a marker of severe necrosis (Jennings and Reimer, 1981). As judged by the rate of fall of ATP, many cells in the severely ischemic zone are destined to die soon, within 30–45 min. Other cells in the ischemic zone may still be viable for hours especially in the infarct edge and peri-infarct border (for criticism of the "critical ATP level" see page 149).

Loss of ATP in the ischemic zone suggests that the ischemic zone should be in a state of contracture like the stone heart. The relaxed state found soon after coronary ligation is explained by Kübler and Katz (1977) as the result of an accumulation of inorganic phosphate (derived from the breakdown of creatine phosphate via ATP) effectively depleting the heart of calcium, thereby causing a relaxed state. Depending on the relative degree of depletion of ATP or accumulation of inorganic phosphate, there may be either contraction or relaxation of the heart.

Sodium and edema

The "pump-leak" hypothesis of McKnight and Leaf (1977) states that inhibition of the sodium pump leads to accumulation of sodium within the cell as potassium leaks out. Similar disruptive effects on cells are found when the pump is markedly inhibited by very high concentrations of digitalis glycosides. Formation of edema, limited by the collagen network of the heart, is concomitant with sodium retention. The relatively mild nature of tissue edema even when ischemic damage has become irreversible (Dalby et al., 1981) shows that edema formation is not the critical event in developing infarction. In contrast, reperfusion can greatly accelerate edema formation, which then becomes an important cause of reperfusion damage (Whalen et al., 1974). When the sarcolemma stretches there is increased permeability to macromolecules.

Intracellular acidosis

Once the buffer systems of the body are overcome by excess proton production, intracellular acidosis may play an important part not only in contractile failure, but also in the inhibition of glycolysis and in the production of irreversible ischemic damage (Armiger et al., 1975). The rate of fall of intracellular pH will depend on the severity of the ischemia. In the pig model, where collateral flow is very low, the pH can fall to 5.5 within 50 min. In the dog, where the collateral flow is quite high, pH 6.20 is reached after only 4–6 hours.

One major source of acidosis in ischemia is continued anaerobic glycolysis with ATP breakdown; it is the ATP that releases the protons. Another source is formation of respiratory CO_2 in those mitochondria still respiring oxidatively. A third factor is impaired oxidation of $NADH_2$ with a rise of NADH and H^+. A fourth factor is the theoretical operation of proton-producing cycles (triglyceride-fatty acid; glycogen synthesis and breakdown); ATP is continuously broken down in such cycles to yield protons.

Lysosomes

For lysosomal acid hydrolases to act in the cytosol requires damage to the lysosomal membrane for their liberation and a very acid pH (5.0 or below) for their optimal activity. Some workers think that a low pH reached in ischemic muscle could both release the acid hydrolases into the cytoplasm and then activate the enzymes. In reality, isolated cardiac lysosomes are rather resistant to even extreme changes of pH (Romeo et al., 1966). Thus the low pH of 5.5–6.5 reached in severe ischemia is unlikely to cause much liberation of lysosomal enzymes. Rather, the low pH will render active the enzymes released by other factors which labilize lysosomal membranes such as lack of ATP, osmotic changes, accumulation of membrane-active fatty acids and increased phospholipase activity. The source of the phospholipases may be in the damaged lysosomal membranes. Whether lysosomes really play a critical role in irreversible ischemic damage is still being debated (Wildenthal, 1978).

Calcium

Calcium accumulates in the cells damaged by prolonged ischemia, especially after reperfusion. The overall cellular content of calcium does not change over the first 40 min of ischemia, by which time many cells are already irreversibly damaged. Hypoxia or ischemia has to be prolonged for 1–3 hours before an increased uptake of calcium can be detected by the uptake of lanthanum (Burton et al., 1977) or calcium-seeking isotopes (Chien et al., 1981). Therefore a net gain of cellular calcium cannot be the critical event

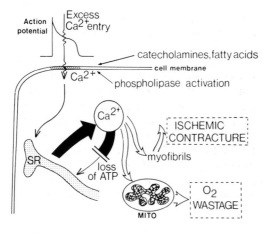

Fig. 25-4 Proposed role of accumulated calcium ions in irreversible injury, as found in early reperfusion. Note that the source of the calcium is intracellular, possibly being calcium that is not taken back into the sarcoplasmic reticulum. SR = sarcoplasmic reticulum; MITO = mitochondria.

in ischemic irreversibility. Rather, the source of the increased cytosolic calcium ions recently found by direct measurement is intracellular (Allen and Orchard, 1983; Fig. 25-4); this rise in internal calcium may have important electrophysiological consequences (pages 95, 321). It is in reperfusion damage that the net gain of calcium is most striking. The uptake of excess calcium by mitochondria requires energy and occurs before total energy depletion; hence reperfusion damage is greatest when the blood supply is restored in the pre-necrotic phase, before 40–90 min of ischemia (Jennings and Ganote, 1976). Once taken up into mitochondria, calcium can participate in the formulation of intramitochondrial dense bodies which are a feature of irreversible injury.

Accumulated lipid intermediates

In ischemia the rate of uptake of fatty acids exceeds the rate of disposal and intermediates of lipid metabolism such as intracellular free fatty acid, acyl CoA and acyl carnitine accumulate (Fig. 25-3); these changes occur despite the major effect of ischemia in decreasing fatty acid uptake. At least some of the lipid intermediates might be derived from endogenous lipolysis. The exact mechanism whereby these lipid intermediates exert their "toxic" effect still remains

to be clarified, but their low water-solubility and highly detergent properties may be relevant. In the case of accumulated lysophosphoglycerides (derived from membrane phospholipids), an arrhythmogenic potential has been found (page 321). Derangements of fatty acid metabolism are, therefore, of considerable potential importance in the evolution of ischemic injury. These concepts, although experimentally valid, are still at the state of clinical evaluation.

Phospholipases

Phospholipases potentially have a doubly harmful effect. First, breakdown of membrane phospholipids increases sarcolemmal permeability to calcium (Chien et al., 1981). Secondly, the lysophosphoglycerides produced have destructive effects on cell membranes. Lysophosphoglycerides may also damage the mitochondrial membrane and can uncouple oxidative phosphorylation. The critical question now becomes: does ischemia activate the various phospholipases and, if so, how? As yet there is no clear evidence for such activation; possible mechanisms are an increased concentration of calcium ions or an accumulation of cyclic AMP (Fig. 25-3).

Catecholamines, beta-adrenergic receptors and cyclic AMP

The rise of cyclic AMP in the first minutes of developing infarction (Podzuweit et al., 1978) is followed later by a fall. Catecholamine activation of the beta-receptor may explain the early rise, especially as there is some evidence suggesting that there is local release of catecholamines in the ischemic zone. Such a rise of cyclic AMP may contribute to the postulated early rise of internal calcium in ischemia with the potential for development of arrhythmias (page 321). The later fall of cyclic AMP presumably indicates that adenylate cyclase is damaged, because the beta-adrenergic receptor density actually increases in the first hour of developing infarction (Mukherjee et al., 1982).

Lipid peroxidation and free radicals

When hearts are re-oxygenated after an anoxic period there is peroxidation of polyunsaturated lipids of the membranes. The consequences of such peroxidation are potentially serious and depend on the membrane involved. The decreased availability of reduced glutathione is an important event in the lipid peroxidation of membranes. In the case of reoxygenation after anoxia, the reduced glutathione is used up and less is available to keep membrane sulfhydryl groups in a reduced state. Lipid peroxidation may therefore occur after cardioplegic arrest, to the detriment of cardiac survival, or in reperfusion (page 359). The key enzyme protecting against lipid peroxidation is glutathione reductase which utilizes reduced glutathione for H donation to the membrane lipids, thereby keeping them reduced. Once membranes are damaged by lipid peroxidation, increased permeability follows. Free oxygen radicals could also be generated by the xanthine oxidase reaction. In regional ischemia early formation of free radicals and lipid peroxides (Rao et al., 1983) may contribute to membrane damage.

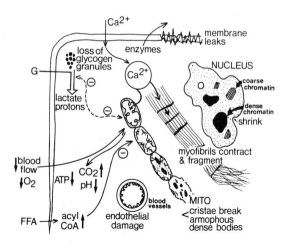

Fig. 25-5 Proposed role of multiple metabolic abnormalities, including true accommodation of calcium within the injured cell, in causing irreversible ischemic damage — that is, infarction. MITO = mitochondria; FFA = free fatty acids.

Increased permeability to proteins

Greatly increased rates of enzyme release are found in the presence of various insults to the cell membrane —catecholamine stimulation, fatty acid perfusion, ischemia and especially cell necrosis. The greatly increased membrane permeability found when ischemia progresses to infarction can be viewed as a continuum of damage, initially no different from the transient damage of transient ischemia (Poole-Wilson, 1984). A series of progressive events occurs (Fig. 25-2). The balance of life versus death is reflected by the failure of those reactions requiring ATP, while the degradation reactions set in motion by ischemia take over and tip the balance decisively in favor of irreversiblity. Once the sarcolemmal structure is severely damaged, intracellular enzymes pour out (Fig. 25-5) which indicates to the clinician the severity of the necrosis.

Amorphous matrix densities (= intramitochondrial dense bodies) contain both lipid and calcium and are indicative of irreversible injury. Small amorphous densities start after 40 min of ischemia; later they grow to 60–150 μm. They are probably formed as a result of the effect of detergent-active lipid compounds on the mitochondrial membrane (Feuvray and Plouet, 1981). Links between irreversible damage and mitochondrial dense bodies could explain why perfusion of infarcting hearts with free fatty acids gives a much

higher incidence of dense bodies than perfusion with glucose, thus showing that extreme loading of the heart with fatty acids can promote irreversible damage. It has not yet been proven that such mitochondrial derangements are the critical changes which convert reversible ischemia to irreversible cell necrosis and infarction.

Time scale of events

The time scale of irreversibility is important. The major events have been traced out in dog or pig hearts with developing infarction and it is assumed that such studies are relevant to man. Particular importance has been laid on the early transition stage of damage 20–60 min after the onset of ischemia. Because of the "advancing wave front" phenomenon, whereby damage spreads from endocardium to epicardium (see Fig. 12-8), it would be wrong to place an arbitrary limit on the "maximal tolerance to ischemia" such as 45 min. Rather, ischemia marches on to infarction over hours (Table 25-1). The final point of irreversibility is beyond 4–6 hours as shown both in animals and in patients in whom early intervention by beta-blockade or by reperfusion has been undertaken.

Table 25-1

Projected time scale of events in developing myocardial infarction

Phase of infarction	Time from onset	Metabolic events	Time of first detection	Ultrastructural and histological changes	Contractile events	Clinically detectable events
Acute ischemic injury	Seconds and minutes; up to 20–30 min	Intracellular effects of anoxia: tissue pO_2 falls breakdown of ATP and CP anaerobic glycolysis decreased glycogen gain of Na^+; K^+ loss cyclic AMP rise Intracellular retention of metabolites: lactate, NADH, CO_2, H^+ fatty acyl CoA phospholipids Extracellular events: loss of K, P_i, lactate release of inosine and hypoxanthine rise of pCO_2 fall of pH	30 sec–5 min[1] 10–30 sec[2] 15–30 sec[2] 5 min[4] 5 min[5] Minutes[6] As above 15–30 min[7] ? scale As soon as coronary venous blood sampled[8]	Myofibrils relax and particulate glycogen lost (15 min)[3]	Decreased contractility within 30 sec[1] failure	ST elevation Acute LV regional function ↓ Decreased thallium perfusion
Transition phase	20–60 min	Progressive increase in above changes except that cAMP reverts to normal	20–45 min[9]	Foci of coagulation necrosis (20 min) progressing to major subendo-cardial necrosis by 60 min[3]	Decreased contractility	Progressive loss of R-wave
		Impaired mitochondrial function	20–30 min[10]	Amorphous dense bodies in mito-chondria (30 min)[3]		
		Release of lysosomal enzymes	30 min[11]	Mitochondrial swelling and increased matrix space[3]		
		Early change in tissue Ca^{2+} level	60 min[12]	Disruption of cell membrane[3]		
Progressive infarction	1–6 hours	Progressive loss of tissue enzymes	60–120 min[3]	Spread of necrotic zone from endo-cardium to epi-cardium (6 hours)[3]	Stiffness	Appearance of enzymes in circulation
		Decreased protein synthesis ([14C]-glycine-incorporation)	4 hours[13]	Increased lipid drops and autolysis[14]		Uptake of 99mTc-gluco heptonate by infarct[16]
		Progressive intracellular accumulation of calcium	2–3 hours of hypoxia[15]			
Early catabolic phase repair	5 hours onwards	Increased activities of exogenous lysosomal enzymes such as N-acetyl-β-glucosaminidase	5 hours[17]	Infiltration with leukocytes. Earliest changes in routine light microscopy at 6 hours[18]		Increased lysosomal enzymes in circulation[17]

(continued)

Table 25-1 *(continued)*

Late synthetic repair	Hours to days	Increased protein synthesis	1 day;[19] could be sooner	Fibroblasts proliferate and collagen forms	None
		Increased activity of pentose shunt		Infiltration by monocytes with phagocytic capacity	
		Increased lipid synthesis			
		No generation of myofibrils		Main part of removal of cell debris (2–6 days)[20]	
Completed infarct	Up to 1 week	Normal metabolic activity except that oxygen requiring myofibrils replaced by fibrous tissue with very little O$_2$ requirement		Dead cells replaced by fibrous tissue	New stable state

[1]Sayen et al. (1958). Circ Res 6: 779–798.
[2]Gudbjarnason (1971/72). Cardiology 56: 240.
[3]Jennings and Reimer (1979). In: Enzymes in Cardiology, pp 21–57.
[4]Opie et al. (1973). Europ J Clin Invest 3: 419–435.
[5]Nayler et al. (1971). J Molec Cell Cardiol 2: 125–143.
[6]Krause and Wollenberger (1980). Adv Cycl Nucl Res 12: 49–61.
[7]Shrago et al. (1976). Circ Res 38: Suppl 1, 75–78.
[8]Opie et al. (1973). Amer J Cardiol 32: 295–305.
[9]Opie et al. (1979). Amer J Cardiol 43: 131–148.
[10]Lochner et al. (1975). J Molec Cell Cardiol 7: 203–217.
[11]Decker et al. (1977). J Clin Invest 59: 911–921.
[12]Lee et al. (1967). Circ Res 21: 439–444.
[13]Gudbjarnason (1963). J Lab Clin Med 62: 880.
[14]Bryant et al. (1958). Circ Res 6: 699–709.
[15]Burton et al. (1977). J Clin Invest 60: 1289–1302.
[16]Jacobstein (1977). J Nucl Med 18: 413–418.
[17]Welman et al. (1978). Cardiovasc Res 12: 99–105.
[18]Rose et al. (1976). AMA Arch Pathol 100: 516–571.
[19]Bing (1971/72). Cardiology 56: 314–324.
[20]Ravens and Gudbjarnason (1969). Circ Res 24: 851–856.

Role of Reperfusion Damage

When the blood supply to the ischemic myocardium is restored ischemic damage may temporarily be exaggerated. The possibility of reperfusion damage has two practical implications: (i) in the recovery of hearts arrested by ischemia for surgical purposes; (ii) in cases of myocardial infarction, when acute revascularization is now being attempted. The cellular events involved in reperfusion damage can at least in part be explained by the calcium and the oxygen paradoxes.

Calcium paradox

Depriving the heart of its normal extracellular calcium and then re-introducing the same component leads not to normality but to severe cellular damage. Zimmerman and Hulsmann (1960) perfused hearts for short periods with calcium-free solutions; re-introduction of the normal solution with calcium then caused massive tissue disruption, marked enzyme release and severe contracture of the muscle. The

explanation is that these massive mitochondrial uptakes of calcium are associated with a sudden fall of cardiac contents of ATP and creatine phosphate. The phenomenon is energy-dependent and the phenomenon does not occur until oxygen is also re-admitted and mitochondrial activity restarts (Ruigrok et al., 1978).

Oxygen paradox

The oxygen paradox is closely related. In isolated hearts arrested by a high potassium medium, deprivation of oxygen leads to two phases of enzyme release. First, there is a relatively low rate of release. Thereafter follows a sustained large-scale release of enzyme until virtually all intracellular enzymes are lost. Re-introduction of oxygen during the first phase leads to a decrease in the rate of release; introduction of oxygen in the second phase leads to greatly exaggerated rates of release (Fig. 25-6). The proposed explanation is that with re-oxygenation, the sudden commencement of mitochondrial activity causes abrupt uptake of

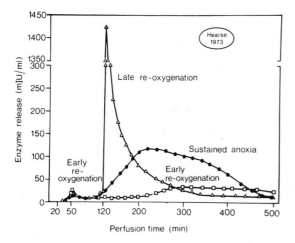

Fig. 25-6 Patterns of release of lactate dehydrogenase from isolated perfused heart. With sustained anoxia 240 units of enzyme are released over 6 hours; with early reoxygenation 141 units; with late reoxygenation 138 units. Although late reoxygenation temporarily exaggerated the rate of enzyme release, the total amount released was reduced. From Hearse et al. (1973). J Molec Cell Cardiol 5: 402, with permission.

calcium, energy provision fails and enzymes are released. An important point is that the effects of late re-oxygenation are not entirely harmful because total enzyme release is decreased (Fig. 25-6).

Reperfusion damage and calcium

The prototype experiments on reperfusion damage and calcium were performed by Jennings et al. (1960) who found that upon reperfusion of a coronary artery, tissue cation changes were much more marked than if coronary occlusion were maintained. Reperfusion caused a 10-fold increase in the uptake of radio-calcium with the appearance of contraction bands and intramitochondrial dense bodies (probably deposits of calcium phosphate). These phenomena are strikingly similar to those of the calcium paradox and show a major role for calcium overloading in reperfusion damage (Jennings and Ganote, 1976). Apparently reperfusion with re-introduction of calcium leads to excess uptake of calcium into the cytosol with subsequent mitochondrial overloading of calcium. A new proposal is that re-introduction of oxygen during reperfusion may result in the formation of lipid peroxides (page 356) with enhanced damage to membranes.

Reperfusion arrhythmias are ill-understood. It is possible that they are associated with accumulation of cyclic AMP and hence intracellular calcium during the ischemic period (Bricknell and Opie, 1978). Numerous other metabolic changes could equally well be responsible, such as washout of potassium from the previously ischemic cells during the early phase of reperfusion, or the formation of toxic oxygen radicals.

No-reflow is found when removal of coronary occlusion does not lead to restoration of coronary flow. There are two possible explanations for the no-reflow phenomenon. First, microvascular damage can lead to endothelial cell edema. Secondly, ischemic contracture of the myocardium can "squeeze" the coronary arteries and prevent normal flow. Some agents protecting the ischemic myocardium can also prevent microvascular damage: an example is pro-pranolol. Some agents can counter the no-reflow phenomenon, but do not decrease ischemic damage: an example is mannitol.

In the dog, massive **myocardial hemorrhage** may occur with reperfusion of infarcts, causing hemor-rhagic necrosis. This is presumably the result of the sudden re-introduction of blood under pressure into vessels with microvascular damage.

Metabolic recovery in the reperfusion period

After the initial period of exaggerated ischemic damage caused by reperfusion there is uptake of potassium and inorganic phosphate by the heart. These changes probably indicate restoration of normal cellular potassium and resynthesis of adenine nucleotides. However, the ATP level does not recover rapidly and total adenine nucleotide values also stay depressed for some hours. The rate of synthesis of adenine appears to be rate-limiting. Whether reperfusion damage could be decreased by provision of an adenine precursor such as ribose, or a substrate for the salvage pathway such as inosine, remains to be tested.

From the above complexities it is apparent that reperfusion does not always benefit the heart, and that there must be risks attached to early revascularization. In the case of surgical cardiac arrest, reperfusion damage is recognized increasingly as an undesirable entity, to be minimized by (i) a low external calcium concentration; (ii) calcium antagonist agents; and (iii) avoiding catecholamine stimulation in the reperfusion period. In the case of acute myocardial infarction transient reperfusion arrhythmias are taken as a sign of successful reperfusion during coronary thrombolysis. The possibility of enhanced cell damage during the reperfusion period has not yet received critical evaluation. Whether or not the benefits outweigh the risks remain to be shown, although recent clinical opinion increasingly favors the benefits of early revascularization.

Effects of reperfusion on hypokinetics and dyskinetic segments

As experimental infarction develops, impaired contraction of specific segments of the ischemic myocardium can be registered by ultrasonic crystals implanted in the myocardium. Mildly ischemic zones lose part of their ability to contract (hypokinetic segments). Severely ischemic segments not only fail to contract and become **akinetic,** but actually bulge in systole as the intraventricular pressure rises with a paradoxical **dyskinetic** movement. During reperfusion, hypokinetic segments recover most of their function in contrast to the poor recovery of dyskinetic segments

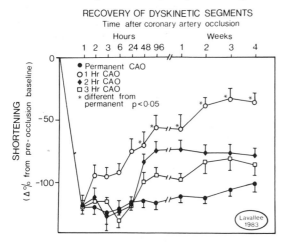

RECOVERY OF DYSKINETIC SEGMENTS
Time after coronary artery occlusion

Fig. 25-7 Effects of reperfusion of ischemic myocardium after varying duration of coronary artery occlusion (CAO). In these severely ischemic segments there is systolic expansion because the depression of systolic shortening exceeds 100 percent. Note that prolonged reperfusion combined with a short period of coronary occlusion (ideally no longer than 1 hour) is required for even partial restoration of systolic shortening. Data from Lavallee et al. (1983). Circ Res 53: 235, with permission from the authors and the American Heart Association.

(Fig. 25-7). The duration of regional ischemia that can be tolerated is short — even 1 hour of severe ischemia with dyskinesia means that there is very poor recovery during reperfusion, whereas mild ischemia allows some recovery even after 3 hours of coronary occlusion.

Not all the recovery occurs rapidly after reperfusion; full recovery may take 1–3 weeks. Part of the delay can be accounted for by a metabolic factor (delayed synthesis of adenine nucleotides, page 149). Soon after reperfusion the ischemic segment swells (Bush et al., 1983), possibly the combined result of edema, reperfusion hemorrhage and metabolic damage. This mechanical factor may account for the slow delayed recovery over weeks after reperfusion.

Can Infarct Size be Measured?

The benefits of any possible therapy in acute myocardial infarction can be assessed by (i) the effect on complications such as arrhythmias or left ventricular failure; (ii) the extent of necrotic damage — the "infarct size"; (iii) myocardial function in the post-infarct period and (iv) the long-term clinical prognosis. Strong experimental evidence that "infarct size" can be reduced (Maroko et al., 1970) has been difficult to translate into clinical practice because the only way to quantify infarct size exactly is by pathological measurements of the excised heart. The great variability of "infarct size" from patient to patient also requires large numbers of patients to judge the clinical effects of any given intervention.

From the clinical point of view, there are three hallmarks of the infarction process — formation of Q waves in the electrocardiogram, large-scale release of cardiac enzymes and the uptake of calcium-seeking isotopes.

The **typical infarction pattern of the electrocardiogram** starts off in the hyperacute phase as a pattern of ST-segment deviation reflecting the localized extracellular transfer of potassium ions (see Fig. 24-2). Depending on whether the lesion is subepicardial or subendocardial, there will be ST-elevation or ST-depression in the hyperacute phase of myocardial infarction (Fig. 25-8). The more severe the ischemia, the greater the potassium loss and the greater the ST-deviation. Experimentally, agents decreasing early ST-elevation also decrease ultimate infarct size (Maroko et al., 1970). Theoretically, the efficacy of an intervention reducing experimental infarct size can be tested in man by its capacity to lessen the development

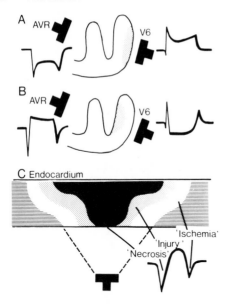

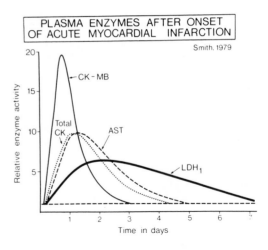

Fig. 25-9 In patients with acute myocardial infarction a number of enzymes are released including creatine kinase (CK), its MB isoenzyme, aspartate transaminase (AST) and lactate dehydrogenase (LDH). The cardiac isoenzyme of LDH is LDH_1. Taken from Smith (1979). Enzymes in Cardiology. Eds DJ Hearse, J De Leiris, p 223, John Wiley, Chichester, with permission.

Fig. 25-8 Electrocardiographic changes of hyperacute myocardial infarction are those of ST-segment deviation which is a positive deflection in the case of epicardial damage (A), and a negative deflection in the case of endocardial damage (B). The ST changes represent the current of injury, largely caused by potassium ion shifts (see Fig. 24-2). The next step is loss of the R wave with formation of a Q wave (C). Hypothetically, the electrocardiographic changes of the typical infarction pattern (C) correspond to zones of necrosis, injury and ischemia. In reality this differentiation is probably not justified although it is a useful electrocardiographic concept. The extent of change of the typical electrocardiographic pattern from early ST-elevation (panel A) to Q wave formation (panel B) over 4–12 hours provides an indirect index of myocardial necrosis. From Schamroth (1983) An Introduction to Electrocardiography, pp 22–23, Blackwell Scientific Publications, Oxford, with permission.

of electrocardiographic signs of necrosis such as loss of frontal forces (fall of R waves) and formation of Q waves, which occurs over about 4–12 hours. Using this approach, early intravenous beta-blockade diminishes the electrocardiographic features of infarction (Yusuf et al., 1980). The major factors preventing widespread use of the electrocardiographic technique are (i) the great individual variation in the evolution of the typical infarction pattern and (ii) the difficulty of following the changes in inferior infarction, which requires special siting of the precordial electrodes.

Changes in the blood levels of **cardiac enzymes**, such

as creatine kinase, are another index of infarct size. In experimental situations, where the heart muscle is available for analysis, the extent of depletion of tissue enzymes such as the **MB isoenzyme of creatine kinase** closely reflects the extent of tissue necrosis and is therefore an index of infarct size. By making certain assumptions about the volume of distribution into which the enzyme is released and the factors governing the rate of removal of the enzyme, it is possible to extrapolate form the rate of release of creatine kinase (Fig. 25-9) to the cumulative loss of creatine kinase, to the mass of heart tissue that has suffered enzyme depletion and thereby to estimate infarct size. The high rate of destruction of the enzyme in the infarct zone (only about 15 percent is released) is an obvious potential source of error unless the fraction released is known to be constant. Another problem is the variable rate of decay (K_D) of the enzyme in the blood from patient to patient. The infarct size cannot accurately be predicted by the initial rate of rise of enzymes in the circulation. Because of these problems, large numbers of patients must be studied. Hence the current thrust is towards the use of radionuclide tracers to quantify infarction.

Technetium-99M-pyrophosphate is the prototype agent used to image myocardial infarction in man. It is selectively taken up by the infarct, probably because the pyrophosphate adsorbs to an excess of intra-myocardial calcium; the mechanism of this complex process is still controversial. A recent proposal is that the passage of labeled pyrophosphate through the sarcolemma is closely related to the development of a permeability defect for calcium ions after 1–3 hours of ischemia (Chien et al., 1981) and to an increased tissue calcium content (Buja et al., 1977). Such data strengthen the hypothesis that cytosolic calcium overloading is an important feature of irreversible ischemic damage. Once inside the cell the radionuclide adsorbs on to various tissue stores of calcium. A defect of this technique is that the label is found chiefly in the severely damaged or necrotic cells in the border zone and in the peripheral infarct zone to create a "doughnut" effect; presumably the blood flow to the central infarct zone is too low to carry the label.

That the uptake of labeled pyrophosphate could be specific to the infarction process is suggested by the good correlation of such uptake with the rise of serum MB creatine kinase. Although the techniques are not yet sufficiently sensitive to give an exact measure of infarct size, the patients with small foci of uptake have a good prognosis and those with large foci have a high incidence of complications and mortality (Coleman et al., 1977).

Palmitate carbon-11 is a positron-emitting fatty acid isotope. In the normally oxygenated heart the rate of clearance of ^{11}C-palmitate is proportional to the rate of carbon dioxide production (Klein et al., 1979). In the ischemic myocardium the clearance of ^{11}C is correspondingly reduced, independently of the decreased myocardial blood flow (Lerch et al., 1982). The effects of ischemia in decreasing oxidation of fatty acids must far exceed the small increase of recovery of label in accumulated products of lipid metabolism such as acyl CoA, acyl carnitine and triglyceride. Thus when fatty acids are not oxidized a "cold area" develops and can be used for assessment of "infarct size". Because the cold area develops very soon after the onset of the reduction of blood flow, and because the half-life of the isotope is so short, repetitive measurements are theoretically possible to estimate the rate of development of the infarction process in any given patient. Considerable practical problems must still be overcome before this procedure could be widely applied. Fatty acids can also be labeled with iodine-123 or tellurium-123m (Okada et al., 1982); both are gamma emitters and hence are easier to analyze than positron emitters. With the latter isotopes it is not the direct oxidation of the fatty acid that is monitored and so interpretation of data is not easy.

Comment: No current technique is ideal for "infarct sizing". In anterior infarction a rough guide can be obtained from the rate of evolution of electrocardiographic changes in the standard 12-lead electrocardiogram. If intervention really decreases infarct size there should be accompanying clinical benefits such as fewer arrhythmias, less development of heart failure and improved post-infarct myocardial function as well as improved long-term prognosis. These are the real criteria by which the possible benefits of agents such as beta-blockade are being assessed.

Principles of Therapy in Myocardial Infarction

Since myocardial infarction is ultimately the consequence of an imbalance between myocardial oxygen supply and demand it is logical and prudent to employ measures aimed at regressing the imbalance (Table 25-2). These include the treatment of pain,

Table 25-2

Principles of therapy of acute myocardial infarction

1. **Acute general care**
   — relief of pain
   — therapy of arrhythmias including bradycardia (atropine) and tachycardia
   — check cardiac output clinically and rule out heart failure

2. **Within first 4 hours of onset of symptoms**
   (i) consider intravenous beta-blockade to limit infarct size
   (ii) intravenous streptokinase (or intracoronary if facilities available)
   (iii) consider percutaneous transluminal coronary angioplasty
   (iv) consider glucose–insulin–potassium

3. **Prophylactic lidocaine** — consider need which is most logical when patient is seen very early, as above

4. **Treat complications**
   (i) congestive heart failure with **pulmonary congestion** — nitrates; furosemide
   (ii) congestive heart failure and **low cardiac output** — nifedipine (avoid hypotension) or sometimes nitroprusside (watch for rebound)
   (iii) **poor peripheral perfusion or cardiogenic shock** — intravenous dobutamine or dopamine

arrhythmias, heart failure, hypertension and tachy-cardia. **Morphine** combines a potent analgesic effect with hemodynamic actions that are particularly beneficial in reducing myocardial oxygen demand, namely a marked venodilator action reducing the ventricular preload, an ability to decrease the heart rate and a mild arterial vasodilator action that may reduce the afterload. At least some of these effects are mediated by central opiate receptors (see Fig. 20-3). However, in the presence of hypovolemia (sometimes caused by excess diuretic therapy) morphine may cause profound hypotension and must therefore be given while the patient is under careful observation (morphine dose: 5–10 mg intravenously at 1 mg/min).

Relief of enhanced wall stress

If the infarcting myocardium dilates, wall stress will increase as will the oxygen demand (Fig. 25-10). Therefore left-sided heart failure represents a considerable hazard to the ischemic zone besides causing severe discomfort to the patient. Reduction of preload and afterload as well as the cautious use of inotropic agents all merit evaluation so that the left ventricular filling pressure may be reduced. The standard initial measure frequently used is the intravenous administration of **furosemide** (20–80 mg intravenously or orally) which acts beneficially both by venodilation and by diuresis. Sublingual nitrates (sublingual nitroglycerin 0.5 mg every 5–10 min for 20 min; sublingual isosorbide dinitrate 20 mg) are given to relieve the preload and to decrease wall stress. When there is associated hypertension, afterload reduction

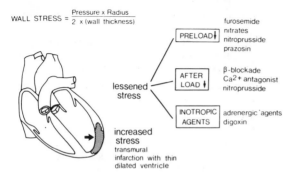

Fig. 25-10 Beneficial effects of agents reducing wall stress, thereby improving oxygen balance in acute myocardial infarction.

by nifedipine is undergoing evaluation. In the presence of combined backward and forward failure, intravenous nitroprusside (with careful monitoring of the blood pressure, see Fig. 17-6) or oral prazosin is usual. In the presence of cardiac failure and dilation the aim is to reduce the heart size by inotropic therapy using agents such as intravenous dopamine or dobutamine (Chapter 19). Digoxin is best avoided in the early stages until the effect of diuretic therapy and load reduction can be assessed (Chapter 19). Although all these procedures are theoretically sound in individual patients, it is probably the use of the various **nitrates** that has received most adequate evaluation. It is not certain, for example, that intravenous nitroprusside really improves the outlook although it may well bring acute symptomatic relief.

Forward failure in acute infarction

When cardiac output is low in the absence of an elevated wedge pressure or clinical and radiographic evidence of left ventricular failure, it is crucial to exclude **hypovolemia** (again possibly diuretic-induced) or right ventricular infarction. In either of these two cases volume loading is required. In the absence of these factors combined vasodilator and inotropic therapy is the most potent method of increasing cardiac output in severe heart failure. Under hemodynamic monitoring, dobutamine may be combined with nitroprusside. Nitrates as sole therapy are usually contra-indicated because their main effect is to reduce the preload. Nitroprusside is the vasodilator commonly used because of the rapid circulatory response which allows titration of the needs of the patient to the dose given, and because forward failure is usually combined with backward failure (nitroprusside acts on both the preload and the afterload).

Optimal heart rate

The slower the heart rate the better because oxygen demand is lower. However, an excessively slow heart rate might have harmful effects by decreasing the cardiac output too much (hypotension) or by pre-disposing to arrhythmias. An excessively slow heart rate can result from reflex vagal overactivity (page 214). The rational therapy is by atropine, which is given particularly when there is sinus bradycardia or atrioventricular block in the setting of hypotension or ventricular ectopy (dose: atropine 0.3 mg slowly intravenously, repeated if needed to a maximum of 2.0 mg).

Conversely when the heart rate is too fast, the myocardial oxygen demand is increased and should be lessened. The probable mechanism is sympathetic overactivity causing an **inappropriate tachycardia**. Before using intravenous beta-blockade (propranolol 0.5 mg increments up to total dose of 0.1 mg/kg with careful monitoring), the first step is to treat any underlying cause such as pain, anxiety, hypovolemia or pump failure. A particular indicator for beta-blockade is sinus tachycardia with associated hypertension; an intravenous infusion of labetalol with its added alpha-blocking activity will reduce the blood pressure more rapidly than will propranolol.

Ventricular arrhythmias in acute infarction

"Lidocaine is used widely in the prophylaxis and therapy of early infarction arrhythmias. The role of prophylactic lidocaine therapy in abolishing "warning arrhythmias" and consequently ventricular fibrillation is controversial. Because lidocaine is reasonably safe and may be beneficial many argue that it should be given to all patients suspected of acute infarction, provided that there are no obvious contra-indications such as allergy to lidocaine." (Gersh et al. 1984). Others argue that the incidence of primary ventricular fibrillation is very low in a well-run coronary care unit and lidocaine should only be given when the arrhythmias actually require therapy (i.e. therapeutic and not prophylactic use). The recommended dosages are 75 mg as a bolus followed by an infusion of 2–4 mg/min (page 328). Because lidocaine is metabolized by the liver, the dose should be reduced in patients with congestive heart failure, shock, liver disease or those receiving cimetidine. If lidocaine fails the blood potassium should be checked because lidocaine works best at a high normal potassium level. Otherwise a number of other intravenous agents may be used, including procainamide or mexilitine (Singh et al., 1984; Table 23-6).

Supraventricular arrhythmias in acute infarction

Atrial fibrillation, flutter or paroxysmal supraventricular tachycardia are usually transient but may be recurrent and troublesome. In the absence of left ventricular failure, verapamil or intravenous propranolol in conjunction with digoxin is acceptable and effective, particularly in controlling the ventricular rate. Cardioversion is limited to resistant cases with hemodynamic compromise. Recurrent atrial flutter may require atrial overdrive pacing.

Anticoagulation

"While still a source of debate, common practice is to treat patients on admission to the coronary care unit with full dose heparin unless there are contra-indications, e.g. advanced age or uncontrolled hypertension. A decrease in the incidence of both pulmonary and systemic thrombo-embolism results from anticoagulation following acute myocardial infarction. **Heparin** is generally discontinued when the patient is either ambulatory or is discharged". (Gersh et al., 1984). Heparin might be expected to increase ischemic injury by its side-effects of increasing blood free fatty acids (heparin stimulates the enzyme breaking down circulating triglycerides). In reality, experimental ischemic injury is reduced showing that the beneficial effects on thrombus-formation outweigh the presumed harmful side-effects. Long-term anticoagulation is no longer employed routinely, but as non-invasive techniques increase the diagnosis of those at risk for the development of intraventricular thrombosis, practice may change. The antiplatelet agent **aspirin** can beneficially influence experimental arterial thrombosis (Moschos et al., 1972), but this approach has not been tested clinically. The routine use of platelet-inhibitors in survivors of acute myocardial infarction is not supported by current data (exception: aspirin for unstable angina; see page 347).

Blood oxygen

A simple procedure to enhance the oxygen supply to the patient is by intranasal oxygen. Occasionally there are unexpected hemodynamic effects. Synthetic oxygen-carrying compounds, such as the perfluorocarbons, are under experimental evaluation to further improve the oxygen-carrying capacity of blood and reduce features of ischemia (Glogar et al., 1981). If the blood oxygen tension is low (chronic pulmonary disease) then nitrates should be used with care because they cause methemoglobinemia and pulmonary shunting of blood.

Relief of coronary spasm

In some patients coronary spasm is thought either to be the initial cause of the infarction process or to be secondary to release of vasoactive amines or thromboxane. Yet in others (the majority, it seems) spasm plays no critical role. The possibility of relief of coronary artery spasm is another argument for the early administration of nitrates.

Role of Beta-adrenergic Receptor Antagonists

The arguments for using beta-blockade in acute ischemia are similar to those advanced in the case of angina pectoris — a reduction of the oxygen demand by a decreased heart rate and decreased afterload as the arterial pressure falls. Such arguments are considerably strengthened by the increased blood catecholamine concentrations found in the acute stage, and by the evidence that catecholamine stimulation can increase the severity of infarction (Fig. 25-11). Debate about the benefit of beta-adrenergic blockade in acute infarction is still not settled, although the clinical benefits achieved by the early administration of atenolol (Yusef et al., 1980), metoprolol (Hjalmarson et al., 1981) or timolol (International Collaborative Study, 1984) are convincing. Most indices of infarction such as development of Q waves or release of creatine kinase are reduced provided that the beta-blocker is given early enough (4–6 hours after onset of chest pain). It is also rational to use beta-blocking agents (provided there is no serious left ventricular failure or any other contra-indication) for the treatment of ventricular arrhythmias related to persistent or recurrent ischemia, or when there is overt evidence of sympathetic overactivity. Two studies have shown that intravenous beta-blockers (atenolol or metoprolol) have wider antiarrhythmic use in acute myocardial infarction and can prevent serious arrhythmias (Rossi et al., 1983) including ventricular fibrillation (Ryden et al., 1983). **Contra-indications** to the use of beta-blockade include a low cardiac output,

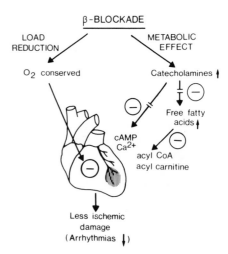

Fig. 25-11 Possible mechanism of beneficial sites of action of beta-blocking drugs in very early hours of acute myocardial infarction. Early intravenous beta-blockade is able to reduce signs of ischemic damage and the incidence of ventricular arrhythmias (see text) but requires careful monitoring and attention to contra-indications.

excess bradycardia or hypotension, clinical left ventricular failure, or lack of experience on the part of the attending physician. The effect of early and continued beta-blockade on the mortality at 3 months is beneficial (Hjalmarson et al., 1981); longer term effects of early beta-blockade have still to be proved.

In the **post-infarct period** propranolol, timolol and metoprolol all protect against long-term mortality after acute myocardial infarction, so that therapy with these beta-blockers in the follow-up stages of myocardial infarction is becoming common. In the case of oxprenolol, data are conflicting. Careful clinical judgement with due respect for selection of patients, contra-indications and side-effects must be maintained. Beta-blockade is seldom indicated in post-infarct patients with good left ventricular function and a correspondingly good prognosis even if untreated. In others, beta-blockade is one of several strategies (possible revascularization, antiarrhythmic agents or anti-failure therapy).

Experimental Procedures

Calcium antagonists

The potential benefit of calcium antagonist agents (Fig. 25-10) can be seen in much the same light as that of beta-blockers—a "direct" effect in ameliorating the process of ischemic damage and an "indirect" effect in reducing the load on the heart. The direct effect argues that calcium entry through the damaged sarcolemma is one of the harmful effects of ischemia; such enhanced calcium entry may play a role in "oxygen-wastage" by increasing the mitochondrial oxygen demand without increasing ATP production (Fig. 25-12). A further possible benefit is relief of coronary artery spasm, which is thought to play a contributory role in the early infarction process (at least in some patients). A novel concept is that verapamil selectively depresses contractility of the ischemic zone (Smith et al., 1976) perhaps because acidosis enhances the uptake of verapamil by the myocardium. Although substantial animal evidence supports the use of calcium antagonists in the limitation of ischemia, it must be stressed that clinical trials are still at a much earlier stage than with beta-adrenergic blockade. Indeed, preliminary results of recent trials cast doubt on the ability of nifedipine or verapamil to benefit patients with acute infarction (in a subgroup with left heart failure, nifedipine increases cardiac output with a fall in atrial filling pressure). An important difference between calcium antagonists and beta-blockers may be that only the latter can be expected to inhibit the excess sympathetic drive at the start of acute myocardial infarction and thereby to exert an effect on the prevention of ventricular fibrillation.

Glucose and ischemic injury

It should be emphasized that the metabolic approach is not yet generally accepted although theoretically sound. In hearts which are anoxic but well-perfused, an increased supply of glucose helps the anoxic heart to survive by increasing the **synthesis of glycolytic anaerobic ATP**, which may help to maintain membrane integrity (page 147). In anoxic cultured heart cells, inhibition of glycolysis by a low–medium glucose or by the glycolytic inhibitor 2-deoxyglucose or by lactate all increase enzyme release (Higgins et al., 1981). An increase of glycolytic flux in isolated hearts with coronary ligation decreases enzyme release (Opie and Bricknell, 1979). Conversely, deprivation of glucose by hypoglycemia increases ischemic injury after coronary ligation (Libby et al., 1975). The major problem with this concept is that glycolytic flux in the severely ischemic zone is limited by products of glycolysis (see Figs 10-3 and 10-4). Hence provision of glucose is most likely to be effective in models where collateral flow to the ischemic zone is high (Apstein et al., 1983) or in the "border zone" of infarcts or in small infarcts with high collateral flow (Dalby et al., 1981). In the non-ischemic zone, glucose may limit the progression of ischemia (Liedtke et al., 1982).

The use of **glucose–insulin–potassium** has gone through several phases. Some early clinical trials were poorly designed and soon discredited. Then emphasis changed from replacement of tissue potassium to the benefits of enhanced glucose utilization and the effect of glucose and insulin in lowering blood free fatty acids (Opie and Owen, 1976). Theoretically added benefit could be derived from the effects of insulin, bearing in mind that patients with acute infarction go through a temporary diabetic process. In general, all experimental studies have shown benefit from glucose–insulin–potassium — with one exception in which low-dose infusions were used and the blood glucose was raised only temporarily (see Dalby et al., 1981). The sobering feature of the "GIK story" is that Sodi-Pallares' proposals were first made in 1962; yet it was not until 17 years later that the results of the first randomized trials on patients became available (Mantle et al., 1981). The major results thus far are that left

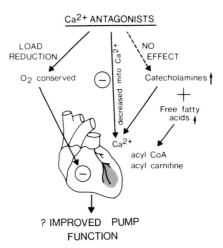

Ca²⁺ ANTAGONISTS

LOAD REDUCTION

decreased mito Ca²⁺

NO EFFECT

O₂ conserved

Catecholamines ↑

Free fatty acids ↑

Ca²⁺

acyl CoA
acyl carnitine

? IMPROVED PUMP FUNCTION

Fig. 25-12 Possible beneficial sites of action of calcium antagonists in acute stages of myocardial infarction. Pump function may be improved by unloading the ischemic myocardium. There is the danger of a direct negative inotropic effect, and as yet no clinical evidence of reduction of mortality with these agents. The use of these agents is still under investigation.

ventricular function improves and infarct size assessed angiographically decreases (Rackley et al., 1981). In practice, the conflicting early data on GIK have discouraged its general use.

Fatty acids and ischemic injury

The second main proposal linking metabolic events to ischemic injury has been that **increased circulating free fatty acids** can exaggerate the severity of ischemia. Oliver's group proposed that the increase of blood free fatty acids could trigger ventricular arrhythmias in developing infarction (Chapter 10). Other workers failed to repeat their findings which led to a temporary eclipse of the concept. Numerous recent studies have defined intracellular abnormalities of lipid metabolism in ischemic tissue—such as accumulation of acyl compounds and lysophosphoglycerides, or products of lipid peroxidation. The Oliver hypothesis can now be restated in broad terms: abnormalities of lipid metabolism play an important role in exaggerating the severity of myocardial ischemia.

Can the administration of **carnitine** (Chapter 10) help to remove the accumulation of lipid metabolites such as acyl CoA in ischemic cells? This possibility seems unlikely. In ischemia intramitochondrial acyl CoA cannot be further oxidized and must accumulate; the transport system for ATP across the mitochondrial membrane is sensitive to an accumulation of acyl CoA on either side. Provision of carnitine might merely convert acyl CoA to acyl carnitine, which is also thought to have harmful effects. It is more likely that the additional properties of carnitine, such as inhibition of uptake of fatty acids (Liedtke et al., 1981) are responsible. L-Carnitine, the biologically active isomer, has greater anti-ischemic potential than *dl*-carnitine, which occurs naturally.

Membrane stabilization

An even more experimental approach is that of membrane stabilization. Abnormally enhanced movement of component phospholipids and proteins leads to destruction of the membranes or to severe ischemia. A reasonable approach to the problem of limiting the effects of ischemia would be to administer agents which could "stabilize" the membranes. Originally the concept arose to describe the effects of multivalent ions and drugs which could alter the shape of the action potential in nerves, leading to the idea that the quinidine-like drugs have membrane-stabilizing properties. Other potential membrane stabilizers in ischemic damage are the steroids, alpha-tocopherol, some beta-adrenergic blocking agents such as propranolol, and possibly ATP itself. **Lysosomotropic agents,** such as chlorpromazine, specifically protect lysosomal membranes. Coenzyme Q_{10}, a normal component of the respiratory chain, has an elongated structure which might function by stabilizing the mitochondrial membrane. Thus far no conclusive benefits of any such agents have been shown in experimental myocardial infarction. Even the effect of propranolol in reducing infarct size is controversial; in all probability it acts chiefly through antagonism of the beta-adrenergic receptors and not as a membrane stabilizer.

Limitation of Infarct Size versus Early Revascularization

Despite much experimental evidence that pharmacologic agents such as beta-blockers, hyaluronidase and nitrates, or metabolic agents such as glucose–insulin–potassium will reduce infarct size (Opie, 1980), clinical proof has been difficult to obtain chiefly because of the lack of a suitable method of assessing the effect of therapy on ultimate infarct size in any given patient. However, preliminary data would suggest that the early administration of intravenous beta-blockade or intravenous nitroglycerin may influence infarct size favorably in specific subgroups of patients. Hyaluronidase is currently under evaluation.

"An increase in blood supply remains the most effective mode of preservation of ischemic myocardium and the concept of intracoronary thrombolysis or thrombus recanalization has the potential to alter profoundly the management of acute infarction. The results of this approach are currently a major focus of investigation. Whether or not the procedure should be combined, or followed by, percutaneous transluminal coronary angioplasty or coronary bypass grafting requires further evaluation, as does the optimal timing of these interventions. In summary, progress in preserving ischemic myocardium is encouraging but further data are required before firm guidelines can be given." (Gersh et al., 1984).

Early revascularization

Reperfusion has to be started sufficiently soon to avoid the irreversible phase of ischemic damage which occurs, at the latest, by about 4 hours after the onset of symptoms (Schwarz et al., 1983). It should theoretically be possible to protect the heart from some aspects of reperfusion damage by the use of calcium antagonist agents. Because the severity of ischemic damage predisposes to that of reperfusion damage, an approach that warrants testing is the preservation of the ischemic myocardium by agents thought to limit infarct size, while awaiting reperfusion. Revascularization by intracoronary or even intravenous enzymes such as streptokinase can apparently be undertaken in patients without serious immediate risks and with probable benefit (Schwarz et al., 1983).

Therapy of Cardiogenic Shock

Cardiogenic shock is a variety of shock in which the basic cause is a very low cardiac output. Its most frequent cause is pump failure resulting from a very large acute myocardial infarction, or a repetitive series of infarctions involving 40 percent or more of the ventricular mass. The consequences of the severe underperfusion are both cardiac and peripheral. The decreased coronary perfusion pressure leads to further myocardial ischemic and contractile failure. The decreased blood flow to skeletal muscle and other tissues may cause a secondary lactic acidosis (severe stimulation of anaerobic metabolism as a result of tissue hypoxia). Release of a vasodepressive substance from the underperfused liver has been described. Blood platelets may become overcoagulable so that there is disseminated intravascular coagulation. Renal underperfusion may cause oliguria or anuria. By these multiple mechanisms, cardiogenic shock is likely to make itself worse so that the cardiovascular system is caught in a vicious downward circle.

The principles of therapy are those of preservation of the ischemic myocardium, including the use of peripheral vasodilators such as sodium nitroprusside. Frequently added inotropic support by dobutamine is given. Blood electrolytes and pH changes must be recorded. **Intra-aortic balloon pumping** improves diastolic perfusion because the balloon is blown up in diastole and collapsed in systole. None of these measures is entirely successful, being without proven effect on the long-term outcome. Hence the real hope lies in prevention by limitation of infarct size or by reperfusion in the early stages.

Summary

Basically energy in the form of ATP is required to maintain ionic gradients. In some way not yet understood, **energy depletion** may lead to an early redistribution of calcium ions in the cell, which may activate phospholipases to damage the sarcolemma. Membrane changes also result from the accumulation of unmetabolized lipid products such as acyl CoA and acyl carnitine. These processes increase sarcolemmal damage. Once membrane disruption occurs beyond a certain point there is a net gain of cellular calcium, associated with irreversible damage, and large-scale release of enzymes which indicates the clinical point-of-no-return. Hence the factors controlling permeability of the cell membranes would appear to be of prime importance.

In sustained coronary occlusion, numerous metabolic and hemodynamic factors contribute to the development of **cellular necrosis**. Whereas severely or totally ischemic cells probably die after 30–45 min, the situation in the development of acute myocardial infarction is much more dynamic, so that various therapies applied up to 4–8 hours following experimental coronary occlusion are still effective. It is possible that therapy started even later is effective in some patients. Such discrepancies in the time taken to reach the point-of-no-return are ill-understood, but may reflect progressive or slowly evolving infarction in patients, where continued high levels of catecholamines and free fatty acids could play an important role.

In the **therapy** of acute myocardial infarction attention is first directed towards those procedures which yield symptomatic or hemodynamic benefit. The use of intravenous morphine, the therapy of arrhythmias and the correction of left ventricular failure all fall in this category. The principle of infarct size limitation is still controversial and under evaluation. Evidence favors the use of cautious beta-blockade as soon as possible after the onset of symptoms of acute myocardial infarction, provided that left ventricular failure is excluded. Much evidence favors post-infarction protection by beta-blockade in selected patients. Vasodilators are used increasingly to reduce the preload or afterload in the presence of heart failure when beta-blockade is contra-indicated.

Reperfusion of the ischemic myocardium within 4–6 hours of the onset of symptoms by early revascularization procedures is under intense clinical investigation; thus far results are encouraging.

References

Allen DG, Orchard CH (1983). Intracellular calcium concentration during hypoxia and metabolic inhibition in mammalian ventricular muscle. J Physiol (Lond) 339: 107–122.

Apstein CS, Gravino FN, Haudenschild CC (1983). Determinants of a protective effect of glucose and insulin on the ischemic myocardium: effects on cardiac contractile function, diastolic compliance, metabolism and ultrastructure during ischemia and reperfusion. Circ Res 52: 515–526.

Armiger LC, Herdson PB, Gavin JB (1975). Mitochondrial changes in dog myocardium induced by lowered pH in vitro. Lab Invest 32: 223–226.

Bricknell OL, Opie LH (1978). Effects of various substrates on lactate dehydrogenase release and on arrhythmias in the isolated rat heart during underperfusion and reperfusion. Circ Res 43: 102–115.

Buja LM, Tofe AJ, Kulharni PV, Mukherjee A, Parkey RW, Francis MD, Bonte FJ, Willerson JT (1977). Site and mechanisms of localization of technetium-99m phosphorous radiopharmaceuticals in acute myocardial infarcts and other tissues. J Clin Invest 60: 724–740.

Burton KP, Hagler HK, Templeton GH, Willerson JT, Buka LM (1977). Lanthanum probe studies of cellular pathophysiology induced by hypoxia in isolated cardiac muscle. J Clin Invest 60: 1289–1302.

Bush LR, Buja LM, Samowitz W, Rude RE, Wathen M, Tilton GD, Willerson JT (1983). Recovery of left ventricular segmental function after long-term reperfusion following temporary coronary occlusion in dogs. Circ Res 53: 248–263.

Chien KR, Reeves JP, Buja LM, Bonte F, Parkey RW, Willerson JT (1981). Phospholipid alterations in canine ischemic myocardium. Temporary and topographical correlations with Tc-99m-PPi accumulation and an in vitro sarcolemmal Ca²⁺ permeability defect. Circ Res 48: 711–719.

Coleman RE, Klein MS, Ahmed SA, Weiss ES, Buchholz WM, Sobel BE (1977). Mechanisms contributing to myocardial accumulation of technetium-99m stannous pyrophosphate after coronary artery occlusion. Am J Cardiol 39: 55–59.

Dalby AJ, Bricknell OL, Opie LH (1981). Effect of glucose–insulin–potassium infusions on epicardial ECG changes and on myocardial metabolic changes after coronary artery ligation in dogs. Cardioivasc Res 15: 588–598.

Feuvray D, Plouet J (1981). Relationship between structure and fatty acid metabolism in mitochondria isolated from ischemic rat hearts. Circ Res 48: 740–747.

Gersh B, Opie LH, Kaplan N (1984) Which drug for which disease? In: Drugs for the Heart, Ed. LH Opie, pp 153–191, Grune & Stratton, Orlando, New York and London.

Glogar D, Rude RE, Khuri S, Karaffa S, Kloner RA, Clark LC Jr, Muller JE, Kaindl F, Braunwald E (1981). Protective effect of perfluorocarbons and supplemental O₂ in acute myocardial ischemia as assessed by intramyocardial mass spectrometry (Abstract). J Molec Cell Cardiol 13: Suppl 1, 32.

Gorman MW, Sparks HV Jr (1982). Progressive coronary vasoconstriction during relative ischemia in canine myocardium. Circ Res 51: 411–420.

Grayson J, Lapin BA (1966). Observations on the mechanism of infarction in the dog after experimental occlusion of the coronary artery. Lancet i: 1284–1288.

Higgins TJ, Allsopp D, Bailey PJ, D'Souza EDA (1981). The relationship between glycolysis, fatty acid metabolism and membrane integrity in neonatal myocytes. J Molec Cell Cardiol 13: 599–615.

Hjalmarson A, Elmfeldt D, Herlitz J, Holmber S, Malek I, Nyberg G, Ryden L, Swedberg K, Vedin A, Waagstein F, Waldenstrom A, Waldenstrom J, Wedel H, Wilhelmsen L, Wilhelmsson C (1981). Effect of metoprolol on mortality in acute myocardial infarction. Lancet ii: 823–827.

International Collaborative Study Group (1984). Reduction of infarct size with the early use of timolol in acute myocardial infarction. New Engl J Med 310: 9–15.

Jennings RB, Ganote C (1976). Mitochondrial structure and function in acute myocardial ischemic injury. Circ Res 38: Suppl 1, 80–91.

Jennings RB, Reimer KA (1981). Lethal myocardial ischemic injury. Am J Path 102: 241–255.

Jennings RB, Sommers H, Smyth G, Flack H, Linn H (1960). Myocardial necrosis induced by temporary occlusion of a coronary artery in the dog. Arch Path 70: 83–92.

Klein MS, Goldstein KA, Welch MJ, Sobel BE (1979). External assessment of myocardial metabolism with (¹¹C)-palmitate in rabbit hearts. Am J Physiol 237: H51–H58.

Kübler W, Katz AM (1977). Mechanism of early "pump" failure of the ischemic heart: possible role of adenosine triphosphate depletion and inorganic phosphate accumulations. Am J Cardiol 40: 467–471.

Lerch RA, Bergmann SR, Ambos HD, Welch MJ, Ter-Pogossian MM, Sobel BE (1982). Effect of flow-independent reduction of metabolism on regional myocardial clearance of ¹¹C-palmitate. Circulation 65: 731–738.

Libby P, Maroko PR, Braunwald E (1975). The effect of hypoglycaemia on myocardial ischemic injury during acute experimental coronary artery occlusion. Circulation 51: 621–626.

Liedtke AJ, Nellis SH, Whitesell LF (1981). Effects of carnitine isomers on fatty acid metabolism in ischemic swine hearts. Circ Res 48: 859–866.

Liedtke AJ, Nellis SH, Whitesell LF (1982). Effects of regional ischemia on metabolic function in adjacent aerobic myocardium. J Molec Cell Cardiol 14: 195–206.

McKnight ADC, Leaf A (1977). Regulation of cell volume. Physiol Rev 57: 510–573.

Mantle JA, Rogers WJ, Smith LR, McDaniel HG, Papapietro SE, Russell RO, Rackley CE (1981). Clinical effects of glucose-insulin-potassium on left ventricular function in acute myocardial infarction: results from a randomized clinical trial. Am Heart J 102: 313–324.

Maroko PR, Kjekshus JK, Sobel BE, Watanabe T, Covell JW, Ross J Jr, Braunwald E (1970). Factors influencing infarct size following experimental coronary artery occlusions. Circulation 43: 67–82.

Moschos CB, Lahiri K, Peter A, Jerani MU, Regan TJ, Newark NJ (1972). Effect of aspirin upon experimental coronary and non-coronary thrombosis and arrhythmia. Am Heart J 84: 525–530.

Mukherjee A, Bush LR, McCoy KE, Duke RJ, Hagler H, Buja LM, Willerson JT (1982). Relationship between beta-adrenergic receptor numbers and physiological responses during experimental canine myocardial ischemia. Circ Res 50: 735–741.

Okada RD, Knapp FF, Elmaleh DR, Yasuda T, Boucher CA, Strauss HW (1982). Tellurium-123m-9-telluraheptadecanoic acid: a possible cardiac imaging agent. Circulation 65: 305–310.

Opie LH (1980). Myocardial infarct size. Part 2. Comparison of anti-infarct effects of beta-blockade, glucose–insulin–potassium, nitrates, and hyaluronidase. Am Heart J 100: 531–522.

Opie LH, Bricknell OL (1979). Role of glycolytic flux in effect of glucose in decreasing fatty acid-induced release of lactate dehydrogenase from isolated coronary ligated rat heart. Cardiovasc Res 13: 693–702.

Opie LH, Owen P (1976). Effect of glucose–insulin–potassium infusions on arteriovenous differences of glucose and of free fatty acids and on tissue metabolic changes in dogs with developing myocardial infarction. Am J Cardiol 38: 310–321.

Podzuweit T, Dalby AJ, Cherry GW, Opie LH (1978). Cyclic AMP levels in ischaemic and non-ischaemic myocardium following coronary artery ligation. Relation to ventricular fibrillation. J Molec Cell Cardiol 10: 81–94.

Poole-Wilson PA (1984). Enzyme ions and calcium exchange in ischemic or hypoxic myocardium. In: Calcium antagonists and cardiovascular disease. Ed. LH Opie, pp 97–104, Raven Press, New York.

Rackley CE, Russell RO, Rogers WJ, Mantle JA, McDaniel HG, Papapietro SE (1981). Clinical experience with glucose–insulin–potassium therapy in acute myocardial infarction. Am Heart J 102: 1038–1049.

Rao RS, Cohen MU, Mueller HS (1983). Production of free radicals and lipid peroxides in early experimental myocardial ischemia. J Molec Cell Cardiol 15: 713–716.

Romeo D, Stagni N, Sottocasa GL, Pugliarello MC, de Bernard B, Vittur F (1966). Lysosomes in heart tissue. Biochim Biophys Acta 130: 64–80.

Rossi PRF, Yusuf S, Ramsdale D (1983). Reduction of ventricular arrhythmias by early intravenous atenolol in suspected acute myocardial infarction. Brit Med J 286: 506–529.

Ruigrok TJC, Boink ABTJ, Spies F, Blok FJ, Mass AHJ, Zimmerman ANE (1978). Energy dependence of the calcium paradox. J Molec Cell Cardiol 10: 991–1002.

Ryden L, Ariniego R, Arnman K, Herlitz J, Hjalmarson A, Holmberg S, Reyes C, Smedgard P, Svedberg K, Vedin A, Waagstein F, Waldenstrom A, Wilhelmsson C, Wedel H (1983). A double-blind trial of metoprolol in acute myocardial infarction: effects on ventricular tachy-arrhythmias. N Engl J Med 308: 614–618.

Schwarz F, Faure A, Katus H, von Olshausen K, Hofmann M, Schuler G, Manthey J, Kübler W (1983). Intracoronary thrombolysis in acute myocardial infarction: an attempt to quantitate its effect by comparison of enzymatic estimate of myocardial necrosis with left ventricular ejection fraction. Am J Cardiol 51: 1573–1578.

Singh BM, Opie LH, Marcus FI (1984). Antiarrhythmic agents. In: Drugs for the Heart. American edition, pp 65–98, Grune & Stratton, Orlando, New York and London.

Smith HJ, Goldstein RA, Griffith JM, Kent KM, Epstein SE (1976). Regional contractility. Selective depression of ischemic myocardium by verapamil. Circulation 54: 629–635.

Steenbergen C, De Leeuw G, Barlow C, Chance B, Williamson JR (1977). Heterogeneity of the hypoxic state in perfused rat heart. Circ Res 41: 606–615.

Whalen DA Jr, Hamilton DG, Ganote CE, Jennings RB (1974). Effect of transient period of ischemia on myocardial cells. Am J Path 74: 381–397.

Wildenthal K (1978). Lysosomal alterations in ischemic myocardium: result or cause of myocellular damage. J Molec Cell Cardiol 10: 595–603.

Yusef S, Ramsdale D, Peto R, Furse L, Bennett D, Bray C, Sleight P (1980). Early intravenous atenolol treatment in suspected acute myocardial infarction: preliminary report of a randomized trial. Lancet ii: 273–276.

Zimmerman ANE, Hülsmann WC (1960). Paradoxical influence of calcium ions on the permeability of the isolated rat heart. Nature 211: 646–647.

New References

McCord JM (1985). Oxygen-derived free radicals in post-ischemic tissue injury. New Engl J Med 312: 159–163.

Index

Tables and figures are given in italic